Handbook of Clinical Laboratory Testing During Pregnancy

CURRENT CLINICAL PATHOLOGY

IVAN DAMJANOV, MD
SERIES EDITOR

HANDBOOK OF CLINICAL LABORATORY TESTING DURING PREGNANCY

Edited by

ANN M. GRONOWSKI, PhD, DABCC

*Departments of Pathology and Immunology and Obstetrics
and Gynecology, Washington University School of Medicine,
and Clinical Chemistry and Serology Laboratories,
Barnes-Jewish Hospital, St. Louis, MO*

Foreword by

Gillian Lockitch, MBChb, MD, FRCP(C)
*Department of Pathology and Laboratory Medicine, Children's
and Women's Health Centre of British Columbia and University
of British Columbia, Vancouver, British Columbia, Canada*

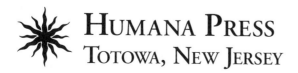 **HUMANA PRESS**
TOTOWA, NEW JERSEY

© 2004 Humana Press Inc.
999 Riverview Drive, Suite 208
Totowa, New Jersey 07512

www.humanapress.com

The content and opinions expressed in this book are the sole work of the authors and editors, who have warranted due diligence in the creation and issuance of their work. The publisher, editors, and authors are not responsible for errors or omissions or for any consequences arising from the information or opinions presented in this book and make no warranty, express or implied, with respect to its contents.

Due diligence has been taken by the publishers, editors, and authors of this book to assure the accuracy of the information published and to describe generally accepted practices. The contributors herein have carefully checked to ensure that the drug selections and dosages set forth in this text are accurate and in accord with the standards accepted at the time of publication. Notwithstanding, as new research, changes in government regulations, and knowledge from clinical experience relating to drug therapy and drug reactions constantly occurs, the reader is advised to check the product information provided by the manufacturer of each drug for any change in dosages or for additional warnings and contraindications. This is of utmost importance when the recommended drug herein is a new or infrequently used drug. It is the responsibility of the treating physician to determine dosages and treatment strategies for individual patients. Further it is the responsibility of the health care provider to ascertain the Food and Drug Administration status of each drug or device used in their clinical practice. The publisher, editors, and authors are not responsible for errors or omissions or for any consequences from the application of the information presented in this book and make no warranty, express or implied, with respect to the contents in this publication.

Production Editor: Robin B. Weisberg.
Cover design by Patricia F. Cleary.
Cover illustration: (Background) From Fig. 1 in Chapter 3, "Biological Markers of Preterm Delivery," by Stephen F. Thung and Alan M. Peaceman. (Foreground) From Fig. 5 in Chapter 5, "Maternal Prenatal Screening for Fetal Defects," by Andrew R. MacRae and Jacob A. Canick; Fig. 1 in Chapter 6, "Chromosome Analysis in Prenatal Diagnosis," by Syed M. Jalal, Adewale Adeyinka, and Alan Thornhill; Fig. 1 in Chapter 9, "Thyroid Disease During Pregnancy: Assessment of the Fetus," by Pratima K. Singh and Ann M. Gronowski; and Fig. 32, in Chapter 11, "Hemolytic Disease of the Newborn," by David G. Grenache.

This publication is printed on acid-free paper. ∞

ANSI Z39.48-1984 (American National Standards Institute) Permanence of Paper for Printed Library Materials.

Printed in the United States of America. 10 9 8 7 6 5 4 3 2 1

E-ISBN 1-59259-787-4

Library of Congress Cataloging-in-Publication Data

Handbook of clinical laboratory testing during pregnancy / edited by Ann
M. Gronowski.
   p. ; cm. -- (Current clinical pathology)
Includes bibliographical references and index.
 ISBN 1-58829-270-3 (alk. paper)
 1. Obstetrics--Diagnosis--Handbooks, manuals, etc. 2. Prenatal diagnosis--Handbooks, manuals, etc.
   3. Fetus--Diseases--Diagnosis--Handbooks, manuals, etc. 4. Pregnancy--Complications--
   Diagnosis--Handbooks, manuals, etc. 5. Diagnosis, Laboratory--Handbooks, manuals, etc.
 [DNLM: 1. Prenatal Diagnosis--methods--Handbooks. 2. Fetal
Diseases--diagnosis--Handbooks. 3. Laboratory Techniques and Procedures--Handbooks.
   4. Pregnancy Complications--diagnosis--Handbooks. WQ 39 H23552 2004]
   I. Gronowski, Ann M. II. Series.
 RG527.5.L3H36 2004
 618.2'075--dc22
                                                      2003023726

DEDICATION

This book is dedicated to Alexander and Zachary

FOREWORD

Laboratory medicine is a fundamental component of antenatal care and risk assessment in pregnancy. From preconception counseling to postpartum followup of mother and infant, laboratory testing is used to diagnose, screen, and monitor maternal and fetal health and well-being. However, outside of specialized obstetric or perinatal centers, testing during pregnancy is often performed in community laboratories or hospitals where pregnancy testing may not be a major focus. The need for all laboratories to use appropriately determined gestation-specific reference ranges for correct interpretation of tests in pregnancy cannot be emphasized enough.

The opening chapter of this book discusses the physiological adaptations that occur in pregnancy profoundly change biochemical and biophysical characteristics of the pregnant woman. Reference ranges for many laboratory tests change significantly from the normal values seen in the healthy nonpregnant woman. These changes are influenced by mechanisms that impact different stages of gestation. The direction, magnitude, and duration of reference range changes differ between different organ systems, and for different tests. Maternal disease during pregnancy, whether pregnancy-specific or other medical disorders, further complicates interpretation of tests in pregnancy and may profoundly alter the biochemistry of the infant.

This comprehensive handbook will assist physicians, nurses, midwives, and others who provide care to pregnant women to understand the effect of pregnancy on laboratory testing. *Handbook of Clinical Laboratory Testing During Pregnancy* will especially be useful to laboratory physicians and scientists who may be required to interpret test results in pregnancy. Obstetric residents, medical students, and laboratory technologists will find this handbook invaluable.

Throughout *Handbook of Clinical Laboratory Testing During Pregnancy,* the focus is on the appropriate use of laboratory tests during pregnancy. Currently used test methodologies, as well as new technologies, are clearly explained for the nontechnical reader but provide useful details for laboratory professionals. Topics include the physiological effect on laboratory tests, changes in reference ranges, test selection for diagnosis, and monitoring and interpretation of test results.

A key strength of *Handbook of Clinical Laboratory Testing During Pregnancy* is the authors. Chosen from practicing specialists in pathology, laboratory medicine and obstetrics, they bring a practical expertise to each section, to complement their comprehensive theoretical reviews of the basis of laboratory testing in pregnancy.

An overview of physiological mechanisms of human pregnancy provides a framework for the later chapters. A comprehensive appendix sets out a compilation of published reference ranges by first, second, and third trimester. It is important for laboratory physicians to realize that these ranges are population, method, and instrument dependent.

Although they can serve as guidelines, it is incumbent on each laboratory to ensure that the reference ranges they use for pregnancy are validated for their own methods and equipment and their referral populations.

Other works on laboratory reference ranges have focused on testing in one or two disciplines of laboratory medicine or on medical disorders in pregnancy. The comprehensive range of this book makes it a valuable addition to the reference shelf of professionals caring for the pregnant woman.

Gillian Lockitch, MBChb, MD, FRCP(C)
Department of Pathology and Laboratory Medicine
Children's and Women's Health Centre of British Columbia
and University of British Columbia
Vancouver, British Columbia, Canada

PREFACE

During pregnancy, a woman undergoes a multitude of normal physiological changes and is subject to a variety of pregnancy-specific diseases. Furthermore, there are a number of diseases that can affect the unborn fetus and the physiological status of the fetus can in turn affect the mother. Taken together, laboratory testing during pregnancy can be complicated and confusing.

The aim of *Handbook of Clinical Laboratory Testing During Pregnancy* is to aid clinicians and laboratorians in the art of diagnosis during pregnancy using laboratory testing. Currently, there is not a comprehensive text available that focuses exclusively on clinical laboratory testing in the pregnant patient. The focus of this handbook is on the use of laboratory tests during pregnancy, including the effects of normal physiological changes on test results; the proper use of laboratory tests; interpretation of results; changes in reference ranges; monitoring the pregnant patient; methodologies; and such new technologies as molecular diagnostics. Topics are not limited to clinical chemistry, but also include molecular biology, serology, immunology, and hematology. Included is a comprehensive appendix of normal reference ranges in pregnant women. These ranges are compiled from the literature, which should prove an excellent resource for any medical professional.

Laboratorians, medical directors, physicians, medical technologists, students, clinical chemists, nurses, physician's assistants, and researchers from the in vitro diagnostics and pharmaceutical industries should find *Handbook of Clinical Laboratory Testing During Pregnancy* to be a useful reference.

Ann M. Gronowski, PhD, DABCC

ACKNOWLEDGMENTS

I would like to acknowledge my mentors—Jack Ladenson, Mitchell Scott, and Sam Santoro. They have created a unique environment at Washington University that fosters critical thought. Their guidance and confidence have made this book possible. Thank you to David Grenache and Joan Nelson, who were instrumental in editing, formatting, and providing novel ideas. Thank you to Wm. Michael Dunne for serving as an ad hoc editor. Additionally, thank you to my assistant and "right hand," Linda Dickey, for limitless technical support. Finally, the support of my husband, Scott, cannot go unrecognized. This book has stolen many nights, weekends, and much sleep. He has been there through it all.

CONTENTS

CONTRIBUTORS

ADEWALE ADEYINKA, MBBS, PhD • *Cytogenetics Laboratory, Mayo Clinic and Mayo Foundation, Rochester, MN*

EDWARD R. ASHWOOD, MD • *ARUP Laboratories, University of Utah School of Medicine, Salt Lake City, UT*

WILLIAM A. BENNETT, PhD • *Department of Obstetrics and Gynecology, University of Mississippi Medical Center, Jackson , MS*

ISAAC BLICKSTEIN, MD • *Department of Obstetrics and Gynecology, Kaplan Medical Center, Rehovot and the Hadassah-Hebrew University School of Medicine, Jerusalem, Israel*

LYNN BRY, MD, PhD • *Clinical Laboratories, Department of Pathology, Brigham and Women's Hospital and Lymphocyte Biology Section, Harvard Medical School, Boston, MA*

JACOB A. CANICK, PhD, FACB • *Division of Prenatal and Special Testing, Women and Infants Hospital and Department of Pathology, Brown Medical School, Providence, RI*

ALBERT C. CHEN, BS • *Sansum Medical Research Institute, Santa Barbara, CA*

LAURENCE A. COLE, PhD • *Department of Obstetrics and Gynecology and Biochemistry and Molecular Biology; Division of Women's Health Research; USA hCG Reference Service, University of New Mexico, Albuquerque, NM*

CAROLYN B. COULAM, MD • *Millenova Immunology Laboratories and Sher Institute for Reproductive Medicine/RPL, Chicago, IL*

JONATHAN W. DUKES, BS • *Sansum Medical Research Institute, Santa Barbara, CA*

CHARLES S. EBY, MD • *Department of Pathology and Immunology, Washington University School of Medicine and Department of Hematology, Barnes-Jewish Hospital, St. Louis, MO*

CORINNE R. FANTZ, PhD • *Department of Pathology and Laboratory Medicine, Emory University, Atlanta, GA*

SEBASTIAN FARO, MD, PhD • *The University of Texas-Houston Health Science Center and Associates in Infectious Diseases on OB/GYN, Houston, TX*

DAVID G. GRENACHE, PhD • *Department of Pathology and Laboratory Medicine, University of North Carolina and Clinical Chemistry Laboratory, UNC Hospitals, Chapel Hill, NC*

ANN M. GRONOWSKI, PhD, DABCC • *Departments of Pathology and Immunology and Obstetrics and Gynecology, Washington University School of Medicine, and Clinical Chemistry and Serology Laboratories, Barnes-Jewish Hospital, St. Louis, MO*

SYED M. JALAL, PhD, FACMG • *Cytogenetics Laboratory, Mayo Clinic and Mayo Foundation, Rochester, MN*

LOIS JOVANOVIC, MD • *Sansum Medical Research Institute and Department of Medicine, University of Southern California and Department of Biomolecular Science and Engineering, University of California-Santa Barbara, Santa Barbara, CA*

LOUIS G. KEITH, MD, PhD • *Department of Obstetrics and Gynecology, The Feinberg School of Medicine, Northwestern University and Prentice Women's Hospital and Maternity Center of the Northwestern Memorial Hospital, The Center for Study of Multiple Birth, Chicago, IL*

KEE-HAK LIM, MD • *Obstetrics, Gynecology and Reproductive Biology, Harvard Medical School, Beth Israel Deaconess Medical Center, Boston, MA*

GARY LIPSCOMB, MD • *Division of Gynecologic Specialties, Department of Obstetrics and Gynecology, University of Tennessee Health Science Center, Memphis, TN*

GILLIAN LOCKITCH, MBChb, MD, FRCP(C) • *Department of Pathology and Laboratory Medicine, Children's & Women's Health Centre of British Columbia and University of British Columbia, Vancouver, British Columbia, Canada*

ANDREW R. MACRAE, PhD, FCACB • *The Research Institute at Lakeridge Health, Oshawa and Department of Laboratory Medicine and Pathobiology, University of Toronto, Ontario, Canada*

ALAN M. PEACEMAN, MD • *Department of Obstetrics and Gynecology, Northwestern University Feinberg School of Medicine, Chicago, IL*

YOEL SADOVSKY, MD • *Departments of Obstetrics and Gynecology, Cell Biology and Physiology, Division of Maternal-Fetal Medicine and Ultrasound, Washington University School of Medicine, St. Louis, MO*

PRATIMA K. SINGH, MD • *Department of Pathology and Immunology, Washington University School of Medicine and Department of Pathology, Barnes-Jewish Hospital, St. Louis, MO*

ALAN THORNHILL, PHD • *In Vitro Fertilization and Fertility Laboratories, Mayo Clinic and Mayo Foundation, Rochester, MN*

STEPHEN F. THUNG, MD • *Department of Obstetrics and Gynecology, Northwestern University, Chicago, IL*

MELANIE M. WATKINS, MD • *Obstetrics, Gynecology and Reproductive Biology, University of California–San Francisco, San Francisco, CA*

JASON D. WRIGHT, MD • *Department of Obstetrics and Gynecology, Washington University School of Medicine, St. Louis, MO*

VALUE-ADDED eBOOK/PDA

This book is accompanied by a value-added CD-ROM that contains an Adobe eBook version of the volume you have just purchased. This eBook can be viewed on your computer, and you can synchronize it to your PDA for viewing on your handheld device. The eBook enables you to view this volume on only one computer and PDA. Once the eBook is installed on your computer, you cannot download, install, or e-mail it to another computer; it resides solely with the computer to which it is installed. The license provided is for only one computer. The eBook can only be read using Adobe® Reader® 6.0 software, which is available free from Adobe Systems Incorporated at www.Adobe.com. You may also view the eBook on your PDA using the Adobe® PDA Reader® software that is also available free from Adobe.com.

You must follow a simple procedure when you install the eBook/PDA that will require you to connect to the Humana Press website in order to receive your license. Please read and follow the instructions below:

1. Download and install Adobe® Reader® 6.0 software
   You can obtain a free copy of Adobe® Reader® 6.0 software at www.adobe.com
   Note: If you already have Adobe® Reader® 6.0 software, you do not need to reinstall it.
2. Launch Adobe® Reader® 6.0 software
3. Install eBook: Insert your eBook CD into your CD-ROM drive
   PC: Click on the "Start" button, then click on "Run"
   At the prompt, type "d:\ebookinstall.pdf" and click "OK"
   Note: If your CD-ROM drive letter is something other than d: change the above command accordingly.
   MAC: Double click on the "eBook CD" that you will see mounted on your desktop. Double click "ebookinstall.pdf"
4. Adobe® Reader® 6.0 software will open and you will receive the message "This document is protected by Adobe DRM" Click "OK"
   Note: If you have not already activated Adobe® Reader® 6.0 software, you will be prompted to do so. Simply follow the directions to activate and continue installation.
   Your web browser will open and you will be taken to the Humana Press eBook registration page. Follow the instructions on that page to complete installation. You will need the serial number located on the sticker sealing the envelope containing the CD-ROM.

If you require assistance during the installation, or you would like more information regarding your eBook and PDA installation, please refer to the eBookManual.pdf located on your CD. If you need further assistance, contact Humana Press eBook Support by e-mail at ebooksupport@humanapr.com or by phone at 973-256-1699.

---

*Adobe and Reader are either registered trademarks or trademarks of Adobe Systems Incorporated in the United States and/or other countries.

1 Human Pregnancy
An Overview

Ann M. Gronowski, PhD, DABCC

CONTENTS

INTRODUCTION

The average human gestation is 280 d (40 wk), as counted from the first day of the last menstrual period (LMP). During this time, a woman undergoes a multitude of normal physiological changes and can be subject to a variety of pregnancy-specific diseases. Furthermore, there are a number of diseases that can affect the unborn fetus, and the physiological status of the fetus can affect the mother. Taken together, laboratory testing during pregnancy is important but can be complicated and confusing. The aim of this book is to aid clinicians and laboratorians in the use of laboratory testing during pregnancy.

Understanding the normal changes that occur during pregnancy is essential to the correct assessment of a pregnant woman. Additionally, familiarity with pregnancy-specific reference intervals is necessary to avoid incorrect diagnoses. This book provides a comprehensive list of reference intervals for pregnant serum amniotic fluid and urine derived from the literature (see the Appendix). This chapter provides an overview of the normal physiological changes that occur during pregnancy that can impact clinical laboratory testing (Table 1).

From: *Current Clinical Pathology: Handbook of Clinical Laboratory Testing During Pregnancy*
Edited by: A. M. Gronowski © Humana Press, Totowa, NJ

Table 1
Physiological Changes During Pregnancy

Endocrine	Insulin resistance/glucose intolerance
Hepatic	Increased plasma protein synthesis
Renal	Increased glomerular filtration rate
	Net sodium retention
Hemodynamic	Increased plasma volume
	Increased red cell mass
Cardiac	Increased cardiac output
Respiratory	Hyperventilation and mild respiratory alkalosis

ENDOCRINE CHANGES AND METABOLIC ADAPTATIONS

Gestation is associated with profound hormonal and metabolic changes in the mother. These changes are responsible for establishing and maintaining pregnancy, fetal growth and development, and subsequent lactation. The first endocrine changes of pregnancy can be detected as early as 1 wk after ovulation. During the luteal phase of the menstrual cycle, the corpus luteum (CL) produces progesterone and estrogen for approx 12–14 d. Progesterone is required to maintain pregnancy. If fertilization occurs, implantation generally takes place between days 6 and 12 after ovulation (1). The trophoblast cells of the implanting blastocyst then begin to produce human chorionic gonadotropin (hCG).

Human Chorionic Gonadotropin

hCG can be detected in approx 90% of pregnancies by the first day of the missed menstrual period and in 97% by 1 wk after the missed menstrual period (2). Serum hCG concentrations continue to rise exponentially for the first 8 wk, doubling in concentration on average every 2 d (3–6). Concentrations of hCG then decrease for the remainder of pregnancy (see Fig. 3, Chapter 2). The hCG molecule is similar in structure to luteinizing hormone (LH) and therefore binds to LH receptors on the CL. This maintains the CL until weeks 7–9, when the placenta is able to produce progesterone and estrogen independently (see Chapter 2).

Progesterone

Progesterone is required to sustain early embryonic growth. After the initial rapid rise in progesterone concentrations during the luteal phase, progesterone concentrations continue to rise for the remainder of pregnancy (Fig. 1) (7). Progesterone inhibits smooth muscle tone in the uterus, gastrointestinal tract, and renal collecting system. This results in a decrease in uterine contractions, but also increases esophageal reflux, delayed gastric emptying, constipation, gallbladder enlargement, and hydronephrosis. Progesterone inhibits the aldosterone effect on renal tubules, causing a decrease in tubular reabsorption of sodium.

Estrogen

There are more than 25 different estrogens that have been isolated from the urine of pregnant women (8). However, there are three main estrogens that have been studied most extensively: estrone, estradiol, and estriol. These hormones are secreted by the

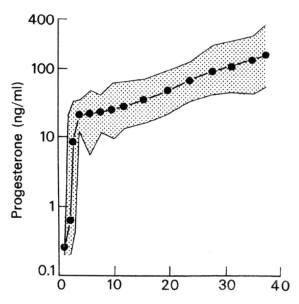

Fig. 1. Geometric mean and range of serum progesterone concentrations from 32 healthy women throughout normal pregnancy. (Reprinted from ref. 7. With permission from Blackwell Publishing.)

placenta, but their precursors are actually fetal in origin. There is an absence of 17-hydroxylase and 17 to 20 desmolase in the placenta. Therefore, by week 20 of pregnancy, the vast majority of the estrogen in maternal blood is derived from dehydroepiandrosterone sulfate (DHEAS) from the fetal adrenal gland. Concentrations of estradiol rise continuously through pregnancy so that by 38 wk the concentration is approx 130 times greater than concentrations at week 4 (Fig. 2) *(7)*. The purpose of estrogen during pregnancy is not entirely clear. It increases angiotensinogen (renin substrate) production from the liver and hence may control blood flow to the uterus, and it also enhances prostaglandin synthetase function *(8)*.

Insulin

In the first few weeks of pregnancy, the rise in serum estrogen and progesterone results in hyperplasia of the pancreatic β-cells. There is also increased secretion of insulin and heightened tissue sensitivity to insulin *(9,10)* (Table 2). These changes are anabolic and stimulate increased storage of tissue glycogen. Fasting blood glucose is reduced 10–20% in the first trimester as a result of the β-cell hyperplasia, increased insulin secretion, and increased peripheral demand (9–11). In contrast, postprandial glucose concentrations are exaggerated to approx 130–140 mg/dL because of the effects of placentally produced anti-insulin hormones. Mean glucose concentrations, however, remain unchanged *(11,12)*.

During the latter part of pregnancy, maternal carbohydrate metabolism is stressed by rising concentrations of placental lactogen and other placental-derived hormones (Table 3). Prolactin, cortisol, and glucagon are also increased in late pregnancy. The sum of these hormonal changes results in modest insulin resistance. Insulin secretion increases by approx 10 wk of pregnancy and by term, fasting insulin concentrations are nearly twofold higher than nonpregnancy concentrations *(11,12)*. The net effect of the metabolic changes in pregnancy is diabetogenic and characterized by a resistance to insulin *(8,9,12)*.

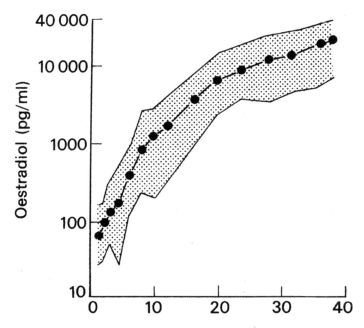

Fig. 2. Geometric mean and range of serum estradiol concentrations from 32 healthy women throughout normal pregnancy. (Reprinted from ref. 7. With permission from Blackwell Publishing.)

Table 2
Carbohydrate Metabolism in Early Pregnancy (to 20 wk)

Hormonal alteration	Effect	Metabolic change
↑ Estrogen and	↑ Tissue glycogen storage	Anabolic
↑ Progesterone	↓ Hepatic glucose production	
β-cell hyperplasia and	↑ Peripheral glucose utilization	↑ Attributed to sex steroids +
↑ insulin secretion	↓ Fasting plasma glucose	Hyperinsulinemia

Data obtained from ref. 9.

Table 3
Carbohydrate Metabolism in Late Pregnancy (20–40 wk)

Hormonal change	Effect	Metabolic change
↑ Human chorionic somatomammotropin	"Diabetogenic" ↓ Glucose tolerance	Facilitated anabolism during feeding
↑ Prolactin	Insulin resistance	Accelerated starvation during fasting
↑ Bound and free cortisol	↓ Hepatic glycogen stores ↑ Hepatic glucose production	Ensure glucose and amino acids to fetus

Data obtained from ref. 9.

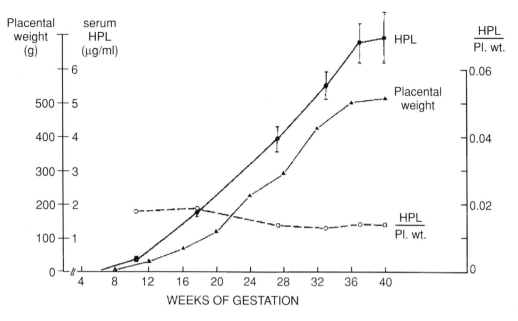

Fig. 3. Serum concentrations of HPL during pregnancy in relation to placental weight. (From ref. *12a*. With permission from Elsevier.)

Human Placental Lactogen

Human placental lactogen (HPL), or human chorionic somatotropin, is produced by the trophoblast and is closely related to growth hormone *(8)*. It is a major mediator of the metabolic changes of pregnancy. HPL becomes detectable in maternal serum by 5–6 wk of gestation, and concentrations continue to rise until 34–40 wk, when they plateau. There is no circadian variation in HPL and very little enters the fetal circulation. Unlike hCG, HPL concentrations rise in parallel to placental weight (Fig. 3) *(12a)*. HPL's growth hormonelike activity is responsible for the maternal glucose-sparing effect during pregnancy. HPL causes mobilization of free fatty acids from maternal fat depots, shifting glucose toward the needs of the growing fetus. It also has an antagonistic effect against insulin. HPL is therefore a key diabetogenic factor during pregnancy. Its concentrations are greatest during the last 4 wk of pregnancy, when the fetus requires the largest amounts of glucose *(8)*. In the past, HPL has been measured as a diagnostic adjunct to follow patients with hypertension, intrauterine growth retardation, diabetes, and fetal demise. However, HPL reflects only fetal size, not fetal status itself. Therefore, today, HPL measurements are rarely used to monitor pregnancy.

Renin–Aldosterone Axis

During normal pregnancy, the rennin–aldosterone axis is upregulated. Plasma renin activity (PRA), plasma renin concentrations (PRC), angiotensinogen (renin substrate), angiotensin, and angiotensin II all increase beginning in the first trimester *(10,13,14)* (Table 4). It is likely that both progesterone and estrogens are responsible for these changes. Estrogen stimulates increased production of angiotensinogen from the liver. This ultimately results in increased aldosterone production, and sodium reabsorption.

Table 4
Changes in the Renin–Aldosterone Axis During Pregnancy

	Fold increase
Plasma renin activity	2.4–9.4
Plasma renin concentration	1.5–6
Angiotensinogen (renin substrate)	3–5
Angiotensin	2–6
Angiotensin II	2–10
Aldosterone	4

Data obtained from refs. *13,51*.

Progesterone has also been shown to increase both PRA and urinary aldosterone secretion *(15)*. This shift in the renin–angiotensin–aldosterone axis may play an important role in the increase in plasma volume seen during pregnancy *(16)*.

Calcium Homeostasis

Pregnancy places a tremendous demand on calcium homeostasis because the growing fetus requires significant calcium for normal growth (30 g of calcium and 15 g of phosphorus by term *[10]*) yet maternal bone and plasma concentrations of calcium have to be maintained. The major changes that occur to keep these needs in balance involve an increase in plasma concentrations of 1,25-dihydroxyvitamin D [1,25-(OH)2-D] and calcitonin *(17)*. At the same time, concentrations of parathyroid hormone, 25-hydroxyvitamin D, and ionized calcium remain unchanged. The major action of 1,25-(OH)2-D is to maintain plasma calcium concentrations by increasing absorption from the gut and accelerating bone resorption. Alternatively, calcitonin, opposes 1,25-(OH)2-D's bone-resorbing activities. Therefore, the combined result is to obtain calcium for the fetus from the maternal gut and not from the maternal skeleton while maintaining maternal serum-ionized calcium concentrations *(17)*.

HEPATIC SYSTEM

The size and histology of the liver is largely unchanged during pregnancy. Absolute blood flow through the liver is also unchanged. Therefore, because cardiac output increases, the liver actually receives a smaller percentage of the total cardiac output *(10)*. The relative decrease in blood volume through the liver, combined with the increase in volume of distribution, may affect the clearance of some drugs during pregnancy.

Liver function tests are frequently misinterpreted in normal pregnancy and may be incorrectly associated with liver disease because of the considerable changes that occur in some enzymes and proteins (Table 5). The most important effect of pregnancy on liver function is the estrogenic stimulation of protein synthesis causing marked changes in the plasma concentrations of coagulation factors, angiotensinogen, hormone-binding proteins, and some acute phase reactants such as ceruloplasmin and α-1-antitrypsin. Serum alkaline phosphatase concentrations can be as much as twofold greater than nonpregnant concentrations by the third trimester and therefore cannot be used as a reliable marker of hepatic function *(11,18–21)*. Because concentrations of γ-glutamyl transferase are not changed to the same extent (decreased 10–20%) *(11,21,22)*, this enzyme serves as a better

Table 5
Changes in Liver Function Tests During Pregnancy

α-1-Antitrypsin	↑ 30–90%
Albumin	↓ 10–20%
Alkaline phosphatase	↑ 100%
Alanine amniotransferase	↓ 10–20%
Angiotensinogen	↑ 300–500%
Aspartate aminotransferase	↓ to unchanged
Bilirubin (unconjugated)	↑ 30–40%
Bilirubin (conjugated)	↑ 40–60%
Ceruloplasmin	↓ 50–100%
Cholesterol	↓ 30–50%
Fibrinogen	↓ 20–60%
γ-Glutamyl transferase	↑ 10%–20%
5'-Nucleotidase	Unchanged
Immunoglobulins	↑ 10–20%
Lactate dehydrogenase	Unchanged
Protein (total)	↑ 20%
Prothrombin	Unchanged
Sex hormone binding globulin	↓ 400%
Thyroxine-binding globulin	↓ 50%

Data obtained from refs. *11,13,52,53.*

marker of liver disease in pregnancy than does alkaline phosphatase. The increased concentrations of alkaline phosphatase result, in part, from placental production of heat-stable alkaline phosphatase isoenzyme that can account for up to two-thirds of the enzyme activity *(10,18,23)*. The liver is also likely producing more alkaline phosphatase enzyme because similar changes have been observed when estrogen is administered to nonpregnant women *(24)*. Serum concentrations of the transaminases (alanine amniotransferase and aspartate aminotransferase) and lactate dehydrogenase are largely unchanged during pregnancy *(11)*, whereas concentrations of conjugated, unconjugated, and total bilirubin are significantly decreased. Hemodilution is likely responsible for part of the decrease as is the decrease, in plasma albumin, the main transport protein for unconjugated bilirubin *(11,23)*. For more detail on pregnancy-related liver changes, *see* Chapter 19.

RENAL FUNCTION

During pregnancy, both kidneys increase in size and mass, becoming 1–1.5 cm longer *(10)*. This change is thought to be the result of, in part, the increase in renal vascular volume. By mid-gestation, renal plasma flow and glomerular filtration rate (GFR) are 50% greater than in the nonpregnant state and they remain elevated until late in pregnancy *(25)*. Renal plasma flow, estimated by *p*-aminohippurate (PAH) clearance, increases from 500 mL/min in the nonpregnant patient to 700 mL/min. GFR, estimated by 24-h creatinine clearance, increases from 100 to 110 mL/min to 140 to 170 mL/min (Fig. 4) *(11,25)*. Owing to the increase in GFR without significant change in production of urea or creatinine, the serum concentrations of these substances decrease. Renal changes during pregnancy are summarized in Table 6.

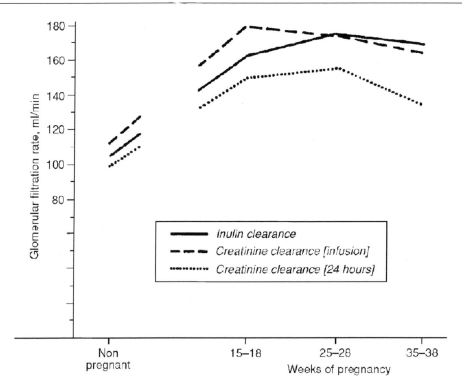

Fig. 4. Mean GFR measured by three methods in 10 healthy women at 15–18, 25–28, and 35–38 wk of pregnancy, and again at 8–12 wk postpartum (nonpregnant). (Reprinted from ref. 25, with permission from Elsevier.)

Table 6
Changes in Renal Function Tests During Pregnancy

Inulin clearance	↑ 50%
Creatinine clearance	↑ 50%
Serum urea	↓ 30–40%
Blood urea nitrogen	↓ 30–40%
Serum creatinine	↓ 30%
Serum cystatin-C	↑ 30%

Data obtained from refs. 10,11,21.

One of the most dramatic changes during pregnancy is the increase in tubular sodium reabsorption. The increase in GFR, the increase in plasma progesterone concentrations, and the decrease in plasma albumin concentrations all affect this change (10). The positive sodium balance occurs gradually over gestation. The increased tubular absorption is promoted by the increase in aldosterone, as well as estrogen, deoxycortisone, and placental lactogen. However, the water retention that occurs during pregnancy is proportionally greater than the sodium retention. Therefore, plasma sodium concentrations actually decrease.

HEMODYNAMIC CHANGES

In addition to sodium retention, water retention is also a key pregnancy-induced change. Plasma osmolality decreases as early as 5 wk *(14)*. The relative hypotonicity of the plasma is maintained by an approx 10 mosmol/kg decrease in the osmotic threshold for both thirst and vasopressin (antidiuretic hormone) release. Lowering the threshold to drink stimulates water intake and dilution of body fluids. Vasopressin is not suppressed at the usual osmolality, therefore, it continues to circulate and water is retained *(26)*. Water is a major component of the weight gained during pregnancy and approx 6 L are retained. Seventy percent (4200 mL) of the water is contained in the extracellular compartment and nearly 20% (1100 mL) is located in plasma *(27)*.

An average increase in blood volume of approx 1500 to 1600 mL (40–50%) occurs in the normal singleton pregnancy, with 300 to 400 mL (20–30%) attributed to increased red cell mass. Iron supplementation may influence the increase in red cell mass. The increase in plasma volume is positively correlated with the size of the fetus; thus, women carrying multiple gestations have proportionally higher increases in plasma volume.

Expansion of plasma volume results in an apparent decrease in concentration of sodium, albumin, and hemoglobin, despite the fact that there is effectively a net increase in the total circulating mass of each analyte. The disproportionate increase in plasma volume relative to red cell volume results in a decrease in hematocrit by the third trimester. This is termed the "physiologic anemia of pregnancy" and is not a true anemia, but a normal physiological hemodilution. The increase in total blood volume during pregnancy serves to protect the mother against late pregnancy hypertension and peripartum hemorrhage. The average blood loss during pregnancy is 500 mL *(14)*. For more detail on the hemodynamic changes during pregnancy, *see* Chapter 10.

The risk of deep vein thrombosis (or venous thrombosis) during pregnancy is estimated to be five times greater than in similar nonpregnant patients *(28)*. This hypercoaguable state has been attributed to increased venous stasis in the legs and pelvis during pregnancy and to changes in the balance between coagulation and fibrinolytic systems that are prothrombotic *(29)*.

CARDIAC CHANGES

Maternal heart rate increases significantly by week 5 of pregnancy and continues to rise until approx week 32, when it is 17% higher than nonpregnant rates *(30)*. Cardiac output increases 34–39% by 12 wk of gestation and by 24 wk is increased 43–48%. The increased cardiac output is maintained until term *(30–32)*. This increased output is distributed among several organ systems. The uteroplacental circulation exhibits a tenfold increase in blood flow and receives approx 17–20% of the total maternal cardiac output, or 500–800 mL/min at term. The renal system also receives a significant percentage of maternal cardiac output, with absolute renal blood flow increasing approx 50% by midpregnancy. The breast and skin are also recipients of an increased percentage of cardiac output during pregnancy. Increased blood flow to the skin helps dissipate heat.

RESPIRATORY SYSTEM

Relative hyperventilation occurs during the luteal phase of the menstrual cycle, resulting from the presence of progesterone. This causes alveolar and arterial tensions of carbon dioxide to fall. When pregnancy is established, the hyperventilation continues and by term, end-tidal partial pressure carbon dioxide (PCO_2) and arterial PCO_2 decline to below 30 torr *(14,33)*. The magnitude of this decrease is proportional to progesterone concentrations *(14)*. The mechanism by which progesterone causes hyperventilation is unclear. The hyperventilation in pregnancy is accompanied by a decrease in plasma bicarbonate, which partially compensates for respiratory alkalosis; however, a small increase (approx 0.02) in blood pH is observed *(34)*.

AMNIOTIC FLUID

Amniotic fluid is a body fluid that is unique to pregnancy. The volume of amniotic fluid increases progressively through gestation until approx 34 wk, when the volume begins to decrease. It is approx 200 to 300 mL at 16 wk, 400 to 1400 mL at 26 wk, 300 to 2000 mL at 34 wk, and 300 to 1400 mL at 40 wk *(35)*. The volume of amniotic fluid at term is approx 800 mL and constitutes only 6% of the total maternal weight gain by fluids (27) (Table 7). During gestation, a woman with a single fetus will gain, on average, 12.5 kg (27.5 lb), of which 4.85 kg (10.7 lb) constitute the fetus, placenta, and amniotic fluid *(27)*. As a percent of the total weight gained by the mother, the products of conception rise from about 10% at 10 wk to 20% at 20 wk, 30% at 30 wk, and 40% at term (Table 7).

In the first trimester, the origin of amniotic fluid is uncertain. Beginning in the second trimester, the origin and dynamics of amniotic fluid are better understood. Amniotic fluid volume is maintained by a balance of fetal fluid production (lung liquid and urine) and fluid reabsorption (fetal swallowing and flow across the amniotic membranes). Alterations in the volume of amniotic fluid are associated with a variety of pathological conditions. Oligohydramnios, or abnormally low amniotic fluid volume, is associated with intrauterine growth restriction and abnormalities of the fetal urinary tract. Polyhydramnios, or increased amniotic fluid volume, is associated with maternal diabetes mellitus, severe Rh isoimmunization disease, fetal esophageal atresia, multifetal pregnancy, enencephaly, and spina bifida *(36)*.

During gestation, concentrations of glucose, urea nitrogen, and creatinine increase, whereas concentrations of sodium and osmolality decrease *(19,37)*. These changes are not unexpected as, late in gestation, the primary source of amniotic fluid is fetal urine (*see* the appendix). The urine is normally hypotonic, and this low osmolality accounts for the relative hypotonicity of amniotic fluid (compared to maternal and fetal plasma). Early in pregnancy, there is little particulate matter in the amniotic fluid. As gestation progresses, fetal cells and hair are shed into the amniotic fluid, which can increase the turbidity of the fluid. As the fetal lung matures, production of phospholipid-containing lamellar bodies also increases the fluid turbidity. Finally, at term, amniotic fluid contains gross particles of vernix caseosa, the oily substance composed of sebum and desquamated epithelial cells covering the fetal skin *(36)*.

Because amniotic fluid is derived from substances of fetal origin, it is often sampled and tested in order to monitor fetal development or detect fetal disease. Amniotic fluid is sampled routinely to obtain fetal cells for chromosomal analysis and detection of Down syndrome, trisomy 18, and a variety of other chromosomal abnormalities and to measure α-fetoprotein and acetylcholinesterase to detect neural tube defects (*see* Chapters 5 and 6 for more detail). It is also sampled later in pregnancy for the analysis of fetal lung-

Table 7
Average Weight of Products of Conception, Plasma, Red Cells, Extracellular Fluid,
and Maternal Body by Gestational Age (in Grams)

Weeks of pregnancy				
	10	*20*	*30*	*40*
Total maternal weight gain	650	4000	8500	12,500
Fetus	5	300	1500	3400
Placenta	20	170	430	650
Amniotic fluid	30	250	750	800
Total product of conception	55	820	2680	4850
(% of total weight gain from products of conception)	(10)	(20)	(30)	(40)
Plasma	550	1150	1200	
Red cells	50	150	250	
Extravascular fluid (no edema)	0	30	80	1,496

Modified from ref. *27*.

derived phospholipids, as an estimation of fetal lung maturity (*see* Chapter 4). Amniotic fluid bilirubin is measured as an assessment of Rh isoimmunization reactions (*see* Chapter 11).

In addition to these more traditional measurements, a variety of biochemical markers have been examined to detect a whole assortment of conditions, with varied success. A few are listed here: steroid hormones have been measured as a predictor of fetuses at risk of congenital adrenal hyperplasia *(38)*; concentrations of androgens and estrogens have been measured in an attempt to predict fetal sex; fetal thyroid status has been examined by measuring amniotic fluid thyroid-stimulating hormone and thyroid hormones as an alternative to fetal cord blood sampling *(39–43)*; amniotic fluid concentrations of various liver enzymes have been examined to help confirm echochoriographic evidence of bowel disorders *(44)*; a variety of cytokines in amniotic fluid have been examined as a predictor of impending delivery and infection *(45–48)*; amniotic fluid amino acid concentrations have been measured as an aid in the diagnosis of amnioacidopathies *(49)*; and neuron-specific enolase has been examined in cases of fetal neurological injury *(50)*.

SUMMARY

Pregnancy is associated with numerous changes to maternal physiology. These changes often result in altered reference intervals for commonly measured compounds in serum. It is important to understand these normal changes in order to properly detect and diagnose disease during pregnancy.

REFERENCES

1. Wilcox AJ, Baird DD, Weinberg CR. Time of implantation of the conceptus and loss of pregnancy. N Engl J Med 1999;340:1796–1799.
2. Wilcox AJ, Baird DD, Dunson D, McChesney R, Weinberg CR. Natural limits of pregnancy testing in relation to the expected menstrual period. JAMA 2001;286:1759–1761.
3. Daya S. Human chorionic gonadotropin increase in normal early pregnancy. Am J Obstet Gynecol 1987;156:286–290.

4. Pittaway DE, Reish RL, Wentz AC. Doubling times of human chorionic gonadotropin increase in early viable intrauterine pregnancies. Am J Obstet Gynecol 1985;152:299–302.
5. Pittaway DE, Wentz AC. Evaluation of early pregnancy by serial chorionic gonadotropin determinations: a comparison of methods by receiver operating characteristics. Fertil Steril 1985;43(4):529–533.
6. Batzer FR, Schlaff S, Goldfarb AF, Corson SL. Serial b-subunit human chorionic gonadotropin doubling times as a prognostic indicator of pregnancy outcome in an infertile population. Fertil Steril 1981; 35(3):307–312.
7. Aspillaga MO, Whittaker PG, Taylor A, Lind T. Some new aspects of the endocrinological response to pregnancy. Br J Obstet Gynaecol 1983;90:596–603.
8. Kase NG, Reyniak JV, Bergh PA. Endocrinology of pregnancy. In: Cherry SH, Merkatz IR, eds. Complications of Pregnancy: Medical, surgical, gynecologic, psychosocial, and perinatal. Baltimore: Williams & Wilkins, 1991;916–939.
9. Hollingsworth DR. Maternal metabolism in normal pregnancy and pregnancy complicated by diabetes mellitus. Clin Obstet Gynecol 1985;28(3):457–472.
10. Royek AB, Parisi VM. Maternal biological adaptations to pregnancy. In: Reece EA, Hobbins JC, eds. Medicine of the Fetus and Mother. Philadelphia: Lippincott-Raven, 1999;903–920.
11. Lockitch G. Handbook of Diagnostic Biochemistry and Hematology in Normal Pregnancy. Boca Raton: CRC Press, 1993.
12. Lind T, Billewicz WZ, Brown G. A serial study of changes occuring in the oral glucose tolerance test during pregnancy. J Obstet Gynecol Br Commonw 1973;80(12):1033–1039.
12a. Selenkow HA. Saxena BN, Dana CL, et al. Measurement and pathophysiologic significance of human placental lactogen. In: Pecile A, Finzi C, eds. The Foeto-Placental Unit. Amsterdam: Excerpta Media, 1969;340–362.
13. Chesley LC. The renin-angiotensin system in pregnancy. J Reprod Med 1975;5:173–180.
14. Stock MK, Metcalfe J. Maternal physiology during gestation. In: Knobil E, Neill JD, eds. The Physiology of Reproduction. New York: Raven, 1994;947–983.
15. Sundsfjord JA. Plasma renin activity and aldosterone excretion during prolonged progesterone administration. Acta Endocrinol 1971;67:483–490.
16. Longo LD. Maternal blood volume and cardiac output during pregnancy: a hypothesis of endocrinologic control. Am J Physiol 1983;245:R720–R729.
17. Whitehead M, Lane G, Young O, et al. Interregulations of calcium-regulating hormonees during normal pregnancy. Br Med J 1981;283:10–12.
18. Valenzuela GJ, Munson LA, Tarbaux NM, Farley JR. Time-dependent changes in bone, placental, intestinal, and hepatic alkaline phosphatase activities in serum during human pregnancy. Clin Chem 1987;33(10):1801–1806.
19. Benzie RJ, Doran TA, Harkins JL, et al. Composition of the amniotic fluid and maternal serum in pregnancy. Am J Obstet Gynecol 1974;119:798–810.
20. Ardawi MSM, Nasrat HAN, BA'Aqueel HS. Calcium-regulating hormones and parathyroid hormone-related peptide in normal human pregnancy and postpartum: a longitudinal study. Eur J Endocrinol 1997;137:402–409.
21. van Buul EJA, Steegers EAP, Jongsma HW, Eskes TKAB, Thomas CMG, Hein PR. Haematological and biochemical profile of uncomplicated pregnancy in nulliparous women; a longitudinal study. Netherland J Med 1995;46:73–85.
22. Girling JC, Dow E, Smith JH. Liver function tests in pre-eclampsia: importance of comparison with a reference range derived for normal pregnancy. Br J Obstet Gynaecol 1997;104:246–250.
23. Bacq Y, Zarka O, Brechot J-F, et al. Liver function tests in normal pregnancy: a prospective study of 103 pregnant women and 103 matched controls. Hepatology 1996;23:1030–1034.
24. Mueller MN, Kappas A, Damgaard E. Estrogen pharmacology. I. The influence of estradiol and estriol on hepatic disposal of sulfobromophthalein (BSP) in man. J Clin Invest 1964;43(10):1905–1914.
25. Davison JM, Hytten FE. Glomerular filtration during and after pregnancy. J Obstet Gynecol 1974;81:588–595.
26. Lindheimer MD, Barron WM, Davison JM. Osmoregulation of thirst and vasopressin release in pregnancy. Am J Physiol 1989;257:F159–F169.
27. Hytten FE. Weight gain in pregnancy. In: Hytten FE, Chaimberlain G, eds. Clinical Physiology in Obstetrics. London: Blackwell Scientific, 1991:173–203.
28. Anonymous. Prevention of venous thrombosis and pulmonary embolism. NIH consensus conference. JAMA 1986;256(6):744–749.

29. Toglia MR, Weg JG. Venous thromboembolism during pregnancy. N Engl J Med 1996;335(2):108–114.
30. Robson SC, Hunter S, Boys RJ, Dunlop W. Serial study of factors influencing changes in cardiac output during human pregnancy. Am J Physiol 1989; 256:H1060-H1065.
31. Ueland K, Novy M, Peterson EN, Metcalfe J. Maternal cardiovascular dynamics. Am J Obstet Gynecol 1969;104(6):856–864.
32. Lees MM, Taylor SH, Scott DB, Kerr MG. A study of cardiac output at rest throughout pregnancy. J Obstet Gynecol Br Commonw 1967;74(3):319–328.
33. Lim VS, Katz AI, Lindheimer MD. Acid-base regulation in pregnancy. Am J Physiol 1976;231(6): 1764–1770.
34. Sjostedt S. Acid-base balance of arterial blood during pregnancy, at delivery, and in the puerperium. Am J Obstet Gynecol 1962;84(6):775–779.
35. Queenan JT, Thompson W, Whitfield CR, Shah SI. Amniotic fluid volumes in normal pregnancies. Am J Obstet Gynecol 1972;114(1):34–38.
36. Ashwood ER. Clinical Chemistry of Pregnancy. In: Burtis CA, Ashwood ER, eds. Tietz Textbook of Clinical Chemistry. Philadelphia: W.B. Saunders, 1999: 1736–1775.
37. Lind T, Billewicz WZ, Cheyne GA. Composition of amniotic fluid and maternal blood through pregnancy. J Obstet Gynecol Br Commonw 1971;78:505–512.
38. Wudy SA, Dorr HG, Solleder C, Djalali M, Homoki J. Profiling steroid hormones in amniotic fluid of midpregnancy by routine stable isotope dilution/gas chromatography-mass spectrometry: reference values and concentrations in fetuses at risk for 21-hydroxylase deficiency. J Clin Endocrinol Metab 1999;84(8):2724–2728.
39. Singh PK, Parvin CA, Gronowski AM. A case of fetal goiter and establishment of reference intervals for markers of fetal thyroid status in amniotic fluid. Clin Endocrinol Metab 2003;88:4175–4179.
40. Kourides IA, Heath CV, Ginsberg-Fellner F. Measurement of thyroid-stimulating hormone in human amniotic fluid. J Clin Endocrinol Metab 1982;54:635–637.
41. Chopra IJ, Crandall BF. Thyroid hormones and thyrotropin in amniotic fluid. N Engl J Med 1975;293:740–743.
42. Klein AH, Murphy BEP, Artal R, Oddie TH, Fisher DA. Amniotic fluid thyroid hormone concentrations during human gestation. Am J Obstet Gynecol 1980;136:626–630.
43. Yoshida K, Sakurada T, Takakashi T, Furruhashi N, Kaise K, Yoshinaga K. Measurement of TSH in human amniotic fluid: diagnosis of fetal thyroid abnormality in utero. Clin Endocrinol 1986;25:313–318.
44. Burc L, Guibourdenche J, Luton D, et al. Establishment of reference values of five amniotic fluid enzymes: analytical performances of the Hitachi 911: aplication to complicated pregnancies. Clin Biochem 2001;34:317–322.
45. Wennerholm U-B, Holm B, Mattsby-Baltzer I, et al. Interleukin-1[α], interleukin-6 and interleukin-8 in cervico/vaginal secretion for screening of preterm birth in twin gestations. Acta Obstet Gynecol Scand 1998;77:508–514.
46. Rizzo G, Capponi A, Rinaldo D, Tedeschi D, Arduini D, Romanini C. Interleukin-6 concentrations in cervical secretions identify microbial invasion of the amniotic cavity in patients with pre-term labor and intact membranes. Am J Obstet Gynecol 1996;175:812–817.
47. Inglis SR, Jeremias J, Kuno K, et al. Detection of tumor necrosis factor-alpha, interleukin-6, and fetal fibronectin in the lower genital tract during pregnancy: relation to outcome. Am J Obstet Gynecol 1994;171:5–10.
48. Hitti J, Hillier SL, Agnew KJ, Krohn MA, Reisner DP, Eschenbach DA. Vaginal indicators of amniotic fluid infection in preterm labor. Obstet Gynecol 2001;97:211–218.
49. Rabier D, Chadefaux-Vekemans B, Oury J-F, et al. Gestational age-related reference values for amniotic fluid amnio acids: a useful tool for prenatal diagnosis of aminoacidopathies. Prenatal Diag 1996;16:623–628.
50. Elimian A, Figueroa R, Patel K, Visintainer P, Sehgal PB, Tejani N. Reference values of amniotic fluid neuron-specific enolase. J Maternal Fetal Med 2001;10:155–158.
51. Brown MA, Zammit VC, Mitar DA, Whitworth JA. Renin-aldosterone relationships in pregnancy-induced hypertension. Am J Hypertens 1992;5:366–371.
52. O'Leary P, Boyne P, Flett P, Beilby J, James I. Longitudinal assessment of changes in reproductive hormones during normal pregnancy. Clin Chem 1991;37(5):667–672.
53. Cheng CY, Bardin CW, Musto NA, Gunsalas GL, Cheng SL, Ganguly M. Radioimmunoassay of testosterone-estradiol-binding globulin in humans: a reassessment of normal values. J Clin Endocrinol Metab 1983;56:68–75.

2 Human Chorionic Gonadotropin

Laurence A. Cole, PhD

CONTENTS

INTRODUCTION

Human chorionic gonadotropin (hCG) is a glycoprotein composed of two dissimilar subunits, α- and β-subunit, held together by charge interactions. hCG is produced by trophoblastic cells of the placenta in both pregnancy and gestational trophoblastic diseases. It is a remarkable glycoprotein in that up to 35% of the molecular weight (MW) is from oligosaccharide side chains. hCG is sometimes considered a mucopolysaccharide, like collagen, because of the large carbohydrate component. There is wide variation in hCG structure throughout normal and abnormal pregnancies, and in gestational trophoblastic diseases. In addition to "regular" hCG (hCG with intact subunits and the midtrimester pregnancy-like complement of oligosaccharides), at least six other key variants are present in serum samples: hyperglycosylated hCG, nicked hCG, hCG missing the β-subunit C-terminal peptide, free β-subunit, hyperglycosylated free β-subunit, and nicked free β-subunit as well as multiple combinations of these variants (i.e., nicked hyperglycosylated hCG missing the β-subunit C-terminal peptide). The same seven molecules plus the β-core fragment can be detected in urine samples *(1–9)*. Table 1 and Fig. 1 summarize the structures of these key hCG-related molecules, which vary in size from β-core fragment (MW 9000–10,000) to hyperglycosylated hCG (MW 38,000–42,000). hCG and related molecules may vary widely in charge because of differences in sialic acid content. As shown in Fig. 2, multiple charge isoforms in the range pI 3–7 are found in serum and urine samples, and in the range of pI 3–8 in hyperglycosylated hCG.

From: *Current Clinical Pathology: Handbook of Clinical Laboratory Testing During Pregnancy*
Edited by: A. M. Gronowski © Humana Press, Totowa, NJ

Table 1

Structure of hCG-Related Molecules Detected in Serum and Urine Samples in Normal and Abnormal Pregnancies and Trophoblastic Diseases (1–9)

Molecule	α-subunit structure	β-subunit structure	Occurrence
Regular hCG (MW 37,000)	92 amino acids, no cleavages mono- and biantennary N-linked oligosaccharides	145 amino acids, no cleavages biantennary ± fucose N-linked, and mostly tri- and tetrasaccharide O-linked oligosaccharides	Principal form of βhCG in serum, 6–40 wk of gestation
Hyperglycosylated hCG (MW 41,000)	92 amino acids, no cleavages mono- and biantennary + fucose N-linked oligosaccharides	145 amino acids, no cleavages bi-, short tri-, and triantennary ± fucose N-linked and hexasaccharide O-linked oligosaccharides	Principal βhCG form produced at 3–5 wk of gestation, and in choriocarcinoma
Nicked hCG[1] (MW 36,000)	92 amino acids, no cleavages mono- and bi-antennary N-linked oligosaccharides	145 amino acids, cleaved at β47–48, β43–44 or β44–45 biantennary ± fucose N-linked, and mostly tri- and tetrasaccharide O-linked oligosaccharides	Low concentrations in pregnancy, major hCG in weeks following termination or parturition
hCG missing β-subunit C-terminal peptide[1] cancer (MW 29,000)	92 amino acids, no cleavages mono- (8 sugars) and biantennary N-linked oligosaccharides	Residues 1–92, C-terminal peptide absent biantennary ± fucose N-linked, and mostly tri- and tetrasaccharide O-linked oligosaccharides	Primarily detected in gestational trophoblastic diseases and
Free β-subunit[1] (MW 22,000)	No α-subunit	145 amino acids, no cleavages biantennary ± fucose N-linked, and mostly tri- and tetrasaccharide O-linked oligosaccharides	Dissociation product of nicked hCG. Low levels in serum and urine in pregnancy

continued

Table 1 (continued)

Molecule	α-subunit structure	β-subunit structure	Occurrence
Hyperglycosylated free β-subunit[1] (MW 26,000)	No α-subunit	145 amino acids, no cleavages bi-, short tri- and triantennary ± fucose N-linked and hexasaccharide O-linked oligosaccharides	Significant production at 3–5 wk of gestation, and in choriocarcinoma
Nicked free β-subunit[1] (MW 22,000)	No α-subunit	145 amino acids, cleaved at β47–48, β43–44 or β44–45 biantennary ± fucose N-linked, and mostly tri- and tetrasaccharide O-linked oligosaccharides	Most free β-subunit is nicked in serum or is dissociated from nicked hCG
Urine β-core fragment (MW 10,000)	No α-subunit	Two peptides β-subunit residues 6–40 linked to 55–92 degraded biantennary N-linked and no O-linked side chains	Cleared from circulation rapidly. Principal of β-hCG in urine from 7–40 wk of gestation

[1]Variations of these hCG variants are present in serum and urine, such as hyperglycosylated nicked hCG, nicked hCG missing β-subunit C-terminal peptide, nicked hyperglycosylated free β-subunit, nicked free β-subunit missing the C-terminal peptide, and others.

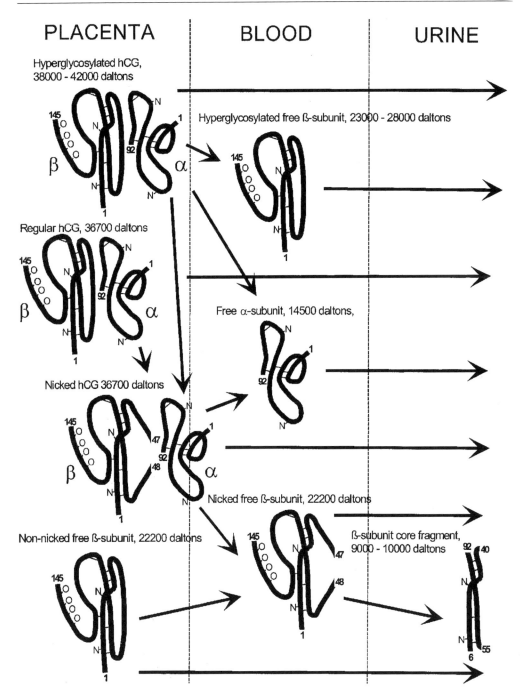

Fig. 1. Two-dimensional representation of structure and molecular weights of hCG forms produced by the placenta and present in serum and urine samples. Dark black lines represent peptide
with numbers indicating N- and C-terminal residues. The letters *N* and *O* indicate sites of *N*- and
O-linked oligosaccharides, and the thin lines indicate sites of disulfide linkages. Representations
are based on the βcore fragment sequence as shown by Birken et al. *(40)*, amino acid sequences
as reported by Morgan et al. *(41)*, disulphide bonds as shown by Lapthorn et al. *(42)*, and the
nicking sites as indicated by Elliott et al. *(7)*.

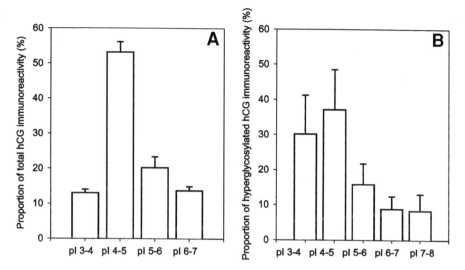

Fig. 2. Charge isoforms of hCG and hyperglycosylated hCG. Pregnancy urine samples were separated into 20 fractions by preparative isoelectric focusing using a Bio-Rad. Panel A shows total hCG isoforms in six samples (Rotofor DPC Immulite hCG assay); Panel B shows hyperglycosylated hCG isoforms in eight further samples (Nichols Advantage hyperglycosylated hCG [ITA] test). All results are distribution of isoforms (% ± standard error).

hCG PRODUCTION DURING PREGNANCY

hCG production does not begin until the developing blastocyst implants into the uterus. Circulating hCG can first be detected (following implantation of the fertilized egg) in serum and urine, with an ultrasensitive hCG test (detection limit 0.13 mIU/mL) as early as day 21 of the menstrual cycle (approx 7 d after fertilization) (10). Total hCG concentrations in serum and urine samples increase exponentially, doubling approximately every 40–48 h, and reach a peak between 8 and 12 wk of pregnancy (Fig. 3) (10a,10b). Total hCG production decreases between the 10th and 20th wk of pregnancy to between one-fifth and one-twentieth of peak hCG concentrations and then plateaus close to this concentration until term. Pregnancy hCG concentrations vary widely among individuals, probably more than any other hormone measurement. This is complicated further by interassay variation in quantitative serum hCG tests (see "Interassay Variation"). Table 2 illustrates the range of serum hCG results we have observed with the DPC Immulite (Diagnostic Products Corp., Los Angeles, CA) test in 300 serum samples. Table 2 is limited to hCG measurements over 4-wk periods and to ranges of concentrations; therefore, it is used only to illustrate the wide range of hCG results during pregnancy and not as a reference interval for different hCG tests or for patient care. As shown in Table 2, for any 4-wk period of pregnancy there is anywhere from a 10- to 200,000-fold variation in interindividual serum hCG concentrations.

Table 3 illustrates median concentrations and ranges for urine total β-hCG concentrations throughout the course of pregnancy, as determined using the DPC Immulite test. In our experience, first morning urine total β-hCG concentrations (including hyperglycosylated hCG and β-core fragment) are approximately one-half of serum total β-hCG concentrations. As shown in Table 3, for any one period of pregnancy there is approximately a 10- to 4000-fold variation in interindividual urine hCG concentrations.

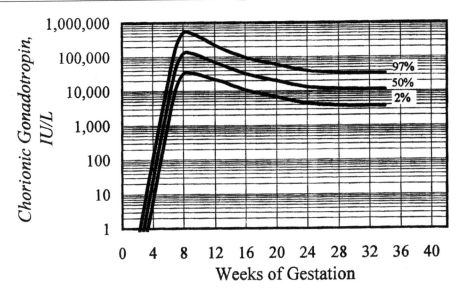

Fig. 3. Concentration of chorionic gonadotropin in maternal serum as a function of gestational age. Lines represent the 2nd, 50th, and 97th percentiles. The maternal serum values from 14 to 25 wk are medians calculated from 24,229 pregnancies from testing performed at ARUP Laboratories, Inc., from January to October 1997. Evaluating health and maturation of the unborn: the role of the clinical laboratory. Clin Chem, 1992;38:1523–1529. Reprinted with permission from W.B. Saunders Co. Aswood, ER. Clinical chemistry of pregnancy. In Burtis CA, Ashwood, ER, eds. Tietz Textbook of Clinical Chemistry. 3rd ed. Philadelphia: W.B. Saunders, 1998, pp. 1736–1775. (Redrawn from ref. *10a*: Reprinted with permission from W.B. Saunders [*10b*].)

Table 2
Range of Total β-hCG Concentrations in 300 Serum Samples Collected
During the Course of Pregnancy, as Determined
in the DPC Immulite hCG Assay

Gestational age (wk)	Total β-hCG range (mIU/mL)
4–7	0–233,200
8–11	11,440–465,300
12–15	14,300–510,400
16–19	6490–337,700
20–23	550–72,930
24–27	9240–107,470
28–31	12,760–152,900
32–35	12,980–128,480
35–39	5390–114,730

Table 3
Median and Range of Total β-hCG and Hyperglycosylated hCG Concentrations in Urine

Gestational age (wk)[a]	Number of samples	Total β-hCG[b] mIU/mL	Range	H-hCG[c] mIU/mL	Range	Proportion H-hCG[d] (% of hCG)	Range
4	63	454	(23–4653)	282	(5–7513)	68%	(7–100%)
5	45	1615	(114–45,800)	779	(35–17,479)	50%	(10–100%)
6	14	2678	(187–20,439)	483	(37–5931)	25%	(7.9–53%)
7	5	16,649	(1608–59,277)	1871	(333–14,055)	13%	(2–24%)
11	20	24,550	(5534–100,222)	1997	(180–13,152)	10%	(0.8–55%)
15	92	8371	(2298–43,932)	290	(28–2906)	3%	(0.2–48%)
19	12	4452	(2278–24,228)	125	(25–797)	2.5%	(0.4–17%)
23	13	3702	(1129–20,725)	32	(11–411)	1.1%	(0.1–12%)
27	12	4600	(840–10,266)	41	(17–473)	2.0%	(0.2–7.5%)
31	7	4449	(1651–39,549)	55	(11–446)	2.0%	(0.1–8.7%)
35	16	5430	(1399–62,500)	78	(17–587)	1.5%	(0.3–14%)
39	16	2379	(276–13,321)	34	(6–260)	1.9%	(0.5–7.4%)

[a]Weeks since last menstrual period.
[b]Determined using DPC Immulite.
[c]Determined using the Nichols Advantage, Invasive Trophoblstic Antigen (ITA) assay.
[d]The proportion of hyperglycosylated hCG was determined as the concentration of hyperglycosylated hCG divided by the total β-hCG result.

While regular hCG is produced by highly differentiated multinucleated syncytiotrophoblast cells during pregnancy, hyperglycosylated hCG, also called invasive trophoblast antigen (ITA), is produced by the poorly differentiated, invasive cytotrophoblast cells *(2,11)*. Invasive cytotrophoblasts are the cells of implantation and the primitive cells of early pregnancy. Therefore, as illustrated in Table 3, hyperglycosylated hCG is responsible for most of the total hCG immunoreactivity in the third, fourth and fifth weeks of pregnancy *(1,3)*. This is true for both serum and urine samples. This early period of pregnancy is the most frequent time for hCG testing, yet, as described in "Interassay Variation," assays vary greatly in their ability to detect hyperglycosylated hCG. Underestimation and overestimation of this critical pregnancy marker occurs frequently *(3,4)*.

PRINCIPALS OF hCG TESTS

More than 40 quantitative serum hCG assays, approx 30 qualitative urine/serum point-of-care tests, and 25 qualitative urine home pregnancy tests are available in the United States for detecting pregnancy *(4,12)*. These assays are all "sandwich"-type immunoassays that utilize capture and detection antibodies that recognize different sites on hCG and hCG-related molecules.

Quantitative hCG Tests

In quantitative serum tests, a capture antibody directed against one site on hCG is immobilized on or linked to a tube, vial, well, or bead. Patient serum is added. The antibody binds and immobilizes the hCG in the serum sample (hCG + immobilized antibody). A second ("detection" or "tracer") antibody directed against a distant site on hCG is linked to a tracer molecule (such as a radioisotope or an enzyme). This forms an immobilized "sandwich" complex (tracer-antibody + hCG + immobilized antibody. In most commercial hCG assays, both antibodies are directed against different portions of the β chain. Therefore, the assays measure total β-hCG (i.e., free β and intact $\alpha\beta$ molecules). After washing, the amount of tracer is measured (in the case of enzyme assays, incubation with substrate is required). The amount of signal is directly proportional to the amount of hCG in the sample. Quantitative hCG tests are either one step or two step. In a one-step assay, the serum is incubated with both immobilized and tracer antibodies simultaneously. In a two-step assay, the serum is first incubated with the immobilized antibody and then washed before the addition of the tracer antibody. The one-step protocol is by far the most common protocol used. It is the fastest and the least complicated. The slower two-step protocol, however, avoids problems with hook effect and limits false positive hCG results caused by heterophilic antibodies. Both of these issues are discussed later in this chapter under "Limitations of hCG Tests."

Qualitative hCG Tests

Qualitative hCG assays, whether home pregnancy tests or point-of-care hCG tests, work on a very similar principal to the quantitative assays. Urine is placed on a single-use assay cassette. The urine is absorbed through changing densities of nitrocellulose. This concentrates the antigens into a narrow band. The urine mixes with a colored-dye-labeled anti-hCG antibody ("tracer" antibody) stored in a sponge at the proximal end of the device. The combination of urine and colored-dye-labeled anti-hCG antibody slowly moves distally through the absorbent nitrocellulose. A complex is formed (hCG + antibody dye). The complex reaches a stationary band of immobilized secondary "capture" antibody in the nitrocellulose matrix. This antibody is directed against an alternative binding site on the hCG molecule. These devices are designed to recognize intact hCG, so one antibody is against the α chain, the other against the β chain. An antibody dye + hCG + immobilized antibody complex is formed that generates a colored line at the site of the "capture" hCG antibody. This is referred to as the "test band." The appearance of a colored line indicates a positive test result (generally at concentrations >20 mIU/mL). Remaining antibody dye migrates further through the device to a second stationary band referred to as the "control band." What is immobilized on the control band varies from test to test. The optimal control band is coated with all or part of the hCG molecule. Excess antibody dye will bind the immobilized hCG, indicating that there was both enough volume to carry the sample across the nitrocellulose and that the antibody dye is working correctly. Unfortunately, not all devices contain this type of control. Some devices have a control band coated with anti dye antibody. This type of control merely indicates that there was enough volume to carry the antibody dye to that distal point.

Antibody Selection

All of these tests, whether quantitative or qualitative, employ at least two different antibodies, whether monoclonal or polyclonal. These are generated against a combination of any of seven established epitopes on hCG. These are the outer section of the β-subunit C-terminal peptide (CTP outer: residues 123–145 plus other hCG three-dimensional [3D] folded structures), the inner section of the CTP (CTP inner: residues 93–122 plus hCG 3D folded structures), at least two separate sites in the core 3D folded structure of the β-subunit (core β-subunit sites 1 and 2), the interface of the α- and β-subunits (anti-hCG, 3D structures on both subunits), and a specific site in the core 3D folded structure of α-subunit (core α-subunit site) (Table 4). In addition, there are specific antibody binding sites for hyperglycosylated hCG only, free β-subunit only, free β-subunit plus β-core fragment β-core fragment only, nicked hCG only, and free α-subunit only. Examining the different antibody combinations used in today's hCG tests shows that manufacturers are effectively using almost all combinations of these seven epitopes on hCG and the seven epitopes plus free subunit antibodies for their tracer and immobilized antibody *(12)*. As a result, there is very large number of different types of hCG assays, whether quantitative or qualitative. These vary widely in their detection of the eight key variants of hCG. Whereas some tests in each category measure only regular hCG, others detect all eight key variants from hyperglycosylated hCG to β-core fragment (Table 4). This is a major source of interassay variation in the results of quantitative serum tests and in the sensitivities and utilities of qualitative tests (*see* "Interassay Variation").

All tests use at least one antibody directed against one of the sites on the β-subunit of hCG to differentiate hCG from luteinizing hormone, thyroid-stimulating hormone, and follicle-stimulating hormone. Some assays use a secondary antibody against the α chain, others utilize two β chain antibodies. Thus, the term βhCG test is commonly used for an hCG test. For the purpose of this chapter, an hCG test and a βhCG test are the same.

hCG STANDARDS

All hCG tests, whether quantitative or qualitative, are standardized with World Health Organization (WHO) international hCG standards. WHO standards are calibrated in

Table 4
Antigenic Determinants on hCG, Freeβ, Freeα, and β-Core and Derivatives

Antigenic determinant	Description	Regular hCG	Hyperglycosylated hCG	Nicked hCG	hCG missing β C-terminal	Regular free β	Hyperglycosylated free β	Nicked free β-subunit	β-core fragment	Free α-subunit
Anti-hCG dimer	A site involving the interface of α- and β-subunit	±	+							
Anticore β1	Mutual site found on hCG, free β, and β-core	+	+	+	+	+	+	+	+	
Anticore β2	Alternate mutual site on hCG, free β and β-core	+	+	+	+	+	+	+	+	
Anti-β C-terminal-1	Site on hCG and free β (needs β C-terminal peptide)	+	±	+		+	±	+		
Anti-β C-terminal-2	Site on hCG and freeβ (needs β C-terminal peptide)	+	±	+		+	±	+		
Anticommonα	Mutual site on hCG and freeα	+	+	±	+					+
Antinicked hCG	Nicked hCG site between β44 and 48			+				+		
Anti-H-hCG	Hyperglycosylated hCG site on β C-terminal peptide		+				+			
Antifreeβ	Free subunit-specific site, hidden on hCG					+	+	±		
Antifree β + β-core	Mutual site on free β and β-core					+	+	+	+	
Anti-β core	Core fragment-specific site, hidden on freeβ							±	+	
Antifreeα	Free subunit-specific site, hidden on hCG									+

+ indicates recognized by all polyclonal and monoclonal antibody against this antigenic determinant.

± indicates recognized poorly or recognized by some polyclonal and monoclonal antibodies to this determinant.

international units (IU). The use of international units dates back to the rabbit biological test of the 1940s *(12)*. The first WHO international standard for hCG was the First International Standard (1st IS), released in 1938. This was followed by the 2nd IS, released in 1964. These were both crude hCG preparations, made from pregnancy urine extracts, and contained a mixture of biologically active hCG, free subunits, and other substances. In 1978, the 2nd IS was replaced by the First International Reference Preparation (1st IRP, also known as hCG preparation 75/735), prepared from a highly purified hCG preparation (CR119) from the National Institutes of Health *(13)*. The 1st IRP contained a defined mass concentration of hCG but the designation of international units was kept for compatibility with the 2nd IS (1 µg hCG = 9.3 IU; *14*). On a weight basis, the 2nd IS has approximately one-half the biological activity of the 1st IRP The CR119 preparation was later used to make the 3rd IS in 1986 (hCG preparation 75/537) and, more recently, the 4th IS (hCG preparation 75/589), released in 1999. Currently, all tests are calibrated with either the 3rd IS or the 4th IS.

The CR119 series of standards was purified from crude pregnancy urine preparation that was collected and stored at ambient temperature, which allowed for aberrant cleavage or nicking of hCG. Research shows that 9% of the 1st IRP, 3rd IS and 4th IS hCG molecules are nicked or damaged in the region of β-subunit residues 43–48 *(15)*. This presented a problem with assays that failed to recognize or poorly detected nicked hCG molecules *(12,16)*. A new hCG standard was released in 2003, isolated from a new commercial crude pregnancy urine extract. This will be referred to as the 1st reference reagent (1st RR, hCG preparation 99/688). To improve assay recognition and reduce interassay variation, this standard has been further purified to remove enzyme impurities and the small proportion of nicked hCG molecules that were present in previous standard hCG preparations *(16)*.

As discussed under "Interassay Variation," the availability of WHO standards to normalize hCG test results and cutoff values is important. All manufacturers purchase WHO standards for calibrating tests. The quantities, however, are very limited and not sufficient to provide calibrators and quality control material for qualitative products. As such, almost all manufacturers purchase crude or partially purified urine-derived hCG either from Scripps Laboratories (La Jolla, CA), Organon (West Orange, NJ), or other suppliers. These preparations are calibrated with the WHO standard and subsequently used as calibrators and/or standards. This is problematic as these preparations are not nearly as well characterized as the WHO standards and may contain a mixture of hCG, nicked hCG, free β-subunit, and β-core fragment. As a result, they are recognized differently by different quantitative hCG tests and may calibrate qualitative pregnancy tests differently. This is likely a major cause of interassay variation and may explain why two serum hCG tests can give different results and why one qualitative test may be positive and another negative with the same urine sample *(17)*.

INTERASSAY VARIATION

Interassay variation between different quantitative serum tests and between different qualitative urine tests can cause confusion and misdiagnosis of pregnancy. Most clinical laboratories participate in external proficiency testing through the College of American Pathologists (CAP). CAP surveys have been the biggest indicator of interassay variation. The five most recent CAP surveys (each with a single hCG preparation) of 2307 to 2324 testing laboratories showed 1.50- to 1.59-fold variations from the mean in results for the 16 most commonly used hCG assays in the United States *(18)*. In 1990, Bock wrote an article titled "hCG Assays: A Plea for Uniformity," strongly criticizing the wide variation in CAP survey hCG results and demanding that manufacturers resolve these differences *(19)*. Clearly, the plea was not effective and the problem, although slightly less pronounced, still exists today. Because of the differences between assays, individual assay-specific reference intervals must be established and should not be interchanged. This can be a source of confusion when hCG is measured at different medical centers.

Figure 4a illustrates the interassay variation in the 10 most commonly used hCG tests from the most recent CAP survey report *(18)*. We recently requested that 11 laboratories quantitate the 1st RR, the newest, purest, and supposedly the most homogenous WHO hCG standard available *(16)*, using the same 10 hCG tests (each calibrated against the current 3rd IS). As shown in Fig. 3, Panel B, wide variation in results was recorded between assays (1.6-fold variation). Interestingly, the tests giving the highest and lowest results with the 1st RR standard [the Bayer Centaur (Bayer, Medfield, MA) and Roche Elecsys (Roche Diagnostics, Indianapolis, IN) tests, respectively] are completely different than those giving the highest results and lowest results with CAP proficiency test material [the DPC Immulite and Beckman Access-2 (Beckman Coulter, Fullerton, CA), respectively]. Similarly, when the same 10 assays were calibrated directly with the 1st RR, 1.6-fold variation remained (data not shown), with the Dade Dimension RXL (Dade Behring, Newark, DE) yielding the highest and the Bayer Centaur the lowest result *(17)*. All of these observations indicate the complexity of interassay variation.

We attribute much of the interassay variation to two main factors: (1) differences in assay specificity, and (2) standardization material. Each will be discussed in more detail below.

Assay Specificity

One of the causes of interassay variation between hCG measurements is the use of antibodies that recognize different hCG molecules and degradation products (Table 4). The manufacturer's choice of antibodies will significantly affect results because antibody specificity will determine the number of different hCG molecules the assay will be able to detect. For instance, the reason the DPC Immulite hCG test consistently gives the highest result with the CAP proficiency test material, and not with the pure 1st RR, is that it is the only commercial hCG test that detects β-core fragment (Fig. 5). Whereas the 1st RR is pure and free of such contaminants, the CAP hCG proficiency test material is derived from a crude urine preparation (CAP technical service; Northfield, IL; personal communication), which likely contains significant β-core fragment, recognized only by the DPC Immulite hCG test. In addition, serum hCG assays differ in their ability to recognize hyperglycosylated hCG (Fig. 5). Quantification of a purified hyperglycosylated hCG standard ranged from 468 IU/L (Dade Dimension RXL) to 1544 IU/L (Roche Elecsys) *(9,12,17)*. This is a 3.3-fold variation. Similarly, serum hCG assays differ in their ability to recognize hCG free β-subunit (2.2-fold variation) and nicked hCG (1.5-fold variation). For a comprehensive list of comercially available hCG immunoassays and their specificity, see Cole *(12)*.

Significant interassay variation is also observed with home pregnancy tests and urine point of care tests. These tests are all approved for use with urine, yet in a recent study, we found that only 2 of 14 home pregnancy tests and a similar low proportion of urine

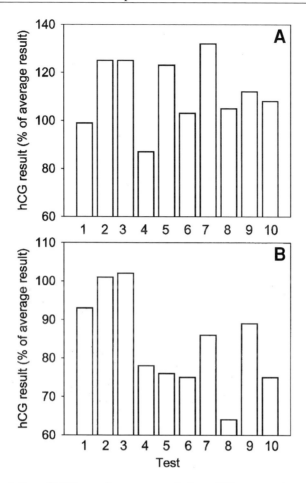

Fig. 4. Interassay variation of hCG tests. Interassay variation of 10 tests was investigated, the Abbott AxSym (test 1), Bayer ACS-180 (test 2), Bayer Centaur (test 3), Beckman Access-2 (test 4), Dade Dimension (test 5), Dade Stratus (test 6), DPC Immulite (test 7), Roche Elecsys (test 8), Tosoh A1A600 (test 9), and Vitros Eci (test 10). Panel A shows interassay variation as reported as part of ongoing CAP interlaboratory comparisons, involving 2307 laboratories *(18)*. Panel B shows a blind 11-laboratory comparison with the same 10 assays and the new 1st RR hCG standard.

point-of-care devices detect β-core fragment, the principal immunoreactive subunit in pregnancy urine throughout gestation *(3)*. These tests are intended for use in early pregnancy detection. However, in a study of 14 home pregnancy test devices, 3 (Rite Aid, Long's, and Inverness Medical One-Step) had poor detection or completely failed to detect hyperglycosylated hCG, the principal hCG molecule produced in the first weeks of gestation. In a more recent study, three other products (Sav-Osco, Target, and CVS one-step tests) were also shown to either not recognize or poorly recognize hyperglycosylated hCG (Cole L, Khanlian S, Sutton J, and Davies S, unpublished data). It was also observed that two products, Answer and Answer Quick and Simple, preferentially detected hyperglycosylated hCG.

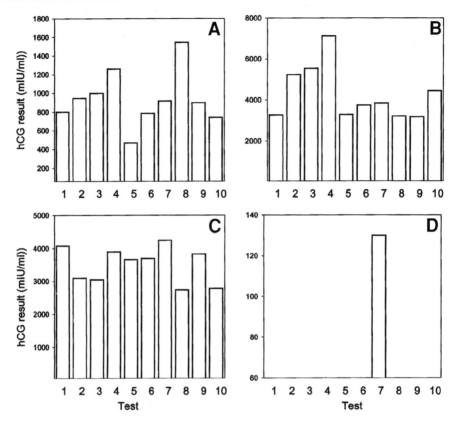

Fig. 5. Interassay variation of hCG tests. Interassay variation of 10 tests was investigated, the Abbott AxSym (test 1), Bayer ACS-180 (test 2), Bayer Centaur (test 3), Beckman Access-2 (test 4), Dade Dimension (test 5), Dade Stratus (test 6), DPC Immulite (test 7), Roche Elecsys (test 8), Tosoh A1A600 (test 9), and Vitros Eci (test 10). All were determined blindly in 11 laboratories *(17)*. Panel A is pure hyperglycosylated hCG, calibrated by mass as 100 µg/L. Panel B is pure free β-subunit (250 µg/L). Panel C is pure nicked hCG, nicked only at β47–48 (7) (400 µg/L). Panel D is pure β-core fragment (50 µg/L).

Standardization Material

The second factor that impacts interassay variation is the supply of pure WHO standards *(20)*. As stated earlier, the quantities of WHO standards are limited and are not sufficient for the provision of calibrators for all laboratories or standards for quality controls. As such, manufacturers purchase crude or partially purified urine-derived hCG and calibrate these with the WHO standard for use as calibrators and quality control material. This can greatly affect the hCG result. If a test manufacturer, for instance, uses a WHO-calibrated commercial hCG standard that contains significant nicked hCG, and the test does not detect nicked hCG, it will appear as if the assay gives lower results than it actually should *(9,12,17)*. However, even if WHO standards were available in larger quantities, as stated earlier, they are based on urine-based material, which may be inappropriate as a calibrator for serum-based assays.

LIMITATIONS OF DETECTING PREGNANCY
Urine-Based Tests

One of the principal uses of an hCG assay is to aid in the early detection of pregnancy. Home pregnancy and point-of-care urine tests are often the first indication of pregnancy during the third, fourth, and fifth weeks following the last menstrual period. Most home pregnancy and point of care test devices have manufacturer claims of "over 99% accurate" and "use as early the first day of missing a period." How valid are these claims?

Production of hCG does not begin until the blastocyst implants in the uterus. A study by Wilcox et al. reported that 10% of the 136 pregnancies they examined had not yet implanted by the first day of the missed menses *(10)*. Therefore, the highest possible screening sensitivity for an hCG test on the first day of the missed menses is 90% (95% confidence interval [CI] 84–94%). By 1 wk after the day of the missed menses, the highest sensitivity was estimated to be 97% (95% CI 94–99%). In addition, once hCG production has begun, urine hCG concentrations vary greatly between individuals at the same gestational age. A recent study by our group showed that to detect 95% of pregnancies with urine tests the day of the missed period, and at days 1, 2, and 3 after missing menses, would require test detection limits as low as 12.4, 21, 35, and 58 mIU/mL, respectively *(21)*. Although most urine point of care tests have claimed detection limits of 25–100 mIU/mL, we found that only 1 of 18 home pregnancy tests (First Response Early Result) had a detection limit as low as 12.5 mIU/mL *(21)*. A urine concentration of 100 mIU/mL hCG was needed, together with extended incubation times beyond the time suggested by manufacturers for 18 of 18 devices to yield positive results. At a detection limit of 100 mIU/mL it was estimated that only 16% of pregnancies would be detected on the day of the missed menses *(21)*. Based on these recent studies, we determined that a detection limit of 25 mIU/mL should detect 95% of pregnancies somewhere between 1 and 2 d after missing menses, and approx 74% of pregnancies at the time of missed menses *(21)*.

How can manufacturers claim such a high accuracy in very early gestation? The answer relates to an arcane Food and Drug Administration (FDA) 510(k) regulation. The manufacturer needs to demonstrate only that its test results agree with those of an existing test more than 99% of the time in order to advertise "greater than 99% accuracy." A new product is compared to an older FDA-approved test and evaluated with more than 100 urine samples supplemented with hCG at a concentration close to claimed sensitivity of the old test and with more than 100 urine samples containing no added hCG. The suggested use at the time of the missed menses and the 25 mIU/mL cutoff all come from studies performed with serum samples in the 1960s and 1970s and the now-proven erroneous assumption that serum and urine hCG concentrations are the same *(3)*. These FDA guidelines and 510(k) evaluations, however, have no bearing on the ability of a product to detect early pregnancy. New guidelines are required for both home and point-of-care pregnancy tests that would require determination of the proportion of pregnancies detected by the product on a specific day of gestation (i.e., time of missed menses).

A word of caution should be given about the use of urine in general. Urine hCG concentrations can vary significantly depending on fluid intake. Therefore, a serum hCG-positive individual may test negative on a urine hCG test because of very dilute urine. This is one of the limitations of urine testing to confirm pregnancy, especially on random samples. A positive result is useful, but a negative result must be interpreted with caution.

Serum-Based Tests

Most quantitative serum hCG tests have a lowest detection limit of greater than 1 mIU/mL. Considering that there can be background hCG of pituitary origin in serum *(22)*, most manufacturers recommend reporting negative results as less than 5 mIU/mL and using 5 mIU/mL as a cutoff for detecting pregnancy. Clearly, serum hCG tests are many times more sensitive than home pregnancy and point of care tests, and can detect more than 95% of pregnancies on or before the time of the missed menses. For this reason, quantitative serum hCG tests are the test of choice for pregnancy confirmation or for accurate early pregnancy detection.

Between one-quarter and one-third of naturally fertilized pregnancies and a much higher proportion of in vitro fertilized or assisted reproductive technology pregnancies fail to implant properly and result in early pregnancy losses. These lead to a transient increase in serum and urine hCG concentrations that diminish by the time of menses. An early pregnancy loss may also postpone menses 2 d *(23)*. This transient production of hCG can potentially cause a so-called false-positive pregnancy test result with urine or serum tests at or around the time of the missed menses. This is referred to as a "biochemical pregnancy." Repeat testing 2 to 3 d later will yield a true negative test result *(13,23,24)*. Recent studies by O'Connor and colleagues indicate minimal hyperglycosylated hCG production by early pregnancy losses, and specific measurement of hyper-glycosylated hCG may avoid the false detection of early pregnancy losses *(13)*.

In summary, it is clear that no test, serum or urine, can detect pregnancy with 99% accuracy at the first day of the missed menses. However, taking into account all of the above factors, it is estimated that urine or serum tests can detect pregnancy with 99% accuracy by 5 wk of gestation, or 1 wk following a missed menses.

LIMITATIONS OF hCG TESTS

Manufacturing Defects

Home pregnancy and point-of-care urine hCG tests are inexpensive disposable devices. Some poorly made devices can give false positive results in the absence of hCG, others can fail to function properly resulting in false negatives. These devices incorporate a test window and a control window. The test window indicates a positive or negative result and the control window indicates that the device is functioning properly (see "Principals of hCG Tests" above). Invalid tests fail to show a band in the control window. In a recent study examining home pregnancy tests *(21)*, two devices (Confirm and Clear Choice home pregnancy tests) gave one or more false-positive results with a urine solution containing 0 mIU/mL hCG. Similarly, 9 of 30 tests using the Clear Choice and 10 of 30 tests using the Confirm were invalid because they lacked the proper formation of a band in the control window. It is important to confirm all home pregnancy and point-of-care urine test results with quantitative serum hCG tests. Qualitatitive and semi-quantitative serum point-of-care tests are calibrated and somewhat better controlled products. Although they offer an improvement over urine point-of-care products, they are still a "second best choice" and positive results need to be confirmed using a quantitative serum test.

The Hook Effect

The "hook effect" is a major limitation of all serum and urine one-step immunometric assays (see "Principals of hCG Tests" section). The hook effect occurs when extremely high concentrations of an analyte such as hCG occupies all the sites on both the capture and detection antibodies and prevents the formation of a so called "sandwich." The end result is that few or no tracer antibody + hCG + immobilized-antibody complexes will be formed, yielding a false negative result. The "hook effect" does not occur with two-step quantitative assays because excess analyte is washed away before the tracer antibody is added. This problem has been documented for both quantitative and qualitative hCG assays *(25–29)*. As a rule, if a physician finds that the hCG result is inconsistent with the clinical presentation (e.g., patient is clearly at 8–10 wk of pregnancy, and a quantitative hCG is 10 mIU/mL, or a point-of-care test is negative), the qualitative or quantitative test should be repeated with 10- and 100-fold diluted sample *(9,22,30)*.

Heterophilic Antibodies

Heterophilic antibodies are human antibodies against other antibodies (human or animal) that can link a capture and tracer antibody in the absence of specific analyte and give a false-positive hCG result *(30–33)*. Because antibodies are large glycoproteins and generally do not cross the glomerular basement membrane and enter urine, this is only a problem in serum, not urine, assays *(30–33)*. The USA hCG Reference Service is a reference facility consulting with physicians in cases of conflicting or nonrepresentative hCG test results. In the last 5 yr, the USA hCG Reference Service has identified 54 cases of women who were erroneously treated for gestational trophoblastic disease, choriocarcinoma, or ectopic pregnancy because of false-positive hCG results *(4,22,32–38)*. In the first few months of operation, the USA hCG Reference Service investigated three unusual cases *(22)*. In all three cases, the women had an incidental pregnancy test that was positive. The positive hCG persisted with small apparent changes in concentrations. Ultrasound, dialation and curetlage, and laparoscopy ruled out pregnancy or ectopic pregnancy. The diagnosis of gestational trophoblastic disease or choriocarcinoma was assumed. In two of the three cases, chemotherapy was started, and in one case a hysterectomy was carried out. At this time, the reported hCG concentrations were 17, 53, and 110 IU/L, respectively. In all three cases, the presence of hCG was not confirmed and it was shown that these assays were subject to interference by heterophilic antibodies. To date, approx 145 individuals have been referred to the USA hCG Reference Service for investigating potential false positive hCG results. Fifty-four subjects were confirmed to have true false-positive results. False-positive results were identified by the following criteria *(22,32–36)*:

1. the finding of more than a fivefold difference in serum hCG results when tested with an alternative immunoassay (critical criterion)
2. the presence of hCG in serum and absence of detectable hCG or hCG-related molecule immunoreactivity in a parallel urine sample (critical criterion)
   Note: Where possible, urine testing should be performed using a quantitative hCG test with high sensitivity (sensitivity 2 mIU/mL). Even though this is an "off-label" application, it is the most appropriate and quickest confirmation of real or false-positive hCG. Point-of-care urine tests are limited to a sensitivity of 25 mIU/mL. We have found that

a qualitative urine test is not certain to confirm a serum hCG result unless that result exceeds at least 100 mIU/mL. In addition, because most qualitative assays currently detect intact hCG, they will not detect free β-hCG in the urine in cases of β-hCG-producing germ cell tumor. Germ cell tumors that produce only free β chain can present a similar clinical picture as heterophile antibodies (i.e., unexpected positive quantitative serum hCG, no clinical signs of pregnancy, and a negative qualitative urine hCG test).

3. the observation of false-positive results in other tests for molecules not normally present in serum, such as urine β-core fragment (confirmatory criterion)
4. the finding that a heterophilic antibody blocking agent (such as HBR, produced by Scantibodies Inc.) prevents or limits false positive (confirmatory criterion)

In all 54 confirmed false-positive cases, there was no prior history of trophoblastic disease or other tumors. Patients were treated for a diagnosis of ectopic pregnancy, gestational trophoblastic disease, or choriocarcinoma. Each case started with an incidental pregnancy test. Forty-five of 54 received needless surgery or single-agent chemotherapy; many received an unnecessary hysterectomy or other major surgery, or cytotoxic combination chemotherapy (32–38). To the best of our knowledge, in all cases, after false-positive hCG was identified, all treatment was halted, even though the quantitative test remained positive. Women having false-positive hCG results may also have falsely elevated results in other unrelated tests such as CEA, CA125, PSA, thyroid hormones, troponin, and other tumor and cardiac markers (39).

In most cases, false positive hCG results (in the USA hCG Reference Service assays) were eliminated by pretreatment of serum with a heterophilic antibody blocking agent, HBT (Scantibodies Inc., San Diego, CA) (36). It is noteworthy that certain hCG assays seem to have a propensity for producing false-positive results. All of the 53 false-positive cases arose from physicians who were monitoring patients with the Abbott AxSym hCGβ assay, Bayer Centaur test, Bayer ACS180, Bayer Immuno-1, Roche Elecsys, J&J Vitros ECI, Tosoh Nexia, and Dade Dimension RXL quantitative serum tests or with the Beckman Icon 2 serum point of care hCG test. It is noteworthy that 43 of the 53 false-positive cases detected by the USA hCG Reference Service arose from centers monitoring patients with the Abbott AxSym hCGβ assay. This has been observed by other centers (38). The Abbott AxSym test appears to be particularly prone to giving false-positive hCG results. An examination of the instruction sheet shows that animal serum is added in the Abbott AxSym test to just the diluent, rather than to the antibody preparation. As such, undiluted samples may not be protected from heterophilic antibody interference. This may explain the preponderance of false-positive results with this test (36,37).

Many of the clinicians who managed the 54 false-positive cases were misled by transient decreases in the hCG values after chemotherapy or surgery. This is because the decreases in hCG falsely suggested the presence of disease or indicated the success of therapy. The transient decreases were likely an interim weakening of the immune system after chemotherapy or surgery, reducing circulating heterophilic and antianimal antibody concentrations, leading to decreased false-positive hCG results.

SUMMARY

hCG is a complex glycoprotein that is produced by the trophoblastic cells of the placenta during pregnancy and in gestational trophoblastic diseases. Concentrations of hCG rise very rapidly during early pregnancy and peak at approx 8 and 12 wk. Numerous quantitative and qualitative assays for detecting hCG in serum or urine are available. All of these assays are two-site "sandwich"-type immunoassays. Although immunoassays for hCG have existed for more than 25 yr, many problems still exist, causing considerable interassay variation. The problems can be traced to two fundamental factors: (1) differences in assay specificity, and (2) standardization material. Assay specificity problems are caused by the use of a variety of different antibodies that recognize any combination of the different molecular forms of hCG. To further compound the problem, good standarization material does not exist, and the material that does exist is not available in sufficient quantities. Pregnancy detection is itself problematical because of variation in the timing of initial hCG production by individuals, wide variation in the extent of hCG production, and hCG production by early pregnancy losses. Further limitations of the hCG assays themselves include manufacturing defects, the hook effect, and heterophilic antibodies. Considering these observations, great care is needed in the use and interpretation of pregnancy tests. Home pregnancy tests and point-of-care pregnancy tests should be considered as indicators of pregnancy, and confirmation of pregnancy should be obtained using a quantitative serum assay.

REFERENCES

1. Kovalesvskaya G, Birken S, Kakuma T, O'Connor JF. Early pregnancy human chorionic gonodotropin (hCG) isoforms measured by immunometric assay for choriocarcinoma-like hCG. J Endocrinol 1999;161:99–106.
2. Cole LA, Shahabi S, Oz UA, Bahado-Singh RO, Mahoney MJ. Hyperglycosylated hCG (invasive trophoblastic antigen) immunoassay: a new basis for gestational down syndrome screening. Clin Chem 1999;45:2109-2119.
3. Butler SA, Khanlian SA, Cole LA. Detection of early pregnancy forms of hCG by home pregnancy test devices. Clin Chem 2001;47:2131–2136.
4. Cole LA, Shahabi S, Butler SA, et al. Utility of commonly used commercial hCG immunoassays in the diagnosis and management of trophoblastic diseases. Clin Chem, 2001;47:308–315.
5. Cole LA, Kohorn EI, Kim GS. Detecting and monitoring trophoblastic disease: new perspectives in measuring human chorionic gonadotropin levels. J Reprod Med 1994;39:193–200.
6. Kohorn EI, Cole LA. Nicked human chorionic gonadotropin in trophoblastic disease. Intl J Obstet Gynecol 2000;10:330–335.
7. Elliott M, Kardana A, Lustbader JW, Cole LA. Carbohydrate and peptide structure of the α- and β-subunits of human chorionic gonadotropin from normal and aberrant pregnancy and choriocarcinoma. Endocrine 1997;7:15–32.
8. Cole LA, Kardana A, Park S-Y, Braunstein GD. The deactivation of hCG by nicking and dissociation. J Clin Endocrinol Metab 1993;76;704–713.
9. Cole LA, Kardana A. Discordant results in human chorionic gonadotropin assays. Clin Chem 1992;38:263–270.
10. Wilcox AJ, Baird DD, Dunson D, McCheaney R, Weinberg CR. Natural limits of pregnancy testing in relation to the expected menstrual period. J Am Med Assoc 2001;286:1759–1761.
10a. Aswood ER. Evaluating health and maturation of the unborn: the role of the clinical laboratory. Clin Chem 1992;38:1523–1529.
10b. Aswood ER. Clinical chemistry of pregnancy. In; Burtis CA, Aswood EK, eds. Tier Textbook of Clinical Chemistry, 3rd ed. Philadelphia, Saunders, 1998;1736–1775.
11. Kovaleskaya G, Genbacev O, Fisher SJ, Caceres E, O'Connor JF. Trophoblast origin of hCG isoforms: cytotrophoblasts are the primary source of choriocarcinoma-like hCG. Mol Cell Endocrinol 2002;94:147–155.
12. Cole, LA, Immunoassay of hCG, its free subunits and metabolites. Clin Chem 1997;43:2233–2243.
13. O'Connor JF, Ellish N, Kakuma T, Schlatterer J, Kovalevskaya G. Differential urinary gonadotrophin profiles in early pregnancy and early pregnancy loss. Prenatal Diagnosis 1998;18:1232–1240.
14. Storring PL, Gaines-Das RE, Bangham DR. International reference preparation of human chorionic gonadotrophin for immunoassay: potency estimates in various bioassay and protein binding assay

systems; and international reference preparations of the α and β subunits of human chorionic gonadotrophin for immunoassay. J Endocr 1980;84;295–310.

15. Cole LA, Cermik D, Bahado-Singh R. Oligosaccharide variants of hCG-related molecules: potential screening markers for Down syndrome. Prenat Diagn 1997;17:1188–1190.

16. Birken S, Berger P, Bidart J-M, et al. Preparation and characterization of new W.H.O. reference reagents for human chorionic gonadotropin (hCG) and metabolites. Clin Chem 2002;49:144–154.

17. Sutton JM, Higgins TN, Cembrowski GS, Cole LA. Source of inter-assay variations in hCG test results. Clin Chem submitted 2003 (to be updated at proof).

18. College of American Pathologists, Ligand Assay Series, CA-B 2002 Survey, 2002; p. 32.

19. Bock JL. hCG assays: a plea for uniformity. Am J Clin Path 1990;93:432–433.

20. Canfield RE, Ross GT. A new reference preparation of human chorionic gonadotrophin and its subunits. Bull World Health Organization 1976;54:463–72.

21. Khanlian S, Davies S, Sutton JM, Cole LA, Rayburn WF. Utility of home pregnancy test kits at the time of missed menses. Am J Obstet Gynecol, submitted, 2004. In press.

22. Cole LA. Phantom hCG and phantom choriocarcinoma. Gynecol Oncol 1998;71:325–329.

23. Wilcox AJ, Weinberg CR, O'Connor JF, et al. Incidence of early loss of pregnancy. N Engl J Med 1988;319:189–194.

24. Bjercke S, Tanbo T, Dale PO, Morkrid L, Abyholm T. Human chorionic gonadotrophin concentrations in early pregnancy after in-vitro fertilization. Human Reprod 1999;14:1642–1646.

25. Yoo A, Zaccaro J. Falsely low hCG level in a patient with hydatidiform mole caused by the "high-dose hook effect." Lab Med 2000;31:431–435.

26. Witherspoon LR, Schuler SE, Joseph GF, Baird GF, Neely HR, Sonnemaker RE. Immunoassay for quantifying choriogonadotropin compared for assay performance and clinical application. Clin Chem 1992;38:887–894.

27. Forest JC, Masse J, Lane A. Evaluation of the analytical performance of the Boehringer Mannheim Elecsys 2010 immunoanalyzer. Clin Biochem 1998;31:81–88.

28. Levavi H, Neri A, Bar J, Regev D, Nordenberg J, Ovadia J. "Hook effect" in complete hydatidiform molar pregnancy: a falsely low level of beta-hCG. Obstet Gynecol 1993;82:720–721.

29. Stickle DF, Gronowski AM, Olsen GA, Fellows PA, Avery MB, Studts DJ. Decreased signal intensity of Sure-Vue serum/urine qualitative hCG test at very high [hCG]. Clin Chem 2000;46:A3.

30. Hussa RO, Rinke ML, Schweitzer PG. Discordant human chorionic gonadotropin results: causes and solutions. Obstet Gynecol 1985;65:211–219.

31. Vladutiu AO, Sulewski JM, Pudlak KA, Stull CG. Heterophilic antibodies interfering with radioimmunoassay: a false-positive pregnancy test. J Am Med Assoc 1982;248:2489–2490.

32. Ward G, McKinnon L, Badrick T, Hickman PE. Heterophillic antibodies remain a problem for the immunoassay laboratory. Am J Clin Path 1997;108:417–421.

33. Rotmensch S, Cole LA. False diagnosis and needless therapy of presumed malignant disease in women with false-positive human chorionic gonadotropin concentrations. Lancet 2000;355:712–715.

34. Cole LA, Butler SA. False positive or phantom hCG result: a serious problem. Clin Lab Intl 2001; 25:9–14.

35. Cole LA, Rinne KM, Shababi S, Omrani A. False positive hCG assay results leading to unnecessary surgery and chemotherapy and needless occurrence of diabetes and coma. Clin Chem 1999;45:313–314.

36. Butler SA, Cole LA. The use of heterophilic antibody blocking agent (HBT) in reducing false positive hCG results. Clin Chem 2001;47:1332–1333.

37. Cole LA, Butler SA. hCG, its free subunits and metabolites in trophoblastic diseases. J Reprod Med 2002;47:433–444.

38. Olsen TG, Hubert PR, Nycum LR. Falsely elevated human chorionic gonadotrophin leading to unnecessary therapy. Obstet Gynecol 2001;98:843–845.

39. Covinsky M, Laterza O, Pfeifer JD, Farkas-Szallasi T, Scott MG. An IgM antibody to E. coli produces false positive results in multiple immunometric assays. Clin Chem 2000;46:1157–1161.

40. Birken S, Armstrong EG, Kolks MAG, et al. Structure of human chorionic gonadotropin β-subunit core fragment from pregnancy urine. Endocrinology 1988;123;572–580.

41. Morgan FJ, Birken S, Canfield RE. The amino acid sequence of human chorionic gonadotropin: the α subunit and β-subunit. J Biol Chem 1975;2250;5247–5257.

42. Lapthorn AJ, Harris DC, Littlejohn A, et al. Crystal structure of human chorionic gonadotropin. Nature 1994;369;455–460.

3

Biological Markers of Preterm Delivery

Stephen F. Thung, MD
and Alan M. Peaceman, MD

INTRODUCTION

Preterm birth is a major public health problem in the United States. It is the most common reason for both neonatal mortality and serious long-term morbidity after congenital birth defects *(1)*. Preterm birth, as defined by the World Health Organization (WHO), is the delivery of an infant prior to 37 wk and greater than 20 wk gestational age. Preterm birth arises from three major problems: 50% arise from spontaneous preterm labor with intact membranes, another 30% are the result of preterm premature rupture of membranes (PPROM), and the remaining 20% of preterm births are indicated deliveries because of declining fetal status, such as fetal growth restriction, or worsening maternal status, such as hypertension *(2)*. It is the first two categories, spontaneous preterm labor and PPROM, that research on biological markers of preterm delivery has focused on.

The preterm delivery rate in the United States has steadily climbed upward from 9.4% in 1981 to 11.6% in 2000, a 26% increase *(3)*. During this interval, the preterm birth rate before 32 wk gestation has remained unchanged at approx 2% *(3)*. Many factors have contributed to this overall increase. The rate of multiple gestations has risen 19% during the period 1989 to 1996, primarily because of increased utilization of infertility treatments. Preterm birth is the norm in multiple gestations, with 49.5% of twins and 90.1% of triplets affected *(4)*. The increase in preterm births has also been attributed to increased

From: *Current Clinical Pathology: Handbook of Clinical Laboratory Testing During Pregnancy*
Edited by: A. M. Gronowski © Humana Press, Totowa, NJ

intervention before term for medical indications, increased intervention for fetal indications, and improved determination of gestational age by ultrasound with greater recognition of preterm deliveries.

Although all preterm births are concerning, the approx 2% that occur prior to 32 wk gestation are the greatest concern because the bulk of perinatal mortality occurs in births before this gestational age. In fact, approx 50% of all long-term neurological morbidity and 60% of perinatal mortality occurs in these preterm infants (5). A large prospective study by Lemons et al. (6) followed 4438 infants with birth weights between 501 and 1500 g that survived long enough to be brought to the neonatal intensive care unit. At 24 wk gestation, there was approx 50% mortality, 20% at 26 wk, 8% at 28 wk, and 3% at 32 wk, with little improvement with each additional week. These findings are consistent with previous studies examining similar outcomes (6–8).

Short-term morbidities are also a major problem that improves with advancing gestational age. Although the incidence of respiratory distress syndrome decreases until 36 wk, necrotizing enterocolitis, intraventricular hemorrhage, and sepsis are virtually absent after 32 wk of gestation (9). Lemons et al. (6) also identified an association between gestational age at birth and neonatal complications. Morbidities included chronic lung disease, severe intracranial hemorrhage, and necrotizing enterocolitis. At the smallest infant birth weights (501–750 g), only 36.9% of survivors were discharged without obvious morbidity, whereas at 1251–1500 g birth weight, 90.1% survived without obvious morbidity (6).

Other groups have examined long-term morbidities with results suggesting that increases in both birth weight and gestational age decrease the incidence of long-term morbidities. Vohr et al. (10) examined 1151 infants (between 1993 and 1994) who had a birth weight of 401–1000 g. They evaluated the developmental, sensory, and functional outcomes at 18–22 mo and found that 25% had an abnormal neurological exam, 37% had delayed mental development, and 29% had delayed motor development. Furthermore, 9% had vision impairment and 11% had hearing impairment.

Wood et al. (11) followed 283 infants born before 25 wk gestation and demonstrated, at a median of 30 mo of age, that 49% of the cohort had some form of neurological or developmental dysfunction. The trend once again showed that morbidities decreased with gestational age. Survival without disability was 5% at 23 wk gestation, 12% at 24 wk, and 23% at 25 wk.

Hack et al. (12) followed two cohorts to elementary school age. The first study group was composed of 68 survivors who had birth weights less than 750 g. The second group consisted of 65 survivors with birth weights between 750 and 1499 g. They assessed both groups at a median of 6.9 yr of age for growth, sensory status, motor function, academic performance, and behavioral function at school age and found an IQ score less than 70 in 21% and 8%, respectively, compared to 2% in term gestation controls. The incidence of cerebral palsy was 9% and 6% for the two study groups and 0% for the term control. Limitations in academic performance were identified in 27% and 9% of the study cohorts compared with 2% in the control group.

Hack et al. (13) later evaluated a cohort of 242 individuals in young adulthood who were born between 1977 and 1979 and who had birth weights less than 1500 g. When compared to normal birth weight controls, they found that at 20 yr of age, these children had lower IQ scores, were less likely to enter high school (74 vs 83%), and had higher rates of neurosensory impairments such as blindness, deafness, or cerebral palsy (10 vs <1%).

The problem of preterm delivery and low birth weight is associated with increased mortality and morbidity in neonates. The initial attempts at identifying individuals at high risk of preterm delivery involved risk assessment systems based on information readily available to clinicians, including historical information, demographic data, and symptoms. Unfortunately, these systems are neither sensitive nor specific for predicting preterm delivery. Quantitative biological markers, such as cervicovaginal fetal fibronectin (fFN) and transvaginal cervical length studies, are now the most commonly used methods for assessing the preterm birth risk, with improved predictive values over traditional risk assessment systems.

RISK ASSESSMENT

The greatest obstacle to predicting which patients will deliver preterm is our incomplete understanding of what initiates preterm labor and subsequent preterm birth. Much of our knowledge of labor physiology comes from animal models in the mouse, sheep, and monkey, and is often not applicable to the human labor model. Available risk-based, rather than biologically based, scoring systems took advantage of known historical, physical, and behavioral risk factors that are readily available to physicians. In essence, they determine a high-risk patient by identifying the presence of risk factors that have been known to be associated with increased preterm birth risk. Some of the risk factors commonly evaluated are listed in Table 1.

The best-known risk-based system was developed by Creasy (14). This system scored patients at their first prenatal visit and again at 26–28 wk in four categories, and assigned a rank between 1 and 10, with higher scores given to patients with higher risk. This system utilized many of the factors noted earlier. However, risk-based systems have been shown to lack sensitivity and specificity to identify a patient who will deliver prematurely (14–16). Mercer et al. (15) examined a risk-based system for predicting spontaneous preterm delivery in a low-risk population. He assessed risk factors for 2929 patients at 23–24 wk and found that the risk-based system identified a minority of patients who ultimately delivered preterm. A sensitivity of 24.2% and a positive predictive value of 28.6% for preterm birth were calculated for nulliparous patients, with slight improvement for multiparous patients.

FETAL FIBRONECTIN

Adult fibronectins are ubiquitous glycoproteins that are found in plasma and the extracellular matrix. They play major roles in many fundamental biologic processes including cell adhesion and migration, maintenance of normal cell physiology, cell differentiation, embryogenesis, and tumor genesis. fFN, also known as oncofetal fibronectin, is a unique glycosylated form expressed only in fetal tissue and cancer lines and is recognized by the FDC-6 murine antibody that recognizes the IIICS domain (17). The fibronectin molecule consists of repeating modules known as type I-III modules. The III-CS domain resides in a type III module adjacent to the carboxyl terminus. fFN, as shown by immunohistochemical studies, localizes to the uterine–placental and decidual–chorionic extracellular matrices. In cell culture, native fFN shows adhesive properties suggesting that fFN may be "trophoblast glue" that results in physiologic cellular adhesion. It is believed that fFN is released into the cervix and vagina when the interface between the chorion and decidua is interrupted prior to the initiation of labor (18).

Table 1
Risk Factors Associated With Preterm Delivery

History of preterm birth
Black race
Multiple gestation
Women under 17 and over 35 yr of age
Lower socioeconomic status
Poor or excessive weight gain
Smoking
Substance abuse

Data from ref. *36*.

fFN in cervicovaginal secretions is present during the first 16–20 wk of gestation *(19,20)* but drops to undetectable levels in nearly all patients after 24 wk. fFN concentrations remain low in normal pregnancies until approx 34 wk, when fFN concentrations typically increase prior to delivery *(20)*.

One of the earliest studies evaluating elevated fFN as a marker for preterm delivery *(20)* determined a discriminatory cutoff of 50 ng/mL, in a post hoc analysis, for predicting the likelihood of preterm delivery. This concentration was chosen because it maximized the sensitivity and the specificity of predicting a preterm birth. Based on receiver operating curves (ROC) constructed from cervical and vaginal fFN concentrations in 2926 women, Goepfert et al. *(21)* demonstrated that this 50 ng/mL discriminatory cutoff was reasonable for screening from 24 to 30 wk gestation. This concentration has been commonly accepted for studies examining the fFN assay. Elevated concentrations of fFN after 20 wk have uniformly been associated with delivering preterm in symptomatic *(22–24)* and asymptomatic patients *(25–29)*. Elevated concentrations of fFN are also associated with the onset of term labor *(30,31)*.

Symptomatic Patients

Attention has been given to the predictive value of fFN in the preterm patient with symptoms consistent with preterm labor. Prospective studies have consistently shown that a positive fFN test (>50 ng/mL) is significantly associated with preterm delivery with relative risk values of 38.8, 31.3, and 3.2 for delivery prior to 7 d, 14 d, and less than 37 wk respectively *(22–24)*. However, the positive predictive value of fFN for imminent preterm delivery is low, ranging from 13 to 29% in the largest studies *(22,24,25)*. This makes the utility of a positive test unclear, because the majority of patients who test positive will actually deliver at term. Conversely, the test has a high negative predictive value, and the true value of fFN may be with its ability to rule out preterm labor in symptomatic patients with a negative test *(22,24)*.

Peaceman et al. *(22)* performed the largest prospective study in this population. Their data are summarized in Table 2. They screened 763 symptomatic patients between 24 and 34 wk and found negative predictive values for preterm birth of 99.5% within 7 d, 99.2% within 14 d, and 84.5% at less than 37 wk. These findings suggest that fFN testing should improve the accuracy of diagnosing preterm labor in symptomatic patients when testing is negative. A negative result provides reassurance that the patient will have a less than 1% chance of delivering within the next 7 to 14 d. However, in this study, 127 of the patients received tocolysis within 7 d of enrollment. It is possible that withholding tocolysis treatment in those patients would have lowered the negative predictive value of fFN.

Table 2
Predictive Accuracy of Cervicovaginal fFN in 725 Symptomatic Singleton Pregnancies
for Delivery <7 D, <14 D, <37 Wk

Delivery	Relative risk	95% Confidence	Sensitivity	PPV	NPV
<7 d	38.8	(9.1–165)	90.5%	13.4%	99.7%
<14 d	31.3	(9.5–103)	88.5%	16.2%	99.5%
<37 w	3.2	(2.4–4.3)	43.9%	43.0%	86.6%

NPV, negative predictive value; PPV, positive predictive value.
Data from ref. 22.

Table 3
Predictive Accuracy of Fetal Fibronectin for Delivery <34 Wk
Gestation From Either Cervical or Vaginal Swabs in 2929
Asymptomatic Patients

Gestational age of screening	Sensitivity	Specificity	PPV	NPV
22–24 wk	23%	97%	25%	96%
26 wk	22%	97%	20%	
28 wk	20%	97%	17%	
30 wk	29%	96%	18%	

NPV, negative predictive value; PPV, positive predictive value. Data
from refs. 21,25.

Asymptomatic Patients

In asymptomatic patients, fFN has also been shown to predict preterm birth with
relative risks of 59.2, 39.9, 21.2, 8.9, and 3.8 for deliveries occurring between 24 and 27
wk, 24 and 29 wk, 24 and 31 wk, 24 and 34 wk, and 24 and 36 wk, respectively (25). The
largest study to date was completed by the National Institute of Child Health and Human
Development Maternal Fetal Medicine Units Network (25), which screened 2929 asymptomatic patients with fFN at 22–24, 26, 28, and 30 wk gestation. These data are summarized in Table 3. For deliveries prior to 34 wk gestation, the sensitivity for a positive test
ranged from 20 to 29% depending on the gestational age at testing. The specificity for a
negative test remained more than 96%, despite the timing of screening. The positive
predictive value, similar to symptomatic patients, was low (18–25%).

For deliveries prior to 28 wk gestation where neonatal morbidity and mortality is
greatest, fFN screening demonstrated its highest sensitivity, specificity, and relative risk
at 63%, 98%, and 59, respectively. This suggests that fFN was most successful at predicting early preterm birth (<28 wk) and less successful at later gestational ages (<34 wk),
a significant advantage to the use of fFN because of worsening neonatal mortality and
morbidity at these early gestational ages.

A meta-analysis by Leitich et al. (32) evaluated the ability of fFN to predict preterm
births for both symptomatic and asymptomatic patients. For predicting preterm deliveries less than 34 wk in asymptomatic patients, a value greater than 50 ng/mL had a
sensitivity of 61% and a specificity of 83%. When patients with preterm labor symptoms

were evaluated, the sensitivity was 85% and the specificity was 68%. The test performed best when predicting a delivery within 7 d in symptomatic patients, with a sensitivity of 89% and a specificity of 86%.

Multiple Gestations

Although there are a disproportionate number of preterm births in pregnancies with more than one fetus, there have been few studies evaluating the utility of fFN screening in these individuals. The small studies performed have consistently found an association of premature deliveries with a positive fFN test *(33–35)*. Wennerholm et al. *(35)* screened 101 asymptomatic twin pregnancies from 24 wk to 34 wk. For twin gestations delivering before 35 wk, screening at 24 wk had a sensitivity, specificity, positive predictive value, negative predictive value, and relative risk of 36.8%, 91.3%, 53.8%, 84%, and 4.2 (95% confidence interval [CI] 1.6–11.1). The accuracy of screening was improved at 28 wk: 50.0%, 92%, 62.5%, 87.3%, 6.3 (95% CI 2.6–15.1). Positive screening at 26 and 30 wk gestation was not associated with increased risk for preterm birth.

The fFN Assay

The cervicovaginal fFN assay is approved by the Food and Drug Administration (FDA) for use in pregnant patients who display symptoms of preterm labor. However, patients must conform to certain criteria as stated by the manufacturer (Adeza Biomedical, Sunnyvale, CA), which include gestational age between $24\frac{0}{7}$ and $34\frac{6}{7}$ wk, singleton pregnancy, intact fetal membranes, cervical exam less than 3 cm dilatation, no history of placenta previa, no cervical manipulation from pelvic exam or ultrasound exam for 24 h, and no use of lubricants or recent sexual intercourse within 24 h.

Once an appropriate patient has been identified for fFN testing, a speculum should be placed in the vagina (prior to any cervical exam). A Dacron® polyester swab, supplied by Adeza, should be placed in the posterior vaginal fornix (asymptomatic or symptomatic patients) or the ectocervical region of the external cervical os (asymptomatic patients) for 10 s to absorb vaginal or cervical secretions. The sample should be placed immediately into the collecting tube provided by the manufacturer and refrigerated until the fFN assay is performed.

Prior to the availability of the rapid fFN assay (described later), all samples were frozen and sent to Adeza Biomedical for analysis. fFN concentrations were determined by a fFN enzyme immunoassay. After the cervicovaginal samples of interest were incubated in microtiter wells coated with FDC-6 antibody, the antibody–antigen complex was washed and reacted with an enzyme-labeled antibody against fFN. Following formation of this antigen–antibody complex, the microtiter well was cleared of all unbound labeled antibody. It was then incubated with an enzyme substrate, allowing the amount of fFN in the specimens to be calculated spectrophotometrically at a wavelength of 550 nm.

Two rapid assays for fFN are currently marketed by Adeza Biomedical. The first assay is a membrane immunogold assay that utilizes an antihuman fibronectin–gold colloid conjugate that binds to fFN in the specimen. Detection of the fFN–gold colloid complex is accomplished by passing the specimen through a membrane containing the monoclonal antibody FDC-6, which is specific for fFN. The gold complexes are then immobilized and produce a visible spot within 5 min. Specimens with an fFN concentration greater than 50 ng/mL will produce a positive result within a control ring and are interpreted visually. This assay is not available in the United States and its use in the literature has been reported only from countries outside the United States. The second assay is the rapid fFN cassette and is available in the United States. It was approved by the FDA for marketing in 1998. It is also a membrane immunoassay and uses the monoclonal FDC-6 anti-fFN antibody coupled to a blue microsphere and an immobilized polyclonal goat anti-fibronectin antibody. The intensities of the test and control lines on the device are interpreted with the TLi$_{IQ}$™ analyzer. Concentrations of fFN greater than 50 ng/mL are reported as positive. The majority of studies regarding fFN have been performed using the microtiter plate enzyme immunoassay, and very few have examined the utility of the rapid fFN tests.

Summary

A negative fFN test in the symptomatic patient is reassuring because it suggests that the patient has a less than 1% chance of delivering within the next week. Most of these patients should be safe to return home, reassured that they are not in preterm labor *(5)*. The best use of fFN screening may be in these symptomatic patients, when a negative test may result in a more accurate exclusion of preterm labor and decreased utilization of hospital stays and pharmacological interventions, such as tocolysis and corticosteroid use. The American College of Obstetricians and Gynecologists states that "fetal fibronectin testing may be useful in women with symptoms of preterm labor to identify those with negative values and a reduced risk of preterm birth, thereby avoiding unnecessary intervention" *(36)*. Screening the general obstetrical population is not recommended until effective interventions to improve maternal and neonatal health are identified.

CERVICAL ULTRASOUND

The cervix changes throughout gestation, with the most dramatic changes occurring soon before delivery. The cervix shortens, softens, takes a more anterior position, and finally begins to dilate *(5)*. Although digital exams are used to assess these cervical changes and to stratify which patients are at high risk for preterm delivery, manual cervical examinations by clinicians are subject to significant variation between observers, making digital exams of questionable accuracy and reproducibility *(37,38)*.

Transvaginal cervical ultrasonography has gained popularity because of its greater reliability in assessing the status of the cervix when compared to digital examination *(39,40)* and transabdominal cervical ultrasonography *(41)*. Critical to the popularity is the inverse association of decreasing ultrasound measured cervical length and increasing risk of preterm birth *(42)*. Cervical length by ultrasound has been found to be more sensitive at predicting preterm delivery than digital examination *(39)*. However, despite the ability of cervical length to predict preterm birth, routine screening of low-risk patients is not currently recommended because of the lack of demonstrated benefit from detecting shortened length.

Once a patient has been selected for cervical length measurements, it becomes important to perform the test properly to minimize error and variability. The length of the cervix is measured using a real-time transvaginal ultrasound probe. After the subject empties her bladder, she is placed in the dorsal lithotomy position. Ultrasound gel is placed in a condom or other sterile covering prior to inserting the ultrasound probe. The ultrasound probe is then placed into the vaginal anterior fornix until a sagittal view of the cervix is appreciated. The view should include the internal cervical os, the external cervical os, and the endocervical canal.

The image of the cervix, from the internal os to the external os should fill the ultrasound screen prior to measurement. The probe is then withdrawn to minimize the pressure of the probe on the cervix, because excess pressure can distort the measured cervical length. Once the entire cervix is visualized, the sonographer may freeze the image and measure the distance between the internal and external cervical os as the cervical length (Fig. 1). Several measurements should be taken and averaged. Occasionally, the cervical canal is not linear. In these cases, the sum of the two shortest linear measurements that best follow the endocervical canal should be used *(42)*.

In the largest prospective study to date *(42)*, the cervix, when measured with transvaginal ultrasound, has a median length of 35.2 mm ± 8.3 mm between 22 and 24 wk gestation. The 10th percentile is 25 mm and the 90th percentile is 45 mm. The cervix normally shortens as gestation advances. The median cervical length decreases to 33.7 ± 8.5 mm between 26 and 28 wk gestation. Zilanti et al. *(43)* qualitatively characterized the process of cervical shortening on ultrasound. As cervical development and shortening occurs, the internal os of the cervix progresses through a variety of appearances. As seen in Fig. 2, the internal os is typically closed and looks like a T. As the lower uterine segment develops and thins, the internal os opens and initially resembles a Y, a V, and finally a U *(43)*.

Asymptomatic Patients

There have been several prospective studies evaluating the use of cervical ultrasound as a screening tool to predict subsequent preterm birth in asymptomatic low-risk patients screened in the early second trimester *(44)*, high-risk patients screened in the early second trimester *(45,46)*, and low-risk patients in the late second trimester *(42,47)*. All of these studies have confirmed an association between preterm birth and short cervical length. A meta-analysis by Leitich *(48)* summarized 35 studies of cervical length for preterm delivery prediction and found that the sensitivity ranged from 68 to 100% and the specificity from 44 to 79%.

The largest prospective multicenter trial by Iams et al. *(42)* included 2915 women who had cervical ultrasounds at 22–24 wk gestation and again 4 wk later; 2513 patients were available for study. The group found that there was an inverse relationship between the cervical length and the gestational age at delivery, with the highest risk in the group below the 10th percentile of cervical length. Compared to the preterm birth rates of women above the 75th percentile (40 mm), the relative risks of preterm birth before 35 wk for cervical lengths performed between 22 and 24 wk were less than 75th percentile (40 mm) 1.98, less than 50th percentile (35 mm) 2.35, less than 25th pecentile (30 mm) 3.79, less than10th percentile (26 mm) 6.19, less than 5th percentile (22 mm) 9.57, and less than 1st percentile (13 mm) 13.99. At 26–28 wk gestation, the corresponding relative risks were 2.80, 3.52, 5.39, 9.57, 13.88, and 24.94.

The Iams study *(42)* evaluated different cervical lengths as a marker for preterm delivery before 35 wk gestation. Table 4 summarizes the sensitivity, specificity, positive predictive value, and negative predictive value for each cervical length. Data on funneling and Bishop scores are also included for comparison. Bishop scores are used to assess the "ripeness" of the cervix and the success of a multiparous patient for vaginal delivery. Categories assessed are cervical dilatation, cervical effacement, fetal head station, cer-

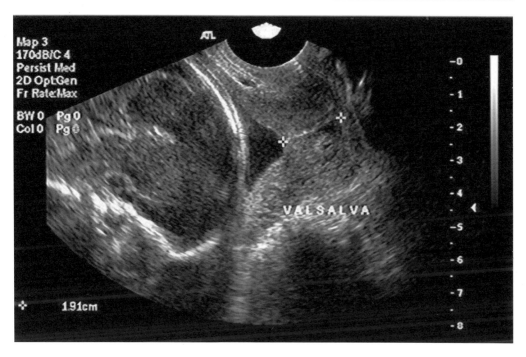

Fig. 1. Example of transvaginal ultrasound of a shortened cervix. This cervix measures 1.91 cm (distance between crosshairs +). (Courtesy of Edmund Funai.)

vical consistency, and cervical position (posterior, anterior, etc). Higher scores are associated with more advanced cervical changes.

Owen et al. *(45)* performed a blinded cohort study in 183 women who were at high risk, defined as a history of spontaneous preterm birth before 32 wk. Screening ultrasounds were started as early as 16–18 wk and were repeated biweekly until $23^{6}/_{7}$ wk. In this high risk population, the initial median cervical length measurement was 37 mm. The lowest 10th percentile measured at 26 mm and the lowest 5th percentile was at 23 mm. Cervical lengths measuring less than 30 mm were associated with preterm delivery before 35 wk as summarized in Table 5. The relative risks for less than 15 mm, less than 20 mm, less than 25 mm, less than 30 mm were 4.1, 3.4, 3.3, and 2.5, respectively. Funneling of the internal os was not an independent risk factor for preterm delivery.

Improved sensitivity for preterm birth was noted beyond the first 16- to 18-wk ultrasound if serial ultrasounds were performed or if dynamic cervical shortening, defined as spontaneous cervical shortening or cervical shortening with application of fundal pressure, was noted. The sensitivity, specificity, positive predictive value, negative predictive value, and relative risks for a cervical length of less than 25 mm on the first ultrasound were 19%, 98%, 75%, 77%, 3.3 (95% CI 2.1–5.0). Any cervical length less than 25 mm on serial ultrasounds improved the test with values 58%, 81%, 53%, 85% and 3.4 (95% CI 2.1–5.5). If dynamic change was identified on serial exams, the values were 69%, 80%, 55%, 88%, and 4.5 (95% CI 2.7–7.6).

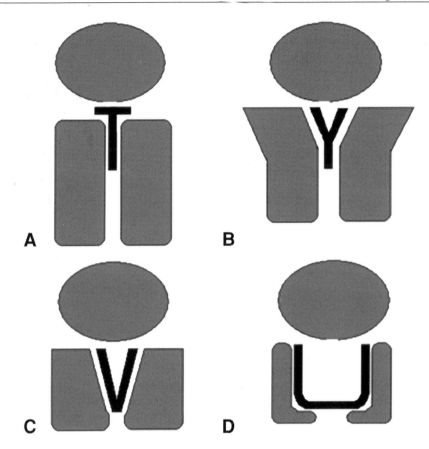

Fig. 2. Illustration of progressive cervical effacement with fetal head. (**A**) Normal cervix. (**B**) Cervix with early effacement at internal os. (**C**) Cervix with progressive effacement at the internal os. (**D**) Cervix with progressive effacement to the external os.

Symptomatic Patients

Unlike fFN testing, only small studies have demonstrated the utility of transvaginal ultrasonography in the setting of symptomatic preterm contractions for predicting imminent preterm birth *(49–52)*. The largest study to date, by Crane et al. *(49)*, prospectively performed transvaginal cervical ultrasound on 136 women with singleton pregnancies and 26 women with twin pregnancies admitted between 23 and 33 wk for suspected preterm labor. A cervical length was measured after preterm uterine contractions resolved, with tocolytic therapy in some cases. A cervical length of less than 30 mm was found to be the optimal length for predicting a preterm delivery before 37 wk gestation. In singleton pregnancies, this discriminatory cutoff had a sensitivity of 81%, specificity of 65%, positive predictive value of 46%, and negative predictive value of 90%. For twins, cervical length was not as predictive, with values 75%, 30%, 63%, and 43%, respectively.

Table 4
Predictive Accuracy of Cervical Length Assessment
by Ultrasound and Physical Exam at 24 Wk in Asymptomatic
Patients for Preterm Birth <35 Wk

	Sensitivity	Specificity	PPV	NPV
< 20 mm	23.0	97.0	25.7	96.5
< 25 mm	37.3	92.2	17.8	97.0
< 30 mm	54.0	76.3	9.3	97.4
Funneling	25.4	94.5	17.3	96.6
Bishop > 6	7.9	99.4	38.5	96.0
Bishop > 4	27.6	90.9	12.1	96.5

NPV, negative predictive value; PPV, positive predictive value.
Data from ref. *42.*

Table 5
Predictive Accuracy of Cervical Length Measurements at 16–18 Wk in Asymptomatic Women
at High Risk for Preterm Birth <35 Wk

	<15 mm	*<20 mm*	*<25 mm*	*<30 mm*
Sensitivity %	10	10	19	38
Specificity %	100	99	98	87
Positive Predictive Value %	100	83	75	77
Negative Predictive Value %	76	76	77	80
Relative Risk (95% CI)	4.1 (3.2–5.4)	3.4 (2.2–5.3)	3.3 (2.1–5.0)	2.5 (1.6–3.9)

Data from ref. *45.*

Summary

Transvaginal cervical length studies can be used to identify patients at increased risk of preterm birth. The risk of a shortened cervix for preterm birth increases in a continuous fashion as the cervical length decreases. Although many studies have identified a discriminatory cervical length of 25 mm as the ideal length in the asymptomatic patient and 30 mm in the symptomatic patient to place a patient at high risk or low risk for preterm delivery, this length is to some degree an arbitrary cutoff.

SALIVARY ESTRIOL

Estriol is one of three major estrogens found in humans (estriol, estradiol, and estrone). During pregnancy, it is present at concentrations 10–20 times higher than other estrogens and is produced almost exclusively by fetal tissue rather than maternal tissue *(53)*. In humans, the fetal adrenal gland produces dehydroepiandrosterone sulfate (DHEAS), the primary substrate for estradiol synthesis in the placenta. DHEAS is converted to 16-OH-DHEAS in the fetal liver and to estriol in the placenta. Estriol easily crosses from the placenta into the maternal circulation. Therefore, estriol concentrations in the maternal serum and saliva are direct markers of the activity of the fetal hypothalamic–pituitary–adrenal axis, which is thought to be activated prior to the initiation of spontaneous labor *(54)*.

Estriol is detectable as early as 9 wk gestation and generally increases after 30 wk, with a rapid rise in estriol concentrations prior to labor (55,56). This estriol surge occurs approx 3–5 wk prior to the onset of preterm or term labor (56,57) but does not occur in patients who require induction of labor or whose pregnancies are complicated by premature rupture of membranes without the onset of labor (59).

One of the strengths of performing salivary estriol screening is the simplicity. Collecting saliva is noninvasive and may be performed at home, rather than in the hospital or in a physician's office. Protocols in prospective studies (58,59) have instructed patients to rinse their mouths with water and to wait 10 min prior to collecting 2–3 cc of freely flowing saliva in a container every week. Patients are told to avoid brushing teeth, eating, drinking, smoking, or gum chewing, for 1 h prior to collecting samples. Collection is performed weekly and only between 9 AM and 8 PM because of possible diurnal variations (60). After collection, samples must be assayed within 17 h of collection, or they may be frozen at –20°C (61).

Prospective trials evaluating salivary estriol concentrations as a screening test for preterm delivery were inspired by the predictable rise in estriol concentrations before spontaneous labor. McGregor et al. (59) screened 241 women with singleton pregnancies weekly from as early as 22 wk gestation. They found that salivary estriol concentrations increased with gestational age and that there was a more rapid increase, or surge, in estriol concentrations about 3 wk prior to delivery in patients who delivered preterm and term. A concentration greater than 2.3 ng/dL, determined by ROC curve analysis, was the most sensitive and specific discriminatory concentration for identifying a patient at risk for preterm birth. This discriminatory value had a sensitivity of 71% and a specificity of 77%.

Heine et al. (58) completed a multicenter prospective trial of 956 women with singleton pregnancies that screened asymptomatic women with weekly salivary estriol concentrations from 22 wk until delivery. Estriol concentrations above the discriminatory cutoff set at 2.1 ng/mL were considered positive. If the estriol concentration was persistently elevated in the following week, the specificity and positive predictive value improved. The data are summarized in Table 6. In patients who had symptoms of preterm labor evaluated, it was found that estriol concentrations greater than 2.1 ng/mL in the 2 wk prior to symptoms had a sensitivity and specificity of 29 and 92% for a delivery within 2 wk.

A single salivary estriol concentration greater than 2.1 ng/mL was significantly associated with preterm delivery (relative risk 4.2). A second positive test, performed the following week, increased the relative risk to 7.8. A higher specificity (92%) and positive predictive value (19%) were also noted with two consecutive positive tests, with a modest loss of sensitivity. Although estriol was successful in identifying preterm delivery, elevated estriol concentrations were not identified in patients that were destined to deliver before 30 wk, pregnancies at highest risk for morbidity and mortality associated with severe prematurity.

Similar to other screening tests for preterm birth that we have discussed, salivary estriol has low sensitivity, low positive predictive value, and a high negative predictive value. An additional weakness of salivary estriol, not present in more commonly used biomarkers of preterm birth, is the inability to identify pregnancies at risk for extreme preterm birth (<30 wk). As with other forms of screening, salivary estriol is not recommended for routine use. At this time, the American College of Obstetricians and Gynecologists does not suggest measuring salivary estriol concentrations except for research purposes (36).

Table 6
Predictive Accuracy of Salivary Estriol for Preterm Delivery <37 Wk
If One Test >2.1 ng/mL and If Repeat Test Also >2.1 ng/mL

	Sensitivity	Specificity	PPV	NPV	RR
Single test +	57%	78%	9%	98%	4.2 (1.9–9.4)
Repeat test +	44%	92%	19%	98%	7.8 (3.6–16.9)

NPV, positive predictive value; PPV, positive predictive value; RR, relative risk with 95% confidence interval.
Data from ref. *58*.

RESEARCH MARKERS

Corticotropin-Releasing Hormone

Corticotropin-releasing hormone (CRH) is a 41 amino acid peptide that was initially found in the plasma of third-trimester pregnant subjects *(62)*. The CRH gene is expressed in the human placenta *(63)* and is produced in cytotrophoblasts, amniocytes, and decidual cells *(64–67)*. CRH, typically found in low concentrations in nonpregnant subjects, rises during the second and third trimester of pregnancy and rises exponentially in the last weeks prior to delivery *(68–73)*.

What initiates the rise of CRH is unclear, but maternal stress has been implicated as a possible mechanism *(74)*. In vitro studies have shown that glucocorticoids stimulate trophoblast cells to produce CRH *(75)*. In abnormal pregnancies complicated by preeclampsia, intrauterine growth restriction, and preterm birth, CRH concentrations are higher when compared to their normal pregnancy controls *(68,76–78)*.

Multiple studies have shown increases in CRH concentrations in symptomatic pregnancies that deliver preterm *(72,78–80)*. However, interest in CRH has been focused on utilizing this screening marker in the asymptomatic patient in the second trimester and early third trimester. MacLean et al. *(73)* developed the idea of CRH as a "placental clock" that controls the length of gestation, with higher concentrations being the harbinger for labor and ultimate delivery weeks later. They studied CRH and CRH-binding protein (CRH-BP) in a prospective cohort of 485 pregnant women and demonstrated that women destined to deliver prematurely had higher concentrations of CRH when compared to women who deliver at term. This finding was noted as early as 16–20 wk. They also showed that CRH-BP concentrations drop in the third trimester and return to normal by 5 d postpartum, leading to increased bioactivity of CRH before delivery *(73)*.

McLean et al. *(81)* then compared CRH, α fetoprotein, and a risk-factor scoring system in 819 low-risk women for predicting preterm birth. Each marker performed similarly with a sensitivity range of 37–39% and a specificity of 87%. When combined, they showed an improved sensitivity of 54% and a stable specificity of 87%.

Leung et al. *(82)* performed the largest prospective cohort study, following 1047 low-risk patients between 15 and 20 wk gestation. They showed that elevated CRH concentrations in the second trimester are associated with preterm birth (<34 wk). With a cutoff of 1.9 MoM, the sensitivity, specificity, postive predictive value, negative predictive value, and relative risk for preterm birth before 34 wk were 72.7%, 78.4%, 3.6%, 99.6%, and 9.4.

At this time, CRH may be helpful in our comprehension of maternal stress as a mechanism for preterm birth. However, before CRH can be used as a routine marker for preterm birth, larger prospective studies are necessary.

Interleukin-6

Intrauterine infection has been shown to be associated with preterm delivery (83–85). Interleukin (IL)-6 has received the most attention as a marker for infection and hence an increased risk for preterm birth. IL-6 is part of the inflammatory pathway and is produced by endometrial stromal cells, decidual cells, and macrophages as a response to interleukin-1, tumor necrosis factor-α, and endotoxic lipopolysaccharide in tissue culture (86–88). IL-6, in turn, stimulates prostaglandin production, which predisposes subjects to preterm labor and premature rupture of membranes (89).

An elevated concentration of IL-6 in amniotic fluid is a reliable marker of intra-amniotic infection in patients with either preterm labor or PPROM (90,91). Increased IL-6 concentrations are associated with an increased risk for spontaneous preterm birth when measured at the time of preterm labor (85,92) and as early as the second trimester, when measured from samples obtained at genetic amniocentesis (93). Unfortunately, amniotic fluid can be obtained only by amniocentesis, which has inherent risks of fetal death, PPROM, and iatrogenic infections, making amniotic fluid IL-6 an impractical biomarker for routine screening.

Elevated concentrations of IL-6 in cervical secretions are associated with elevated amniotic fluid IL-6 concentrations and histologically confirmed chorioamnionitis in patients with preterm labor (94). Lockwood et al. (95) measured IL-6 concentrations every 3–4 wk between 24 and 36 wk of gestation in a cohort of 161 women. They found a 4.2-fold increase and a 3.4-fold increase in the maximal cervical and vaginal IL-6 concentrations in patients who delivered preterm, compared with the term subjects. ROC curves identified a cutoff of greater than 250 pg/mL of sample buffer as the optimal concentration for predicting preterm birth in cervical samples, with a sensitivity, specificity, positive predictive value, and negative predictive value of 50, 85, 47.2, and 86.4%, respectively. Vaginal IL-6 was less predictive of preterm birth than cervical IL-6 (95).

Goepfert et al. (96) conducted a nested case-control study to evaluate the utility of cervical IL-6 concentrations measured at 22–24$^6/_7$ wk in preterm delivery prediction. From the original cohort of 2929 patients, there were 125 cases that delivered before 35 wk. When compared to matched controls, these cases had significantly elevated IL-6 concentrations (247 vs 84 pg/mL; $p = < 0.005$). When cases that delivered before 32 wk were examined (49 cases), IL-6 concentrations remained significantly higher than controls (212 vs 111 pg/mL; $p = 0.008$). They also found that elevated IL-6 concentrations were highest within 4 wk of delivery, with a median of 159.7 pg/mL. Subjects who delivered between 4 and 8 wk from testing had a median IL-6 of 53.0 pg/mL.

Elevated maternal IL-6 concentrations in symptomatic patients (preterm labor or PPROM) are associated with subsequent preterm birth in some studies (97,98). Murtha et al. (98) performed a case-control study with 89 symptomatic study subjects and 41 asymptomatic control subjects. An IL-6 concentration greather than 8 pg/mL was considered elevated. The study divided patients into three groups: study subjects with an IL-6 greater than 8 pg/mL, study subjects with IL-6 less than 8 pg/mL, and control subjects with (IL-6 less than 8 pg/mL). Sixteen of the 89 study patients were found to have elevated IL-6 concentrations. In these patients, the median time to delivery was statistically shorter (5.5 h) and the gestational age at delivery was significantly earlier (29.6 wk). Study subjects with an IL-6 less than 8 pg/mL had a median time to delivery of 240 h and a median gestational age at delivery of 33.4 wk. Control subjects had a median time to delivery of 1801 h and a median gestational age at delivery of 39 wk. Bihar et al. *(99)* performed a small cross-sectional study that did not confirm the increase of IL-6 concentrations in maternal serum in patients who delivered preterm.

The data concerning IL-6 as a marker of preterm birth are compelling through an inflammatory mechanism. However, studies examining IL-6 concentrations in the setting of cervicovaginal secretions and maternal serum are insufficient to suggest that these markers be used for screening the general population. Other markers of inflammation have been studied with positive associations with preterm birth including cervical lactoferrin *(100,101)* and plasma granulocyte colony stimulating factor *(102)*.

Other Markers

Other placental products have been evaluated as markers for preterm birth including alkaline phosphatase *(103,104)*, human chorionic gonadotropin *(105,106)*, and α-fetoprotein *(107–109)*.

CONCLUSIONS

Biological markers for predicting preterm delivery, such as cervicovaginal fFN, cervical length measurements, and salivary estriol measurements, have all been shown to be more effective at identifying increased risk of preterm birth than traditional risk-based methods. Screening low-risk patients with the intent of providing a proven intervention to improve the health of neonate and mother, however, is the ultimate goal. At this time, interventions are limited and their efficacies are questionable at prolonging gestation. Furthermore, no studies have confirmed that use of biological markers in clinical practice improves neonatal outcomes. Routine screening of the asymptomatic low-risk population with any of these biologic markers cannot be recommended at this time. Screening the symptomatic population with either fFN or cervical length may be useful because negative tests could improve our accuracy at diagnosing true preterm labor and potentially reduce the use of unneeded interventions. The significance of positive tests in the symptomatic population remains unclear.

REFERENCES

1. Matthews TJ. Infant mortality statistics from the 1999 period linked birth/infant death data set. Natl Vital Stat Rep 2001;50(4).
2. Tucker JM, Goldenberg RL, Davis RO, Copper RL, Winkler CL, Hauth JC. Etiologies of preterm birth in an indigent population: is prevention a logical expectation? Obstet Gynecol 1991;77(3):343–347.
3. Martin J. Births: final data for 2000. Natl Vital Stat Rep 2002;50(5).
4. Kiely JL. What is the population-based risk of preterm birth among twins and other multiples? Clin Obstet Gynecol 1998;41(1):3–11.
5. Goldenberg RL. High-risk pregnancy series: an expert's view, the management of preterm labor. Obstet Gynecol 2002;100(1):1020–1037.
6. Lemons JA, Bauer CR, Oh W, et al. for the NICHD Neonatal Research Network. Very low birth weight outcomes of the National Institute of Child Health and Human Development Neonatal Research Network, January 1995 through December 1996. Pediatrics 2001;107(1):E1.
7. Bottoms SF, Paul RH, Iams J, Mercer BM, Thom EA, Roberts JM for the National Institute of Child Health and Human Development Network of Maternal-Fetal Medicine Units. Obstetric determinants of

neonatal survival: influence of willingness to perform cesarean delivery on survival of extremely low-birth-weight infants. Am J Obstet Gynecol 1997;176:960–966.

8. Copper RL, Goldenberg RL, Creasy RK, et al. A multicenter study of preterm birth weight and gestational age-specific neonatal mortality. Am J Obstet Gynecol 1993;168(1):78–84.

9. Robertson CM, Hrynchyshyn GJ, Etches PC, Pain KS. Population based study of the incidence, complexity, and severity of neurologic disability among survivors weighing 500 through 1250 grams at birth: a comparison of two birth cohorts. Pediatrics 1992;90(5):750–755.

10. Vohr BR, Wright LL, Dusick AM, et al. Neurodevelopmental and functional outcomes of extremely low birth weight infants in the National Institute of Child Health and Human Development Neonatal Research Network, 1993–1994. Pediatrics 2000;105:1216–1226.

11. Wood NS, Marlow N, Costeloe K, Gibson AT, Wilkinson AR for the EPICure Study Group. Neurologic and developmental disability after extremely preterm birth. N Engl J Med 2000;343:378–384.

12. Hack M, Taylor HG, Klein N, Eiben R, Schatschneier C, Mercuri-Minich N. School-age outcomes in children with birth weights under 750g. N Engl J Med 1994;331:753–759.

13. Hack M, Flannery DJ, Schluchter M, Carter L, Borawski E, Klein N. Outcomes in young adulthood for very low birth weights. N Engl J Med 2002;346:149–157.

14. Creasy RK, Gummer BA, Liggins GC. System for predicting spontaneous preterm birth. Obstet Gynecol 1980;55:692–695.

15. Mercer BM, Goldenberg RL, Das A, et al. The preterm prediction study: a clinical risk assessment system. Am J Obstet Gynecol 1996;174(6):1885–1893.

16. Main DM, Gabbe SG, Richardson D, Strong S. Can preterm deliveries be prevented? Am J Obstet Gynecol 1985;151(7):892–898.

17. Matsuura H, Takio K, Titani K, et al. The oncofetal structure of human fibronectin defined by monoclonal antibody FDC-6: unique structural requirement for the antigen specificity provided by a glycosylhexapeptide. J Biol Chem 1988;263:3314–3322.

18. Feinberg RF, Kliman HJ, Lockwood CJ. Is oncofetal fibronectin a trophoblast glue for human implantation? Am J Pathol 1991;138(3):537–543.

19. Goldenberg RL, Klebanoff M, Carey JC, et al. Vaginal fetal fibronectin measurements from 8–22 weeks gestation and subsequent spontaneous preterm birth. Am J Obstet Gynecol 2000;183(2):469–475.

20. Lockwood CJ, Senyei AE, Dische MR, et al. Fetal fibronectin in cervical and vaginal secretions as a predictor of preterm delivery. N Engl J Med 1991;325(10):669–674.

21. Goepfert AR, Goldenberg RL, Mercer BM, et al. for the National Institute of Child Health and Development Maternal-Fetal Medicine Units Network. The preterm prediction study: quantitative fetal fibronectin values and the prediction of spontaneous preterm birth. Am J Obstet Gynecol 2000;183(6):1480–1483.

22. Peaceman AM, Andrews WW, Thorp JM, et al. Fetal fibronectin as a predictor of preterm birth in patients with symptoms: a multicenter trial. Am J Obstet Gynecol 1997;177(1):13–18.

23. Morrison JC, Naef RW, Botti JJ, Katz M, Belluomini JM, McLaughlin BN. Prediction of spontaneous preterm birth by fetal fibronectin and uterine activity. Obstet Gynecol 1996;87(5):649–655.

24. Iams JD, Casal D, McGregor JA, et al. Fetal fibronectin improves the accuracy of diagnosis of preterm labor. Am J Obstet Gynecol 1995;173(1):141–145.

25. Goldenberg RL, Mercer BM, Meis PJ, Copper RL, Das A, McNellis D for NICHD Maternal Fetal Medicine Units Network. The preterm prediction study: fetal fibronectin testing and spontaneous preterm birth. Obstet Gynecol 1996;87(5 pt 1):643–648.

26. Bartnicki J, Casal D, Kreaden US, Saling E, Vetter K. Fetal fibronectin in vaginal specimens predicts preterm delivery and very-low-birth-weight infants. Am J Obstet Gynecol 1996;174(3):971–974.

27. Nageotte MP, Casal D, Senyei AE. Fetal fibronectin in patients at increased risk for premature birth. Am J Obstet Gynecol 1994;170 (1 pt 1):20–25.

28. Morrison JC, Albert JR, McLaughlin BN, Whitworth NS, Roberts WE, Martin RW. Oncofetal fibronectin in patients with false labor as a predictor of preterm delivery. Am J Obstet Gynecol 1993;168(2):538–542.

29. Lockwood CJ, Wein R, Lapinski R, et al. The presence of cervical and vaginal fetal fibronectin predicts preterm delivery in an inner-city obstetric population. Am J Obstet Gynecol 1993;169(4):798–804.

30. Ahner R, Kiss H, Egarter C, et al. Fetal fibronectin as a marker to predict the onset of term labor and delivery. Am J Obstet Gynecol 1995;172(1 pt 1):134–137.

31. Lockwood CJ, Moscarelli RD, Wein R, Lynch L, Lapinski RH, Ghidini A. Low concentrations of vaginal fetal fibronectin as a predictor of deliveries occurring after 41 weeks. Am J Obstet Gynecol 1994;171(1):1–4.

32. Leitich H, Egarter C, Kaider A, Hohlagschwandtner M, Berghammer P, Husslein P. Cervicovaginal fetal fibronectin as a marker for preterm delivery: a meta-analysis. Am J Obstet Gynecol 1999;180(5):1169–76.
33. Goldenberg RL, Iams JD, Miodovnik M. The preterm prediction study: risk factors in twin gestations. Am J Obstet Gynecol 1996;175(4):1047–1053.
34. Oliveira T, de Souza E, Mariani-Neto C. Fetal fibronectin as a predictor of preterm delivery in twin gestations. Intl J Obstet Gynecol 1998;62:135–139.
35. Wennerholm UB, Holm B, Mattsby-Baltzer I. Fetal fibronectin, endotoxin, bacterial vaginosis, and cervical length as predictors of preterm birth and neonatal morbidity in twin pregnancies. Br J Obstet Gynecol 1997;104:1398–1404.
36. ACOG Practice Bulletin No. 31: Assessment of risk factors for preterm birth: clinical management guidelines for obstetricians-gynecologists. Obstet Gynecol 2001;98(4):709–716.
37. Phelps JY, Higby K, Smyth MH, Ward JA, Arredondo F, Mayer AR. Accuracy and intraobserver variability of simulated cervical dilatation measurements. Am J Obstet Gynecol 1995;173(3 pt 1):942–945.
38. Holcomb WL, Smeltzer JS. Cervical effacement: variation in belief among clinicians. Obstet Gynecol 1991;78(1):43–45.
39. Berghella V, Tolosa JE, Kuhlman K, Weiner S, Bolognese RJ, Wapner RJ. Cervical ultrasonography compared with manual examination as a predictor of preterm delivery. Am J Obstet Gynecol 1997;177:723–730.
40. Sonek JD, Iams JD, Blumefeld M, Johnson F, Landon M, Gabbe S. Measurement of cervical length in pregnancy: comparison between vaginal ultrasonography and digital examination. Obstet Gynecol 1990;76:172–175.
41. Andersen HF. Transvaginal and transabdominal ultrasonography of the uterine cervix during pregnancy. J Clin Ultra 1991;19:77–83.
42. Iams JD, Goldenberg RL, Meis PJ, et al. The length of the cervix and the risk of spontaneous premature delivery. N Engl J Med 1996;334:567–572.
43. Zilanti M, Azuaga A, Calderon F, Pages G, Mendoza G. Monitoring the effacement of the uterine cervix by transperineal sonography: a new perspective. J Ultra Med 1995;14:719–724.
44. Hibbard JU, Tart M, Moawad A. Cervical length at 16–22 weeks' gestation and risk for preterm delivery. Obstet Gynecol 2000;96(6):972–978.
45. Owen J, Yost N, Berghella V, et al. Mid-trimester endovaginal sonography in women at high risk for spontaneous preterm birth. JAMA 2001;286(11):1340–1348.
46. Andrews WW, Copper R, Hauth JC, Goldenberg RL, Neely C, Dubard M. Second-trimester cervical ultrasound: associations with increased risk for recurrent early spontaneous delivery. Obstet Gynecol 2000;95(2):222–226.
47. Tongsong T, Kamprapanth P, Srisomboon J, Wanapirak C, Piyamongkol W, Sirichotiyakul S. Single transvaginal sonographic measurement of cervical length early in the third trimester as a predictor of preterm delivery. Obstet Gynecol 1995;86(2):184–187.
48. Leitich H, Brunbauer M, Kaider A, Egarter C, Husslein P. Cervical length dilatation of the internal cervical os detected by vaginal ultrasonography as markers for preterm delivery: a systematic review. Am J Obstet Gynecol 1999;181:1465–1472.
49. Crane JM, Van den Hof M, Armson BA, Liston R. Transvaginal ultrasound in the prediction of preterm delivery: singleton and twin gestations. Obstet Gynecol 1997;90:357–363.
50. Timor-Tritsch IE, Boozarjomehri F, Masakowski Y, Monteagudo A, Chao CR. Can a "snapshot" sagittal view of the cervix by transvaginal ultrasonography predict active preterm labor? Am J Obstet Gynecol 1996;174(3):990–995.
51. Iams J, Paraskos J, Landon MB, Teteris JN, Johnson FF. Cervical sonography in preterm labor. Obstet Gynecol 1994;84(1):40–46.
52. Murakawa H, Utumi T, Hasegawa I, Tanaka K, Fuzimori R. Evaluation of threatened preterm delivery by transvaginal ultrasonographic measurement of cervical length. Obstet Gynecol 1993;82(5):829–32.
53. Speroff L, Glass RH, Kase NG. Clinical Gynecologic Endocrinology and Infertility. Baltimore: Lippincott Williams & Wilkins, 1999, pp. 275–335.
54. Goodwin TM. A role for estriol in human labor, term and preterm. Am J Obstet Gynecol 1999;180:S208–S213.
55. Darne J, McGarrigle HH, Lachelin GC. Saliva oestriol, oestradiol, oestrone and progesterone levels in pregnancy: spontaneous labour at term is preceded by a rise in the saliva oestriol:progesterone ratio. Br J Obstet Gynecol 1987;94:227–235.
56. Lachelin GC, McGarrigle HH. A comparison of saliva, plasma unconjugated and plasma total oestriol levels throughout normal pregnancy. Br J Obstet Gynaecol 1984;91:1203–1209.

57. Hedriana HL, Munro CJ, Eby-Wilkens EM, Lasley BL. Changes in the rates of salivary estriol increases before parturition at term. Am J Obstet Gynecol 2001;184:123–130.

58. Heine PR, McGregor JA, Goodwin TM, et al. Serial salivary estriol to detect an increased risk of preterm birth. Obstet Gynecol 2000;96(4):490–497.

59. Moran DJ, McGarrigle HH, Lachelin GC. Lack of normal increase in saliva estriol/progesterone ratio in women with labor induced at 42 weeks gestation. Am J Obstet Gynecol 1992;167:1563–1564.

60. McGregor JA, Hastings C, Roberts T, Barrett J. Diurnal variation in salivary estriol level in pregnancy. Am J Obstet Gynecol 1999;180:S223–S225.

61. Voss HF. Saliva as a fluid for measurement of estriol levels. Am J Obstet Gynecol 1999;180:S226–S231.

62. Sasaki A, Liotta AS, Luckey MM, et al. Immunoreactive corticotropin-releasing factor is present in human maternal plasma during the third trimester of pregnancy. J Clin Enocrinol Metab 1984;59:812–814.

63. Grino M, Chrousos GP, Margioris AN. The corticotropin releasing hormone gene is expressed in human placenta. Biochem Biophys Res Commun 1987;148(3):1208–1214.

64. Petraglia F, Sawchenko PE, Rivier J, et al. Evidence for local stimulation of ACTH secretion by corticotropin-releasing factor in human placenta. Nature 1987(6132);328:717–719.

65. Saijonmaa O, Laatikainen T, Wahlstrom T. Corticotropin-releasing factor in human placenta: localization, concentration and release in vitro. Placenta 1988;9(4):373–385.

66. Jones SA, Challis JRG. Local stimulation of prostaglandin production by corticotropin-releasing hormone in human fetal membranes and placenta. Biochem Biophys Res Commun 1989;159(1):192–199.

67. Riley SC, Walton JC, Herlick JM, et al. The localization and distribution of corticotropin-releasing hormone in the human placenta and fetal membranes throughout gestation. J Clin Endocrinol Metab 1991;72(5):1001–1007.

68. Campbell EA, Linton EA, Wolfe CDA, et al. Plasma corticotropin-releasing hormone concentrations during pregnancy and parturition. J Clin Endocrinol Metab 1987;64(5):1054–1059.

69. Goland RS, Wardlaw SL, Stark RI, et al. High levels of corticotropin-releasing hormone immunoactivity in maternal and fetal plasma during pregnancy. J Clin Endocrinol Metab 1986;63(5):1199–1203.

70. Laatikainen T, Virtanen T, Raisanen I, et al. Immunoreactive corticotropin-releasing factor and corticotropin during pregnancy, labor, and puerperium. Neuropeptides 1987;10(4):343–353.

71. Sasaki A, Shinkawa O, Margioris AN, et al. Immunoreactive corticotropin releasing hormone in human plasma during pregnancy, labor, and delivery. J Clin Endocrinol Metab 1987;64(2):224–229.

72. Wolfe CD, Patel SP, Campbell EA, et al. Plasma corticotropin-releasing factor (CRF) in normal pregnancy. Br J Obstet Gynaecol 1988;95(10):997–1002.

73. McLean M, Bisits A, Davies J, et al. A placental clock controlling the length of human pregnancy. Nature Med 1995;1(5):460–463.

74. Hobel CJ, Dunkel-Schetter C, Roesch SC. Maternal plasma corticotropin-releasing hormone associated with stress at 20 weeks' gestation in pregnancies ending in preterm delivery. Am J Obstet Gynecol 1999;180:S257–S263.

75. Jones SA, Brooks AN, Challis JRG. Steroids modulate corticotropin-releasing hormone production in human fetal membranes and placenta. J Clin Endocrinol Metab 1989;68(4):825–830.

76. Kurki T, Laatikainen T, Salminen-Lappalainen K, et al. Maternal plasma corticotrophin-releasing hormone elevated in preterm labour but unaffected by indomethacin or nylidrin. Br J Obstet Gynaecol 1991;98(7):685–691.

77. Laatikainen T, Virtanen T, Kaaja R, et al. Corticotropin-releasing hormone in maternal and cord plasma in preeclampsia. Eur J Obstet Gynecol Reprod Biol 1991;39(1):19–24.

78. Warren WB, Patrick SL, Goland RS. Elevated maternal plasma corticotropin-releasing hormone levels in pregnancies complicated by preterm labor. Am J Obstet Gynecol 1992;166(4):1198–1204.

79. Korebrits C, Ramirez MM, Watson L, et al. Maternal corticotropin-releasing hormone is increased with impending preterm birth. J Clin Endocrinol Metab 1998;83(5):1585–1591.

80. Wadhwa P, Porto M, Garite TJ, et al. Maternal corticotropin-releasing hormone levels in the early third trimester predict length of gestation in human pregnancy. Am J Obstet Gynecol 1998;170(4):1079–1085.

81. McLean M, Bisits A, Davies J, et al. Predicting risk of preterm delivery by second-trimester measurement of maternal plasma corticotropin-releasing hormone and alpha-fetoprotein concentrations. Am J Obstet Gynecol 1999;181(1):207–215.

82. Leung TN, Chung TK, Madsen G, et al. Elevated mid-trimester maternal corticotrophin-releasing hormone levels in pregnancies that delivered before 34 weeks. Br J Obstet Gynaecol 1999; 106(10):1041–1046.

83. Gibbs RS, Romero R, Hillier SL, et al. A review of premature birth and subclinical infection. Am J Obstet Gynecol 1992;166(5):1515–1528.

84. Romero R, Sirtori M, Oyarzun E. Infection and labor: V. Prevalence, microbiology, and clinical significance of intraamniotic infection with preterm labor and intact membranes. Am J Obstet Gynecol 1989;161(3):817–824.

85. Hillier SL, Witkin SS, Krohn MA, et al. The relationship of amniotic fluid cytokines and preterm delivery, amniotic fluid infection, histologic chorioamnionitis, and chorioamnion infection. Obstet Gynecol 1993;81(6):941–948.

86. Dudley DJ, Trautman MS, Araneo BA, et al. Decidual cell biosynthesis of interleukin-6: regulation by inflammatory cytokines. J Clin Endocrinol Metab 1992;74(4):884–889.

87. Romero R, Avila C, Santhanam U, et al. Amniotic fluid interleukin 6 in preterm labor: association with infection. J Clin Invest 1990;85(5):1392–1400.

88. Fortunado SJ, Menon RP, Swan KF, et al. Inflammatory cytokine (interleukins 1, 6 and 8 and tumor necrosis factor-alpha) release from cultured human fetal membranes in response to endotoxic lipopolysaccharide mirrors amniotic fluid concentrations. Am J Obstet Gynecol 1996;174(6):1855–1862.

89. Mitchell MD, Dudley DJ, Edwin SS. Interleukin-6 stimulated prostaglandin production by human amnion and decidual cells. Eur J Pharmacol 1991;192(1):189–191.

90. Romero R, Yoon BH, Mazur M, et al. The diagnostic and prognostic value of amniotic fluid white blood cell count, glucose, interluekin-6, and Gram stain in patients with preterm labor and intact membranes. Am J Obstet Gynecol 1993;169:805–816.

91. Romero R, Yoon BH, Mazur M, et al. A comparative study of the diagnostic performance of amniotic fluid glucose, white blood cell count, interleukin-6, and Gram stain in the detection of microbial invasion in patients with preterm premature rupture of membranes. Am J Obstet Gynecol 1993;169:839–851.

92. Andrews WW, Hauth JC, Goldenberg RL, et al. Amniotic fluid interleukin-6: correlation with upper genital tract microbial colonization and gestational age in women delivered after spontaneous labor versus indicated delivery. Am J Obstet Gynecol 1995;173(2):606–612.

93. Wenstrom KD, Andrews WW, Tamura T, et al. Elevated amniotic fluid interleukin-6 levels at genetic amniocentesis predict subsequent pregnancy loss. Am J Obstet Gynecol 1996;175(4 pt 1):830–833.

94. Rizzo G, Capponi A, Rinaldo D, et al. Interleukin-6 concentrations in cervical secretions identify microbial invasion of the amniotic cavity in patients with preterm labor and intact membranes. Am J Obstet Gynecol 1996:175(4 pt 1):812–817.

95. Lockwood CJ, Ghindini A, Wein R, et al. Increased interleukin-6 concentrations in cervical secretions are associated with preterm delivery. Am J Obstet Gynecol 1994;171(4):1097–1102.

96. Goepfert AR, Goldenberg RL, Andrews WW, et al. for the National Institute of Child Health and Human Development Maternal-Fetal Medicine Units Network. The Preterm Prediction Study: association between cervical interleukin 6 concentration and spontaneous preterm birth. Am J Obstet Gynecol 2001;184:483–488.

97. Greig PC, Murtha AP, Jimmerson CJ, et al. Maternal serum interleukin-6 during pregnancy and during term and preterm labor. Obstet Gynecol 1997;90(3):465–469.

98. Murtha AP, Greig PC, Jimmerson CE, et al. Maternal serum interleukin-6 concentration as a marker for impending preterm delivery. Obstet Gynecol 1998;91(2):161–164.

99. Bahar AM, Ghalib HW, Moosa RA, et al. Maternal serum interleukin-6, interleukin-8, tumor necrosis factor-alpha and interferon-gamma in preterm labor. Acta Obstet Gynecol Scand 2003;82(6):543–549.

100. Goldenberg RL, Andrews WW, Guerrant RL, et al. The Preterm Prediction Study: cervical lactoferritin concentration, other markers of genital tract infection, and preterm birth. Am J Obstet Gynecol 2000;182(3):361–365.

101. Ramsey PS, Tamura T, Goldenberg RL, et al. The Preterm Prediction Study: Elevated cervical ferritin levels at 22 to 24 weeks of gestation are associated with spontaneous preterm delivery in asymptomatic women. Am J Obstet Gynecol 2002;186(3):458–463.

102. Goldenberg RL, Andrews WW, Mercer BM, et al. for the National Institute of Child Health and Human Development Maternal-Fetal Medicine Units Network. The Preterm Prediction Study: granulocyte colony-stimulating factor and spontaneous preterm birth. Am J Obstet Gynecol 2000; 182(3):625–630.

103. Meyer RE, Thompson SJ, Addy CL, et al. Maternal serum placental alkaline phosphatase level and risk for preterm delivery. Am J Obstet Gynecol 1995;173(1):181–186.

104. Goldenberg RL, Tamura T, DuBard M, et al. Plasma alkaline phosphatase and pregnancy outcome. J Matern Fetal Med 1997;6(3):140–145.

105. Bernstein PS, Stein R, Lin N, et al. Beta-human chorionic gonadotropin in cervicovaginal secretions as a predictor of preterm delivery. Am J Obstet Gynecol 1998;179(4):870–873.

106. Gonen R, Perez R, David M, et al. The association between unexplained second-trimester maternal serum hCG elevation and pregnancy complications. Obstet Gynecol 1992;80(1):83–86.

107. Waller DK, Lustig LS, Cunningham GC, et al. The association between maternal serum alpha-fetoprotein and preterm birth, small for gestational age infants, preeclampsia, and placental complications. Obstet Gynecol 1996;88(5):816–822.

108. Davis RO, Goldenberg RL, Boots L, et al. Elevated levels of midtrimester maternal serum alphafetoprotein are associated with preterm delivery but not fetal growth retardation. Am J Obstet Gynecol 1992;167(3):596–601.

109. Weiner CP, Grant SS, Williamson RA. Relationship between second trimester maternal serum alphafetoprotein and umbilical artery Doppler velocimetry and their association with preterm delivery. Am J Perinatol 1991;8:263.

4 Markers of Fetal Lung Maturity

Edward R. Ashwood, MD

CONTENTS

INTRODUCTION

Fetal organ development occurs in the first trimester of pregnancy and major growth occurs in the second. In the third trimester, the fetal organs mature, although at differing rates. The production of adequate pulmonary surfactant is one of the last developments. This critical process, termed fetal lung maturity (FLM), can be accelerated or delayed by a number of fetal and maternal conditions.

FLM testing has declined since 1995. Neonatal surfactant therapy and clinical adherence to obstetrical guidelines *(1)* have lessened demand. Still, clinicians use FLM tests to assess whether the best infant survival will be achieved in utero or following an early delivery. Knowing that the fetal lung is producing adequate surfactant may persuade the use of labor-inducing drugs for an immediate delivery. On the other hand, delivery can be delayed by using tocolytic agents. Another option is accelerating fetal surfactant production by administering steroids to the mother.

LUNGS AND PULMONARY SURFACTANT

Normal Surfactant Development and Production

Surfactant coats the alveolar epithelium in normal air-breathing lungs. Without surfactant, the surface tension in the airway is inversely proportional its radius. Thus, small alveoli have a propensity to collapse during expiration. Surfactant responds to alveolar volume changes by reducing the surface tension in the alveolar wall during expiration and thereby prevents airway collapse.

Type II granular pneumocytes synthesize pulmonary surfactant packaged into laminated storage granules called lamellar bodies *(2,3)*. These particles are from 1 to 5 µm in diameter *(4)*. Specific phospholipids and surfactant proteins, but not sphingomyelin, are components of lamellar bodies. The pneumocytes begin producing lamellar bodies at 28

From: *Current Clinical Pathology: Handbook of Clinical Laboratory Testing During Pregnancy*
Edited by: A. M. Gronowski © Humana Press, Totowa, NJ

wk gestation *(3)*, but the quantity is inadequate. At about 36 wk gestation, most fetuses experience a surge in surfactant production. As compared to the adult lung, the newborn lung contains 100 times more surfactant per cm^3. This excess surfactant enables the transition from liquid breathing, with zero alveolar air radii, to air breathing, with radii from 10 to 50 μm.

Composition of Surfactant

Pulmonary surfactant lamellar bodies contain phospholipids and specific proteins. The lipids comprise about 90% of the lameller bodies, while the proteins comprise 10%.

PULMONARY PHOSPHOLIPIDS

The most abundant phospholipid is lecithin (phosphatidylcholine [PC]). Unlike lecithin from nonpulmonary sources, this phospholipid commonly has two saturated fatty acid subgroups, usually palmitoyl groups. Three other lipids are present: phosphatidylglycerol (PG), phosphatidylinositol (PI), and phosphatidylethanolamine. The structures of these compounds are shown in Fig. 1. Sphingomyelin is nearly absent, representing less than 2% of the composition.

Most tissues synthesize PC using cytidine diphosphate diacylglycerol and serine to form phosphatidylserine, which is decarboxylated to yield the intermediate phosphatidylethanolamine. Three successive *S*-adenosylmethionine-mediated methyl group transfers form PC. Type II pneumocytes use an alternate pathway, which uses choline phosphotransferase to transfer phosphocholine from cytidine diphosphocholine onto diacylglycerol, forming PC *(5)*.

While present as early as 28 wk, the production of PC surges at about 36 wk and continues to increase until delivery. In contrast, phosphatidylinositol peaks at about 35 wk and then declines. Onset of PG production is about 36 wk in normal pregnancy *(6)*. Little is known of the role of phosphatidylethanolamine in pulmonary surfactant.

PULMONARY SURFACTANT PROTEINS

The surfactant-specific proteins are named SP-A (248 aa), SP-B (381 aa), SP-C (197 aa), and SP-D (375 aa) *(7,8)*. SP-B and SP-C are hydrophobic, and SP-A and SP-B are hydrophilic. Although the hydrophobic proteins are essential to the surface tension ability of surfactant *(9)*, SP-A and SP-D play an important role in the immune defense of the lung *(10)*. An autosomal recessive inherited disorder of SP-B has been described that causes surfactant deficiency in term newborns *(11,12)*. This often fatal condition was first called congenital alveolar proteinosis but is more properly described as hereditary SP-B deficiency. In this condition, the lamellar bodies missing or are in very low numbers.

RESPIRATORY DISTRESS SYNDROME

A common critical problem encountered in the clinical management of preterm newborns is respiratory distress syndrome (RDS), which is caused by surfactant deficiency. This disorder occurs in 10–15% of infants born before 37 wk gestation *(13)*. The risk of RDS is strongly affected by the gestational age at the time of birth: 1% at 37 wk, 20% at 34 wk, and 60% at 29 wk *(14)*. In the United States, RDS was recorded as the cause of death in 1000 infants in 2000 *(15)*. Affected infants are treated with supplemental oxygen and mechanical ventilation. When surfactant is not present, smaller alveoli collapse and larger alveoli are overinflated. This leads to stiff (noncompliant) lungs and alveoli that

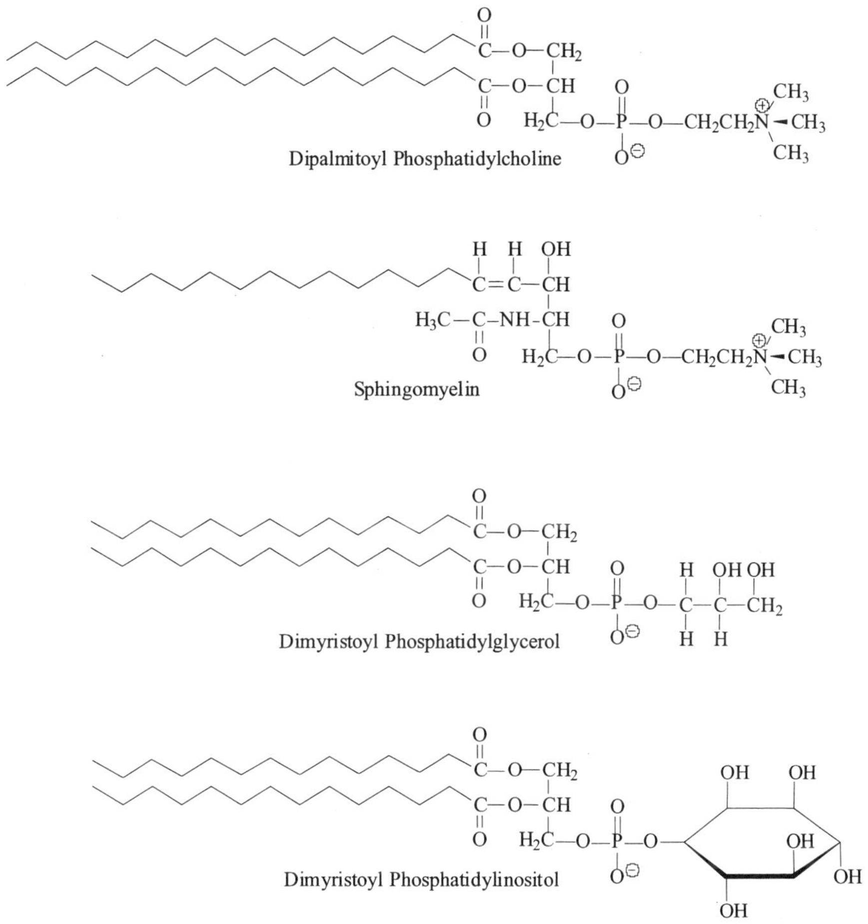

Fig. 1. Chemical structures of dipalmitoyl phosphatidylcholine (the most common surfactant lecithin), sphingomyelin (a convenient internal standard), dimyristoyl phosphatidylglycerol (a late-appearing surfactant lipid), and dimyristoyl phosphatidylinositol (a transitional-phase surfactant lipid).

are perfused with blood but not aerated, a process termed ventilation perfusion mismatch (V/Q mismatch). The infant cannot fully oxygenate and becomes progressively cyanotic. RDS is usually worse on the third or fourth day of life.

Delaying birth until pulmonary maturation occurs can prevent RDS. Maternal steroid treatment accelerates surfactant development (16). New evidence suggests that 11β-hydroxylsteroid dehydrogenase type 1 is necessary for this induction (17,18). When early delivery is necessary or cannot be prevented, newborns can be treated with exogenous surfactant administered intratracheally immediately at birth (19).

TESTS FOR EVALUATING FLM

Six tests of amniotic fluid (AF) are used by nine or more US laboratories to predict FLM and are therefore reviewed in this chapter. They include surfactant/albumin ratio (TDx FLM), fluorescence polarization (FPol) of NBD-phosphatidylcholine (NBD-PC),

Table 1
Use of Fetal Lung Maturity Testing Methods (2002)

Method	Number of laboratories [a]
Surfactant/albumin ratio (TDx FLM II)	462
Phosphatidylglycerol (AmnioStat-FLM)	447
Lecithin/sphingomyelin ratio	138
Phosphatidylglycerol (1-dimensional TLC)	92
Phosphatidylglycerol (2-dimensional TLC)	18
Lamellar body counts	59 [b]
Foam stability	Fewer than 50[c]
Fluorescence polarization (NBD-PC)	9

[a]Data from ref. *20*, unless stated otherwise.
[b]Data from ref. *21*.
[c]Author's estimate.

PG, lecithin/sphingomyelin ratio (L/S ratio), lamellar body counts (LBC), and foam stability. The number of laboratories using each method is listed in Table 1 *(20,21)*.

In the past 30 yr, a number of FLM tests have been proposed. Only those that measure surfactant directly or a biophysical property of surfactant have proven to be useful. Among those tests that correlate with gestational age but are not direct surfactant indicators are AF creatinine *(22)*, AF urea *(23)*, lipid-staining AF cells *(24)*, and AF acid protease *(25)*. Ultrasound techniques are under investigation *(26)*, but the only one used is a biparietal diameter of at least 9.2 cm in an otherwise normal fetus *(27)*. This measurement correlates with a term pregnancy.

SP-A concentrations in newborn sera have been evaluated as a predictor of RDS development, but the results were disappointing *(28)*. Measurement of SP-A and SP-B concentrations in AF did not predict RDS as well as L/S ratio and PG *(29)*. None of the other surfactant proteins have been evaluated as FLM tests.

Several surfactant-based tests are used in a small number of laboratories or have been reported under investigation. These include disaturated PC *(30)*, dipalmitoyl PC *(31)*, refractive index-matched anomalous diffraction *(32)*, turbidity at 400 nm *(33)* or 650 nm *(34)*, the drop volume test *(35)*, capillary filter paper flow rate *(36)*, and surface tension of lipid extract *(37)*. The tap test *(38)* can be used directly by clinicians, but the extent of its use is unknown.

TDx FLM II

The first-generation test, TDx FLM, was developed by Russell *(39)* at Abbott Laboratories, Inc., in collaboration with Tait et al. *(40)* as an attempt to improve on the original work of Shinitzky and colleagues *(41)*. The original Shinitzky method used diphenylhexatriene (DPH) and an ultraviolet fluorescence spectrophometer. The results were reported in polarization units. Because DPH is very unstable and the instrument was difficult to maintain, this method never achieved widespread use. Tait's method uses a laboratory instrument common to most US laboratories, the Abbott TDx, and a fluorescent dye, NBD-PC. Russell's assay, TDx FLM, uses a more stable fluorescent dye, PC-16. In the early 1990s, Abbott Laboratories modified the first-generation test to produce the second-generation TDx FLM II.

METHOD DESCRIPTION

The TDx FLM II method uses uncentrifuged AF that is passed through a glass filter. While the TDx FLM method used 0.5 mL of filtered AF, the TDx FLM II method uses only 0.25 mL. The filtration step, however, usually requires 1 mL. The method is calibrated with six solutions containing differing ratios of surfactant to albumin. The results are reported in units of mg of surfactant to g of albumin. The analytical measurement range is 0 to 160 mg/g. The method has excellent precision of 4% at 20 mg/g and 5% at 160 mg/g. The transition from TDx FLM to TDx FLM II apparently lowered the results, although no direct comparison can be found in the published or manufacturer literature.

The NBD-PC method, known simply as FPol, has a very strong nonlinear correlation to PC-16. The FPol results are reported in mPol units and vary from 160 mPol to 350 mPol. Unlike the TDx FLM II, the values decrease with increasing maturity. The FPol method uses mild centrifugation at $400g$ for 2 min. The strong correlation ($r = 0.95$) permits outcome studies by FPol to be converted into the units of the TDx FLM (42). From unpublished work in my research laboratory, the equation for converting from FPol to TDx FLM II results is

$$\text{TDx FLM II (in mg/g)} = -139.48 \ln(\text{FPol in mPol}) + 817.1$$

The FPol decision limits are mature, less than 260; transitional, 260 to 290; and immature, greater than 290 mPol. Note that 260 mPol is equivalent to 41.5 mg/g and that 290 mPol is equivalent to 26.2 mg/g.

PREANALYTICAL VARIABLES

Although uncentrifuged AF should be used, laboratories can resuspend fluids that have been accidentally centrifuged (43). Either mild vortexing or thorough mixing for 5 min on a tube rocker suffices.

Blood contamination tends to lower results greater than 55 mg/g and increase results less than 39 mg/g $(43,44)$. Although blood contamination changes the results, an immature result will not erroneously be classified as mature; 5% blood contamination increased an immature result of 18 mg/g to 32 mg/g, whereas an indeterminate result of 48 mg/g was unchanged (43).

A 2002 study reported that TDx FLM of AF were unchanged following 16 h at room temperature and 24 h at 4°C (43). Freezing at –20°C for up to $1\frac{1}{2}$ yr introduced an average negative bias, but, more importantly, showed a large random error. Results were ±30% of their baseline values. This is a striking contrast to the stability of FPol in samples stored at –20°C (45).

The use of specimens collected vaginally has been shown to produce results that are on average 35% lower than those collected by amniocentesis (46). Thus, a mature result from a vaginal pool specimen can be trusted, but an immature result may be falsely lowered.

INTERPRETATION

Abbott Laboratories recommends three interpretation categories for TDx FLM II: immature ($\leq$39 mg/g), intermediate (40–54 mg/g), and mature ($\geq$55 mg/g). The maturity decision limit for the first-generation TDx FLM was higher; 70 mg/g (47). Several studies of the first-generation test suggested that the upper decision limit could be lowered without reducing the sensitivity for RDS $(48–50)$. The second-generation TDx FLM II also appears to have a conservative upper decision limit *(51–55)*. Therefore, contrary to the manufacturer's recommendation, an upper decision limit of greater than or equal to 45 mg/g is recommended because it will improve specificity to about 85% without compromising high sensitivity. Although the exact confidence interval for the sensitivity at this cutoff is difficult to estimate because of the small aggregate number of RDS cases reported (<100), it is probably 95–100%. The 45 mg/g decision limit agrees well with clinical outcome studies of FPol *(56–59)* that show that 260 mPol yields a sensitivity of 95% and specificity of approx 65%.

Several investigators have recommended that TDx FLM II be interpreted after gestational age stratification *(60–62)*. Two recent editorials have also encouraged this practice *(63,64)*. Instead of using differing decision limits at each gestational age, the authors advocate reporting the risk of RDS for the TDx FLM II result in combination with the gestational age. The logistic model recommended by one editorial *(64)* was derived from the first-generation TDx FLM, making its use with TDx FLM II inadvisable *(65)*. Because these risks are essentially predictive values, they will vary with the tested population. Because the studies were conducted at tertiary hospitals that handle high-risk obstetrical cases, use of these models is best restricted to those settings. If the models are applied to hospitals that care for low-risk obstetrical populations, the risks reported should be disclaimed as maximum risks.

Almost half of all twins are delivered preterm. If complications other than preterm are excluded, twins appear to have the same incidence of RDS as do gestational age-matched singletons *(66)*. Yet after 31 wk gestation, the average TDx FLM II results from twin pregnancies are 22 mg/g higher than those from singleton pregnancies *(67)*. The ability of TDx FLM II to predict RDS in twins may be different than its predictability in singletons. If testing prior to 32 wk gestation, sampling both sacs is recommended *(68)*.

Several studies have shown that the TDx FLM II is reliable when used in diabetic pregnancies without changing the reference values *(69–71)*.

L/S Ratio

Marie Kulovich and Louis Gluck developed the L/S ratio in the early 1970s *(72,73)*. The major component of AF lecithin is dipalmitoyl PC, the best biologically derived surfactant. Sphingomyelin has no pulmonary surfactant role and therefore serves as a convenient internal control. Kulovich and Gluck expanded the technique to include PG and PI by two-dimensional chromatography and called this procedure the lung profile *(74,75)*. In 2002, only 18 laboratories perform the lung profile *(20)*. Because most laboratories performing L/S ratio testing do not offer the full lung profile, this discussion excludes that version of the test. While some laboratories continue to use L/S methods developed in their own laboratories (so called "home-brew), most laboratories have switched to a commercially available procedure (Fetal Tek 200 available from Helena, Beaumont, TX).

METHOD DESCRIPTION

The L/S ratio involves an initial light centrifugation to remove debris, a lipid extraction, separation by thin-layer chromatography (TLC), lipid staining, and quantitative measurement of the lecithin relative to the sphingomyelin. The procedure can be performed in about 3 h in an emergency, but most laboratories perform a single run per day (e.g., starting analysis by 1 PM and reporting results to the clinics by 5 PM).

The ideal debris-removing centrifugation step is short (2 min) and at low speed (400g) to prevent excessive loss of phospholipids *(76)*. The spun AF is decanted into a glass test tube and mixed well. Two milliliters of the AF is combined with 2 mL of methanol and mixed. Then 2 mL of chloroform is added. The lipids are extracted into the chloroform layer. The tubes are centrifuged to assist solvent separation. A pipet is used to remove 1 mL of the chloroform, which is then completely evaporated. The original method then dissolved the lipid fraction in ice-cold acetone. The acetone precipitation was thought to separate the saturated phospholipids from the unsaturated phospholipids. As originally used, this step was incomplete *(77,78)*, difficult to control *(79)*, and highly variable *(80)*. Acetone precipitation can be omitted without adversely affecting the clinical utility of the test *(79,81)*.

The lipid extract is dissolved in 40 µL of chloroform and painted onto a TLC plate as a band. Two or three of the lanes on the plate are used for controls that will mark the position of the lipids. After applying all the samples, the TLC plate is developed in a solvent system of chloroform, methanol, triethylamine, 2-propanol, and water. The plate is removed, dried, and dipped into a solution of phosphoric acid and cupric acetate. Warming the plate to 180°C chars the lipids, developing dark bands whose size and intensity are proportional to the lipid concentration. The plate is scanned on a densitometer at 525 nm. The area of the lecithin peak is divided by the area of the sphingomyelin peak.

The interlaboratory variation of L/S ratio results on proficiency testing is 15–20% for mean ratios of 1.0–2.0 and, paradoxically, 22–31% for mean ratios about 4.0 *(82)*. The within-laboratory precision is much better. The quality control specimens analyzed in the past 165 L/S ratio runs in my laboratory yielded the following statistics (mean, SD, and CV): low control, 1.03, 0.185, 18%; borderline control, 2.18, 0.205, 9.4%; and high control, 3.10, 0.225, 7.2%. Thus, trends of results from a single laboratory will be more reliable than those from multiple laboratories.

PREANALYTICAL VARIABLES

Specimens obtained from the vagina are frequently contaminated with blood, bacteria, and mucus. These specimens are adequate only when the fluid has been in the vagina a short time and the specimen is chilled immediately after collection *(83,84)*. For patients with ruptured membranes, physicians should consider amniocentesis for specimen collection *(76)*.

Blood contamination changes the L/S ratio result because serum contains high concentrations of lecithin and sphingomyelin. High results are depressed and low results are raised. In heavy contamination, final results can be in the transitional decision zone *(85)*.

Specimens contaminated with meconium are not interpretable *(86)*. Even though meconium-contains no lecithin or sphingomyelin, the method produces erroneous values from 1.1 to 3.6 when meconium contaminated buffer is used.

INTERPRETATION

As originally described *(72)*, an L/S ratio of 2.0 or greater indicates maturity. Although many laboratories continue to use this decision limit, the methodology used can affect the results. Some laboratories use a decision limit as high as 3.5 *(87)*. Many laboratories omit the acetone precipitation step, which raises the L/S ratio *(79)*. Most of these laboratories use a decision limit of 2.5 or greater. The prediction is not, of course, perfect. Most clinical outcome studies report a sensitivity of about 95% and a specificity of about 65%. Given an RDS prevalence of 15, the predictive value of a mature result is 98–99%, but the predictive value of an immature result is about 33%. An inherent value of the L/S ratio is the quantitative nature of the result—1.1 translates to a higher RDS risk than does 1.9, yet both are immature results.

Before the development of tight glycemic control, RDS developed much more frequently in the diabetic pregnancy (88). The newer treatment algorithms have led to a marked decrease in RDS incidence in diabetes (89). Some investigators report that infants of diabetic mothers develop RDS more frequently despite mature L/S ratio results (90), whereas others disagree that L/S ratio produces more false predictions of maturity (91,92). Both a delay in the appearance of mature L/S ratio results (93) and no delay (6) have been reported for poorly controlled diabetic cases. Investigators appear to agree that well-controlled diabetic patients have L/S ratio to gestational age characteristics that are not statistically different from nondiabetic subjects (6,94). Separate L/S ratio reference intervals for diabetic pregnancies are not recommended (76).

PG

In 1976, Hallman et al. reported that PG was useful for predicting fetal lung maturity, especially when the specimen was contaminated with blood (95). The surfactant composition is thought to be important to its function (96). Even though PG has much less surfactant activity than PC, it may assist with surfactant spreading (97). Using a sensitive method, PG can be detected at concentrations of approx 0.05 μmol/L even early in gestation when L/S ratio is approx 1.0 (98). Most methods are insensitive, detecting down to only approx 2 μmol/L, a concentration achieved much later in pregnancy (36 wk or later).

METHOD DESCRIPTION

The original clinical method for PG determination was two-dimensional TLC (95). In 2002, only 18 of 557 reporting CAP proficiency test results for PG were using this method; 92 laboratories reported using one-dimensional TLC and 447 used a rapid immunologic, semiquantitative agglutination test for PG (AmnioStat-FLM, Irvine Scientific, Santa Ana, CA). Although a specific enzymatic PG method has been reported, no laboratories are using this method for clinical testing (98).

The AmnioStat-FLM uses PG-antibodies to clump the PG-containing lamellar bodies to form macroscopic clusters. In a test tube, 25 μL of AF is mixed with 25 μL of a solution containing lecithin and cholesterol in ethanol; 250 μL phosphate buffer is added and mixed. Then, on a glass slide, 10 μL of this solution is mixed with 25 μL of anti-PG for 9 min. The agglutination in the sample is compared to three controls. The test has three possible results: negative, low positive (0.5 μg/mL), and high positive (2 μg/mL) (99). In the CAP proficiency surveys from 1992 to 1995, the performance of AmnioStat-FLM at detecting PG 97.9% of the time when present or not detecting it 98.4% when absent was at least as good as TLC (82).

PREANALYTICAL VARIABLES

Although several studies report excellent results for PG in contaminated vaginal pool samples (100,101), vaginal flora have been shown to produce PG and rarely cause false positives (102–104). Blood and meconium do not interfere (105,106).

INTERPRETATION

All of the currently used PG tests report the results as negative or positive. Several clinical outcome studies of the AmnioStat-FLM have been conducted (107–111). Although positive AmnioStat-FLM results are between 99 and 100% predictive of FLM, negative results are highly unpredictive (about 25%) and are not clinically helpful. These performance characteristics are very similar to PG by TLC (112). Many investigators report miscalculated positive predictive values because the result nomenclature (negative/positive) is inherently opposite that of medical decision-making nomenclature (positive for disease vs negative for disease).

Many clinicians use PG whenever they are assessing a diabetic patient for FLM (82,111). The literature contains no modern studies to support this practice. PG detection by TLC or AmnioStat-FLM in normal pregnancies occurs at approx 35 wk gestation. In diabetic patients, regardless of glucose control, PG detection is about 1.5 wk later (6,113,114). Many diabetic patients will deliver term infants with mature surfactant status before any PG is detected (115). The method of detection is unaffected by the diabetic status of the patient (116).

LBC

The haziness of mature AF is a result of the light-scattering characteristics of lamellar bodies (32). Dubin reported that these particles can be counted directly using most whole blood cell counters. This technique is known as LBC (117) or lamellar body number density (LBND) (118). The LBC method is a direct reflection of surfactant concentration. Thus, it differs from L/S ratio and TDx FLM II, which are inherently ratios. Fetal urination should lower LBC but does not affect the other two methods.

METHOD DESCRIPTION

The surfactant-containing particles in AF range from 0.2 to 10 fL in size (119). Most whole blood cell counters designed to count platelets (5 to 15 fL in volume) use a size gate from 2 to 20 fL. Thus, a portion of the lamellar bodies will be enumerated in the platelet channel of these instruments. This analysis can be performed in under 10 min.

Prior to analysis, the AF should be mixed well but not centrifuged (76,82). Two min on a tube rocker or at least 20 inversions just before analysis suffices (120). The counter should be flushed with saline twice just before analysis. When sampled, the instrument aspirates approx 200 μL amniotic fluid, dilutes it with electrolyte buffer, and then pulls a portion of the solution through a 50 μm orifice. Particles entering the orifice produce sudden increases in electrical resistance across the orifice. The resistance increase is proportional to the size of the particle. The instrument counts the number of particles within various size ranges. LBC results vary from 0 to 150,000/μL.

A comparison of four common instruments used for LBC showed poor agreement but a high correlation for three instruments, Coulter Gen-S, Cell-dyn 3500, and Sysmex XE-2100 (121). The Advia 120, the only flow cytometer of the group, produced results that did not correlate with the other three, all resistive pulse counters. Among these three instruments, the proportional bias was from –32% to +76%. The authors advocated instrument-specific LBC decision limits. Because of the high degree of correlation, I theorize that instrument harmonization is possible by applying a correction factor to the results.

LBC precision, as accessed by using dilute platelet control specimens, is typically 6–8% at a mean of 35,000/μL (122).

PREANALYTICAL VARIABLES

Specimens containing obvious mucus will produce erratic results *(120)*. Blood contamination greater than 1% will initially increase LBC because of addition of platelets, but as clotting occurs, the lamellar bodies will be trapped and LBC will decline up to 20% *(120)*. Moderate meconium contamination (0.5 A at 390 nm) increases LBC by less than 5000/μL *(118)*.

INTERPRETATION

All LBC clinical outcomes studies have shown that this test is a strong predictor of FLM *(118,119,122–130)*, but, like other FLM methods, is a weak predictor of lung immaturity. A meta-analysis *(131)* reported that receiver-operating characteristic curve for LBC was slightly better than that for L/S ratio: at a fixed sensitivity of 95%, the LBC specificity was 80% whereas the L/S ratio specificity was 70%. The variation in the maturity thresholds reported (19,000–50,000/μL) can be explained by differences in centrifugation protocols *(82)* and differences in analyzers *(121)*. Laboratories that use LBC should not use centrifugation *(120)* and should consider using decision limits adjusted for instrument bias *(121)*. As an alternative, results from specific instruments could be adjusted to agree with instruments used in clinical outcome studies.

There are no clinical outcome studies reported having enough RDS cases from diabetic mothers to directly determine the sensitivity and specificity of LBC in this population. A 7-yr study reported good agreement between LBC compared to L/S ratio and PG in 90 diabetic subjects *(132)*.

Foam Stability

In 1972, Clements and colleagues *(133)* described a foam test that used amniotic fluid to predict FLM. This was modified by Sher et al. *(134)* in 1978 into a foam stability index that was commercialized by Beckman Instruments (Lumadex) in 1982. Unfortunately, this rapid commercial test was discontinued in 1997.

METHOD DESCRIPTION

The foam stability test uses the principle that surfactant is required to maintain a stable foam in the presence of a high concentration of ethanol. A recipe for a "home-brew" method is available *(5)*. Briefly, 0.5 mL of AF that has been centrifuged at 1000g for 3 min is added to six separate tubes containing from 0.43 to 0.55 mL of 95% ethanol. The solutions are shaken for 30 s, then examined for foam after settling for 15 s. The result is then expressed as the highest fraction of ethanol that supports a stable complete ring of foam at the meniscus.

PREANALYTICAL VARIABLES

Blood and meconium contamination as well as test temperatures below 20°C interfere with foam stability by producing falsely mature results *(135)*. Test temperatures greater than 30°C produce falsely immature results.

The hydroscopic nature of ethanol must be considered when performing this test. The cleanliness of the tubes used is also very important.

INTERPRETATION

Several clinical outcome studies have shown that foam stability results of 0.47 or greater indicate maturity *(134,136–140)*. The sensitivity appears to be approx 95% and the specificity about 65%. There are insufficient outcome studies to draw conclusions about the utility of foam stability testing in diabetic mothers.

CASCADE TESTING

Each FLM test has a high sensitivity for RDS (~95%), but a poor specificity for no respiratory distress (~65%). The tests are generally used between 34 and 37 wk gestation when the RDS prevalence is 5–10%. Thus, the predictive value of a mature test (~99%) will be much better than the predictive value of an immature test (20–40%). This has led many investigators to suggest the use of a testing cascade *(122,130,141–145)*. These algorithms are designed to use rapid, inexpensive tests first. LBC is the least expensive of the tests, followed by FPol, TDx FLM II, PG by AmnioStat, foam stability, and L/S ratio. If a clearly mature or immature result is obtained, then testing is stopped. For immature results close to the decision threshold, however, the next test in the cascade is used. The usefulness of an FLM cascade depends on the medical setting and especially on the medical politics of prenatal care. Clinicians who put their highest trust the L/S ratio will want that test to be the final arbiter of a cascade. I share Dubin's doubts *(80)* that the L/S ratio should be held in such high regard. It is slow, imprecise, highly variable across laboratories, subject to interference, and expensive.

REFERENCES

1. American College of Obstetricians and Gynecologists, Committee on Educational Bulletins: Assessment of Fetal Lung Maturity. ACOG Educational Bulletin No. 230. Washington, DC: American College of Obstetricians and Gynecologists, 1996.
2. Hook GER, Gilmore LB, Tombropoulos EG, Fabro SE. Fetal lung lamellar bodies in human amniotic fluid. Am Rev Respir Dis 1978;117:541–550.
3. Snyder JM, Mendelson CR, Johnston JM. The morphology of lung development in the human fetus. In: Nelson GH, ed. Pulmonary Development: Transition from Intrauterine to Extrauterine Life. New York: Marcel Dekker, 1985, pp. 19–46.
4. Oulton M, Martin TR, Faulkner GT, Stinson D, Johnson JP. Developmental study of a lamellar body fraction isolated from human amniotic fluid. Pediatr Res 1980;14:722–728.
5. Ashwood ER. Clinical chemistry of pregnancy. In: Burtis CA, Ashwood ER, eds. Tietz Textbook of Clinical Chemistry, 3rd ed. Philadelphia: Saunders, 1999, pp. 1736–1775.
6. Moore TR. A comparison of amniotic fluid fetal pulmonary phospholipids in normal and diabetic pregnancy. Am J Obstet Gynecol 2002;186:641–650.
7. Hawgood S, Clements JA. Pulmonary surfactant and its apoproteins. J Clin Invest 1990;86:1–6.
8. Persson A, Chang D, Crouch E. Surfactant protein D is a divalent cation-dependent carbohydrate-binding protein. J Biol Chem 1990;26510:5755–5760.
9. Cochrane CG, Revak SD. Pulmonary surfactant protein B (SP-B): structure–function relationships. Science 1991;254:566–568.
10. Haagsman HP, Diemel RV. Surfactant-associated proteins: functions and structural variation. Comp Biochem Physiol A Mol Integr Physiol 2001;129:91–108.
11. Nogee LM, Garnier G, Dietz HC, et al. A mutation in the surfactant protein B gene responsible for fatal neonatal respiratory disease in multiple kindreds. J Clin Invest 1994;3:1860–1863.
12. Andersen C, Ramsay JA, Nogee LM, et al. Recurrent familial neonatal deaths: hereditary surfactant protein B deficiency. Am J Perinatol 2000;17:219–224.
13. Nelson GH, McPherson JC Jr. Respiratory distress syndrome in various cultures and a possible role of diet. In: Nelson GH, ed. Pulmonary Development: Transition from Intrauterine to Extrauterine Life. New York: Marcel Dekker, 1985, pp. 159–178.
14. Farrell PM, Avery ME. Hyaline membrane disease. Am Rev Respir Dis 1975;111:657–688.
15. Miniño AM, Arias E, Kochanek KD, Murphy SL, Smith BL. Deaths: Final Data for 2000. National Vital Statistics Reports. Hyattsville, MD: National Center for Health Statistics, 2002;50(15).
16. American College of Obstetricians and Gynecologists, Committee on Obstetric Practice: Antenatal Corticosteroid Therapy for Fetal Maturation. ACOG Committee Opinion No. 147, December 1994. Washington, DC: American College of Obstetricians and Gynecologists, 1994.

17. Hundertmark S, Dill A, Ebert A, et al. Foetal lung maturation in 11beta-hydroxysteroid dehydrogenase type 1 knockout mice. Horm Metab Res 2002;34:545–549.

18. Hundertmark S, Dill A, Buhler H, et al. C. 11betahydroxysteroid dehydrogenase type 1: a new regulator of fetal lung maturation. Horm Metab Res 2002;34:537–544.

19. Hallman M, Merritt TA, Jarvenpaa AL, et al. Exogenous human surfactant for treatment of severe respiratory distress syndrome: a randomized prospective clinical trial. J Pediatr 1985;106:963–969.

20. College of American Pathologists: CAP Surveys, Lung Maturity Survey, Set LM-B. Northfield, IL: College of American Pathologists, 2002.

21. College of American Pathologists. Supplemental questions on lamellar body counts. Surveys 2000;LM-C:4–5.

22. Darling RE, Zlatnik FJ. Comparison of amniotic fluid optical density, L/S ratio and creatinine concentration in predicting fetal pulmonary maturity. J Reprod Med 1985;30:460–464.

23. Almeida OD Jr, Kitay DZ. Amniotic fluid urea nitrogen in the prediction of respiratory distress syndrome. Am J Obstet Gynecol 1988;159:465–468.

24. Wood GP. The evaluation of fetal lung maturity by amniotic fluid analysis. South Med J 1975;68:538–541.

25. Menashe M, Finci Z, Milwidsky A, Mayer M. Amniotic fluid protease activity, protease inhibitory activity, and fetal lung maturity. Am J Perinatol 1987;4:68–71.

26. Prakash KN, Ramakrishnan AG, Suresh S, Chow TW. An investigation into the feasibility of fetal lung maturity prediction using statistical textural features. Ultrason Imaging 2001;23:39–54.

27. Lenke R, Ashwood E. Lung maturity testing. In: Quilligan EJ, Zuspan FP, eds. Current Therapy in Obstetrics and Gynecology. Philadelphia: Saunders, 2000, pp. 418–420.

28. Kaneko K, Shimizu H, Arakawa H, Ogawa Y. Pulmonary surfactant protein A in sera for assessing neonatal lung maturation. Early Hum Dev 2001;62:11–21.

29. Pryhuber GS, Hull WM, Fink I, McMahan MJ, Whitsett JA. Ontogeny of surfactant proteins A and B in human amniotic fluid as indices of fetal lung maturity. Pediatr Res 1991;30:597–605.

30. Delgado JC, Greene MF, Winkelman JW, Tanasijevic MJ. Comparison of disaturated phosphatidylcholine and fetal lung maturity surfactant/albumin ratio in diabetic and nondiabetic pregnancies. Am J Clin Pathol 2000;113:233–239.

31. Alvarez JG, Richardson DK, Ludmir J. Prediction of respiratory distress syndrome by the novel dipalmitoyl phosphatidylcholine test. Obstet Gynecol 1996;87:429–433.

32. Dubin SB. Determination of lamellar body size, number density and concentration by differential light scattering from amniotic fluid: physical significance of A_{650}. Clin Chem 1988;34:938–943.

33. Sbarra AJ, et al. Correlation between amniotic fluid optical density and LS ratio. Obstet Gynecol 1976;48:613–615.

34. Spellacy WN, Buhi WC, Cruz AC, Gelman SR, Kellner KR, Birk SA. Assessment of fetal lung maturity: a comparison of the lecithin/sphingomyelin ratio and the tests of optical density at 400 and 650 nm. Am J Obstet Gynecol 1979;134:528–531.

35. Moawad AH, Ismail MA, River LP. Use of the drop volume of amniotic fluid in predicting fetal lung maturity: clinical experience. J Reprod Med 1991;36:425–428.

36. Sing EJ. Capillary method for assessment of pulmonary maturity in utero with the use of amniotic fluid. Am J Obstet Gynecol 1980;136:228–229.

37. Tiwary CM, Goldkrand JW. Assessment of fetal pulmonic maturity by measurement of the surface tension of amniotic fluid lipid extract. Obstet Gynecol 1976;48:191–194.

38. Socol ML, Sing E, Depp OR. The tap test: a rapid indicator of fetal pulmonary maturity. Am J Obstet Gynecol 1984;148:445–450.

39. Russell JC. A calibrated fluorescence polarization assay for assessment of fetal lung maturity. Clin Chem 1987;33:1177–1184.

40. Tait JF, Franklin RW, Simpson JB, Ashwood ER. Improved fluorescence polarization assay for use in evaluating fetal lung maturity: I. Development of the assay procedure. Clin Chem 1986;32:248–254.

41. Shinitzky M, Goldfisher A, Bruck A, et al. A new method for assessment of fetal lung maturity. Br J Obstet Gynaecol 1976;83:838–844.

42. Ashwood ER, Palmer SE, Lenke RR. Rapid fetal lung maturity testing: commercial versus NBD-phosphatidylcholine assay. Obstet Gynecol 1992;81:1048–1053.

43. Grenache DG, Parvin CA, Gronowski AM. Preanalytical factors that influence the Abbott TDx Fetal Lung Maturity II Assay. Clin Chem 2003;49:935–939.

44. Carlan SJ, Gearity D, O'Brien WF. The effect of maternal blood contamination on the TDx-FLM II assay. Am J Perinatol 1997;14:491–494.

45. Foerder CA, Tait JF, Franklin RW, Ashwood ER. Improved fluorescence polarization assay for use in evaluating fetal lung maturity: II. Analytical evaluation and comparison with the lecithin/sphingomyelin ratio. Clin Chem 1986;32:255–259.

46. Cleary-Goldman J, Connolly T, Chelmow D, Malone F. Accuracy of the TDx-FLM assay of amniotic fluid: a comparison of vaginal pool samples with amniocentesis. J Matern Fetal Neonatal Med 2002;11:374–377.

47. Russell JC, Cooper CM, Ketchum CH, et al. Multicenter evaluation of TDx test for assessing fetal lung maturity. Clin Chem 1989;35:1005–1010.

48. Apple FS, Bilodeau L, Preese LM, Benson P. Clinical implementation of a rapid, automated assay for assessing fetal lung maturity. J Reprod Med 1994;39:883–887.

49. Herbert WNP, Chapman JF, Schnoor MM. Role of the TDx FLM assay in fetal lung maturity. Am J Obstet Gynecol 1993;168:808–812.

50. Steinfeld JD, Samuels P, Bulley MA, Cohen AW, Goodman DB, Senior MB. The utility of the TDx test in the assessment of fetal lung maturity. Obstet Gynecol 1992;79:460–464.

51. McManamon TG, Mandsager N. Clinical outcome of neonates following the use of the FLM-II as the only test for fetal lung maturity [abstract]. Clin Chem 1998;44:A157.

52. Moxness M, Lawson G, O'Brien J, Burritt M. Assessment of fetal lung maturity by the Abbott FLM II assay and three other methods [abstract]. Clin Chem 1995;41:S95.

53. Dunston-Boone R, Chang T, Bernstein LH. Modified TDx assay for surfactant to albumin ratio in the assessment of fetal lung maturity [abstract]. Clin Chem 1997;43:S196.

54. Fantz CR, Powell C, Karon B, et al. Assessment of the diagnostic accuracy of the TDx-FLM II to predict fetal lung maturity. Clin Chem 2002;48:761–765.

55. Kesselman EJ, Figueroa R, Garry D, Maulik D. The usefulness of the TDx/TDxFLx fetal lung maturity II assay in the initial evaluation of fetal lung maturity. Am J Obstet Gynecol 2003;188:1220–1222.

56. Ashwood ER, Tait JF, Foerder CA, Franklin RW, Benedetti TJ. Improved fluorescence polarization assay for use in evaluating fetal lung maturity: III. Retrospective clinical evaluation and comparison with the lecithin/sphingomyelin ratio. Clin Chem 1986;32:260–264.

57. Tait JF, Foerder CA, Ashwood ER, Benedetti TJ. Prospective clinical evaluation of an improved fluorescence polarization assay for predicting fetal lung maturity. Clin Chem 1987;33:554–558.

58. Chen C, Roby PV, Weiss NS, Wilson JA, Benedetti TJ, Tait JF. Clinical evaluation of the NBD-PC fluorescence polarization assay for prediction of fetal lung maturity. Obstet Gynecol 1992;80:688–692.

59. Ruch AT, Lenke RR, Ashwood ER. Assessment of fetal lung maturity by fluorescence polarization in high-risk pregnancies. J Reprod Med 1993;38:133–136.

60. Tanasijevic MJ, Wybenga DR, Richardson D, Greene MF, Lopez R, Winkelman JW. A predictive model for fetal lung maturity employing gestational age and test results. Am J Clin Pathol 1994;102:788–793.

61. Kaplan LA, Chapman JF, Bock JL, et al. Prediction of respiratory distress syndrome using the Abbott FLM-II amniotic fluid assay. Clin Chim Acta 2002;326:61–68.

62. Pinette MG, Blackstone J, Wax JR, Cartin A. Fetal lung maturity indices: a plea for gestational age-specific interpretation: a case report and discussion. Am J Obstet Gynecol 2002;187:1721–1722.

63. Tanasijevic M. Predictive model for fetal lung maturity assessment incorporating Abbott FLM S/A II test results and obstetric estimates of gestational age. Clin Chim Acta 2002;326:1–2.

64. Stubblefield PG. Using the TDx-FLM assay and gestational age together for more accurate prediction of risk for neonatal respiratory distress syndrome. Am J Obstet Gynecol 2002;187:1429–1430.

65. Gronowski AM, Parvin CA. Prediction of risk for respiratory distress syndrome using gestational age and the TDx FLM II assay. Am J Obstet Gynecol 2003;189:1511–1514.

66. Friedman SA, Schiff E, Kao L, Kuint J, Sibai BM. Do twins mature earlier than singletons? Results from a matched cohort study. Am J Obstet Gynecol 1997;176:1193–1196.

67. McElrath TF, Norwitz ER, Robinson JN, Tanasijevic MJ, Lieberman ES. Differences in TDx fetal lung maturity assay values between twin and singleton gestations. Am J Obstet Gynecol 2000;182:1110–1112.

68. Whitworth NS, Magann EF, Morrison JC. Evaluation of fetal lung maturity in diamniotic twins. Am J Obstet Gynecol 1999;180:1438–1441.

69. Del Valle GO, Adair CD, Ramos EE, Gaudier FL, Sanchez-Ramos L, Morales R. Interpretation of the TDx-FLM fluorescence polarization assay in pregnancies complicated by diabetes mellitus. Am J Perinatol 1997;14:241–244.

70. Livingston EG, Herbert WN, Hage ML, Chapman JF, Stubbs TM for the Diabetes and Fetal Maturity Study Group. Use of the TDx-FLM assay in evaluating fetal lung maturity in an insulin-dependent diabetic population. Obstet Gynecol 1995;86:826–829.

71. Tanasijevic MJ, Winkelman JW, Wybenga DR, Richardson DK, Greene MF. Prediction of fetal lung maturity in infants of diabetic mothers using the FLM S/A and disaturated phosphatidylcholine tests. Am J Clin Pathol 1996;105:17–22.

72. Gluck L, Kulovich MV, Borer RC Jr, Brenner PH, Anderson GG, Spellacy WN. Diagnosis of the respiratory distress syndrome by amniocentesis. Am J Obstet Gynecol 1971;109:440–445.

73. Gluck L, Kulovich MV. Lecithin/sphingomyelin ratios in amniotic fluid in normal and abnormal pregnancy. Am J Obstet Gynecol 1973;115:539–546.

74. Kulovich MV, Hallman MB, Gluck L. The lung profile: I. Normal pregnancy. Am J Obstet Gynecol 1979;135:57–63.

75. Kulovich MV, Gluck L. The lung profile: II. Complicated pregnancy. Am J Obstet Gynecol 1979 135:64–70.

76. Ashwood ER. Standards of laboratory practice: evaluation of fetal lung maturity. Clin Chem 1997;43:1–4.

77. Touchstone JC, Levin SS, Dobbins MF, Beers PC. Analysis of saturated and unsaturated phospholipids in biological fluids. J Liquid Chromatogr 1983;6:179–192.

78. Torday J, Carson L, Lawson E. Saturated phosphatidylcholine in amniotic fluid and prediction of respiratory-distress syndrome. N Engl J Med 1979;301:1013–1018.

79. Brown LM, Duck-Chong CG. Methods of evaluating fetal lung maturity. In: Batsakis J, Savory J, eds. Critical Reviews in Clinical Laboratory Science. Boca Raton, FL: CRC Press, 1982; pp. 84–159.

80. Penney LL, Hagerman DD, Sei CA. Specificity and reproducibility of acetone precipitation in identifying surface-active phosphatidylcholine in amniotic fluid. Clin Chem 1976;22:681–682.

81. Hobson DW, Spillman T, Cotton DB. Effect of acetone precipitation on the clinical prediction of respiratory distress syndrome when utilizing amniotic fluid lecithin/sphingomyelin ratios. Am J Obstet Gynecol 1986;154:1023–1026.

82. Dubin SB. Assessment of fetal lung maturity: practice parameter. Am J Clin Pathol 1998;110:723–732.

83. Dombroski RA, Mackenna J, Brame RG. Comparison of amniotic fluid lung maturity profiles in paired vaginal and amniocentesis specimens. Am J Obstet Gynecol 1981;140:461–464.

84. Shaver DC, Spinnato JA, Whybrew D, Williams WK, Anderson GD. Comparison of phospholipids in vaginal and amniocentesis specimens of patients with premature rupture of membranes. Am J Obstet Gynecol 1987;156:454–457.

85. Gibbons JM, Huntley TE, Corral AG. Effect of maternal blood contamination on amniotic fluid analysis. Obstet Gynecol 1874;44:657–660.

86. Longo SA, Towers CV, Strauss A, Asrat T, Freeman RK. Meconium has no lecithin or sphingomyelin but affects the lecithin/sphingomyelin ratio. Am J Obstet Gynecol 1998;179:1640–1642.

87. Lauria MR, Dombrowski MP, Delaney-Black V, Bottoms SF. Lung maturity tests: relation to source, clarity, gestational age and neonatal outcome. J Reprod Med 1996;41:685–591.

88. Robert MF, Neff RK, Hubbell JP, Taeusch HW, Avery ME. Association between maternal diabetes and the respiratory-distress syndrome in the newborn. N Engl J Med 1976;294:357–360.

89. Mimouni F, Miodovnik M, Whitsett JA, Holroyde JC, Siddiqi TA, Tsang RC. Respiratory distress syndrome in infants of diabetic mothers in the 1980s: no direct adverse effect of maternal diabetes with modern management. Obstet Gynecol 1987;69:191–195.

90. Cruz AC, Buhi WC, Birk SA, Spellacy WN. Respiratory distress syndrome with mature lecithin/sphingomyelin ratios: diabetes mellitus and low Apgar scores. Am J Obstet Gynecol 1978;126:78–82.

91. Gabbe SG, Lowensohn RI, Mestman JH, Freeman RK, Goebelsmann U. Lecithin/sphingomyelin ratio in pregnancies complicated by diabetes mellitus. Am J Obstet Gynecol 1977;128:757–760.

92. Tabsh KM, Brinkman CR 3rd, Bashore RA. Lecithin:sphingomyelin ratio in pregnancies complicated by insulin-dependent diabetes mellitus. Obstet Gynecol 1982;59:353–358.

93. Piper JM, Langer O. Does maternal diabetes delay fetal pulmonary maturity? Am J Obstet Gynecol 1993;168:783–786.

94. Berkowitz K, Reyes C, Saadat P, Kjos SL. Fetal lung maturation: comparison of biochemical indices in gestational diabetic and nondiabetic pregnancies. J Reprod Med 1997;42:793–800.

95. Hallman M, Kulovich M, Kirkpatrick E, Sugarman RG, Gluck L. Phosphatidylinositol and phosphatidylglycerol in amniotic fluid: indices of lung maturity. Am J Obstet Gynecol 1976;125:613–617.

96. Spillman T, Cotton DB. Current perspectives in assessment of fetal pulmonary surfactant status with amniotic fluid. Crit Rev Clin Lab Sci 1989;27:341–389.

97. Bangham AD, Morely CJ, Phillips MC. The physical properties of an effective lung surfactant. Biochim Biophys Acta 1979;573:552–556.

98. Jones GW, Ashwood ER. Enzymatic measurement of phosphatidylglycerol in amniotic fluid. Clin Chem 1994;40:518–525.

99. Eisenbrey AB, Epstein E, Zak B, McEnroe RJ, Artiss JD, Kiechle FL. Phosphatidylglycerol in amniotic fluid: comparison of an "ultrasensitive" immunologic assay with TLC and enzymatic assay. Am J Clin Pathol 1989;91:293–297.

100. Brame RG, MacKenna J. Vaginal pool phospholipids in the management of premature rupture of membranes. Am J Obstet Gynecol 1983;145:992–1000.

101. Lewis DF, Towers CV, Major CA, et al. Use of Amniostat-FLM in detecting the presence of phosphatidylglycerol in vaginal pool samples in preterm premature rupture of membranes. Am J Obstet Gynecol 1993;169:573–576.

102. Schumacher RE, Parisi VM, Steady HM, Tsao FHC. Bacteria causing false positive test for phosphatidylglycerol in amniotic fluid. Am J Obstet Gynecol 1985;151:1067–1068.

103. Pastorek JG 2nd, Letellier RL, Gebbia K. Production of a phosphatidylglycerol-like substance by genital flora bacteria. Am J Obstet Gynecol 1988;159:199–202.

104. Lambers DS, Brady K, Leist PA, Setser C, Helmchen R. Ability of normal vaginal flora to produce detectable phosphatidylglycerol in amniotic fluid in vitro. Obstet Gynecol 1995;85:651–655.

105. Farquharson J, Jamieson EC, Berry E, Buchanan R, Logan RW. Assessment of the AmnioStat-FLM immunoagglutination test for phosphatidylglycerol in amniotic fluid. Clin Chim Acta 1986;156:271–277.

106. Benoit J, Merrill S, Rundell C, Meeker CI. Amniostat-FLM: an initial clinical trial with both vaginal pool and amniocentesis samples. Am J Obstet Gynecol 1986;154:65–68.

107. Halvorsen PR, Gross TL. Laboratory and clinical evaluation of a rapid slide agglutination test for phosphatidylglycerol. Am J Obstet Gynecol 1985;151:1061–1066.

108. Weinbaum PJ, Richardson D, Schwartz JS, Gabbe SG. Amniostat FLM: a new technique for detection of phosphatidylglycerol in amniotic fluid. Am J Perinatol 1985;2:88–92.

109. Lockitch G, Wittmann BK, Mura SM, Hawkley LC. Evaluation of the Amniostat-FLM assay for assessment of fetal lung maturity. Clin Chem 1984;30:1233–1237.

110. Garite TJ, Yabusaki KK, Moberg LJ, et al. A new rapid slide agglutination test for amniotic fluid phosphatidylglycerol: laboratory and clinical correlation. Am J Obstet Gynecol 1983;147:681–686.

111. Towers CV, Garite TJ. Uselessness of the phosphatidylglycerol assay for prediction of lung maturity [reply]. Am J Obstet Gynecol 1989;161:1419.

112. Spillman TA, Cotton DB, Golunski E. Detection frequency by thin-layer chromatography of phosphatidylglycerol in amniotic fluid with clinically functional pulmonary surfactant. Clin Chem 1988;34:1976–1982.

113. Tsai MY, Shultz EK, Nelson JA. Amniotic fluid phosphatidylglycerol in diabetic and control pregnant patients at different gestational lengths. Am J Obstet Gynecol 1984;149:388–392.

114. Cunningham MD, McKean HE, Gillispie DH, Greene JW. Improved prediction of fetal lung maturity in diabetic pregnancies: a comparison of chromatographic methods. Am J Obstet Gynecol 1982;142:197–204.

115. Piper JM, Xenakis EM, Langer O. Delayed appearance of pulmonary maturation markers is associated with poor glucose control in diabetic pregnancies. J Matern Fetal Med 1998;7:148–153.

116. Saad SA, Fadel HE, Fahmy K, Nelson GH, Moustafa M, Davis HC. The reliability and clinical use of a rapid phosphatidylglycerol assay in normal and diabetic pregnancies. Am J Obstet Gynecol 1987;157:1516–1520.

117. Ashwood ER, Oldroyd RG, Palmer SE. Measuring the number of lamellar body particles in amniotic fluid. Obstet Gynecol 1990;75:289–292.

118. Dubin SB. Characterization of amniotic fluid lamellar bodies by resistive-pulse counting: relationship to measures of fetal lung maturity. Clin Chem 1989;35:612–616.

119. Ashwood ER, Palmer SE, Taylor JS, Pingree SS. Lamellar body counts for rapid fetal lung maturity testing. Obstet Gynecol 1993;81:619–624.

120. Neerhof MG, Dohnal JC, Ashwood ER, Lee IS, Anceschi MM. Lamellar body counts: a consensus on protocol. Obstet Gynecol 2001;97:318–320.

121. Szallasi A, Gronowski AM, Eby CS. Lamellar body count in amniotic fluid: a comparative study of four different hematology analyzers. Clin Chem 2003;49:994–997.

122. Greenspoon JS, Rosen DJ, Roll K, Dubin SB. Evaluation of lamellar body number density as the initial assessment in a fetal lung maturity test cascade. J Reprod Med 1995;40:260–266.

123. Bowie LJ, Shammo J, Dohnal JC, Farrell E, Vye MV. Lamellar body number density and the prediction of respiratory distress. Am J Clin Pathol 1991;95:781–786.

124. Dalence CR, Bowie LJ, Dohnal JC, Farrell EE, Neerhof MG. Amniotic fluid lamellar body count: a rapid and reliable fetal lung maturity test. Obstet Gynecol 1995;86:235–239.
125. Fakhoury G, Daikoku NH, Benser J, Dubin NH. Lamellar body concentrations and the prediction of fetal pulmonary maturity. Am J Obstet Gynecol 1994;170:72–76.
126. Lee IS, Cho YK, Kim A, Min WK, Kim KS, Mok JE. Lamellar body count in amniotic fluid as a rapid screening test for fetal lung maturity. J Perinatol 1996;16:176–180.
127. Pearlman ES, Baiocchi JM, Lease JA, Gilbert J, Cooper JH. Utility of a rapid lamellar body count in the assessment of fetal maturity. Am J Clin Pathol 1991;95:778–780.
128. Dilena BA, Ku F, Doyle I, Whiting MJ. Six alternative methods to the lecithin/sphingomyelin ratio in amniotic fluid for assessing fetal lung maturity. Ann Clin Biochem 1997;34:106–108.
129. Neerhof MG, Haney EI, Silver RK, Ashwood ER, Lee IS, Piazze JJ. Lamellar body counts compared with traditional phospholipid analysis as an assay for evaluating fetal lung maturity. Obstet Gynecol 2001;97:305–309.
130. Beinlich A, Fischass C, Kaufmann M, Schlosser R, Dericks-Tan JS. Lamellar body counts in amniotic fluid for prediction of fetal lung maturity. Arch Gynecol Obstet 1999;262:173–180.
131. Wijnberger LD, Huisjes AJ, Voorbij HA, Franx A, Bruinse HW, Mol BW. The accuracy of lamellar body count and lecithin/sphingomyelin ratio in the prediction of neonatal respiratory distress syndrome: a meta-analysis. Br J Obstet Gynecol 2001;108:583–588.
132. DeRoche ME, Ingardia CJ, Guerette PJ, Wu AH, LaSala CA, Mandavilli SR. The use of lamellar body counts to predict fetal lung maturity in pregnancies complicated by diabetes mellitus. Am J Obstet Gynecol 2002;187:908–912.
133. Clements JA, Platzker AC, Tierney DF, et al. Assessment of the risk of the respiratory-distress syndrome by a rapid test for surfactant in amniotic fluid. N Engl J Med 1972;286:1077–1081.
134. Sher G, Statland BE, Freer DE, Kraybill EN. Assessing fetal lung maturation by the foam stability index test. Obstet Gynecol 1978;52:673–677.
135. Keniston RC, Noland GL, Pernoll ML. The effect of blood, meconium, and temperature on the rapid surfactant test. Obstet Gynecol 1976;48:442–446.
136. Sher G, Statland BE, Freer DE. Clinical evaluation of the quantitative foam stability index test. Obstet Gynecol 1980;55:617–620.
137. Sher G, Statland BE, Knutzen VK. Diagnostic reliability of the lecithin/sphingomyelin ratio assay and the quantitative foam stability index test: results of a comparative study. J Reprod Med 1982;27:51–55.
138. Sher G, Statland BE. Assessment of fetal pulmonary maturity by the Lumadex foam stability index test. Obstet Gynecol 1983;61:444–449.
139. Lockitch G, Wittmann BK, Snow BE, Campbell DJ. Prediction of fetal lung maturity by use of the Lumadex-FSI test. Clin Chem 1986;32:361–363.
140. Lipshitz J, Whybrew WD, Anderson GD. Comparison of the Lumadex-foam stability index test, lecithin: sphingomyelin ratio, and simple shake test for fetal lung maturity. Obstet Gynecol 1984;63:349–354.
141. Garite TJ, Freeman RK, Nageotte MP. Fetal maturity cascade: a rapid and cost-effective method for fetal lung maturity testing. Obstet Gynecol 1986;67:619–622.
142. Wong SS, Schenkel O, Qutishat A. Strategic utilization of fetal lung maturity tests. Scand J Clin Lab Invest 1996;56:525–532.
143. Bonebrake RG, Towers CV, Rumney PJ, Reimbold P. Is fluorescence polarization reliable and cost efficient in a fetal lung maturity cascade? Am J Obstet Gynecol 1997;177:835–841.
144. Lewis PS, Lauria MR, Dzieczkowski J, Utter GO, Dombrowski MP. Amniotic fluid lamellar body count: cost-effective screening for fetal lung maturity. Obstet Gynecol 1999;93:387–391.
145. Ross GE, Bever FN, Uddin Z, Hockman EM, Herman BA. Decreased laboratory testing for lecithin-to-sphingomyelin ratio and phosphatidylglycerol after fetal lung maturity assessment from lamellar body count in amniotic fluid. J Am Osteopath Assoc 2002;102:423–428.

5

Maternal Prenatal Screening for Fetal Defects

Andrew R. MacRae, PhD, FCACB
and Jacob A. Canick, PhD, FACB

In Memory of H. Allen Gardner

CONTENTS

INTRODUCTION

Even before a woman becomes pregnant, the parents-to-be wonder about the health of their future child. This natural concern is why prenatal screening for fetal disorders has attracted considerable attention over the past two decades or more. The interest is both professional and personal. The promise of foretelling the health of the developing baby puts new demands on laboratorians, clinicians, and patients alike. Laboratorians must be fully cognizant of the clinical implications of their screening service, clinicians must liaise with laboratories to provide accurate clinical information, and patients face new choices in the information that they can now receive about their pregnancy.

In the "diagnostic laboratory," true diagnostic tests are relatively rare. Most test results are used in subjective combination with clinical evidence to indicate the possibility of a disease or disorder. However, the practice of prenatal screening takes that informal and subjective association of information to a more structured, rational, and evidence-based level. Clinical information and laboratory test results are assembled and combined based on scientific evidence to yield a computed risk of the presence of a targeted disorder. The service is complex, and the results are at times counterintuitive.

From: *Current Clinical Pathology: Handbook of Clinical Laboratory Testing During Pregnancy*
Edited by: A. M. Gronowski © Humana Press, Totowa, NJ

Basic Concepts of Screening

The goal of screening is to identify those individuals who are at sufficient risk, or have a sufficient likelihood of a particular targeted disease, to justify consideration of further investigation leading to a diagnosis. Screening is justified only when a diagnostic test exists to confirm the screen but the diagnostic test is associated with an inherent risk to the patient or a significant cost. Screening is a service that is designed for, and available to, an unselected population. It should be offered to all patients who fit a minimum set of inclusion criteria; otherwise, one screening procedure is being used to select patients for a subsequent screen—a process of sequential screening—which decreases the performance of the overall service.

A useful definition of screening has been provided by Wald *(1)*: "Screening is the systematic application of a test or inquiry, to identify individuals at sufficient risk of a specific disorder, to benefit from further investigation or direct preventive action, among persons who have not sought medical attention because of symptoms of that disorder." The key components of this definition are that the test is uniformly applied (without any bias or preselection) to a population that is without symptoms or indicators for the disorder. The purpose is to identify those who are sufficiently at risk of a specifically targeted disorder to justify a follow-up procedure. Indeed, a screen should be offered only if a follow-up procedure exists that is accessible, and of value, to the patients identified by the screen. It should also be noted that the screen also identifies those patients who are at sufficiently low risk to justify not being offered follow-up.

PRENATAL SCREENING

When this definition is applied to the prenatal screening setting, the specific disorders commonly being screened for include open neural tube defects and fetal trisomies of chromosomes 21 and 18. This is not "genetic screening," which implies inheritance, and specific gene tests and disorders; instead, it is the use of biochemical and possibly ultrasound markers for assessing and informing patients about the risk of developmental disorders *(2)*. The term "prenatal screening" does not in itself specify the limited scope of what is being performed or what can potentially be detected. In describing the procedures being offered to patients, the target disorders should be named, such as prenatal screening for open neural tube defects (ONTDs) or prenatal screening for fetal trisomies 21 and 18.

In both of these prenatal screens, the further investigations offered to screen positive patients include a detailed ultrasound examination of the fetus and/or amniocentesis with diagnostic tests performed on the amniotic fluid or fetal cells in that fluid. Amniocentesis is associated with a risk to the pregnancy, usually considered to be 1:200. It is important that patients and health care providers alike have an understanding that,

- the result of any screen is a likelihood of being affected by the disorder, rather than a certainty; therefore, screening is a risk assessment and not a diagnostic test; and
- most screen-positive patients will not actually have the targeted disorder.

The goal of a screen is to increase the prevalence of the targeted disorder within the subpopulation that is offered invasive and/or expensive follow-up diagnostic testing. With that in mind, there are circumstances where a prenatal screen might not be justified because the risk of the disorder is already known or was discovered during clinical inquiry to be substantially increased above the general population prevalence—for instance, when a close relative is affected with the disorder and the disorder has an established and significant inheritable predisposition.

A screening service should provide patients with the best possible understanding about their risk of being affected by a specific disorder. Communicating the best estimate of risk to a patient is a challenge. Because maternal age is a factor in the risk of fetal trisomy, patients are effectively self-screening whenever they link their age with concern (or reassurance) over the possibility of having an affected pregnancy. When that perception is overlaid with another screening test such as a blood test, it is common for the lay public (and media) to assign a higher level of diagnostic power to a screen-positive result than is appropriate *(3)*. The need for public and provider education is continuous; in its absence or neglect, patient and provider satisfaction declines rapidly.

Defining a Screening Cutoff Value

In order to perform a screen there must be a screening test that is uniformly applied. Figure 1 shows how two populations, labeled "Unaffected" and "Affected," might be separated on the basis of an attribute of the populations such as a test result (the "screening variable" on the independent axis). For the test to be of benefit, the two populations must differ with respect to that variable to a sufficient extent. If that condition is met, performing the test in an individual from a mixed population will yield some information about whether the patient is from the unaffected or affected subpopulation.

The greater the separation of the two subpopulations with respect to the screening variable, the greater the power of the screen. If the test is very powerful at discriminating between the two populations, the two curves would have very little overlap and the test would be considered diagnostic for the targeted disorder.

In a screen, a uniformly applied cutoff value divides the mixed population into two—those who are "screen positive" and those who are "screen negative" for the targeted disorder. The selection of the cutoff value will determine the fraction of the affected population that is detected (detection rate of the screen). It will also determine the fraction of the *unaffected* population that is considered to be screen positive (the false-positive rate [FPR]). Moving the cutoff value further into the affected population (to the right in the example shown in Fig. 1) will diminish the detection rate of the target disorder; however, the benefit would be fewer of the unaffected population identified as screen positive. Moving the cutoff value in the other direction (lowering the cutoff in this example) will have the opposite effect—better detection, but at the cost of identifying a larger fraction of the unaffected population for possible expensive or invasive follow-up studies.

The cutoff for a particular screen is selected following a consideration of the targeted disorder, the available resources for follow-up testing, the risk of follow-up procedures, and the public expectation of the screening service. If the resources for follow-up are scarce, associated with high risk, or costly, a higher cutoff is selected to minimize the FPR; the detection rate is reduced correspondingly.

In screening, the focus is usually on the patients who are screen positive, because these patients proceed to have follow-up testing offered. Therefore, a screen is evaluated on the basis of its detection rate (DR) and its FPR. The DR is the same as the sensitivity of the test— the fraction of the affected population that is screen positive—whereas the FPR is the fraction of the unaffected population that is screen positive. The FPR is equal to one minus the specificity of the test; that is, if the specificity is 0.95 or 95%, the FPR is 0.05 or 5%.

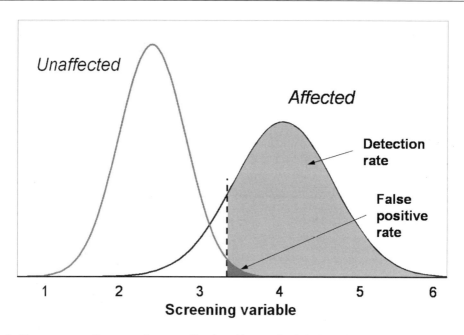

Fig. 1. The concept of a screening cutoff value (the vertical dashed line), and its effect on the detection rate and the false-positive rate.

In prenatal screening, the positive predictive value of the screen is often expressed as the odds of being affected given a positive result (OAPR). This is a useful expression of the prevalence of the target disorder among those who screened positive for the disorder. An OAPR of 1:60 indicates that for every 61 screen-positive patients, one will actually have the target disorder. The power of a screen to increase the prevalence of the targeted disorder can be assessed by comparing the prevalence of the disorder in the general population to the OAPR (the prevalence in the screen-positive subpopulation). If the background prevalence is 1:600 and the OAPR is 1:60, the screening test has increased the prevalence tenfold.

SCREENING FOR OPEN NTDS

NTDs are congenital defects that occur if the developing neural tube fails to close properly during the third or fourth week of embryonic development. Anencephaly is one form of NTD where the cranium fails to form or close, and this results in either miscarriage, stillbirth, or neonatal demise. In the first trimester, before any interventions take place, the incidence of anencephaly and spinal NTDs (spina bifida) is approximately equal. There are conflicting reports concerning a direct but weak association between maternal age and the incidence of NTD *(4)*, and most screening programs do not take maternal age into consideration.

Spina bifida can be either covered by tissue (closed spina bifida, or spina bifida occulta) or open with at most a thin membranous covering (open spina bifida [OSB]). More than 95% of spina bifida cases are open defects *(5)*. The clinical effects of spina bifida range from sensory loss in small closed defects to paralysis below the site of large open defects.

Hydrocephalus is present in approximately one-third of OSB cases because of disrupted cerebrospinal fluid (CSF) circulation. ONTDs include both OSB and anencephaly, and both are detectable with second-trimester maternal serum biochemical screening and carefully targeted ultrasound. Closed spina bifida is not usually detected prenatally and is relatively less serious.

Factors Contributing to the Incidence of NTD

The prevalence of ONTD varies with the geographical region (6), and an additional smaller socioeconomic factor probably relates to the prepregnancy nutritional status of the mother. Most cases of NTDs are sporadic, but some environmental factors are known to increase incidence. Maternal exposure to the anticonvulsants valproic acid (7–9) and carbamazepine (10) increases the risk of NTD. Inheritance is a relatively slight risk factor, although there appear to be associations with specific gene and chromosome disorders (5).

In North America, the overall incidence of NTD is between 0.5 and 2 per 1000 births. The frequency is lower in the western continent and increases to the east, with the highest rates occurring in the southeastern United States and in eastern maritime Canada. In Europe, the incidence of NTD is highest in the western United Kingdom, at approx 2 per 1000 births.

Increased folic acid intake in the preconception time frame has been shown to reduce the incidence of ONTD (11,12). Depending on the folic acid intake, the natural incidence of ONTD can be reduced by 20% at 0.2 mg/d, and up to 85% at 5 mg/d (13). In 1997, both the US and Canadian regulatory bodies mandated folic acid fortification of grain products at the level of 0.14 mg folic acid per 100 g. In a study with ONTD ascertainment at the time of prenatal diagnosis and at birth, this fortification was associated with a 32% decrease in the incidence of ONTD (14). A comparison of the observed and predicted effects of folic acid fortification has concluded that even higher levels of intake would be beneficial (15).

Advent of Prenatal Diagnostic Testing and Screening for ONTD

α-Fetoprotein (AFP) was first reported as a significant component of fetal plasma proteins by Bergstrand and Czar in 1956 (16). AFP is structurally similar to albumin but exhibits a greater binding of polyunsaturated fatty acids compared to albumin, which might indicate a role in embryonic cellular development (17). Nevertheless, a rare congenital absence of fetal AFP production has been reported that was associated with a normal birth outcome (18). Only traces of AFP are present in nonpregnant adults, but serum concentrations increase substantially during hepatocyte regeneration, and in liver and embryonic carcinomas.

The prenatal diagnosis of ONTD became possible with the discovery in 1972 by Brock and Sutcliffe (19) that high concentrations of AFP were present in the amniotic fluid of ONTD-affected pregnancies, primarily in the third trimester of pregnancy. Several confirmatory reports soon followed that extended this observation into the second trimester with AFP measurements in both amniotic fluid and maternal serum (20–22). The UK Collaborative Study on Alpha-Fetoprotein in Relation to Neural-Tube Defects published its findings in 1979 (23) that demonstrated conclusively that amniotic fluid AFP (AFAFP) is elevated during the early second trimester in both anencephaly (20-fold) and in OSB (7-fold). Figure 2 shows the relative frequency distributions of AFAFP in unaffected,

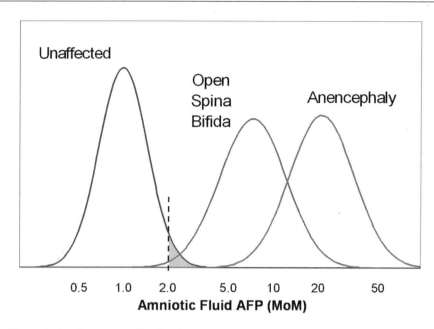

Fig. 2. The relative frequency distributions of AFAFP in unaffected, OSB, and anencephalic pregnancies. The commonly used cutoff value of 2.0 MoM is shown.

OSB, and anencephalic pregnancies. By 1981, a second diagnostic test, acetylcholinesterase (AChE) in amniotic fluid, was also confirmed (24).

Second-trimester AFAFP testing is the first instance of the use of a biochemical test to diagnose a fetal malformation. With the validation of a diagnostic test, a screening program could now be established. Attention then focused on the development of a serum-based screening test. Wald, Brock, and Bonnar reported the first use of maternal serum AFP (MSAFP) as a screening test in 1974 (25). The UK Collaborative Study reported in 1977 that elevated MSAFP, in the early midtrimester of pregnancy could identify 80% of OSB and 90% of anencephaly cases (26) at an FPR of 5%.

The physiological basis for AFAFP as a prenatal diagnostic test for ONTD, and for MSAFP as a prenatal screening marker for increased risk, is very simple: an open defect represents a leak in what is normally the confined circulation of AFP within fetal plasma and CSF. In ONTD, AFP is able to pass from fetal plasma and CSF, where it exists at concentrations of 1–3 g/L, into amniotic fluid, where it normally exists through fetal micturition at concentrations of 10–15 mg/L. AFP from the fetus reaches the maternal compartment (20–50 µg/L) via the placenta and by diffusion across the amniotic membranes (27). The presence of an ONTD represents a breakdown of this normally well-contained concentration gradient, resulting in concentrations 7- to 20-fold higher in amniotic fluid (Fig. 2) and 4-fold higher in maternal serum (Fig. 3).

By 1981, a number of breakthroughs in prenatal screening for ONTD had been achieved: two diagnostic tests had been validated in amniotic fluid (AFP and AChE), both requiring an invasive amniocentesis procedure; a noninvasive screening test— MSAFP, by itself not diagnostic of any condition—had been confirmed to identify at least 80% of ONTD patients within the 3% of the population with the highest MSAFP concentrations (26); and a new method had been developed (25) for reporting concentra-

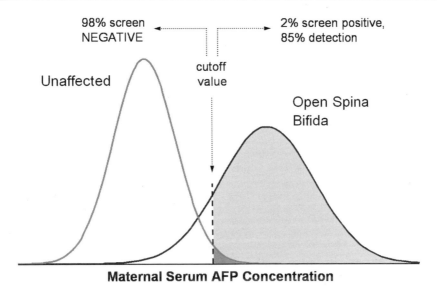

Fig. 3. MSAFP as a screening marker for OSB.

tions as the multiple of the median (MoM) concentration of unaffected patients (see Using the MoM To Adjust for Gestational Age, below). The MoM designation is useful because AFP concentrations in both maternal serum and amniotic fluid change with gestational age, and this is reflected by changes in the median concentrations seen at each gestational week. The use of the MoM designation not only eliminated the concentration effect of different gestational ages, but it also reduced differences between analytical methodologies, allowing the multisite collaboration that is critical for the effective study of relatively rare conditions.

Confounding Variables Influencing AFP Concentration

Several clinical factors, or attributes of the patient, influence the concentration of AFP in maternal serum and amniotic fluid Optimal screening performance for ONTD depends on the collection and uniform application of clinical information about each patient screened.

GESTATIONAL AGE FOR TESTING

AFP concentrations, particularly in maternal serum, are informative about the risk or presence of ONTD only within a specified period of early midtrimester gestation. With MSAFP, the OSB population has the greatest separation from the unaffected population during the 16th to 18th wk of gestation *(26)*. Screening is less effective in week 15 and beyond week 19; performance in weeks 20 to 24 has been estimated as 70% detection for a somewhat elevated 5% FPR *(26,28)*. AFAFP diagnostic testing is best between weeks 16 and 22; detection rates during weeks 13 to 15 are slightly lower *(23,29)*, and given the constraints of MSAFP timing, would be performed only on patients having an amniocentesis for reasons other than an elevated MSAFP result.

Using the MoM to Adjust for Gestational Age. AFP concentrations change throughout pregnancy in the fetus, amniotic fluid, and maternal serum. During the midtrimester, AFAFP concentrations decrease and MSAFP concentrations increase by approx 12–15%

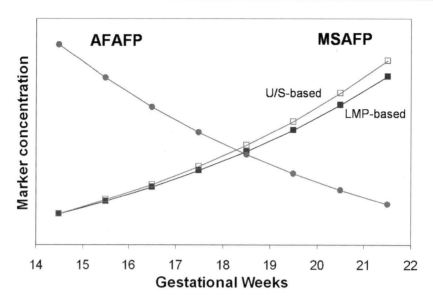

Fig. 4. Relative changes in the median AFP values in maternal serum and AF at each week during the early second trimester of pregnancy.

per week (Fig. 4). In order to eliminate the need to have normative data for each week of gestation, patient results are expressed as the ratio of the median concentration in unaffected pregnancies at that gestational age. The median value is used instead of the mean value to avoid the influence of substantially elevated results that would skew the mean in small population samplings. The MoM result is potentially independent of the gestational age, allowing patients of all gestational ages to be assessed together on the basis of their MoM values. In order to achieve this independence of gestational age, the median values must be selected in a manner that avoids any bias throughout the range of reportable gestational ages.

Obtaining Normative Median Data. Medians are calculated from the AFP concentrations recently measured in a group of specimens that span the gestational age range to be used in screening. If the patient population being served is relatively static, acceptably robust median values can be calculated from 50 to 100 samples for each week of gestation. Knowledge about the normalcy of the pregnancies is not necessary because unusually high concentrations are balanced by low results—an inherent quality of the median rather than the mean of a population. Frozen specimens are also acceptable and particularly useful for establishing AFAFP medians, because AFP is quite stable in both amniotic fluid and serum.

In a screened population, a gestational age of 16 wk is common, whereas 20 wk is uncommon. In order to lessen the inaccuracy of medians at outlying gestational ages, the observed medians are regressed (logarithms of concentration regressed against gestational age, weighted by the number of observations in each category), thus making use of the known natural increasing (MSAFP) or decreasing (AFAFP) pattern of concentration with increasing gestational age. Accuracy in both measures—AFP concentration and gestational age—is required. Gestational ages can be measured in completed weeks (e.g., 16 wk 5 d is 16 completed weeks), but it is preferable to express the gestational age to the nearest day, or in decimal weeks, despite the fact that this implies a greater accuracy than is likely present within any individual patient. The median regression equation is then used to interpolate gestational age medians to the nearest day or decimal weeks for subsequent patients, until such time as the analytical conditions change, requiring a new assessment of medians.

The method of estimating the gestational age in patients should also be known because it imparts a small bias to the median values. Medians for AFAFP are virtually always based on ultrasound biometry. MSAFP medians will differ slightly with different methods of gestational age assignment *(30)*. If the gestational age is inaccurate in a population, the true rise in MSAFP will be partially masked by that inaccuracy. Therefore, medians based on last menstrual period (LMP) rise less steeply than medians based on biometry (Fig. 4). Depending on the size of a screening program and its mix of LMP- and biometry-assigned gestational ages, some programs use different median regressions for these two methods of assignment *(30)*.

Although LMP dating is sufficiently accurate to sustain screening, ultrasound biometry improves performance. At least two pieces of information are required to assign a gestational age: the date of the estimation and the estimated age or biometry measurement. The methods of assigning gestational age ranked in declining accuracy are crown–rump length (CRL) before 12 wk, biparietal diameter (BPD) after 12 wk, age based on composite multiple biometry measurements, and LMP dates. Physical examination and expected date of delivery (EDD) are less reliable. Ultrasound biometry is considered accurate within 8% of the assigned gestational age *(31)* or within 9–10 d at early midtrimester. Because different algorithms exist for converting biometry measurements to gestational age, it is preferable to collect the actual measurements and use an accepted algorithm for the entire screened population. The algorithms by Daya *(32)* for CRL and the 1982 BPD data of Hadlock *(33)* are an example of a pair of biometry algorithms with good concordance that span from 6 to at least 30 wk.

If more than one ultrasound examination is performed, a good first trimester CRL is preferred over a later BPD because biological variation in fetal size will start to become a factor. However, ONTD screening is improved if a BPD is used, for two reasons: first, anencephaly can be ruled out if a BPD measurement is reported by the ultrasonographer; and second, OSB-affected fetuses have smaller BPD measurements *(34)*. A smaller BPD will cause the assignment of a lower than true gestational age and median value. The MSAFP MoM will therefore be, on average, elevated more than if another dating method had been used, increasing the likelihood of a screen-positive result in the presence of OSB.

DEMOGRAPHIC AND CLINICAL FACTORS THAT INFLUENCE THE MoM VALUE

There are a number of patient demographic and clinical factors other than gestational age that influence AFP concentrations and are recommended for adjustments.

Racial Origin. Prenatal screening for fetal ONTD was first developed in largely white populations. Subsequently, it was found that the black (African American) population has 10–22% higher concentrations of AFP in both maternal serum and amniotic fluid in women with and without pregnancies with OSB *(35–38)*. The effects of this racial difference, and possible remedies, will vary with the size of the populations being screened. In a population equally distributed by race, the overall population medians would be higher than those seen strictly in the white women, and lower than those in the black women. Screen-positive rates at any cutoff would be lower, and higher, than expected, respectively. This difference can be compensated either by the use of separate MSAFP median data for the black and white populations, or by the use of a median adjustment factor (commonly 1.10 or 1.15) to modify the white medians for use in black patients. Even though AFAFP concentrations are also 12% higher in the black population *(37)*, adjustment of AFAFP medians is not commonly performed because of the very small overlap between the affected and unaffected populations with this diagnostic test. The Asian population (e.g., Japanese, Chinese, Filipina) have the same, or only slightly higher, weight-corrected MSAFP concentrations compared to the white population *(38,39)*, and median correction for this group is uncommon.

Maternal Weight. A relationship between maternal weight and MSAFP was first reported *(40)* in 1981 and then confirmed in the same year *(41)*. The developing fetus is the source of MSAFP, and because fetal size in early pregnancy does not reflect maternal size, the circulating volume of the mother will indirectly affect the MSAFP concentration. Maternal weight is an easily accessible index of circulating volume. Maternal weight has no effect on AFAFP, nor is maternal weight different between OSB and unaffected pregnancies *(42)*. Two weight correction formulae for MSAFP have been reported: one that fits the observed MSAFP and weight data to a log-linear relationship *(43)*, and one that uses an inverse relationship *(44)*. Published weight correction parameters are appropriate only for screened populations with the same average maternal weight as the published study *(44)*; therefore, individual screening programs should calculate their own weight correction parameters for either of the two formulae. Screening without weight correction will result in a wider distribution of MSAFP MoM values, a higher screen positive rate in lower-weight women, and probably a slight loss in detection of OSB *(42)*.

Number of Fetuses. Multiple gestation pregnancies have MSAFP (but not AFAFP) concentrations that are commensurate with the number of developing fetuses. Twin pregnancies have on average 2.16 times the MSAFP concentration of singleton pregnancies *(45–47)*. Monozygotic twin pregnancies (one-third of all twin pregnancies) probably have slighly higher concentrations than dizygotic pregnancies *(48,49)*. No adjustment is made to the MSAFP medians, but the MoM cutoff for serum samples from known twin pregnancies is selected at a higher value to maintain approximately the same FPR as in singleton pregnancies (see section on Twin Pregnancies).

Insulin-Dependent Diabetes Mellitus. Pregnant patients with a prior diagnosis of insulin-dependent diabetes mellitus have approx 20% lower concentrations of MSAFP *(50,51)*. A factor is usually applied to the MSAFP MoM result to adjust for this. There is insufficient evidence for a similar adjustment in gestational diabetes, even if the patient is receiving insulin. AFAFP concentrations are also decreased in the presence of diabetes mellitus *(52)*; however, adjustment for this is not common for the same reasons as cited for maternal race.

Use of Multiple MoM Correction Factors in Combinations. Although published data are scarce on the coexistence of multiple conditions that affect median MSAFP values, the assumption is that each factor is independent. Factors can therefore be combined—for instance, in a black diabetic pregnancy of a particular weight. Similarly, at present it is assumed that although black patients tend to have larger body frames, and Asians are smaller than whites, it is generally assumed that they all share approximately the same weight correction formula, populating the higher or lower ends of the weight correction curve, respectively.

Calculating Patient-Specific Risks of the Targeted Disorder

With knowledge of the relative frequency distributions of the affected and unaffected populations for a given screening variable (e.g., MSAFP MoM result, see Fig. 3), the risk of the targeted disorder can be calculated from the screening variable result. Although screening for ONTD initially used a MoM cutoff value, as patients become more informed participants in their health care decisions, the pattern of practice is shifting to reporting both the MoM value and its associated patient-specific risk. The most commonly used algorithm to calculate a patient-specific risk utilizes the MoM result (adjusted for variables such as weight and race as discussed above) to calculate a likelihood ratio (LR) based on the overlapping Gaussian distributions defined for the affected and unaffected populations.

GENERAL CONCEPT OF THE LR

The concept of the LR is depicted in Fig. 5. Since the screening variable (MSAFP) distributions span a range of MoM values, any MoM result within that range could be from either a member of the affected population or the unaffected population. The higher the frequency distribution (the curve) at a given MoM value, the more common or likely the result is within that population. If the frequency distribution is known, the height of the distribution (y) can be calculated at any MoM value, such as in the Gaussian distributions in Fig. 5. Because there are two populations, at each MoM value there are two curve heights or distribution heights—one for the affected population (y_a) and one for the unaffected population (y_u). The LR is defined as the ratio of these two heights, affected over unaffected (y_a/y_u). The LR is the relative risk of being affected, and this can be converted to an absolute risk by multiplying by the background prevalence of the disorder in the screened population. In this manner, a risk can be assigned for every MoM value over a finite range.

The calculation of a risk requires knowledge of the frequency distribution parameters for both the affected and unaffected populations, the background prevalence of the disorder, and any specific prevalence factors that might apply for the patient. Then, given a patient's MoM result, a patient-specific risk can be calculated and interpreted. The frequency distributions of both AFAFP and MSAFP conform to the Gaussian distribution if the logarithms of the MoM values are used. Therefore, the distributions can be defined by their mean log MoM values and the log MoM standard deviations (SD). There is a range of MoM values, bordered by truncation limits, over which both distributions can be shown to conform to the Gaussian distribution. Outside of this range, the LR at the truncation limit that was exceeded is used to calculate the risk. The Gaussian distribution parameters (mean and/or SD) vary depending on a number of factors, and the prevalence of the targeted disorder can also vary in assigning patient-specific risks.

Given the complexity of median, MoM, and risk calculations, specialized software is necessary to maintain a database for median calculations, calculate risks, and issue patient-specific interpretive reports including recommended follow-up procedures where indicated.

SPECIFIC FREQUENCY DISTRIBUTION PARAMETER ADJUSTMENTS

Any correction factor that systematically increases the accuracy of MoM values will reduce the variance (SD) of the Gaussian distribution populations and affect the computed risk results. Oddly, long-term analytical precision in the MSAFP assay is not

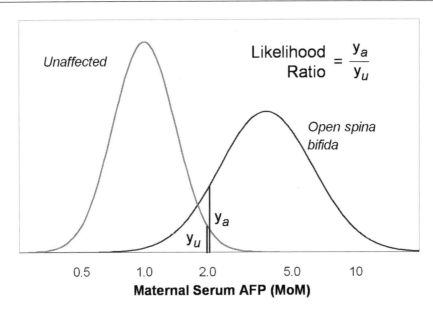

Fig. 5. The LR concept in MSAFP screening for OSB.

frequently used to modify Gaussian distribution parameters. Most laboratories instead opt to use published distribution parameters from large outcome validation studies instead of their own parameters, while maintaining their analytical precision at or below that attained in the published studies (53,54). However, there are two other factors affecting the accuracy of the MoM value that are commonly used independently and together to modify distribution parameters: correction for maternal weight, and the method of assigning gestational age. Twin pregnancies also have their own frequency distributions.

Maternal Weight Correction. Knowledge of the maternal weight and correction of the computed MoM result (see "Maternal Weight") reduces this source of variance in the MoM distribution populations. The lower variance results in a greater separation between the affected and unaffected populations (55) and hence the LR and computed risks for a given MoM are different if weight correction has been performed. OSB screening software applications typically use different Gaussian distribution parameters for weight-corrected and uncorrected patients.

Gestational Age by LMP and Biometry. As indicated earlier (see section on Obtaining Normative Median Data), gestational ages assigned from ultrasound biometry are slightly more accurate on average than LMP-based assignments. The greater accuracy in gestational age is reflected in more accurate median calculation and assignment, and more tightly defined (smaller SD) Gaussian populations. The median MSAFP is also slightly higher in OSB pregnancies when the gestational age is based on biometry. Separate frequency distribution parameters have been established for LMP-based and biometry-based gestational age assignments (55,53). There is no distinction made between the different biometric measurements of CRL, BPD, or composite measurements. In ultrasound-dated pregnancies, the higher mean MSAFP in OSB and the lower SD in both the affected and unaffected populations causes less overlap and improves screening performance. The LR, and hence the assigned risk for a given MoM value, is therefore different depending on the method of gestational age assignment.

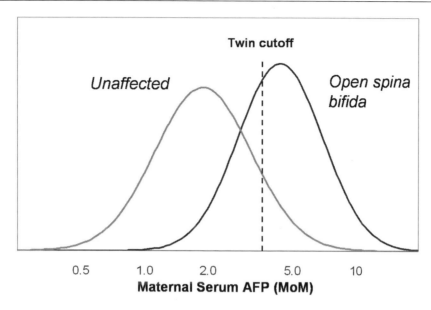

Fig. 6. MSAFP distributions in twin pregnancies, expressed in MoM for unaffected singleton pregnancy. Despite the greater overlap between the unaffected and affected (one twin) pregnancies, a moderately successful OSB screen can be performed.

Twin Pregnancies. Large-scale studies of MSAFP in twin pregnancies have generated sufficient data to construct the frequency distribution of MSAFP in OSB as well as in unaffected twin pregnancies *(47,48,56)*. The distributions are log Gaussian, like their singleton counterparts, but as might be expected, there is more overlap between the affected (one twin) and unaffected populations, which decreases the performance of the OSB screen (Fig. 6). Nevertheless, it is possible to calculate a likelihood ratio for OSB in one twin and to perform a screen using a suitably high MoM cutoff *(56)*, typically 4.0 MoM or higher.

SPECIFIC PREVALENCE ADJUSTMENTS

In ONTD screening, the primary focus is on OSB risk because anencephaly is more easily detected by MSAFP and ultrasound, and survival with anencephaly is limited. Therefore, the local prevalence of OSB is modified by factors discussed below, when appropriate, before multiplying by the patient's LR to achieve the patient-specific risk. OSB prevalence estimates are difficult to achieve for two reasons: the widespread practice of ONTD screening, diagnosis, and intervention has itself reduced the birth prevalence *(57)*; and preconceptual intake of folate might have increased since the time when local prevalence information was obtained *(14)*.

Family History. First-degree relatives of the developing fetus (e.g., siblings of a previous ONTD-affected pregnancy) are at sufficiently elevated risk of ONTD to warrant counseling for diagnostic testing without screening *(5)*. Second-degree relatives have a risk threefold greater than the background prevalence, and this can be factored into a patient's risk calculation *(58)*. More distant relations approach the general prevalence (see Table 1). An unrelated observation is that patients with an elevated MSAFP concen-

Table 1
The Effect of Family History on the Prevalence of Neural Tube Defects (NTDs)

Family history	Recurrence rate[a]	Risk ratio
Background risk; no known history of NTD	0.2%	-
Parent affected with NTD	0.6%	3-fold
Further family history of NTD	0.6%	3-fold
Previous child with NTD	1.4%	7-fold
Two previous children with NTD	5.9%	30-fold

[a]Recurrence rates are based on 100,000 cases of AFAFP analysis as reported by Milunsky (5).

tration in a previous pregnancy are slightly predisposed to having an elevated MSAFP in the next pregnancy (59). The weak correlation does not support any adjustment but might be mentioned during counseling.

Maternal Race. Despite the fact that the black population (African American) has higher MSAFP concentrations in both unaffected and OSB pregnancies (37,38), the prevalence of ONTD is approximately one-half that of the white population. In ONTD screening, cutoffs are set at MSAFP MoM values, usually between 2.0 and 2.5 MoM, and the cutoff value is associated with a particular risk in the white population. The lower prevalence in the black population means that these patients achieve the cutoff risk at higher MoM values. Adjusting the cutoff to this "isorisk" higher MoM value will lower the false positive rate and the detection rate, but all patients who screen positive will have the same minimum risk (37). As an alternative, using the same cutoff as the white population will maintain the detection ("isodetection") and false positive rates unchanged, but the black patients at the cutoff will have half the risk of whites at the same MoM value.

Insulin-Dependent Diabetes Mellitus. Pregnant patients with insulin-dependent diabetes mellitus have a 3- to 10-fold higher risk of ONTD (51,60,61). Most of the increased incidence of ONTD is anencephaly, and for this reason a detailed ultrasound examination is indicated in diabetic pregnancies because of its ability to detect anencephaly. The increase in the risk of OSB in diabetic patients is approx 3- to 4-fold that of nondiabetics. OSB screening is often viewed by practitioners as simply using an MSAFP MoM cutoff value; however, the associated risk of OSB is the more important characteristic of the cutoff. The higher risk in diabetic pregnancies is factored into the selection of the MSAFP MoM cutoff used for OSB screening in these patients. An isorisk approach is used, lowering the MSAFP MoM cutoff and raising detection and FPRs. Diabetic patients at their cutoff have the same risk as nondiabetic patients at their higher MoM cutoff.

Maternal Weight. There have been a number of reports that an increased risk for NTD is associated with prepregnancy maternal obesity (62–64). The most recent report was a population-based case-control study of several selected major birth defects using data from the Atlanta Birth Defects Risk Factor Surveillance Study (65). Nondiabetic mothers with a self-reported prepregnancy body mass index (BMI) greater than 30 ("obese") were 3.5 times more likely than average-weight women (BMI 18.5–24.9) to have an infant with spina bifida. The relative risks of other disorders were also increased, including omphalocele (3.3-fold), heart defects (2-fold), and multiple anomalies (2-fold). Compared to average-weight women, overweight women (BMI 25–30) were twice as likely to have infants with heart defects and multiple anomalies. Screening programs have yet to assess the effect of adjusting the population prevalence of OSB for normal and elevated BMI.

Twin Pregnancies. If a risk is to be quoted in twin pregnancies, it should be the risk of one twin being affected, and this must reflect the fact that twin pregnancies have a higher birth prevalence of OSB. One large study estimated the prevalence to be 2.28 times higher than the local singleton prevalence *(48)*. Follow-up procedures and patient choices should also be considered when assessing the risk of OSB in twins. There might be a greater reliance on detailed ultrasound because of the difficulty in performing amniocentesis in twin pregnancies. There are also difficult choices for the patient, and provider, when one fetus is confirmed as affected.

Combining Prevalence Factors. The prevalence factors of family history, maternal race, diabetes mellitus, and twins are assumed to be independent of each other and therefore can be combined directly in any patient with coincident factors. A black diabetic patient would therefore be assigned a prevalence factor of 1.5 to 2.0, or half of the three- to fourfold increased risk of white diabetics.

Expected Performance of ONTD Screening

The performance of the MSAFP prenatal screen for ONTD, in terms of detection and false positive rates, depends on several factors including long-term analytical precision, the gestational age at which patients are screened and the accuracy of its assignment, the MSAFP cutoff value selected for the screen, and the accuracy of elements of clinical information—the confounding variables in the screen. Table 2 provides the expected performance of ONTD screening using MSAFP.

Conditions other than ONTD that are associated with a screen-positive result include normal variance in a healthy fetus, under-estimated gestational age, an undetected twin or multiple pregnancy, a recent or impending fetal demise, and the presence of open ventral wall defects detectable by ultrasound (e.g., omphalocele, gastroschesis). Complications later in the pregnancy are also significantly more likely in women with a midtrimester MSAFP greater than 2.5 MoM, including preterm birth (<37 wk), small for gestational age (<5th percentile), very low birth weight (<1500 g), and preeclampsia *(66)*.

Follow-Up Activities in MSAFP Screen-Positive Patients

Counseling and follow-up should be offered and implemented as soon as possible after a patient is alerted to a screen-positive result, because of the anxiety that such a report often provokes (see "Psychological Impact of Prenatal Screening" below). Whereas amniocentesis with subsequent AFAFP testing remains the best diagnostic procedure, less invasive ultrasound examinations are now frequently the follow-up procedure of choice. The procedures outlined here may be offered to patients coincidentally.

AMENDING CLINICAL INFORMATION

Any clinical information determined to be in error should be corrected (e.g., weight discrepancies over 10 lbs., maternal race) and a new interpretive report should be issued. A screen-positive situation is a common trigger for an ultrasound-based gestational age estimate if the original report was based on LMP dates. New gestational age estimates that

Table 2
Performance of MSAFP Screening for ONTD
at Three Commonly Selected MoM Cutoff Values

MoM cutoff:	2.00	2.20	2.50
False-positive rate (FPR %):	3–5%	2–3%	1–2%
Detection rate (DR %) for anencephaly:	>95%	>95%	95%
Detection rate (DR %) for open spina bifida:	75–90%	70–85%	65–80%

Factors that would increase detection and lower false positive rates within the indicated ranges include the use of consistent ultrasound biometry to assign gestational age, the fraction of the population screened at 16–18 wk, and maternal weight correction.

are within 9 or 10 d of the original estimate are considered confirmatory of the original because they are within the 2 SD range of the ultrasound biometry measurements (31–33). Amending the gestational age will reduce the false positive rate (e.g., from 2.5 to 2%) but it will also reclassify a few true positive patients as screen negative.

DETAILED ULTRASOUND EXAMINATION IN ONTD

Anencephaly is fully detectable with a successful ultrasound examination. The lesions of OSB are harder to detect, particularly minimal lesions in the caudal spine. The general quality of the ultrasound imaging becomes a factor, as does the gestational age when the examination is performed—examinations at 20–24 wk are better than at 16–20 wk. With modern equipment, detection of OSB in high-risk patients with elevated MSAFP ranges from 80 to 100% (67). In the general population, ultrasound as a screening test for OSB detected only 68% in a recent European study (68). Although the absence of abnormal findings on ultrasound cannot rule out the presence of OSB, it does reduce the likelihood of the disorder by a subjective factor.

REPEAT MSAFP TESTING AS A FOLLOW-UP PROCEDURE

Regression toward the mean is a proven mathematical theorem that states that repeated observations in members of a population at the extremes of that population distribution will return results closer to the mean of the population. In MSAFP screening for ONTD, the cutoff value lies between the means of the unaffected and affected populations (see Fig. 3). Therefore, given sufficient time, unaffected and affected patients above, but close to, the cutoff value will regress to lower and higher MSAFP values respectively. The time between measurements is a factor, and one week is a useful target. Applying a policy of offering repeat testing to patients above the cutoff but below 3.0 MoM (see Table 3) will result in approx 40% of the false-positive patients relapsing to true negative, with 2–3% of OSB patients becoming screen negative (26,69). Some caveats apply to this policy: (1) if the gestational age was revised and the initial sample is now considered to have been taken before 15 wk, the subsequent sample is considered the first interpretable sample; and (2) the risk of OSB in the second sample cannot be assigned ignoring the results of the first sample—the results must be combined according to published methods (69). Repeat MSAFP testing can be useful during the interval awaiting a detailed ultrasound examination.

Table 3
Regression Toward the Unaffected Population Mean
in Repeat MSAFP Specimens[a]

MoM range	Patients	Number and percent with a repeat MSAFP test		Number and percent with a repeat MSAFP <2.20 MoM	
2.20–2.29	659	388	59%	201	52%
2.30–2.39	437	247	57%	100	40%
2.40–2.49	289	168	58%	58	35%
2.50–2.59	225	131	58%	29	22%
2.60–2.69	189	110	58%	21	19%
2.70–2.79	135	67	50%	14	21%
2.80–2.89	114	58	51%	9	16%
2.90–2.99	95	38	40%	8	21%
2.20–2.99	2143	1207	56%	440	36%

[a]From a population of 130,000 patients between weeks 15 and 18, using an MSAFP MoM cutoff for OSB screening of 2.20 MoM and a recommendation for repeat specimen collection between 2.20 and 2.99 MoM (unpublished observations).

Table 4
ONTD Detection Rates for AFAFP Alone at Two Ranges of Gestational Age
and When Combined With AChE

Marker and MoM cutoff:	AFAFP >2.0 at 16–18 wk	AFAFP >2.0 at 19–21 wk	AChE +ve with AFAFP >2.0 MoM[a]
False-positive rate (FPR %):	2%	5%	<0.1%
Detection rate (DR %) for anencephaly:	~100%	~100%	~100%
Detection rate (DR %) for open spina bifida:	96%	99%	97%

[a]Performance in the presence of visible blood contamination: FPR 1.2%; DR 91% for OSB.

Diagnostic Tests for ONTD: AFAFP and AChE

The most accurate diagnosis of ONTD requires amniocentesis with measurement of AF AFP and AChE *(24,70)*. Both of these tests are diagnostic of ONTD, and the existence of two such tests allows for their selected combined application to maximize diagnostic performance. Abnormal AFAFP results are usually defined as greater than 2.0 MoM. In these patients, AChE can add to the diagnostic certainty and reduce false positives to a dramatically low level. AChE can also be performed when a positive family history or ultrasound finding exists despite a normal AFAFP result. Table 4 provides the expected performance of AFAFP and AChE in the diagnosis of ONTD in patients with elevated MSAFP *(71)*.

Conditions other than ONTD that are associated with an elevated AFAFP and/or detectable AChE include normal variance in a healthy fetus (AFAFP only), fetal blood contamination, open ventral wall defects detectable by ultrasound (gastroschesis, and less commonly omphalocele), congenital nephrosis (AFAFP only), and fetal demise.

SCREENING FOR FETAL TRISOMY 21

When prenatal screening for ONTD was introduced in the 1970s, ONTD was the most common birth disorder in some regions of the United Kingdom. Changes in diet and the introduction of screening for ONTD have now reduced its prevalence substantially. At the same time, women have been choosing to have children at a later age, and maternal age-related fetal trisomies have increased in prevalence.

Clinical Aspects of Trisomy 21 (Down Syndrome)

A congenital syndrome of mental retardation associated with specific facial and physical features was first described by J. Langdon Down in 1866 (72). "Down syndrome" is characterized by a moderate to severe learning disability (average IQ approx 40) and congenital heart defects affecting approx 50% of affected individuals. The birth prevalence of Down syndrome ranges from approx 1 in 800 up to 1 in 400, depending on the maternal age distribution of pregnant women in the region. Down syndrome is the most common fetal chromosome disorder compatible with life.

Before the advent of antibiotics, the survival of Down syndrome infants was relatively poor. The life expectancy was only 12 yr in 1947 (73), but the current use of antibiotics and cardiac surgery to repair congenital cardiac anomalies has helped to increase life expectancy. Of those surviving the first 5 yr of life, 85% will have a life expectancy of at least 30 yr with many living to age 50 (74,75). There are medical problems throughout life, including immunodeficiency disorders, thyroid dysfunction, Alzheimer-like disorders, and a substantially increased risk of leukemia.

In 1959, the cause of Down syndrome was discovered to be an extra copy of chromosome 21 (trisomy 21) (76), caused by nondisjunction of this chromosome during meiosis in the oocyte. Rarely, major elements of chromosome 21 are translocated to another chromosome in the oocyte or sperm (translocation Down syndrome).

Diagnostic Testing for Down Syndrome

The diagnosis of fetal trisomy is made by karyotyping fetal cells, typically obtained through amniocentesis. Midtrimester amniocentesis (MTA) is performed between the 15th and 22nd wk of gestation and is by far the most common prenatal procedure leading to a diagnosis of fetal trisomy 21. The first karyotype analysis from human amniocytes was described in 1966 (77) and the first Down syndrome diagnosis following amniocentesis (78) was made in 1968. As an invasive procedure, MTA poses a risk to the pregnancy (79) with fetal loss rates generally accepted as being 1 in 200. For this reason, the diagnostic procedure is offered only to women who have been shown to have an equivalent or greater risk of carrying an affected pregnancy.

Diagnosis earlier in the pregnancy is attractive from a social and obstetrical perspective, and two such first trimester procedures have been proposed in the past decade: chorionic villus sampling (CVS) and early amniocentesis (EA). In CVS, a sample of fetal tissue is obtained by biopsy from the chorionic villi, and this is used for chromosome studies. Transabdominal CVS has a risk of about 1–2% for fetal loss, with progressively fewer losses occurring at gestational weeks 10 through 13 (80,81). EA refers to an amniocentesis procedure performed between 10 and 14 wk. EA was recently shown to have a greater risk to the fetus than MTA (82) in limb deformities, most notably talipes, or club foot. A recent review of 14 randomized studies by the Cochrane Database confirms the excess of risk in EA compared to CVS or MTA (82a). For this reason, EA is rarely performed.

Maternal Age and Down Syndrome Screening

The goal of screening is to raise the prevalence of the targeted disorder in the screen-positive subpopulation, to the point where the risk of the disorder exceeds the risk associated with the diagnostic procedures. In 1933, Penrose first published the association between maternal age and the risk of Down syndrome (83), and women became aware of their "biological clock." Nevertheless, true screening on the basis of maternal age could not be performed until a diagnostic test for fetal trisomy was developed, some 35 yr later (78). The simple act of asking a woman her age became a screening procedure, although it remains largely unrecognized as such, even today.

Patients, and to some extent health care providers, view the association between maternal age and Down syndrome in a binary sense: patients are deemed to be either at low risk or at increased risk, depending on whether the patient will be under or over the age of 35 at delivery. The reality is that maternal age is a continuous risk variable that has been defined through very large combined studies (84) and is independent of geographical location. Recent analyses have suggested minor modifications of the live-born maternal-age associated risk (85–89) primarily at the higher ages (Fig. 7).

Whereas a consensus on the birth prevalence is relatively easy to obtain, determining the antenatal prevalence at various stages of gestation is more difficult. All fetal trisomies are associated with various rates of spontaneous losses during pregnancy. Down syndrome is the least lethal of all the autosomal trisomies, which accounts for its highest birth prevalence. Between the early second trimester and term, an estimated 23% of trisomy 21 pregnancies are lost (84,90), and the rate of loss between the first trimester and term is higher, perhaps 45% (91). In the United States, the prevalence and risks of Down syndrome are usually quoted for the second (or mid) trimester, whereas in Canada and many parts of Europe the risk at term is used. Arguments can be made in support of both practices: the risk at midtrimester is the risk at the usual time of screening, but its calculation is indirect and depends on an estimate of the rate of spontaneous fetal loss; the risk at term is based on more direct evidence and reflects the risk of a liveborn affected newborn.

The Advent of Biochemical Screening for Down Syndrome

In the early 1980s, MSAFP screening for ONTD was becoming fairly common. In 1983, there was a fortuitous observation of a low concentration of MSAFP in a trisomy 18 (T18) pregnancy. This led to an investigation by Merkatz et al. of whether low MSAFP was predictive of fetal trisomies (92). Their study showed that low concentrations of second-trimester MSAFP were not only associated with T18, they were also predictive of trisomy 21, or Down syndrome. This was the first observation that a biochemical marker in a pregnant woman's serum was informative of a chromosomal defect in the fetus. In 1984, Cuckle et al. showed that MSAFP concentrations in Down syndrome

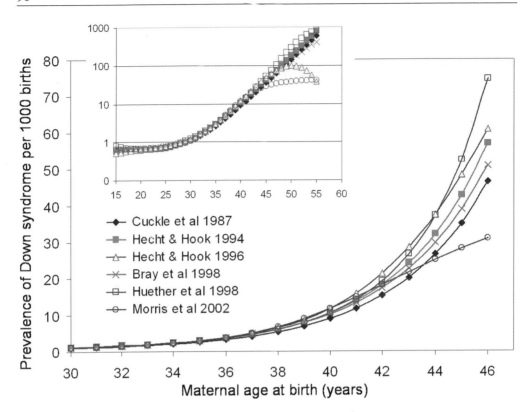

Fig. 7. The association between maternal age at expected date of delivery and the risk of fetal Down syndrome at term. Six studies are shown *(84–89)* that differ only slightly at ages less than 45 yr. Inset represents full dataset up to 55 yr of age.

pregnancies were independent of maternal age, and the two risk factors could be combined *(93)* in women of all ages. MSAFP concentrations are, on average, 25% lower in pregnancies affected with Down syndrome compared to unaffected pregnancies *(94)*.

In 1984, Chard et al. postulated that other fetoplacental biochemical markers might also be informative of the risk of Down syndrome *(95)*. Over the next few years, a number of markers were examined, particularly those biochemical tests that were already associated with pregnancy. For over a decade it had been known that total urinary estriol in the third trimester was substantially lower in Down syndrome pregnancies *(96)*. In 1987, Canick et al. first demonstrated, in a study of 22 Down syndrome cases and 110 matched controls, that the more specific fetoplacental steroid, unconjugated estriol (uE3), was 25–30% lower in second-trimester maternal serum in Down syndrome pregnancies *(97)*. This observation was confirmed the following year in a series of 77 cases of Down syndrome and 385 matched controls *(98)*. The authors postulated that uE3 could be added to maternal age and MSAFP in a prenatal screen for Down syndrome.

Also in 1987, Bogart et al. reported on a series of 25 women with chromosomally abnormal fetuses and 74 unaffected pregnancies between weeks 18 and 25. Concentrations of total human chorionic gonadotrophin (hCG) and its α subunit were significantly higher in the maternal sera from pregnancies with chromosomally abnormal fetuses *(99)*. Combined data from many subsequent studies indicates that hCG concentrations are, on average, twice as high as concentrations in unaffected pregnancies *(94)*. In addition, the free β subunit of hCG in the second trimester is equivalent or better in screening efficiency than hCG itself *(100,101)* and the free β form is used in place of total hCG in some screening programs *(102,103)*.

A number of other biochemical markers were subsequently studied to see whether they could add to, or replace, the "triple markers" of AFP, uE3, and hCG. In 1992, using a relatively nonspecific assay, van Lith first demonstrated that elevated concentrations of "immunoreactive inhibin" were present in maternal serum of Down syndrome pregnancies *(104)*. This observation was subsequently confirmed, and the reported separation between Down syndrome and unaffected pregnancy concentrations continued to improve, driven by improvements in the specificity of assays for this dimeric compound. In the second trimester, the maternal serum concentration of the dimeric inhibin A (DIA) form is approx 2.2 times higher in Down syndrome pregnancies compared to unaffected pregnancies *(103)*.

Second-trimester serum markers that have been reported to be either not sufficiently informative of Down syndrome or not sufficiently easy to measure to displace or add to the triple screen include pregnancy-specific glycoprotein (SP1) *(105)*, placental isoferritin p43 component *(106)*, placental lactogen *(107)*, progesterone *(108)*, the proform of eosinophil major basic protein *(109)*, subtypes of MSAFP bound to lectins *(110)*, dehydroepiandrosterone sulfate (DHEAS) and 16α-hydroxy-DHEAS (16α-OH-DHEAS) *(108)*, urea-resistant neutrophil alkaline phosphatase *(111)*, and different forms of hCG including its degradation products *(112)*.

Combining Multiple Markers Into a Risk-Based Screen

As a marker for risk of Down syndrome, MSAFP by itself measured solely for the purpose of estimating the risk of Down syndrome would not be powerful enough to be justified. However, because MSAFP is widely used for ONTD screening, use of its modest additional information about the risk of Down syndrome is easily justified. Screening for Down syndrome also benefited from screening for ONTD in that the concept of the MoM had already been developed for ONTD screening (see "Using the MoM to Adjust for Gestational Age" above). Like MSAFP, the concentrations of all the markers for fetal trisomy screening are expressed as MoMs. Being a ratio (the patient's concentration divided by the median concentration at that gestational age), the MoM has no units. The MoM compensates for the concentration changes that occur with gestational age and enables combinations of multiple markers on a common scale.

Initially, MSAFP was used in Down syndrome screening in a binary fashion: any value below a fixed cutoff (0.50 MoM) indicated increased risk. However, the fact that the MSAFP distribution in Down syndrome pregnancies was log Gaussian *(55)* soon led to the use of Down syndrome LRs for a range of MSAFP concentrations (Fig. 8), in a manner similar to that used in ONTD screening. With the risk associated with a woman's age as the background prevalence of Down syndrome, patient-specific risks could be generated from the combination of the patient's maternal age and her midtrimester MSAFP result *(113,114)*.

In 1988, the maternal serum concentrations of uE3 and hCG were, like AFP, shown to be independent of maternal age, only weakly correlated to one another, and conforming to Gaussian distributions *(115)* (see Fig. 8). Using the published means and SDs for the unaffected and Down syndrome populations, these three biochemical risk variables were

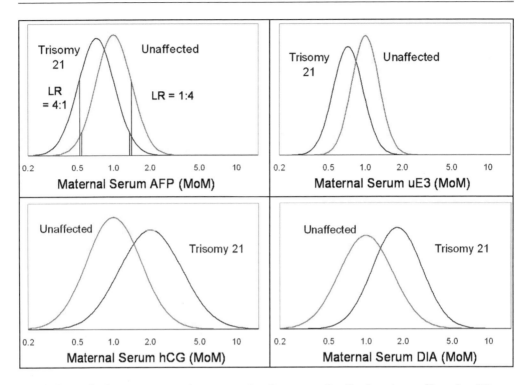

Fig. 8. Second-trimester maternal serum marker frequency distributions in unaffected and Down syndrome pregnancies for AFP, uE3, total hCG, and DIA. For any marker concentration within the limits of the distributions, an LR can be calculated. Two such examples are shown in the figure for MSAFP, with an increased risk (4:1) and a decreased risk (1:4) compared to background.

combined in a trivariate Gaussian LR algorithm: "triple-marker screening" *(116)*. (In 1992, the distributions of the uE3 marker were refined *(55)*, replacing the previous linear MoM values with their log equivalents, which better fit the Gaussian distribution.) In the triple marker screening algorithm, the three LRs are multiplied together, with allowance for the published slight correlations that exist between the various marker pairs. The composite multiple-marker likelihood ratio is then multiplied by the maternal age-related *a priori* risk to yield a patient-specific risk of Down syndrome pregnancy.

In the manner just described, each patient in a screened population will have a calculated risk of the targeted disorder Down syndrome. The population distribution of these risks can be modeled from the underlying marker distributions. Overlapping risk distributions exist for the unaffected and Down syndrome populations, with the Down syndrome population risks being very much higher. The degree of separation of the two populations is sufficient to support screening based on the triple marker Down syndrome risk as the screening variable (see Fig. 9). Modeling the risk distributions has enabled rational decisions for selecting a risk cutoff in Down syndrome screening programs.

When triple marker screening first started, the cutoff from maternal age screening was retained; namely, the term risk of 1:385 (1:290 at midtrimester) was selected because this is the Down syndrome risk at age 35. This choice avoided legal challenges because offering amniocentesis to patients over the age of 35 was deeply embedded in medical

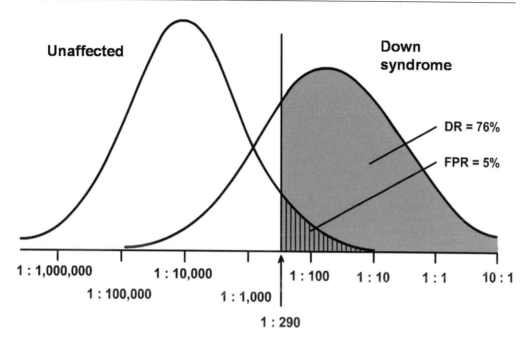

Risk of Down syndrome pregnancy at term

Fig. 9. Down syndrome screening using the combined risk of Down syndrome as the screening variable. The computed risk is based on maternal age and the results of four maternal serum biochemistry tests: AFP, uE3, total hCG, and DIA.

practice and in the minds of the public. Fortuitously, this cutoff achieved the desired increase in Down syndrome detection without increasing the FPR. The new information about Down syndrome risk obtained from the biochemical markers was used to improve detection.

With detection rates at an acceptable level (>70%), attention turned to reducing the FPR from the current 7–10%. DIA was becoming analytically feasible in the late 1990s. The log MoM concentration of DIA conforms to a Gaussian distribution in both the unaffected and Down syndrome populations (Fig. 8), and DIA is essentially independent of AFP and uE3, and only moderately correlated with the concentration of hCG. DIA could therefore be added to the triple marker algorithm by simple mathematical extension of the modeling (Fig. 9) to include the fourth marker *(117–119)*, thereby enabling a four-marker prenatal maternal serum screen for Down syndrome based on AFP, uE3, hCG, and DIA.

Biology of Second-Trimester Serum Biochemical Markers for Down Syndrome

The pathophysiological basis of Down syndrome is unknown, although the sequence of chromosome 21 has now been completed *(120)*. Similarly, the reasons for altered second-trimester maternal serum analytes in Down syndrome pregnancy remain largely unexplained. A current hypothesis for the second trimester is that the serum analyte pattern is related to poorly functioning fetal tissue with compensatory placental hyperfunction. The mechanisms leading to this phenomenon of increased placental and decreased fetal products in second-trimester maternal serum of Down syndrome pregnancy are actively being investigated *(121–126)*.

PLACENTAL-DERIVED DOWN SYNDROME MARKERS: hCG AND DIA

Placental secretory products, such as hCG and DIA are generally increased in the second trimester of Down syndrome pregnancy. None of the genes for these placental products resides on chromosome 21, thereby eliminating a simple higher-dose effect to explain their increased concentrations. Placental size and weight are comparable in Down syndrome and unaffected pregnancies *(127,128)*, although there may be an increase in placental protein synthesis in Down syndrome, as suggested by hCG, inhibin mRNA, and protein extract studies *(121–123)*. Deficient syncytiotrophoblast formation may also have a role in abnormal placental secretion in Down syndrome pregnancies *(124)*.

hCG. The glycoprotein hCG is composed of α and β subunits that also exist in serum in monomeric (free) forms at low concentrations. Biological specificity is imparted by the β subunit, but the β subunit is biologically active only when bound to the α subunit. Analytical specificity for the β subunit can be independent of the presence of the α subunit; hCG can be measured as either the intact hormone, the free β-hCG subunit, or the sum of these. "Total hCG" (bound plus free β-hCG subunits) and "intact β-hCG" (bound β-hCG subunits) are probably equally informative of Down syndrome risk, whereas the free β-hCG concentration appears to be slightly more informative than total or intact hCG *(129)*; however, this form of the molecule is less stable in whole blood specimens, and serum must be separated within 5 h of collection *(130,131)*.

Median concentrations of hCG decrease during the early midtrimester from their peak concentration at 10–12 wk (Fig. 10). hCG decreases in a nonlinear fashion (steeply from 15 to 17 wk and then very gradually from 17 to 22 wk). Free β-hCG concentrations also decrease during the midtrimester.

DIA. The existence of inhibin was predicted (and its name was chosen) on the basis of observations in 1932 of the inhibitory effect of testicular vein serum extracts on anterior pituitary secretion of follicle-stimulating hormone *(132)*. In 1975, an ovarian form of inhibin was also demonstrated, but inhibin and its related opposing hormone activin were not characterized until the mid-1980s *(133)*. Inhibin is a glycoprotein hormone composed of one α and one β subunit. The β subunit exists in two closely related forms (βA and βB), leading to the reference to DIA and dimeric inhibin B. In 1992, Van Lith first demonstrated that in Down syndrome pregnancies the total inhibin concentrations in second-trimester maternal serum were almost twice those of unaffected pregnancies *(104)*. In 1993, Groome *(134,135)* developed more specific antibodies for DIA, using monoclonal antibodies directed against amino acid sequences in the α, βA, and βB forms. These antibodies are the basis of the assays in current use. In 1996, several authors *(117–119)* demonstrated the improved Down syndrome screening potential of this assay, despite a slight correlation between DIA and hCG concentrations. In 2000, an improved assay format for DIA was developed using the Groome antibodies and this product has been validated in two subsequent case-control studies *(136,137)*. The relative frequency distributions of DIA in the unaffected and Down syndrome populations with the current assay format are shown in Fig. 11.

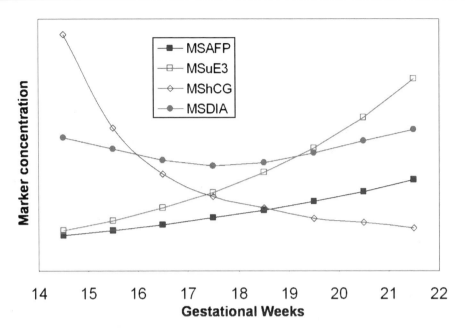

Fig. 10. Relative changes in the median AFP, uE3, total hCG, and DIA concentrations in maternal serum at each week during the early second trimester of pregnancy.

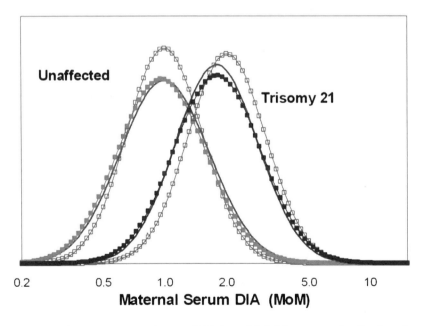

Fig. 11. Agreement between maternal serum DIA $\log_{10}$ MoM frequency distributions from three case-control studies of Down syndrome and matched unaffected controls using the antibodies developed by Groome *(134,135)* in assay systems formatted by Serotec (solid line; ref. *117*) and by DSL (open and closed squares, refs. *136,137*).

During the midtrimester, DIA concentrations are relatively stable in comparison to the other markers at this time (Fig. 10). Median DIA concentrations exhibit a shallow U-shaped curve with its nadir at 17 wk of gestation.

FETAL AND FETOPLACENTAL-DERIVED DOWN SYNDROME MARKERS: AFP AND uE3

In contrast to the placental-sourced markers, secretory products synthesized in the fetus or requiring the combined fetoplacental unit, are low in second-trimester maternal serum from Down syndrome pregnancies. As an example, AFP derived from the fetal liver is reduced, as are the maternal serum and amniotic fluid concentrations of the fetoplacental steroid uE3 *(98,138)* and its fetal androgen precursor molecules, DHEAS *(138)* and 16α-OH-DHEAS *(139)*.

AFP. The cause of the lower maternal serum concentrations of AFP in the presence of a Down syndrome pregnancy remains obscure, with inconclusive results on AFP production in the fetal liver *(125,140)* and a proposed reduction in secretion by the placenta into maternal circulation *(125)*. The concentration of AFP in amniotic fluid is also lower in Down syndrome pregnancies *(141,142)*.

During the midtrimester, AFP concentrations in maternal serum rise at a rate of approximately 15% per wk (Fig. 4). At the same time, the AFAFP concentrations decrease by about 15% per wk, reflecting the pattern of AFP concentrations seen in fetal plasma.

uE3. Maternal serum uE3 is produced by the placenta from precursors synthesized in the fetus; the fetal adrenal secretes large amounts of DHEAS, which is converted to 16-OH-DHEAS by the fetal liver and to uE3 in the placenta. In Down syndrome, the concentrations of uE3 and its DHEAS precursor are lower in the fetal liver, the placenta, and maternal serum *(126)*, suggesting a diminished supply mechanism.

Maternal serum uE3 (MSuE3) concentrations rise rapidly (25% per wk) during the late first trimester and early second trimester of pregnancy (Fig. 10). A simple logarithmic increase model can be used to forecast midtrimester concentrations, although this model slightly overestimates concentrations beyond week 18. A modified exponential method has been proposed as a superior fit to the naturally observed pattern *(143)*.

Confounding Variables of Second-Trimester Markers and Risk

Similar to prenatal screening for ONTD, there are a number of factors that modify the risk of Down syndrome from that derived from the maternal age and optimally measured marker concentrations.

GESTATIONAL AGE

MSuE3 concentrations increase by approx 25% per wk through the early second trimester (Fig. 10), although this rate of rise diminishes slightly beyond week 18 *(143)*. In contrast, maternal serum (MShCG) concentrations decrease from their 10–12 wk maximum, most rapidly during weeks 15–17, reaching relatively stable concentrations by weeks 19–20. DIA concentrations are relatively constant throughout the early second trimester, with a slight nadir at week 16 *(144)*. Regressed median concentrations can be obtained for each week of gestation for each marker in a manner similar to MSAFP, such that all four markers are expressed in MoM units. The optimum gestational age for measuring MSAFP, uE3, hCG, and DIA in terms of the degree of separation between Down syndrome and unaffected pregnancies is between 15 and 22 wk *(145)*. At earlier gestations, the overall performance of this marker combination declines, whereas later gestations leave little time for follow-up diagnostic testing.

METHOD OF ESTIMATION OF GESTATIONAL AGE

Since gestational age is a variable affecting all four biochemical markers, the accuracy of the assignment of gestational age will affect the performance of the biochemical screen, just as it did for MSAFP in ONTD screening *(55,146)*. An error in the estimation of gestational age is the most common reason for a false positive result. If the true gestational age is earlier than reported, MSAFP and uE3 MoM values will be falsely lowered and hCG will be falsely increased, a pattern replicating that seen in Down syndrome pregnancy. In summary: an overestimate of gestational age will overestimate the Down syndrome risk.

The use of ultrasound to estimate gestational age (most commonly the CRL before week 12 and the BPD of the fetal skull thereafter) reduces the population variance of each marker and increases the separation between the Down syndrome and unaffected populations. Therefore, the calculated risk of Down syndrome will change if a gestational age based on LMP is switched to the identical age based on ultrasound, because the tighter distribution curves with ultrasound will change the LRs.

Ultrasound estimation of gestational age increases the detection rate in Down syndrome screening by at least 3% at a fixed 5% FPR, or it can decrease the FPR considerably (e.g., from 3.4% to 2.8%) at a fixed 70% detection rate *(117–119)*. The improved screening performance with use of ultrasound biometry is not caused by any bias in gestational age imparted from the ultrasound, unlike that seen with BPD measurements in ONTD screening *(34)*. At a given gestational age, the median CRL and BPD measurements in Down syndrome and unaffected pregnancies are identical *(30)*.

Although ultrasound biometry is, on average, more accurate than LMP dating, once a screening report has been issued using an LMP date as the basis of the gestational age, it should not be amended unless there is a significant change in the estimated gestational age based on new biometry. Commonly used thresholds are differences greater than 7 or 9 d, which are based on the variance in biometry measurements at 12 wk and 16 wk, respectively *(31)*.

MATERNAL WEIGHT

As with MSAFP, the concentrations of the uE3, hCG, and DIA are all affected by the circulating maternal volume, as indicated by the maternal weight. The maternal weight effect on MSAFP is greater than on hCG and DIA, with uE3 being the least affected. Correcting for the maternal weight reduces the population variance of the marker concentrations and improves Down syndrome screening performance slightly *(55,117,147)*.

RACIAL ORIGIN

After allowing for inherent population differences in maternal weight, the black (African American) population has 10–19% higher concentrations of total hCG and 12% higher free β-hCG concentrations than the white population *(38,147)*. The uE3 concentrations in these two ethnic groups are the same. Separate medians or a median correction factor for hCG in the black population would be appropriate. Fewer data are published on uE3 and hCG concentrations in the Asian population (e.g., Japanese, Chinese, Filipina) *(148,149)*; however, previously unpublished data from 35,000 self-identified Asian pregnancies in Ontario indicate that both uE3 and hCG are higher (14% and 10%) compared to whites. AFP was not different in this dataset. These effects are independent of gestational age, and appropriate methods for adjustment for the Asian population for uE3 and hCG include either racial correction factors for uE3 and hCG, or separate medians. In one study, DIA concentrations were not significantly affected by racial origin *(38)*.

DIABETIC STATUS

Whereas MSAFP concentrations are 20% lower in patients with diabetes mellitus, uE3 and hCG concentrations are only 7–8% lower *(147,150)* and frequently no adjustment is made. Midtrimester DIA concentrations in diabetes have been reported as both greater than *(151)* and less than *(152)* those in nondiabetic pregnancies. There is no consistent evidence that the rate of Down syndrome births in women with insulin-dependent diabetes mellitus is different from that in nondiabetic women.

MULTIPLE GESTATIONS

As expected, maternal serum marker values in multiple gestation pregnancies are approximately proportional to the number of developing fetuses. MSuE3 is slightly less affected by multiple gestations than AFP or hCG, possibly because of its partial reliance on maternal metabolism. In twin pregnancies, concentrations of AFP, uE3, hCG, and DIA are 2.12, 1.68, 2.01, and 1.99 times those seen in singleton pregnancies *(47,147,153)*.

Because one-third of twin pregnancies are monozygotic, genetic models would predict that there would be a 67% increase in the rate of Down syndrome births among twin pregnancies; however, epidemiological studies have reported a much smaller effect, an increase closer to 20% *(154)*. It might be that the coincidence of twin pregnancies and Down syndrome, both associated with an increased rate of fetal loss, causes the lower than expected live birth rate of Down syndrome in twin gestations.

Calculation of a risk of Down syndrome is problematic in twin pregnancies because of the uncertainty about the birth prevalence and the expected greater overlap in the marker distributions for unaffected and Down syndrome pregnancies. Nevertheless, a "pseudorisk" approach has been described for triple *(47)* and double *(155)* marker screening that adjusts for the known higher MoM values in twin pregnancies. This process is likely to rank pregnancies correctly on the basis of their risk, but an absolute risk value should not be quoted in patient reports.

REPEAT TESTING

The phenomenon of regression toward the mean applies to any population-measurement, predicting that an extreme value is likely to regress over time toward the center of its true population. Whereas repeat testing on a subsequent specimen is beneficial in MSAFP screening for ONTD, it is not beneficial in Down syndrome screening, for two reasons. First, patients who are near the Down syndrome screening risk cutoff are likely to have one or more serum markers that are below both the affected and unaffected population means (as opposed to ONTD screening where the cutoff is between the population means). Second, the time constraints for follow-up karyotyping procedures are such that a delay in final screening assessment is clinically less feasible. Therefore, repeat sampling should only be considered when substantial errors in clinical information were present in the original interpretation, such as if the gestational age is revised by more than 10 d to the point where the first sample becomes too early for an interpretable report. In that situation, only the second sample should be considered valid.

MATERNAL SMOKING STATUS

Smoking, maternal age, and risk of Down syndrome are interrelated. There is a greater tendency for younger women to report smoking during a pregnancy compared to older women, whereas older women are at greater risk of Down syndrome. After eliminating maternal age as a confounding variable, smoking has no significant effect on the birth prevalence of Down syndrome *(156)*.

However, smoking does affect individual Down syndrome marker concentrations and could affect screening performance. Patients who report cigarette smoking have 5% higher AFP, 4% lower uE3, 20% lower free β-hCG, and 62% higher DIA concentrations than nonsmokers *(156)*. Total hCG concentrations are also 23% lower in smokers *(108,157,158)*. Although statistically significant, the effects of smoking on AFP and uE3 are small in terms of the calculated risk of Down syndrome. However, failure to adjust the hCG and DIA medians will have significant effects on the calculated risk of Down syndrome. In triple marker screening, risks will be underestimated in smokers. In four-marker screening, the increase in DIA concentration in smokers will surpass the effect of the lower hCG values, and the risk will be overestimated.

From a public health perspective, the overall detection and FPRs are paramount. The issue of smoking becomes a question of the net number of patients who are wrongly placed on one side, or the other, of the screening cutoff. From this perspective, adjustments for smoking have very little effect on screening performance: less than 1% change in the detection rate at a fixed 5% FPR *(156)* depending on the prevalence of smoking. However, if information on smoking can be obtained with little expense, the accuracy of risk information will improve for individual screened patients.

MATERNAL AGE

The maternal age distribution in the screened population will have an effect on the performance of the screening program *(159)*. Those programs that screen a high proportion of older-aged patients will experience a higher detection rate and higher FPR than is usually quoted in the literature. By convention, literature reports of screening algorithms quote detection rates at fixed, comparable, FPRs—most commonly, 5%. Maternal age distributions that yield 5% FPR are currently relatively rare owing to the fact that women are delaying their pregnancies. Therefore, higher FPRs and detection rates are observed; however, the detection rate in the highest 5% of calculated risks should be close to published performance.

Similarly, FPRs and detection rates quoted in publications are for the overall population and reflect performance in women close to the median age of that population (usually 27–30 yr). Older women will have higher FPRs and detection rates, and younger women will experience the opposite. This can be important in individual patient counseling.

PREVIOUS DOWN SYNDROME PREGNANCY

Family history or more correctly stated, prior history of a Down syndrome pregnancy in a patient will have an effect on computed risk. Geneticists generally quote a recurrence risk of aneuploidy of at least 1% if a woman has had a prior Down syndrome pregnancy (nontranslocation type). However, the best estimate of increased risk because of prior history is an excess term risk of 0.34% *(74)*. Therefore, the risk of Down syndrome pregnancy in a woman with a history of Down syndrome in an offspring should be calculated by adding this excess risk to the *a priori* age-specific term risk (e.g., at age 33, the risk of recurrence would be 0.0034 + 0.0016). The risk of recurrence of inherited (i.e., translocation) Down syndrome is usually much higher but depends on the variety of translocation.

OTHER FACTORS WITH LESSER EFFECTS

Factors such as parity *(160)*, fetal gender *(161)*, maternal blood group *(162)*, marker concentrations in a previous pregnancy *(163)*, in vitro fertilization *(164)*, and intrauterine fertilization *(165)* all have lesser or inconsistent effects on certain markers and can be included at the discretion of screening programs.

Full Ascertainment of Pregnancy Outcomes in Screening

Down syndrome detection should be assessed in accordance with the full outcome ascertainment protocol outlined by Palomaki *(166)*. In addition to the Down syndrome outcomes in screen-positive patients (true positives [TP]) and liveborn Down syndrome outcomes in screen-negative patients (false negatives [FN_{LB}]), there must be an allowance made for the screen-negative affected pregnancies that were spontaneously lost before term (FN_{SL}). Otherwise, a substantially overestimated detection rate will be reported *(167)*. The proper detection rate calculation is

$$\text{Detection Rate DR} = TP/(TP + FN_{LB} + FN_{SL}), \text{ or } TP/(TP + FN_{LB}/0.77)$$

where 0.77 is the factor to correct the number of liveborn cases for the expected 23% rate of spontaneous fetal loss *(166)*.

In addition, the expected total number of Down syndrome cases should be calculated from the known maternal age distribution of the study population *(84–87)*, and this should be compared to the number actually ascertained. The calculated fetal loss rates should be similar to literature reports *(84,90,91)*.

Validation of Reported Patient Risks

The risk of fetal Down syndrome calculated and reported to a patient cannot be validated in any individual patient—a patient either has, or does not have, a Down syndrome pregnancy. However, it is possible to group patients with similar estimated risks into clusters and to compare the mean reported risk against the actual prevalence of Down syndrome in the cluster (see Fig. 12). Such an analysis requires close to complete pregnancy outcome ascertainment and a large screened population. At least three such validation studies have been reported for triple marker screening *(168–170)* and one report for first trimester (see below) screening with nuchal translucency (NT), pregnancy-associated plasma protein A (PAPP-A), and free β-hCG *(171)*.

SECOND-TRIMESTER DOWN SYNDROME SCREENING PERFORMANCE

In the 1970s, when Down syndrome screening based on maternal age commenced, the fraction of the pregnant population over the age of 35 (the FPR) was 5%, which is low compared to the present circumstance; however, the detection rate was also low at 25–30%. Coincident with the advent of biochemical screening, the maternal age in the pregnant population was increasing. Despite this, the original focus of the biochemical markers was on increasing detection. Table 5 compares the performance of Down syndrome screening using maternal age and the various combinations of biochemical markers in use from before 1985 to the present triple- and four-marker services. As more

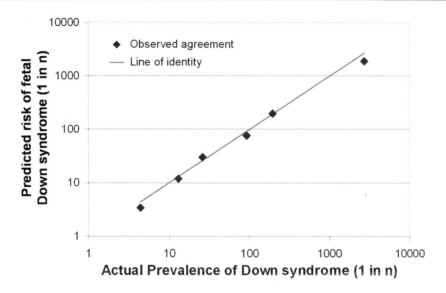

Fig. 12. Agreement between the observed prevalence of fetal Down syndrome and the calculated risk of Down syndrome based on maternal age and maternal serum concentrations of AFP, uE3, and total hCG (see ref. *169*).

Table 5
Down Syndrome Screen Performance at a Risk Cutoff Equivalent
to the Risk at Age 35,Using Past and Present Screening Algorithms[a]

	Maternal age at EDD[b] (>35.5)	Age plus MSAFP	Age, AFP, hCG	Age, AFP, uE3, hCG	Age, AFP, uE3, hCG, DIA[c]
Detection rate:	38%	45%	66%	75%	80%
Screen positive rate:	12%	10%	10%	8%	4%
OAPR:[d]	1:200	1:140	1:100	1:70	1:30

[a]Data are from a study of more than 100,000 women screened between 1993 and 1995, with 94% outcome ascertainment, and 135 Down syndrome cases *(170,173)*.
[b]EDD, expected date of delivery.
[c]Four-marker second-trimester screen performance projected from a composite of several reports.
[d]Positive predictive value expressed as OAPR.

markers were introduced, the detection rate at a given FPR increased. Additionally, since the use of biochemical markers made screening accessible to women under the age of 35, more women were screened and the overall prevalence of Down syndrome among live births has been reduced by as much as 46% *(172)*.

With the triple-screen detection rate at 75%, only one of four cases remains undetected. The opportunity for a new marker such as DIA to detect more is limited—a diminishing returns effect. However, markers add information about both the presence and absence of a high risk—more unaffected patients correctly screen negative *(173)*. With the addition of DIA, a higher risk cutoff can be selected to reduce the false positive rate considerably, while maintaining or slightly increasing the detection rate *(119)*.

The addition of the DIA marker requires no change in the timing of the second-trimester specimen collection, no change in the use of ultrasound to assign gestational age, and a simple update to most commercial software packages. Health care providers are generally quick to endorse the advent of a Down syndrome screen that holds the promise of a lower FPR *(174)*, particularly when the screen poses no change in the logistics of their practice.

Psychological Impact of Prenatal Screening

Patients view a prenatal screen as a test that will provide a result; they rarely appreciate that the result will be expressed as a risk. Screening programs calculate and report the patient's specific risk, and they categorize the patient as either "screen negative" or "screen positive" for the target disorder. The risk cutoff is always established by the service provider from a public health perspective, rather than from a patient perspective. However, risk is a subjective concept. Whereas a triple-marker screening program might describe a risk of 1:250 at midtrimester (1:325 at term) as "increased risk," a 40-yr-old patient might welcome such a "low risk." Similarly, young patients can be concerned by a screen-negative report at a risk of 1:500 (1:650 at term). Screening programs use the terms screen "negative" and "positive" to give overall guidance and structure to the use of follow-up services, but these terms should not carry too much weight in the communication of patient-specific risks.

Screening programs also use different methods to communicate their low-risk (screen-negative) and high-risk (screen-positive) reports. In some practices, screen negative results are never formally communicated to patients; however, in the majority of practices the communication is in the form of a verbal phrase *(175)*, with or without an accompanying risk number. A "low risk" is not always perceived by the patient as being low enough to forego a definitive test result, particularly if the patient previously considered herself to be at high risk because of her age (in effect, a sequential self-screen). In contrast to the sometimes informal communication of low risk, screen-positive results are usually communicated through genetic counseling during which an accurate conveyance of risk is attempted in a nondirective manner.

Patients gain a better understanding of their risk when a numerical probability is provided (e.g., 1:200) compared to when only a verbal probability ("moderate risk") is provided *(176)*. In addition, verbal probability statements are more likely to invoke a "framing effect" that biases decisions (e.g., a discussion of the "risk of the disorder" vs the "chance of an unaffected child"). Framing might occur in the phrasing used to describe the risk of an amniocentesis procedure compared to the description of a patient's risk of Down syndrome. Numerical probability statements are less susceptible to a framing effect *(177)*.

Laboratories should be aware that the risk they calculate and report is an important element of a patient's understanding, her perception of her pregnancy, and her decision making.

The Impetus to Lower the FPR

Screen-positive results cause anxiety *(178–181)* for both the patient and provider *(3,174)*. In a survey assessing provider and patient response to maternal serum screening, half of the physicians responding cited the high screen-positive rate as the aspect they most wanted to change *(174)*. The same majority of physicians also wanted the detection rate to increase. In screening, the screen-positive rate and the detection rate are interrelated for a given set of markers—a decrease in the screen positive rate will also decrease detection. However, adding new screening markers gives the opportunity to improve the screen positive to detection ratio.

From a public health perspective, the cost of follow-up services must be in balance or in proportion to the cost of care related to the disorder. In screening for fetal Down syndrome, the usual panel of follow-up services includes genetic counseling, an ultrasound examination perhaps in the context of an amniocentesis procedure, karyotyping, and further counseling about the result or further services. Because most screen-positive reports are false-positives (Table 5), there is an economic opportunity to invest in a better "front-end" screening procedure and recover the cost from the reduction in volume of follow-up services (Table 6). The overall benefit is a reduction in patient and provider anxiety, and fewer fetal losses from invasive procedures.

New Developments in Down Syndrome Screening

Any attempt to improve the performance of a screen must have one or more of the following as its goal:

- a decrease in the FPR
- an increase in the detection rate
- a decrease in the cost of care
- a reduction in the risk associated with the service

Although health care providers might place equal emphasis on improving detection and reducing the FPR, the improvement that will be noticed first is a reduction in the FPR. Consider that in a busy obstetrical practice of 300 patients per year, one case of Down syndrome will occur on average every 2 yr. An improvement in detection from 70 to 90% would not be perceived for at least a decade. In contrast, a reduction in the FPR from 8 (triple-marker screening) to 4% (adding inhibin) would be noticeable within 1 mo.

With rare exception, there is now no need for a prenatal screening program for fetal Down syndrome to have an FPR greater than 5%. The easiest way to lower the FPR is to measure additional biochemical markers in the existing second-trimester specimen. Second-trimester biochemistry screening programs that rely on two or three markers can justify the cost of adding markers (e.g., uE3 or DIA) to upgrade their service to a four-marker screen *(119,173)*.

Urine Markers for Down Syndrome

Screening for fetal Down syndrome by measuring one or more markers in maternal urine would be less invasive than serum screening. Urine would require the additional step of correction for the varying dilution of the specimens, using creatinine or another dilution marker. The potential urine markers that have been examined include total and free β-hCG, and a degredation product of hCG sometimes called the "β-core fragment." None of these has proved sufficient to displace serum marker screening *(103,112,182)*.

More recently, a variant of hCG, called hyperglycosylated hCG (H-hCG) or invasive trophoblast antigen (ITA), has been proposed as a screening marker superior to hCG itself. H-hCG has more abundant and more branched oligosaccharide side chains than hCG and can be measured using a highly specific monoclonal antibody. Cole et al. have published a series of studies showing that H-hCG measured in second-trimester urine in

Table 6
An Example of the Cost Recovery Potential in Expanded Serum Screening
Algorithms in a Theoretical Population of 10,000 Screened Patients

Screening algorithm[a]	Three[b] marker	Four marker	Five marker
False-positive rate[c] for 75% detection	7.5%	4.0%	2.0%
Number of screen positive patients	750	400	200
Amniocenteses (85% uptake in screen positives)	640	340	170
Reduction in amniocentesis rate compared to triple marker		47%	73%
Amniocentesis procedures avoided		300	470
Reduction in amniocentesis costs		$300,000	$470,000
Additional cost of new serum marker(s)		$250,000	$450,000
Overall screening program cost reduction		$50,000	$20,000
Procedure-related fetal losses avoided		1.5	2.4

[a]Costs used for this projection: Inhibin A, $25; PAPP-A, $20; amniocentesis and related follow-up procedures, $1000 (relative to a triple-marker testing service funded $50 per patient with a total budget of $1.14 millon for screening and follow-up services).
[b]Three marker: AFP, uE3, total hCG; four marker, add DIA; five marker, add PAPP-A.
[c]False-positive rates are a composite of recent publications and will vary with the maternal age frequency distribution but will be proportional to those shown.

Down syndrome pregnancies is markedly elevated (medians ranging from 5 to 9 MoM). Down syndrome detection rates between 75 and 90% were projected at a 5% FPR, far higher detection than any single marker ever described (183–185). Very recently, these authors reported that H-hCG was also markedly elevated in maternal serum, in two case-control series (186). However, two other studies of urinary H-hCG, both of which used stored frozen urine samples, have shown either no improvement (187) or insufficient improvement to warrant the addition of a urine specimen to a serum-based screen (103). Prospective noninterventional studies using fresh serum and urine specimens should provide more definitive information about the potential of H-hCG as a screening marker.

Fetal Cells and DNA in Maternal Serum

Fetal nucleated red cells in the maternal circulation can be identified and concentrated, and such cells have been proposed as a noninvasive source for prenatal diagnosis of chromosome abnormalities and other genetic disorders (188–190). Although the technology has not yet permitted prenatal diagnosis, and may never, a separate finding of a larger number of fetal cells present in the maternal circulation in trisomy 21 and other chromosome abnormalities has raised the possibility of using the concentration of fetal cells as a screening marker (191). However, it is unlikely that such a test would be cost efficient and easy enough to be performed on a large scale basis.

More recently, cell-free fetal DNA has been found in the maternal circulation and, like fetal cells in maternal blood, the concentration of fetal DNA in maternal plasma and serum is higher in Down syndrome pregnancies. Although fetal DNA has been discussed as having potential for noninvasive diagnostics (192,193), similar to what has been noted for fetal cells, a future screening test based on fetal DNA is more likely (194,195). Furthermore, fetal DNA might not be informative about T18 pregnancy (196).

At present, a major impediment to the clinical use of fetal DNA is the inability to measure it when the source is a female fetus. The base sequences currently used to differentiate fetal from maternal DNA are specific to the Y chromosome and found only when the fetus is male. If and when this technical problem is solved, the performance characteristics and methodologic feasibility of measuring this marker should be studied further.

First-Trimester Markers—Biochemistry and Biometry

The focus on the second trimester as the timing for Down syndrome biochemical markers arose from the connection with NTD screening and the fact that the safest diagnostic procedures rely on second-trimester amniocentesis. However, there are perceived advantages and patient preferences for having information about the health of the developing baby earlier in the pregnancy. In addition to the simple preference for an earlier answer, there is increased patient privacy when screening is performed before the pregnancy is announced, and there are safer termination procedures should they be needed. There is also the potential of adding new markers that are informative only in the first trimester *(197)*.

BIOCHEMICAL MARKERS—PAPP-A AND FREE b-hCG

PAPP-A is a glycoprotein derived from the placenta. Despite its name, PAPP-A is also present in serum and plasma in nonpregnant women and men, and recently it has been described as a marker of plaque instability in acute coronary syndromes *(198)*. During pregnancy, PAPP-A circulates in a covalent complex with the proform of eosinophil major basic protein (proMBP), which is itself a potential marker for risk of Down syndrome *(109)*. In pregnancy, the concentration of PAPP-A rises rapidly during the first trimester (Fig. 13); however, concentrations in Down syndrome pregnancies are less than half those in unaffected pregnancies *(199–202)*. PAPP-A in the first trimester is currently the best biochemical marker known for fetal Down syndrome at any gestational age (Fig. 14). PAPP-A is more discriminatory during early gestation *(203–205)*. Detection with PAPP-A and maternal age (at a fixed 5% FPR) decreases from week 10 to week 14 from more than 50% to less than 30% (Table 7) *(205–207)*.

The second-trimester marker hCG first attains its discriminatory character for Down syndrome at about week 11 and gradually increases its power in later gestations (Table 7). The free-β subunit of hCG *(129)* is generally considered to be a better marker than the intact hCG molecule in the first trimester (Fig. 15), although the reverse has also been reported *(204,208,209)*. The gestational age at the time of sampling is a factor in their relative performance *(103,210)*. Although the optimum first-trimester gestation for free β-hCG and PAPP-A differ (Table 7), for practical reasons they are measured in the same specimen usually drawn between 10 and 13 wk. Several studies have shown that the combination of PAPP-A and hCG in the first trimester, together with maternal age, can detect more than 60% of Down syndrome fetuses at a 5% screen-positive rate *(202,204)*. This screening performance is less effective than the second-trimester triple-marker screen *(94,211)*.

The other second-trimester markers AFP and uE3 are also sufficiently informative in the first trimester to add marginally to a first-trimester biochemistry screen, yielding detection rates at 10 wk that rival triple-marker screening in the second trimester *(205,207)*. Nonetheless, first-trimester screening using biochemical markers alone is not performed, perhaps because the standard for detection has been raised by the addition of

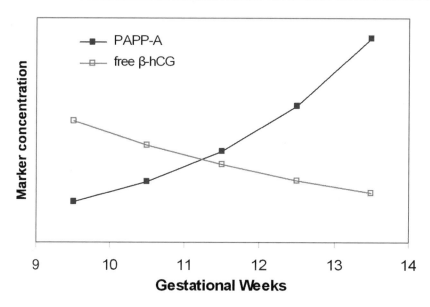

Fig. 13. Relative changes in the median free β-hCG and PAPP-A concentrations in maternal serum during the first trimester of pregnancy.

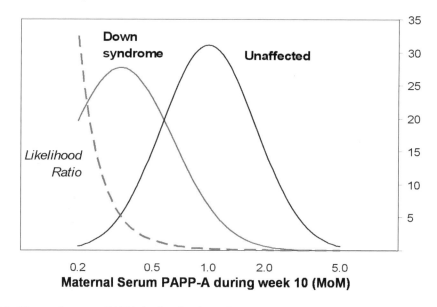

Fig. 14. Maternal serum PAPP-A distributions during the 10th wk of gestation in the Down syndrome and unaffected populations. The LR for the PAPP-A MoM values is shown, with the scale of LR values on the right of the figure.

Table 7
Down Syndrome Marker Performance
at Varying Weeks in the First Trimester[a]

	Detection rate (%) at gestational week:			
Marker	10	11	12	13
Ultrasound NT	51	59	62	62
Serum uE3	13	21	29	37
Serum total hCG	5	15	26	41
Serum free β-hCG	19	28	35	44
Serum DIA	5	16	30	46
Serum PAPP-A	58	45	35	27
Urine ITA	6	16	28	43

[a]Based on the SURUSS *(103)*. Down syndrome detection rates are for a 5% false-positive rate, without the use of maternal age.

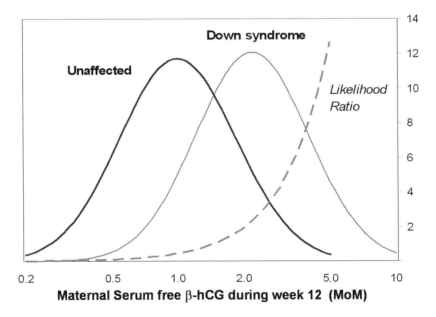

Fig. 15. Maternal serum free β-hCG distributions during the 12th wk of gestation in the Down syndrome and unaffected populations. The LR for the free β-hCG MoM values is shown, with the scale of LR values on the right of the figure.

DIA in the second trimester. PAPP-A, and to a lesser extent free β-hCG, have become important first-trimester markers through their combination with first-trimester ultrasound and/or second-trimester biochemical markers, as described later.

Confounding Variables of PAPP-A and Free β-hCG. As with second-trimester biochemical markers, there is an inverse relationship between maternal weight and observed marker concentrations *(212)*. Black (Afro-Caribbean) patients have been reported to have 57% higher PAPP-A concentrations and 21% higher free β-hCG concentrations compared to white women *(213)*. Asian women had smaller differences. Although corrections for race and weight would have only modest effects on overall screening performance, in individual women such corrections could alter the risk estimate twofold. Smoking appears to reduce PAPP-A by approx 15–20% *(212,214)*; however, in one study of Down syndrome pregnancies, PAPP-A in self-reported smokers was higher than in nonsmokers *(215)*.

The screening performance of all Down syndrome markers is improved when the gestational age of patients is accurate *(30)*. This is particularly true for PAPP-A because its concentration is rising rapidly (50% per wk, see Fig. 13) during the 10 to 13-wk period when testing is performed *(204)*. The concentration of free β-hCG also changes rapidly during this period, decreasing from the hCG peak normally seen between 8 and 10 gestational weeks. In some settings, the potential need for an ultrasound-based gestational age, and its associated cost, could mitigate the cost benefit of the PAPP-A marker, or the marker will be slightly less informative.

BIOMETRY MARKERS—NT AND NASAL BONES

Since 1990, there has been considerable attention paid to specialized ultrasonography in the first trimester as a screening tool for fetal Down syndrome, particularly the measurement of NT *(216)*, and more recently the detection of absent nasal bone *(217)*.

Ultrasound NT. NT is defined as the maximum thickness of the normally occurring subcutaneous space (translucency) between the fetal skin and the soft tissues overlying the cervical spine, when viewed in the sagittal plane *(218,219)*. A typical NT measurement is in the range of 0.5 to 2.0 mm *(220)*, but measurements vary between observers. Increased NT is a nonspecific marker of structural anomalies, in particular cardiac defects *(221-223)*. As with most markers, an increased NT *per se* is not a fetal abnormality *(224)*; NT can be greatly increased in pregnancies with normal outcomes *(225)*. Relative to unaffected fetuses, those with aneuploidies have, on average, increased NT measurements *(216,218,226,227)*. For this reason, NT measurements have been examined for use in Down syndrome screening.

The early reports of an association between fetal aneuploidy and increased NT were from observational studies in selected patient populations at increased risk of a variety of chromosomal defects *(219)*. The aneuploid pregnancies tended to be clustered in the pregnancies with larger NT measurements. Down syndrome was the largest aneuploidy subgroup, reflecting its natural prevalence, but T18, Turner syndrome (45,X0), and trisomy 13 also had increased NT measurements. In the mid-1990s, studies in unselected populations were undertaken to examine NT as a potential general population screening variable. Early studies used fixed NT cutoffs ranging from 2.5 to 3.0 mm, and there was a broad range in the detection and FPRs reported, with an average of 62% detection and a 4% FPR *(219)*. An important finding was the positive correlation between the risk of trisomies and NT size, indicating that LRs and risk of fetal trisomy could be assigned based on the NT measurement *(228–230)*.

Studies with fixed NT cutoffs continued to be published for the rest of the decade, although this method of use of NT as a screening variable was gradually being replaced by a gestational age-adjusted NT measurement. It had been recognized that NT measurements increase in association with fetal growth during the 11- to 13-wk gestational window of measurement *(218,231)*. As with maternal serum markers, the confounding variable of gestational age can be reduced by comparing patient values against the median for the patient's gestational age *(224,231,232)*. The NT measurement has been expressed as either an arithmetic difference from the median for a particular gestational age, the approach taken by Nicolaides et al. *(218)*, or as a ratio of the median in MoM units, the more commonly used method in prenatal risk calculations *(233)*. NT expressed in both manners conforms to a $\log^{10}$ Gaussian distribution (Fig. 16), allowing a calculated risk of Down syndrome based on NT and maternal age *(231)*.

In 1998, Snijders et al. combined the LR from the NT measurement using the offset from the median with the risk associated with maternal age and reported on a large series of patients screened using this combination of NT and maternal age *(234)*. Their study reported that 82% of Down syndrome cases could be detected with an 8% screen-positive rate. However, using the same Snijders data, Haddow recalculated the detection rate to be 60% (at the 8% FPR) if the number of cases was based on the reported maternal age distribution in the study *(167)*—a more reliable method of estimation *(166)*. The effect of this under-ascertainment bias on calculated detection rates can be considerable. In a subsequent review of 15 studies that had no identifiable verification bias, Mol et al. estimated Down syndrome detection to be 63% at a FPR of 5%; whereas, in 10 other studies judged to have a verification bias, the detection was reportedly 77% *(235)*. For a few years, reports with substantially differing performance for NT were published, and the screening community became polarized over this issue *(236)*.

By 1998, it was recognized that even experienced sonographers perform poorly without specialized training *(204)*. In order to lessen the variation in NT measurement techniques and to improve the performance of NT as a screening variable, the Foetal Medicine Foundation in London established a training and quality control program to accredit operators who maintain a record of measurement proficiency. This training program is now being replicated internationally. Despite the increased uniformity that training and certification might impart, discrepant performance persists between studies. An Italian study achieved 77% detection for a 3% FPR *(237)*, whereas a study in Scotland detected only 54% at a 5% FPR *(238)*. Furthermore, the Scottish study found that NT measurements could not be obtained in 27% of women, despite the fact that each of its ultrasonographers received training from the Foetal Medicine Foundation in London. The variation even between trained operators suggests that such performance might represent a practical limitation of the marker.

Confounding Variables of NT. There are clinical and technical factors that affect NT measurements, and reports of these might lead to refinements and adjustments to tighten performance. The use of center-specific medians, and eventually operator-specific medians, is an approach that could reduce variation in the marker *(103,239)*, but the burden of maintaining separate medians each with a small number of observations might make this impractical. The size of the image contributes to the variability between patients, operators, and instruments. One study has reported that larger image magnifications lead to smaller estimates of NT measurements *(240)*. Racial differences have also been reported, with recommendations both for *(241)*, and against *(242)* racial adjust-

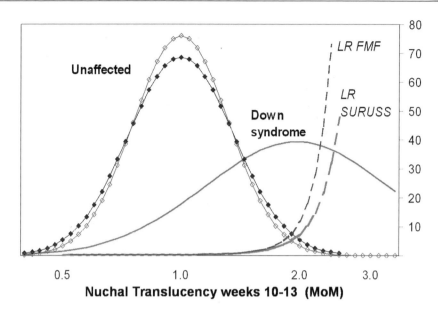

Fig. 16. Frequency distributions of first trimester MoM NT measurements from two studies: the Foetal Medicine Foundation study (open diamond, FMF, ref. *252*) and the SURUSS (closed diamond, ref. *103*). There was good agreement between these studies for the Down syndrome distribution. The LRs from both studies are shown, with the scale of LR values on the right of the figure.

ment. A slight positive correlation in NT measurement in successive pregnancies within individual patients has also been reported *(243)*, and there may also be a small progressive decrease in NT with increasing gravidity and parity that is unlikely to have any effect on screening *(244)*.

Ultrasound Nasal Bone Detection. There have been some quite recent reports that Down syndrome pregnancies have absent nasal bones in the first trimester *(217, 245,246)*. Although not all observers agree *(247)*, the projection is that absent fetal nasal bones could contribute to the detection of Down syndrome, while reducing the screen-positive rate of NT *(217,248)*. The first studies on nasal bones were confined to women who had increased NT measurements, and the authors cautioned that confirmation in a large-scale multicenter trial in the general population is required. They also stressed that ultrasonographers must have "appropriate training and certification in their competence in doing the nasal bone scan" *(217)*. This underscores the specialized training required for ultrasound markers—NT and nasal bones—and the possibility that the general population might have limited access to these markers for the short term at least. A study published in 2001 in the United Kingdom, where ultrasound markers have been most intensively implemented, reported that only 8% of women had access to NT sonography, whereas 71% of women in the United Kingdom used second-trimester serum screening *(249)*.

Potential Biases in First-Trimester Screening

There are two sources of uncertainty and potential bias in the estimated detection rate that are characteristic of all first-trimester screens. Both sources of bias stem from the high rate of spontaneous loss of Down syndrome affected pregnancies (45%) between the first trimester and term *(91)*.

The first source of bias arises because most, if not all, marker-negative Down syndrome pregnancies that are spontaneously lost are not counted (not ascertained) in prospective intervention studies. This was probably true in the NT study of Snijders et al. in 1998 *(234)*. The effect of this ascertainment bias on marker performance can be explained as follows: most unascertained cases have marker values that place them below the screen cutoff, and exclusion of these when calculating the Down syndrome population mean for that marker overestimates the mean and overestimates the detection rate *(103,250,251)*. This source of bias can be approximated, and adjustments can be made *(167,205,250,252)*.

The second source of bias in first-trimester screening is more difficult to estimate and correct; namely, the tendency for the pregnancies with abnormal markers to be preferentially lost. Expressed another way, this is the degree to which a marker preferentially detects those fetuses destined to be lost *(233,253,254)*. A marker that detects only those pregnancies destined to be lost would have no value from a public health perspective.

Combined First-Trimester Biochemical and Ultrasound Screening

The early reports of ultrasound screening in the first trimester were based on NT measurements, with and without maternal age. The debate that arose at the time, and that still persists in some locales, was whether the combination of NT and maternal age was sufficient by itself to support screening. Sometimes the discourse over the power of NT as a marker is confused as dismissing it altogether as a marker, but this is not the intent. NT is a powerful marker for fetal Down syndrome, and the more recent studies have been examining how best to utilize NT and maximize its performance consistency *(255)*.

The first study to combine NT, maternal age, and a biochemistry marker used first-trimester maternal serum PAPP-A *(203)*. There was no significant correlation between the NT and PAPP-A markers, suggesting that this combined ultrasound and biochemistry screen could be useful. A second study used free β-hCG, NT, and maternal age, and reported only modest improvements in detection from the addition of the biochemical marker *(256)*. Multiple urine biochemistry markers in the first trimester were informative on their own and in combination, but failed to add appreciably to overall detection when combined with NT and maternal age *(257)*, although the NT performance had possibly been overestimated.

Wald and Hackshaw took the approach of modeling a combined first-trimester screening algorithm using three separate datasets *(233)*. These authors adjusted the NT dataset of Pandya et al. *(218)* to compensate for a probable ascertainment bias, and then combined it with a similar NT dataset from Schuchter et al. *(231)* in order to construct $\log_{10}$ MoM NT distributions for the Down syndrome and unaffected populations. LRs derived from these overlapping Gaussian NT distributions were then combined with LRs from similar distributions for PAPP-A and free β-hCG *(202)*. It was assumed that the biochemistry and ultrasound markers were not correlated *(203,258)*. This modeled dataset predicted a detection rate of 80% at a 5% FPR using NT, PAPP-A, and free β-hCG *(233)*. This performance was seen as slightly exceeding the four-marker second-trimester serum screen performance estimates at that time—namely, 76% detection.

There were a number of caveats to the Wald and Hackshaw modeled performance of first-trimester screening. First, technical skills in performing the NT measurement would have to be equivalent to those exhibited by Pandya et al. *(218)*. Second, it is important that the ultrasound report be combined with the results of the biochemistry tests rather than acting on an ultrasound report unilaterally; ultrasonographers must be comfortable with this (see "Sequential, or Stepwise, Screening With Ultrasound and Biochemistry" below). Third, the individual performance of these three first-trimester markers is optimal at different times (see Table 7). PAPP-A is most informative at week 10, as is NT at week 12, and hCG improves continually as a marker into the second trimester *(207)*. Nevertheless, in locations where first-trimester screening is offered, it is common for both of the biochemistry markers to be performed on the same serum sample, collected on the same day that the NT measurement is performed. Analysis of the markers and issuing the patient report usually requires 1 or 2 d, although same-day services have been reported *(259)*.

Two trials, one in the United Kingdom and one in the United States, that examine first-trimester combined ultrasound and serum screening have now been reported, and a third trial in the United States will be reported soon. The UK trial is SURUSS, the serum, urine, ultrasound study, supported by the Health Technology Assessment Scheme of the UK National Health Service *(103)*. In that trial, all women who enrolled had a first-trimester blood and urine specimen collected and had an NT measurement attempted. The first-trimester serum markers were not measured and the NT was not used in risk assessment. The same women continued their pregnancies and had a second-trimester serum screen performed, which was acted on in accordance with local practice. The second-trimester serum specimens were frozen, together with coincident urine specimens. After second-trimester ascertainment of all cases in the almost 50,000 women screened, the frozen serum and urine samples from all Down syndrome cases were matched with five control samples each, and all potential and current analytes were measured. Results of this study of almost 100 Down syndrome cases confirmed that combined NT, PAPP-A, and free β-hCG was the best first-trimester screening test, but the second-trimester four-marker screen was unexpectedly almost identical in performance to the first-trimester test. The performance of both tests was 83% detection rate for a 5% FPR. The SURUSS also showed that first- and second-trimester markers combined in an integrated approach to screening was superior to either first- or second-trimester testing (see "The Integrated Test—Combining First- and Second-Trimester Markers" below).

The US study that has been published recently is called the BUN trial *(260)*. In this study, about 8514 women in the first trimester who were candidates for CVS because of age or other risk factors (but not serum screening) were screened using NT, PAPP-A, and free β-hCG. These women did not have second-trimester screening; therefore, comparison with second-trimester tests was not possible. The BUN trial results were similar to, although slightly lower than, those for first-trimester markers in SURUSS. The observed Down syndrome detection rate for a 5% FPR was 79%. A full report of this study will be published later in 2003.

A third trial, called FASTER, will be reported in early 2004. The FASTER Trial (First and Second Trimester Evaluation of Risk of Aneuploidy) is a clinical intervention study in which 36,000 unselected women were offered both first-trimester screening (using NT, PAPP-A, and free β-hCG) and second-trimester four-marker screening. Women who were screen positive by either or both tests were offered diagnostic testing. In this way (and similar to SURUSS), the two screening methods can be compared directly in the same population. In addition, the protocol allows for other combinations of markers to be assessed retrospectively.

All three studies are similar with regard to the need for detailed training in and quality assurance of NT measurement, but only SURUSS and FASTER trial can directly compare earlier and later screening modalities (see "The Integrated Test—Combining First- and Second-Trimester Markers" below).

Sequential, or Stepwise Screening With Ultrasound and Biochemistry

Because ultrasound examinations are performed on patients in "real time," patients have an expectation of immediately receiving some form of report, even if only a brief verbal statement. However, to comment on an ultrasound examination that is only one of several components of a Down syndrome screening algorithm is to issue a partial or stepwise screening report—a practice that diminishes the overall performance of the screen. The need to hold information, even briefly, is not always recognized and accepted by health care providers and patients (224). Favorable ultrasound reports can induce patients to forego subsequent blood tests, whereas removing high-risk patients by screening them positive on the basis of an increased NT measurement will alter the prevalence of the disorder in the patients who go on to have all components of the screen. Calculated second-trimester risks in these latter patients will be over-estimated if the first-trimester results for individual markers are not taken into account (261). Sequential screening using NT has also been challenged on scientific grounds, in that extremely few patients (< 0.1%) would have a sufficiently abnormal NT measurement to cause them to remain screen positive with subsequent "favorable" biochemistry marker concentrations (262). Sequential screening is usually not recognized, particularly where (as is common) the ultrasound and biochemical testing services are performed by different units or at different times (251). It can be safely asserted that all biochemistry laboratories receive specimens, in the first or second trimester, from patient populations that are to some extent biased by previous ultrasound examinations.

Contingency screening is a variant of sequential screening whereby each screening modality is performed separately, with the first stage(s) assigned a low risk cutoff (maximizing detection and greatly increasing the FPR but identifying a fraction of the population as screen negative). Patients who are screen negative at this first stage are at such a low risk that proceeding to the next screening modality is deemed unnecessary. The premise of contingency screening is that some patients will be assigned a risk based on the first marker that is so low that it is very unlikely that subsequent markers could increase the overall risk to the extent that the patient would become screen positive. In effect, contingency screening recognizes and attempts to capitalize on the fact that sequential screening will take place. Although there might be an attractive simplicity to contingency screening—avoiding the need to combine screening elements—the overall detection with such schemes is likely to be less than could be achieved by combining all the screening elements into a single risk (251).

The Integrated Test—Combining First- and Second-Trimester Markers

If first-trimester screening relies on the nondisclosure of the ultrasound results until the first-trimester biochemical markers become available, could screening be further improved by waiting even longer for the second-trimester markers to become available? A screening method called the Integrated Test, first proposed by Wald et al. in 1999, utilizes the potential of both first- and second-trimester screening markers (263). The term "integrated" stems from the concept of combining information from different trimesters. Rather than choosing either first-trimester screening or second-trimester screening, integrated prenatal screening proposed using the best markers of both. The first-trimester serum marker PAPP-A and the ultrasound marker NT would be measured but not disclosed or acted on until the results of the second-trimester AFP, uE3, hCG, and DIA measurements were also available. The measurement of first-trimester free β-hCG (or its total hCG form) is omitted because this analyte will be measured in the second trimester when its discriminatory power is greater. Once all measurements become available in the second trimester, a single risk estimate would be provided for interpretation. The modeling for the proposal predicted a detection rate of 90% with a low 2% screen-positive rate *(263)*.

The SURUSS in the United Kingdom was the first prospective study able to examine the performance of integrated prenatal screening *(103)*. Using several combinations of markers from both the first and second trimesters, the SURUSS essentially confirmed the performance prediction made by Wald et al. in 1999. Specifically, NT plus PAPP-A in the first trimester, followed by AFP, uE3, free β-hCG, and DIA measurements in the second trimester, yielded a detection rate of 90% with an FPR of 3.0%, quite close to the values predicted in the modeling *(263)*. The performance of the integrated screen is compared with earlier algorithms in Fig. 17 and 18.

Proponents of integrated screening cite its maximized detection rate and minimized false positive rate achieved by using all the available markers together. Others refer to this as a two-step strategy (albeit combined into one screen) and point out that the benefit of early markers—namely, early detection and intervention—is lost if first-trimester markers are not reported to patients during the first trimester *(224)*. If absent nasal bone proves to be an achievable and beneficial marker, the performance improvement of the integrated test, as now constituted, over first-trimester screening might not be maintained *(248)*, although nasal bone could also be included in the integrated test to improve its performance.

Some impediments to this screening algorithm need to be mentioned. The full integrated prenatal screening algorithm depends on a reliable NT measurement with its associated issues of access and consistency. Patents have recently been issued in the United States and Australia for the integrated test with and without NT, which will add to the cost of this algorithm. In addition, as mentioned earlier, there is a tendency for the components of the integrated test to segregate into sequential screening when an elevated NT measurement is obtained. Often, sonographers prefer to note NT values that are extreme (usually > 3 mm, or the approximately equivalent 3 MoM), because such elevated NT values are associated with increased risk of structural problems such as cardiac defects *(224)* not specifically related to Down syndrome. These patterns of practice and access challenges will need to be addressed and worked through to local consensus.

OTHER COMBINATIONS OF INTEGRATED SCREENING

The basic concept for integrated screening is to provide patients with as many tests as can be locally provided and justified, while improving the screen with the added information from the expanded testing. There are several combinations of tests possible, and most have not been examined in prospective trials. Different test combinations will have

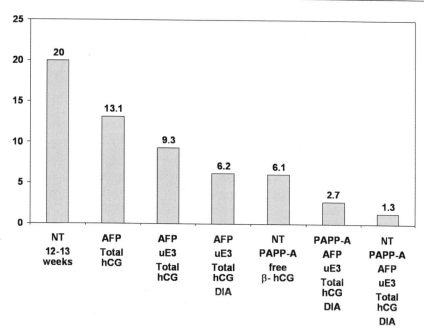

Fig. 17. Summary of the false positive rates associated with a detection rate of 85% for Down syndrome using different combinations of serum and ultrasound markers; data from the SURUSS *(103)*.

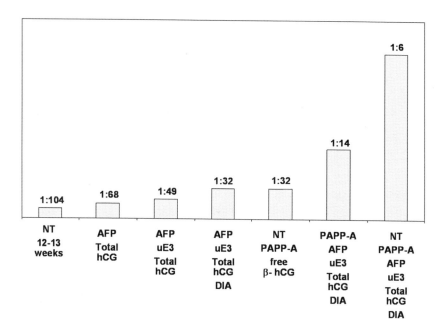

Fig. 18. Summary of the OAPR for the various screening algorithms in the SURUSS *(103)*, at the detection rate of 85%.

inherent economic performances in addition to their performance in detection and screen-positive rates. The reader is referred to the results of the SURUSS *(103)* for a detailed examination of the performance of various marker combinations to date.

Integrated Serum Screening. Much of the benefit of integrating first- and second-trimester screening markers can be realized without the inclusion of NT measurements, thus avoiding the training, sequential screening, and pattern of practice issues cited above. PAPP-A measurement in the first trimester *(263)* can be used in combination with the four second-trimester markers (AFP, uE3, hCG, and DIA). Modeling this algorithm predicts a Down syndrome detection rate of 80–85% with a 3–4% FPR. If true, this would represent a substantial improvement over the current triple-marker screen and a protocol that could be applied in areas where NT measurements are not available. The results of the first prospective trial of integrated screening—the SURUSS *(103)*—are included in Table 8 and in Fig. 19. Several additional studies of these algorithms are under way at present. Table 8 compares the structure and predicted performance of these evolving screening algorithms.

Specimen Logistics for Integrated Screening

Integrated screening, with or without an NT measurement, requires two blood samples collected, on average, about 1 mo apart. The two samples must be matched to the patient for the test results to be correctly combined to yield a single second-trimester risk. Both specimens must be collected within the acceptable first- and second-trimester time frames. For those patients who do not access an NT measurement with its associated gestational age assignment by CRL, a subsequent dating ultrasound scan can indicate that the first-trimester sample was obtained too early or too late. Patients sometimes forget to have their second-trimester sample drawn, or they decide not to continue with the screen after the first specimen, and the laboratory is not informed. Laboratories must determine the correct course of action for each of these: remind the forgetful patient, respect the patient who declined, schedule correctly dated collections, and sometimes interpret results from only one valid specimen. The effort and responsibility of these activities must be considered against the gain in performance of integrated screening over first- or second-trimester screens.

Screening for Down Syndrome—What Are the Choices?

The advent of the new Down syndrome screening algorithms brings the promise of lower false positive rates and higher detection rates. Higher costs for screening can be recovered from the ensuing decrease in the number of patients requiring or requesting expensive follow-up services (see Table 6). Screening programs are constrained to offer only those algorithms for which there is published evidence of efficacy, but increasingly that leaves patients and programs with considerable choice. There are trade-offs between early detection and the small increase in miscarriage rate associated with the early diagnostic procedure, or between maximized detection and the need for two blood collections and holding of ultrasound results. The new algorithms add to the complexity of what patients need to know and choose. It will be necessary to provide information to patients about the choices they can have in their care. The diagram in Fig. 20 is an example of an educative instrument designed to emphasize patient choices and trade-offs between available options.

Table 8
Summary of Potential First-Trimester, Second-Trimester, and Integrated Screening Protocols for
Fetal Down Syndrome, and the Projected Performance of Each Based
on the Results of the SURUSS (103)

Screening protocol	Triple marker	Four marker	First trimester	Integrated serum test	Integrated test
NT	—	—	yes	—	yes
PAPP-A	—	—	yes	yes	yes
Free β-hCG[a] or Total hCG	—	—	yes	—	—
AFP	yes	yes	—	yes	yes
uE3	yes	yes	—	yes	yes
Total hCG[b] or free β-hCG	yes	yes	—	yes	yes
DIA	—	yes	—	yes	yes
Gestational age for collection/ examination (wk)	14–20 wk	14–20 wk	10–13 wk	10 wk & 14–20	10–13 & 14–20
Trimester for interpretation	2nd	2nd	1st	2nd	2nd
FPR at a DR of 80%	7.4%	4.5%	3.4%	2.8%	0.7%
FPR at a DR of 85%	11%	7.1%	6.0%	4.8%	1.4%
FPR at a DR of 90%	17%	12%	11%	8.5%	3.2%

[a]Screening performance quoted for the first-trimester algorithm using free β-hCG.
[b]Performances for second trimester and integrated test with the total hCG marker.

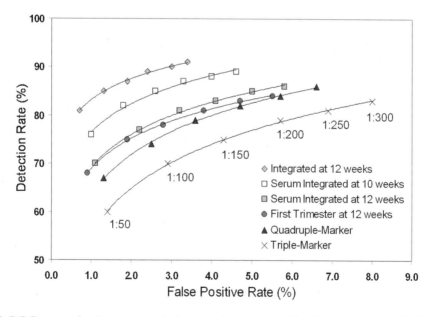

Fig. 19. ROC curves for the serum and ultrasound marker combinations assessed in the SURUSS
(103). The term risk cutoffs that would achieve each point on the curves are shown below the triple-
marker data. Note the relative equivalence in this study between first-trimester screening and the
second-trimester four-marker screen, and the effect of measuring PAPP-A at 10 vs 12 wk on
performance.

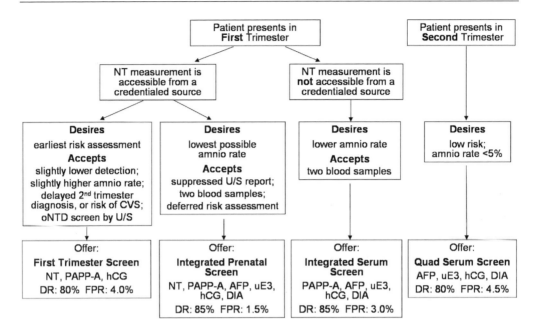

Fig. 20. Current and future prenatal screening algorithms presented from a patient choice perspective.

SCREENING FOR TRISOMY 18 AND OTHER DISORDERS

After Down syndrome, trisomy 18 is the next most common fetal chromosome disorder at birth. Screening for fetal trisomies on the basis of maternal age sometimes persists because of the awareness that there are chromosomal disorders other than Down syndrome that are associated with advanced maternal age, principal among these being trisomy 18.

Trisomy 18

Trisomy 18 (Edwards' syndrome [T18]) is less common and more lethal than trisomy 21. The prevalence of T18 during the first and second trimester is approx 1 in 3000 but spontaneous loss of T18 pregnancies reduces the birth prevalence to approx 1 in 8000. T18 pregnancies miscarry at a rate of 70% between midpregnancy and term *(264,265)*. Like Down syndrome, the prevalence of T18 is correlated with increasing maternal age.

T18 is characterized by severe mental retardation, growth retardation, and hypotonia, with multiple systems affected. Most babies with T18 die within the first weeks after birth, and 90% or more die within 1 yr *(266)*. A major obstetrical issue is that T18 pregnancies tend to be small for their gestational age and are quite often confused for growth-restricted but potentially healthy pregnancies. The ceasarean section rate in T18 pregnancies coming to term is more than 60% *(267)*, and other late pregnancy interventions are common but without long-term benefit. For this reason, it is beneficial to identify T18 early in pregnancy when safe termination can be offered.

SECOND-TRIMESTER MATERNAL SERUM MARKERS FOR T18

The occurrence of a low MSAFP in a T18 pregnancy was the impetus for the first assessment of MSAFP as a marker for fetal trisomy risk *(92)*. Although this earliest study resulted in screening for the more prevalent trisomy, Down syndrome, the correlation

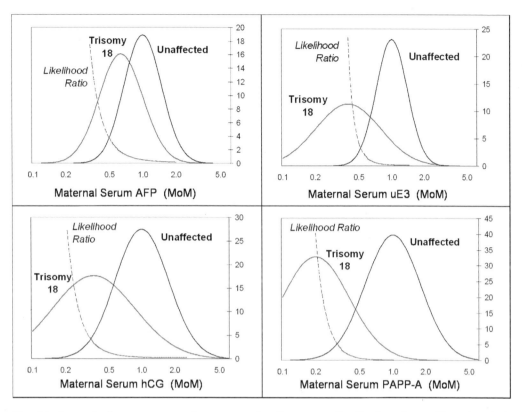

Fig. 21. Second-trimester maternal serum marker frequency distributions in unaffected and tri-somy 18 pregnancies for AFP, uE3, and total hCG *(270)*, together with the recently reported first-trimester distributions of PAPP-A *(278)*. The LR for each marker are also shown within the range of the overlapping distributions for each marker. Note the differing scales for the LR to the right of each figure, showing the relative power of each marker in T18 screening.

between low MSAFP and T18 was not forgotten. As new markers for Down syndrome were discovered and added to screening programs, the markers were assessed for their potential as T18 markers. Within a few years of the advent of triple-marker screening, it was known that T18 pregnancies had a relatively distinctive pattern of suppressed MoM values for all three markers, AFP, uE3, and hCG. A screening algorithm based on all three markers being concurrently low was proposed and implemented for a number of years *(268)* using different fixed low-MoM cutoffs for each marker *(269)*. This algorithm was later improved *(270)* by a trivariate Gaussian risk-based algorithm (see Fig. 21) that projected a detection rate of 60–80% at an extremely low FPR of 0.3%. This performance was subsequently confirmed in prospective trials *(271,272)*. For unknown reasons, con-centrations of DIA are only slightly reduced in T18, and as a consequence, DIA is not used in T18 screening *(273,274)*.

First-Trimester Markers for T18

The concentrations of the first-trimester markers PAPP-A and free β-hCG *(275)* are also considerably reduced in T18 pregnancies, and NT measurements are substantially increased *(276)*. The biochemical markers and, to a slightly lesser extent, the NT marker conform to a log Gaussian distribution *(277)*, enabling a first-trimester risk-based screen that is as effective as the second-trimester screen.

COMBINING FIRST- AND SECOND-TRIMESTER MARKERS FOR T18

The most effective screening algorithm for T18 proposed to date combines the first-trimester biochemical marker PAPP-A with AFP, uE3, and hCG in the second trimester, in a serum integrated screen *(278)*. A detection rate of 90% is projected, with an FPR of only 0.1%.

Smith-Lemli-Opitz Syndrome

Smith-Lemli-Opitz Syndrome (SLOS) is a serious birth defect that arises from an error in cholesterol biosynthesis *(279)* that causes mental retardation, poor growth, and a variety of phenotypic abnormalities in the fetus *(280)*. Maternal serum concentrations of uE3 are very low because the steroid precursors required for estriol synthesis are deficient in the affected fetus. Concentrations of AFP and hCG are also slightly reduced for unknown reasons *(281)*. Although the birth prevalence is quite low (usually given as about 1 in 20,000), prenatal serum screening for SLOS with AFP, uE3, and hCG is expected to be very efficient, with a detection rate of about 60% at a 0.3% FPR *(282)*. A multicenter clinical intervention trial to examine the efficacy of screening for SLOS has just begun.

Other Conditions Identified By Serum

Although not the targets of any formal screening protocol, a number of deleterious conditions and disorders are adventitiously detected through Down syndrome and T18 screening algorithms. In order for this to occur, the conditions must have marker patterns that overlap with those of a targeted disorder, causing the conditions to cluster among the screen positives.

OTHER CHROMOSOME ABNORMALITIES

Other chromosome abnormalities are not screened for specifically, but they may be detected with increased frequency through Down syndrome and T18 protocols and the subsequent karyotype studies. For example, women carrying a fetus affected with hydropic Turner syndrome (45,X) have a maternal serum triple-marker pattern very similar to that observed in cases of Down syndrome *(274,283,284)*. DIA concentrations in Turner syndrome pregnancies are markedly elevated in the presence of fetal hydrops and low in the absence of hydrops *(274)*. Therefore, inclusion of DIA in Down syndrome screening will increase the opportune detection of Turner syndrome with hydrops because the elevated DIA concentrations will further promote a Down syndrome screen-positive situation. Turner syndrome without hydrops has slightly or moderately reduced concentrations of AFP, uE3, and hCG *(274,283,284)* and may be identified by T18 screening protocols.

Cases of triploidy (69,XXX; 69,XXY; 69,XYY) may also be identified through current prenatal serum screening protocols *(285)*. There are two types of triploidy depending on the parental origin of the extra set of chromosomes. Type I triploidy originates from an extra set of paternal chromosomes and is characterized by a large cystic placenta and fetal loss early in gestation. If a fetus survives to the second trimester, low uE3 and elevated hCG *(286)* concentrations in maternal serum may lead to identification through

Down syndrome screening protocols. Type II triploidy originates from an extra set of maternal chromosomes and is characterized by a small fetus, a small placenta, and typical intrauterine survival late into pregnancy. Maternal serum uE3 concentrations tend to be extremely low, usually less than 20% of normal values, and hCG is also reduced *(286)*. These cases are likely to be identified through second-trimester T18 screening protocols.

There appears to be no consistent pattern in the serum markers for cases of trisomy 13, with the exception of a slight reduction in uE3 concentrations *(287)*. Identification of trisomy 13 pregnancies is not expected using current prenatal serum screening protocols.

PREECLAMPSIA

Preeclampsia is defined by hypertension and proteinuria and is a serious obstetrical complication associated with significant maternal and fetal morbidity (see Chapter 18). Although treatments such as aspirin *(288)* and calcium *(289)* have proven ineffective, the ability to identify pregnancies at risk for developing preeclampsia would allow for close monitoring and aid in the development of other treatment strategies. In this regard, the serum markers used for Down syndrome screening have been reported to be altered in pregnancies that later develop preeclampsia. More specifically, concentrations of AFP, hCG, free β-hCG, and DIA are significantly elevated in the second trimester of preeclamptic pregnancies *(290–293)*, whereas concentrations of uE3 are unchanged or reduced *(292,293)*. Not surprisingly, the degree of change in the serum marker values is more marked as the interval between sample collection and clinical onset of disease shortens. Risk of preeclampsia is not currently reported in prenatal serum screening protocols. Current estimates are that a multiple-marker test, including hCG and DIA at about 17 wk gestation, would detect 23% of preeclampsia cases at a 5% FPR *(292)*, whereas a triple-marker test of uE3, free β-hCG, and DIA done at about 24 wk gestation would detect 55% of preeclampsia cases at a 5% FPR *(293)*.

OTHER ADVERSE OUTCOMES

Patients who are screen positive for Down syndrome *(294,295)*, NTD *(294,296)*, or T18 *(272)* pregnancy are also at risk for other adverse outcomes, such as fetal growth restriction, preterm delivery, and fetal demise. However, these are weak associations, and it is not appropriate to follow patients for these complications on the basis of screening results. In fact, a recent study has shown that heightened surveillance of patients with an elevated MSAFP result did not improve assessment of adverse pregnancy outcome as compared to routine management of such pregnancies *(297)*.

PRENATAL SCREENING PROGRAM CONSIDERATIONS

Prenatal screening for ONTD and fetal trisomies is best implemented in the context of a comprehensive program that coordinates preanalytic, analytic, and postanalytic components of the process.

The program should include participants from the testing laboratory, the genetic counseling unit, and the prenatal diagnostic group that will perform interventions (targeted ultrasound, amniocentesis, CVS). Representatives from the family practice and general obstetrics community would be a helpful addition as well, providing useful information about the primary care component in obstetrical care.

The overall direction of a program should be assigned to a professional usually at the doctoral level of training. Adequate specialized training is strongly recommended—two such courses are available.

Health Care Provider and Patient Information

Prenatal screening, by its nature, is associated with ethical, legal, and social issues for the patient, provider, and laboratory. Patients need to be informed partners in the screening process. Laboratories should either develop patient educational materials or be involved in their development and control their distribution. Health care provider education materials should be available at a scientific level that supports the pattern of practice expected of a provider and enables uncomplicated responses to patient questions.

Obtaining informed consent from patients to participate in screening is the responsibility of the provider, but the laboratory has an important role in enabling patient education. Laboratories might wish to document that a process is in place to inform patients about the benefits and risks of screening, about its limitations, and about the implications of a screen-positive report and the need for further testing to make a diagnosis. Patients have the right to end participation at any step without a sense of reprisal. Under some recently introduced guidelines for patient privacy, patients might have the right to withdraw information from screening data banks.

The advent of the new screening algorithms brings new complexity into the healthcare provider and patient relationship. A teaching diagram such as Fig. 20 might assist both parties to achieve an informed patient choice.

REQUISITION FORMS AND INTAKE INFORMATION

Laboratories should have a separate requisition specifically for prenatal screening, in order to solicit the necessary demographic and clinical information for the service. In addition to the usual demographic information, the requisition should provide the following information about the patient:

- Related to the patient:
  - unique identifying number, if available, for outcome follow-up
  - racial origin—at least white or black
  - existence of insulin-dependent diabetes mellitus prior to this pregnancy
  - date of birth (required for fetal trisomy screening only)
- Related to the pregnancy:
  - maternal weight in the late first trimester in pounds or kilograms
  - number of fetuses in the current pregnancy
  - family history of the targeted disorders as it relates to the fetus
  - smoking during the pregnancy
  - gestational age information, including either:
    - date of LMP or,
    - date of ultrasound examination and
      - BPD measurement, and/or
      - CRL measurement, and/or
      - gestational age assigned by the examiner
- Related to the sample:
  - date of specimen collection
  - specimen number(s) assigned at collection
  - ordering health care provider information
  - screening status (any previous screening during this pregnancy)

The requisition should contain information and instructions about specimen collection, instructions for specimen delivery, and stability. A similar or identical requisition can be used for AFAFP samples.

Assay Methodologies

There are several assay methods available for measuring AFP, and some have been approved by the US Food and Drug Administration for an ONTD application. In selecting a method, consideration should be given to the ability of the assay manufacturer to support the additional demands of a prenatal screening service for long-term precision and analytical stability. It is advisable to use the same assay source for both maternal serum and amniotic fluid specimens. Because the latter will require dilution by approximately 100-fold, a stable source of diluent is an important component of the assay.

A number of immunoassays exist for uE3, but not all of them achieve the expected degree of separation between the affected and unaffected populations in prenatal screening, either for Down syndrome *(54,298)* or for T18 *(299)*. A validated assay should be used if the published distribution parameters are to be used in calculating risks.

There have been no reports of differential performance of any intact or total β-hCG assays in Down syndrome screening. Free β-hCG has whole blood specimen stability issues that must be considered; on standing, there is an increase in the apparent free β-hCG concentration caused by the temperature-dependent dissociation of the very large amount of intact hCG present *(300)*. Prompt separation of the serum appears to minimize this problem *(101,131)*. Most intact and total hCG assays are optimized for concentrations found in early pregnancy (up to approx 2000 IU/L). Concentrations of intact and total hCG found in the late first and early second trimesters are much higher (10–100 kIU/L) and prenatal screening serum specimens require dilution with all but one assay *(301)*. If an automated dilution assay is used for hCG, the long-term consistency of the diluent and the dilution ratio are factors to be considered and monitored. Whereas all patient samples will require dilution, typically calibration and quality control materials do not, and patient median values can be affected by a change in diluent (see Fig. 22).

There is only one manufacturer of DIA assays (DSL, Webster, TX) and a stable immunoassay is now available without the originally required specimen pretreatment steps. This DIA assay has been validated in Down syndrome screening programs *(136,137)*. Various patents apply to the assays for, and the diagnostic use of, the inhibins, and these contribute to the cost of testing.

At least four methods are available commercially for PAPP-A measurement, but only two of these (DELFIA, PerkinElmer, Boston, MA; KRYPTOR, Brahms Diagnostica GmbH, Berlin, Germany) have been used in published Down syndrome screening studies. A third assay (DSL, Webster, TX) was used in the FASTER trial, to be published in early 2004. Less is known about the consistency and performance characteristics of other PAPP-A assays.

CALIBRATION, QUALITY CONTROL, AND PATIENT MEDIANS

In prenatal screening, the reported result for the markers is the unitless MoM. From the perspective of screening performance, the mass concentration unit (traditional, activity, or metric) is not as important as in most laboratory tests, nor is the agreement between manufacturers in the assigned calibrator concentrations. External proficiency testing programs can be used to validate the assigned calibrator values. Commercial quality

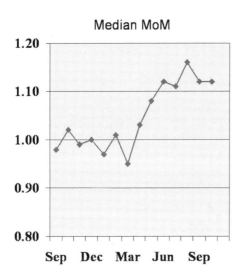

- **7% increase in detection**
- **27% increase in IPR**
  (*e.g.*, from 8.0% to 10.2%)
- **In a 20,000 patient/year service, a 6-month shift causes 180 additional amniocentesis procedures**
  - **~1 procedural fetal loss**
  - **$130,000 added cost**
  - **$13 added cost per screen**

Fig. 22. The effect of a 10% change in the median concentration for second-trimester serum total hCG on the performance, safety, and cost of screening. A shift similar to that shown can be caused by a change in hCG diluent source. IPR, initial positive rate.

control products can assess the analytical precision, but controls from pooled patient sera provide the best check on patient precision; commercial products have sample matrices that can differ from patient samples. Precision should be monitored at two or more clinically significant concentrations, and if commercial controls are used, the assay precision that they indicate should match that of patient pools. Stability in patient median values is more essential than stability of control means; therefore, shifts in median values or in median MoMs take precedence over commercial-quality control sample performance.

NORMATIVE DATA—MEDIAN MARKER CONCENTRATIONS

Because prenatal screening results are expressed as the MoM concentration in the screened population, accurate assignment of the median calculations for all gestational ages is critical. Regressed medians (concentration vs gestational age) are the most robust source of median results, and these must be reassessed periodically for undetected systematic changes in the methodology. Stated simply, the median in a population is constant, whereas the analytical system used to measure the median will vary. Given a static population, any change in the median values will reflect changes in analytical conditions. Marker test results obtained from different reagent lots, even from the same manufacturer, can demonstrate sufficient systematic bias to reflect significantly in the median values, and hence in patient MoM results. For this reason, new reagent lots must be characterized over a period of weeks, with forced extra calibrations if necessary, well in advance of being put into use. Similarly, other analytical sources of systematic bias should be minimized on the testing platforms.

Result Reporting

Final patient screening reports must be clear to a nongeneticist professional and must include all the clinical information used in generating the patient risk(s), the analytic

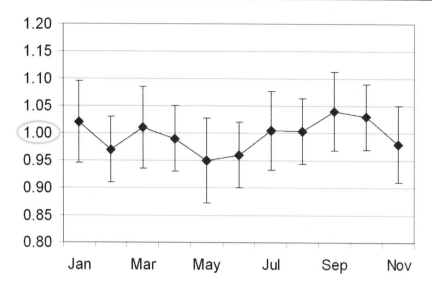

Fig. 23. A median MoM plot as one aspect of epidemiological monitoring to control the performance of screening variables, predominantly but not solely analytical. Median reported MoM values should center at 1.0 within appropriate confidence intervals.

results in both mass units (e.g., ng/mL) and interpretive units (i.e., MoM) on which all adjustments or corrections have been performed. The report should include a clinical interpretation regarding each major screened disorder, including whether the result is screen positive or screen negative, and the patient-specific risk of the targeted disorders.

Epidemiological Monitoring

The use of the patient population as the source of reference or normative data has led to the practice of monitoring the performance of the analytical service in the population being tested. This epidemiological monitoring is additional to, and perhaps more important than, traditional measures of laboratory test performance. Monthly indicators that should be monitored include the median concentrations of each marker at weekly intervals of gestational age, the median MoM concentrations (combined data from all gestational ages, see Fig. 23), and the screen-positive rate for each of the screened disorders. A concentration shift of –10% in a uE3 assay will cause a 40% increase in the screen-positive rate; a shift of +10% in hCG will cause a 27% increase in the number of false-positives (see Fig. 22). If such a shift is detected, either the cause of the shift should be corrected or, if necessary, the median values in use should be adjusted.

Other population-based variables that require periodic monitoring include the patient weight correction factors for each marker, the population MoM SDs for each marker, the detection rate of the targeted disorders (if reliable outcome ascertainment is available), the fraction of patients "dated" by ultrasound, and even the median maternal age.

SUMMARY AND PERSPECTIVE

Prenatal screening using maternal serum biochemical markers and ultrasound biometry represents a major advance in obstetrical care. Beginning with the use of AFP in screening for NTD, the screening methods that were developed were creative and highly rational. With the advances in primary prevention through the increased intake of folic acid in the diet and preconceptional vitamin supplements, and with highly effective secondary prevention through screening with AFP, the prevalence of ONTDs has declined markedly in many countries.

Initially based on maternal age alone, and then linked through AFP to screening for ONTDs, the performance of prenatal screening tests for Down syndrome has improved rapidly during the past 25 yr. With the development of multiple screening markers (both in maternal serum and by using ultrasound) and with the ability to combine these markers into a rational screening algorithm, detection rates are becoming high enough to allow a focus on reducing the FPR. The goal in reducing the FPR is to improve safety in screening because a lower FPR leads to reduced use of invasive diagnostic testing, thus reducing the risk of losing a wanted pregnancy. The goal is a detection rate approaching 100% with an FPR approaching zero. At a point, perhaps not too far in the future, safe, noninvasive diagnostic testing for serious birth defects will have been achieved.

REFERENCES

1. Wald NJ. Guidance on terminology. J Med Screen 1994;1:76.
2. Wald NJ. What is genetic screening anyway? J Med Screen 1996;3:57.
3. Carroll JC, Brown JB, Reid AJ, Pugh P. Womens experience of maternal serum screening. Can Fam Physician 2000;46:614–620.
4. Phillips OP, Elias S. Genetics and epidemiology of neural tube defects. In: Elias S, Simpson JL, eds. Maternal Serum Screening. New York: Churchill Livingstone, 1992, pp. 1–23.
5. Milunsky A. Maternal serum screening for neural tube and other defects. In: Milunsky A, ed. Genetic Disorders of the Fetus: Diagnosis, Prevention and Treatment, 4th ed. Baltimore: Johns Hopkins University Press, 1998, pp. 635–701.
6. Greenberg F, James LM, Oakley GP. Estimates of birth prevalence rates of spina bifida in the United States from computer-generated maps. Am J Obstet Gynecol 1983;145:570–573.
7. Robert E, Guibaud P. Maternal valproic acid and congenital neural tube defects. Lancet 1982;2:937.
8. Guibaud S, Robert E, Simplot A, Boisson C, Francannet C, Patouraux MH. Prenatal diagnosis of spina bifida aperta after first-trimester valproate exposure. Prenat Diagn 1993;13:772–773.
9. Lindhout D, Omtzigt JG, Cornel MC. Spectrum of neural-tube defects in 34 infants prenatally exposed to antiepileptic drugs. Neurology 1992;42:111–118.
10. Rosa FW. Spina bifida in infants of women treated with carbamazepine during pregnancy. N Engl J Med 1991;324:674–677.
11. Milunsky A, Jick H, Jick SS, et al. Multivitamin/folic acid supplementation in early pregnancy reduces the prevalence of neural tube defects. JAMA 1989;262:2847–2852.
12. Wald NJ, Sneddon J, Densem J, Frost C, Stone R. Prevention of neural tube defects: results of the MRC vitamin study. Lancet 1991;338:131–137.
13. Wald NJ, Law MR, Morris JK, Wald DS. Quantifying the effect of folic acid. Lancet 2001;358:2069–2073.
14. Williams LJ, Mai CT, Edmonds LD, et al. Prevalence of spina bifida and anencephaly during the transition to mandatory folic acid fortification in the United States. Terat 2002;66:33–39.
15. Palomaki GE, Williams J, Haddow JE. Comparing the observed and predicted effectiveness of folic acid fortification in preventing neural tube defects. J Med Screen 2003;10:52–53.
16. Bergstrand CG, Czar B. Demonstration of a new protein fraction in serum from the human fetus. Scan J Clin Lab Invest 1956;174:8.
17. Benassayag C, Rigourd V, Mignot TM, et al. Does high polyunsaturated free fatty acid level at the feto-maternal interface alter steroid hormone message during pregnancy? Prostaglandins Leukot Essent Fatty Acids 1999;60:393–399.
18. Greenberg F, Faucett A, Rose E, et al. Congenital deficiency of alpha-fetoprotein. Am J Obstet Gynecol 1992;167:509–511.
19. Brock DJH, Sutcliffe RG. Alpha-fetoprotein in the antenatal diagnosis of anencephaly and spina bifida. Lancet 1972;2:197–199.

20. Hino M, Koki Y, Nishi S. Nimpu ketsu na ka noalpha-fetoprotein [Alpha-fetoprotein in pregnant women]. Igaku No Ayumi 1972;82:512.

21. Leek AE, Ruoss CF, Kitau MJ, Chard T. Raised α-fetoprotein in maternal serum with anencephalic pregnancy. Lancet 1973;2:385.

22. Brock DHJ, Bolton AE, Monaghan JM. Prenatal diagnosis of anencephaly through maternal serum-alphafetoprotein measurement. Lancet 1973;2:923–924.

23. Second Report of the UK Collaborative Study on Alpha-fetoprotein in Relation to Neural-tube Defects: amniotic-fluid alpha-fetoprotein measurement in antenatal diagnosis of anencephaly and spina bifida in early pregnancy. Lancet 1979;2:651–662.

24. Report of the Collaborative Acetylcholinesterase Study: amniotic fluid acetylcholinesterase electrophoresis as a secondary test in the diagnosis of anencephaly and spina bifida in early pregnancy. Lancet 1981;2:321–324.

25. Wald NJ, Brock DJH, Bonnar J. Prenatal diagnosis of spina bifida and anencephaly by maternal serum-alpha-fetoprotein measurement. Lancet 1974;1:765–767.

26. Wald NJ, Cuckle H, Brock JH, Peto R, Polani PE, Woodford FP for the report of the UK collaborative study on alpha-fetoprotein in relation to neural-tube defects. Maternal serum-alpha-fetoprotein measurement in antenatal screening for anencephaly and spina bifida in early pregnancy. Lancet 1977;1:1323–1332.

27. Haddow JE. Biological properties of alpha-fetoprotein in detection of fetal disorders. In: Elias S, Simpson JL, ed. Maternal Serum Screening. New York: Churchill Livingstone, 1992:25–40.

28. Wald NJ, Hackshaw A, Stone R, Densem J. Serum alpha-fetoprotein and neural tube defects in the first trimester of pregnancy. Prenat Diagn 1993;13:1047–1050.

29. Crandall BF, Chua C. Detecting neural tube defects by amniocentesis between 11 and 15 weeks' gestation. Prenat Diagn 1995;15:339–343.

30. Wald NJ, Smith D, Kennard A, et al. Biparietal diameter and crown-rump length in fetuses with Down's Syndrome: implications for antenatal serum screening for Down's syndrome. Br J Obstet Gyneacol 1993;100:430–435.

31. Hadlock FP, Shah YP, Kanon DJ, Lindsey JV. Fetal crown–rump length: reevaluation of relation to menstrual age (5–18 weeks) with high-resolution real-time US. Radiology 1992;182:501–505.

32. Daya S. Accuracy of gestational age estimation by means of fetal crown–rump length measurement. Am J Obs Gyn 1993;168:903–908.

33. Hadlock FP, Deter RL, Harrist RB, Park SK. Fetal biparietal diameter: a critical reevaluation of the relation to menstrual age by means of real-time ultrasound. J Ultrasound Med 1982;1:97–104.

34. Wald N, Cuckle H, Boreham J, Stirrat G. Small biparietal diameter of fetuses with spina bifida: implications for antenatal screening. Br J Obstet Gynaecol 1980;87:219–221.

35. Johnson AM. In: Haddow JE, Wald NJ, eds. Alpha-Fetoprotein Screening: The Current Issues. Scarborough, ME: Foundation for Blood Research, 1981, p. 10.

36. Crandall BF, Lebherz TB, Schroth PC, Matsumoto M. Alpha-fetoprotein concentrations in maternal serum: relation to race and body weight. Clin Chem 1983;29:531–533.

37. Johnson AM, Palomaki GE, Haddow JE. Maternal serum alpha-fetoprotein levels in pregnancies among black and white women with fetal open spina bifida: a United States collaborative study. Am J Obstet Gynecol 1990;162:328–331.

38. Watt HC, Wald NJ, Smith D, Kennard A, Densem J. Effect of allowing for ethnic group in prenatal screening for Downs syndrome. Prenat Diagn 1996;16:691–698.

39. O'Brien JE, Drugan A, Chervenak FA, et al. Maternal serum alpha-fetoprotein screening: the need to use race/ethnic specific medians in Asians. Fetal Diagn Ther 1993;8:367–370.

40. Haddow JE, Kloza EM, Knight GJ, Smith DE. Relationship between maternal weight and serum alpha-fetoprotein concentration during the second trimester. Clin Chem 1981;27:133–134.

41. Wald NJ, Cuckle HS, Boreham J, Terzian E, Redman C. The effect of maternal weight on maternal serum alpha-fetoprotein levels. Br J Obstet Gynaecol 1981;88:1094–1096.

42. Johnson AM, Palomaki GE, Haddow JE. The effect of adjusting maternal serum alpha-fetoprotein levels for maternal weight in pregnancies with fetal open spina bifida: a United States collaborative study. Am J Obstet Gynecol 1990;163:9–11.

43. Palomaki GE, Panizza DS, Canick JA. Screening for Down syndrome using AFP, uE3 and hCG: effect of maternal weight. Am J Hum Genet 1990;7:282a.

44. Neveux LM, Palomaki GE, Larrivee DA, Knight GJ, Haddow JE. Refinements in managing maternal weight adjustment for interpreting prenatal screening results. Prenat Diagn 1996;16:1115–1119.

45. Canick JA, Panizza DS, Palomaki GE. Prenatal screening for Down syndrome using AFP, uE3 and hCG: effect of maternal race, insulin-dependent diabetes and twin pregnancy. Am J Human Genet 1990;47:a270.

46. Wald NJ, Cuckle H, Wu T, George L. Maternal serum unconjugated oestriol and human chorionic gonadotrophin levels in twin pregnancies: implications for Down's syndrome. Br J Obstet Gynaecol 1991;98:905–908.

47. Neveux LM, Palomaki GE, Knight GJ, Haddow JE. Multiple marker screening for Down syndrome in twin pregnancies. Prenat Diagn 1996;16:29–34.

48. Wald NJ, Cuckle HS, Peck S, Stirrat GM, Turnbull AC. Maternal serum alpha-fetoprotein in relation to zygosity. Br Med J 1979;1:455.

49. Thom H, Buckland CM, Campbell AGM, Thompson B, Farr V. Maternal serum AFP in monozygotic and dizygotic twin pregnancies. Prenat Diagn 1984;4:341–346.

50. Wald NJ, Cuckle HS, Boreham J, Stirrat GM, Turnbull AC. Maternal serum alpha-fetoprotein and diabetes mellitus. Br J Obstet Gynaecol 1979;86:101–105.

51. Milunsky A, Alpert E, Kitzmiller JL, Younger MD, Neff RK. Prenatal diagnosis of neural tube defects. VIII. The importance of alpha-fetoprotein screening in diabetic women. Am J Obstet Gynecol 1982;142:1030–1032.

52. Henriques CU, Damm P, Tabor A, Pedersen JF, Molsted-Pedersen L. Decreased alpha-fetoprotein in amniotic fluid and maternal serum in diabetic pregnancy. Obstet Gynecol 1993;82:960–964.

53. Wald NJ, Hackshaw AK, George LM. Assay precision of serum α-fetoprotein in antenatal screening for neural tube defects and Down's syndrome. J Med Screen 2000;7:74–77.

54. MacRae AR, Gardner HA, Allen LC, Tokmakejian S, Lepage N. Outcome validation of the Beckman Coulter Access analyzer in a second-trimester Down syndrome serum screening application. Clin Chem 2003;49:69–76.

55. Wald NJ, Cuckle HS, Densem JW, Kennard A, Smith D. Maternal serum screening for Down's syndrome: the effect of routine ultrasound scan determination of gestational age and adjustment for maternal weight. Br J Obstet Gynaecol 1992;99:144–149.

56. Cuckle H, Wald N, Stevenson JD, et al. Maternal serum alpha-fetoprotein screening for open neural tube defects in twin pregnancies. Prenat Diagn 1990;10:71–77.

57. Palomaki GE, Williams JR, Haddow JE. Prenatal screening for open neural-tube defects in Maine. N Engl J Med 1999;340:1049–1050.

58. Papp Z, Toth Z, Torok O, Szabo M. Prenatal diagnosis policy without routine amniocentesis in pregnancies with a positive family history for neural tube defects. Am J Med Gen 1987;26:103–110.

59. Wax JR, Lopes AM, Benn PA, Lerer T, Steinfeld JD, Ingardia CJ. Unexplained elevated midtrimester maternal serum levels of alpha fetoprotein, human chorionic gonadotropin, or low unconjugated estriol: recurrence risk and association with adverse perinatal outcome. J Matern Fetal Med 2000;9:161–164.

60. Kucera J. Rate and type of congenital anomalies among offspring of diabetic women. J Reprod Med 1971;7:73–82.

61. Mills J, Baker L, Goldman A. Malformations in infants of diabetic mothers occur before the seventh gestational week. Diabetes 1979;28:292–293.

62. Waller DK, Mills JL, Simpson JL, et al. Are obese women at higher risk for producing malformed offspring? Am J Obstet Gynecol 1994;170:541–548.

63. Werler MM, Louik CL, Shapiro S, Mitchell AA. Prepregnant weight in relation to risk of neural tube defects. JAMA 1996;275:1089–1092.

64. Shaw GM, Velie EM, Schaffer D. Risk of neural tube defect-affected pregnancies among obese women. JAMA 1996;275:1093–1096.

65. Watkins ML, Rasmussen SA, Honein MA, Botto LD, Moore CA. Maternal obesity and risk for birth defects. Pediatrics 2003;111:1152–1158.

66. Waller DK, Lustig LS, Cunningham GC, Feuchtbaum LB, Hook EB. The association between maternal serum alpha-fetoprotein and preterm birth, small for gestational age infants, preeclampsia, and placental complications. Obstet Gynecol 1996;88:816–822.

67. Wald NJ, Cuckle HS, Haddow JE, Doherty RA, Knight GJ, Palomaki GE. Sensitivity of ultrasound in detecting spina bifida. N Engl J Med 1991;324:769–772.

68. Boyd PA, Wellesley DG, DeWalle HEK, et al. Evaluation of the prenatal diagnosis of neural tube defects by fetal ultrasonographic examination in different centres across Europe. J Med Screen 2000;7:169–174.

69. Estimating an individual's risk of having a fetus with open spina bifida and the value of repeat AFP testing. Report of the Fourth UK collaborative study on AFP in relation to neural tube defects. J Epidem Comm Health 1982;36:87–95.

70. Smith AD, Wald NJ, Cuckle HS, Stirrat GM, Bobrow M, Lagercrantz H. Amniotic fluid acetylcho-linesterase as a possible diagnostic test for neural-tube defects in early pregnancy. Lancet 1979;1:685–688.

71. Wald N, Cuckle H, Nanchahal K. Amniotic fluid acetylcholinesterase measurement in the prenatal diagnosis of open neural tube defects: second report of the collaborative acetylcholinesterase study. Prenat Diagn 1989;9:813–829.

72. Down JL. Observations on an ethnic classification of idiots. Clinical Lecture Reports, London Hospital 1866;3:259.

73. Wald, N. Down's syndrome. In: Wald N, Leck I, eds. Antenatal and Neonatal Screening. Oxford: Oxford University Press, 2000:85.

74. Noble, J. Natural history of Down's syndrome: a brief review for those involved in antenatal screening. J Med Screen 1998;5:172–177.

75. Torfs CP, Christianson RE. Anomalies in Down syndrome individuals in a large population-based registry. Am J Med Genet 1998;77:431–438.

76. Lejeune J, Gautier M, Turpin R. Etude des chromosomes somatiques de neuf enfants mongoliens. CR Acad Sci Paris 1959;248:1721–1722.

77. Steele MW, Breg WR. Chromosome analysis of human amniotic-fluid cells. Lancet 1966;i:383–385.

78. Valenti C, Schutta EJ, Kehaty T. Prenatal diagnosis of Down's syndrome. Lancet 1968;ii:220.

79. Tabor A, Philip J, Madsen M, Bang J, Obel EB, Norgaard-Pedersen B. Randomized controlled trial of genetic amniocentesis in 4606 low risk women. Lancet 1986;1:1287–1293.

80. Evaluation of chorionic villus sampling safety. WHO/PAHO consultation on CVS. Prenat Diagn 1999;19:97–99.

81. Brun JL, Mangione R, Gangbo F, et al. Feasibility, accuracy and safety of chorionic villus sampling: a report of 10741 cases. Prenat Diagn 2003;23:295–301.

82. The Canadian Early and Mid-Trimester Amniocentesis Trial (CEMAT) Group. Randomized trial to assess safety and fetal outcome of early and midtrimester amniocentesis. Lancet 1998;351:242–247.

82a. Alfirevic Z, Sundberg K, Brigham S. Amniocentesis and chorionic villus sampling for prenatal diag-nosis. Cochrane Database Syst Rev 2003;3:CD0003252.

83. Penrose LS. The relative effects of paternal and maternal age in mongolism. J Genet 1933;27:219–224.

84. Cuckle HS, Wald NJ, Thompson SG. Estimating a woman's risk of having a pregnancy associated with Down's syndrome using her age and serum alpha-fetoprotein level. Br J Obstet Gynaecol 1987;94:387–402.

85. Hecht CA, Hook EB. The imprecision in rates of Down syndrome by 1-year maternal age intervals: a critical analysis of rates used in biochemical screening. Prenat Diagn 1994;14:729–738.

86. Hecht CA, Hook EB. Rates of Down syndrome at livebirth by one-year maternal age intervals in studies with apparent close to complete ascertainment in populations of European origin: a proposed rate schedule for use in genetic and prenatal screening. Am J Med Genet 1996;62:376–385.

87. Bray I, Wright DE, Davies C, Hook EB. Joint estimation of Down syndrome risk and ascertainment rates: a meta-analysis of nine published data sets. Prenat Diagn 1998;18:9–20.

88. Huether CA, Ivanovich J, Goodwin BS, et al. Maternal age specific risk rate estimates for Down syndrome among live births in whites and other races from Ohio and metropolitan Atlanta, 1970–1989. J Med Genet 1998;35:482–490.

89. Morris JK, Mutton DE, Alberman E. Revised estimates of the maternal age specific live birth preva-lence of Down syndrome. J Med Screen 2002;9:2–6.

90. Cuckle H. Down syndrome fetal loss rate in early pregnancy. Prenat Diagn 1999;19:1177–1179.

91. Morris JK, Wald NJ, Watt HC. Fetal loss in Down syndrome pregnancies. Prenat Diagn 1999;19:142–145.

92. Merkatz IR, Nitowsky HM, Macri JN, Johnson WE. An association between low maternal serum alpha-fetoprotein and fetal chromosomal abnormalities. Am J Obstet Gynecol 1984;148:886–894.

93. Cuckle HS, Wald NJ, Lindenbaum RH. Maternal serum alpha-fetoprotein measurement: a screening test for Down syndrome. Lancet 1984;1:926–929.

94. Wald NJ, Kennard A, Hackshaw A, McGuire A. Antenatal screening for Down's syndrome. J Med Screen 1997;4:181–246.

95. Chard T, Lowings C, Kitau MJ. α-fetoprotein and chorionic gonadotrophin levels in relation to Down syndrome. Lancet 1984;2:750.

96. Jergansen PI, Trolle D. Low urinary oestriol excretion during pregnancy in women giving birth to infants with Down's syndrome. Lancet 1972;ii:782–784.

97. Canick JA, Knight GJ, Palomaki GE, Haddow JE, Cuckle HS, Wald NJ. Low second trimester maternal serum estriol in Down syndrome pregnancies. Am J Hum Genet 1987;41:A269.

98. Canick JA, Knight GJ, Palomaki GE, Haddow JE, Cuckle HS, Wald NJ. Low second trimester maternal serum unconjugated oestriol in pregnancies with Down syndrome. Br J Obstet Gynaecol 1988;95:330–333.

99. Bogart MH, Pandian MR, Jones OW. Abnormal maternal serum chorionic gonadotropin levels in pregnancies with fetal chromosome abnormalities. Prenat Diagn 1987;7:623–630.

100. Macri JN, Kasturi RV, Krantz DA, et al. Maternal serum Down syndrome screening: free beta-protein is a more effective marker than human chorionic gonadotropin. Am J Obstet Gynecol 1990;163:1248–1253.

101. Knight GJ, Palomaki GE, Neveux LM, Fodor KK, Haddow JE. hCG and the free beta-subunit as screening tests for Down syndrome. Prenat Diagn 1998;18:235–245.

102. Wald NJ, Densem JW, Smith D, Klee GG. Four-marker serum screening for Down's syndrome. Prenat Diagn 1994;14:707–716.

103. Wald NJ, Rodeck C, Hackshaw AK, Walters J, Chitty L, Mackinson AM. First and second trimester antenatal screening for Down's syndrome: the results of the Serum, Urine and Ultrasound Screening Study (SURUSS). J Med Screen 2003;10:56–104.

104. Van Lith JM, Pratt JJ, Beekhuis JR, Mantingh A. Second-trimester maternal serum immunoreactive inhibin as a marker for fetal Down's syndrome. Prenat Diagn 1992;12:801–806.

105. Qin QP, Christiansen M, Nguyen TH, Sorensen S, Larsen SO, Norgaard-Pedersen B. Schwanger-schaftsprotein 1 (SP1) as a maternal serum marker for Down syndrome in the first and second trimesters. Prenat Diagn 1997;17:101–108.

106. Morez C, Maymon R, Jauniaux E, Traub L, Cuckle H. Screening for trisomies 21 and 18 with maternal serum placental isoferritin p43 component. Prenat Diagn 2000;20:395–399.

107. Ryall RG, Staples AJ, Robertson EF, Pollard AC. Improved performance in a prenatal screening programme for Down's syndrome incorporating serum-free hCG subunit analyses. Prenat Diagn 1992;12:251–261.

108. Cuckle HS, Wald NJ, Densem JW, Royston P. The effect of smoking in pregnancy on maternal serum alpha-fetoprotein, unconjugated oestriol, human chorionic gonadotrophin, progesterone and dehydro-epiandrosterone sulphate levels. Br J Obstet Gynaecol 1990;97:272–276.

109. Christiansen M, Oxvig C, Wagner JM, et al. The proform of eosinophil major basic protein: a new maternal serum marker for Down syndrome. Prenat Diagn 1999;19:905–910.

110. Yamamoto R, Azuma M, Wakui Y, et al. Alpha-fetoprotein microheterogeneity: a potential biochemical marker for Down's syndrome. Clin Chim Acta 2001;304:137–141.

111. Cuckle HS, Wald NJ, Goodburn SF, Sneddon J, Amess JA, Dunn SC. Measurement of activity of urea resistant neutrophil alkaline phosphatase as an antenatal screening test for Down's syndrome. Br Med J 1990;301:1024–1026.

112. Cuckle HS, Canick JA, Kellner LH. Collaborative study of maternal urine beta-core human chorionic gonadotrophin screening for Down syndrome. Prenat Diagn 1999;19:911–917.

113. Cuckle HS, Wald NJ. Thompson SG. Estimating a woman's risk of having a pregnancy associated with Down's syndrome using her age and serum alpha-fetoprotein level. Br J Obstet Gynaecol 1987;94:387–402.

114. Palomaki GE, Haddow JE. Maternal serum α fetoprotein, maternal age, and Down syndrome risk. Am J Obstet Gynecol 1987;156:460–463.

115. Wald NJ, Cuckle HS, Densem JW, et al. Maternal serum unconjugated oestriol as an antenatal screening test for Down's syndrome. Br J Obstet Gynaecol 1988;95:334–341.

116. Wald NJ, Cuckle HS, Densem JW, et al. Maternal serum screening for Down's syndrome in early pregnancy. Br Med J 1988;297:883–887.

117. Wald NJ, Densem JW, George L, Muttukrishna S, Knight PG. Prenatal screening for Down's syndrome using inhibin-A as a serum marker. Prenat Diagn 1996;16:143–153. Erratum: Prenat Diagn 1997;17:285–290.

118. Cuckle HS, Holding S, Jones R, Groome NP, Wallace EM. Combining inhibin A with existing second-trimester markers in maternal serum screening for Down's syndrome. Prenat Diagn 1996;16:1095–1100.

119. Haddow JE, Palomaki GE, Knight GJ, Foster DL, Neveux LM. Second trimester screening for Down's syndrome using maternal serum dimeric inhibin A. J Med Screen 1998;5:115–119.

120. Capone GT. Down syndrome: advances in molecular biology and the neurosciences. J Dev Behav Pediatr 2001;22:40–59.

121. Eldar-Geva T, Hochberg A, deGroot N, Weinstein D. High maternal serum chorionic gonadotropin level in Downs' syndrome pregnancies is caused by elevation of both subunits messenger ribonucleic acid level in trophoblasts. J Clin Endocrinol Metab 1995;80:3528–3531

122. Lambert-Messerlian GM, Luisi S, Florio P, Mazza V, Canick JA, Petraglia F. Second trimester levels of maternal serum total activin A and placental inhibin/activin alpha and betaA subunit messenger ribonucleic acids in Down syndrome pregnancy. Eur J Endocrinol 1998;138:425–429.

123. Dalgliesh GL, Aitken DA, Lyall F, Howatson AG, Connor JM. Placental and maternal serum inhibin-A and activin-A levels in Down's syndrome pregnancies. Placenta 2001;22:227–234.

124. Frendo JL, Vidaud M, Guibourdenche J, et al. Defect of villous cytotrophoblast differentiation into syncytiotrophoblast in Down's syndrome. J Clin Endocrinol Metab 2000;85:3700–3707.

125. Newby D, Aitken DA, Crossley JA, Howatson AG, Macri JN, Connor JM. Biochemical markers of trisomy 21 and the pathophysiology of Down's syndrome pregnancies. Prenat Diagn 1997;17:941–951.

126. Newby D, Aitken DA, Howatson AG, Connor JM. Placental synthesis of oestriol in Down's syndrome pregnancies. Placenta 2000;21:263–267.

127. Golbus MS. Development in the first half of gestation of genetically abnormal human fetuses. Teratology 1978;18:333–335.

128. Shepard TH, FitzSimmons JM, Fantel AG, Pascoe-Mason J. Placental weights of normal and aneuploid early human fetuses. Pediatr Pathol 1989;9:425–431.

129. Wald NJ, Hackshaw AK. Advances in antenatal screening for Down syndrome. Best Prac Res Clin Obstet Gynaecol. 2000;14:563–580.

130. Knight GJ, Cole LA. Measurement of choriogonadotropin free beta-subunit: an alternative to choriogonadotropin in screening for fetal Down's syndrome? Clin Chem 1991;37:779–782.

131. Muller F, Doche C, Ngo S, et al. Stability of free beta-subunit in routine practice for trisomy 21 maternal serum screening. Prenat Diagn 1999;19:85–86.

132. McCullagh DR. Dual endocrine activity of the testis. Science 1932;76:19–20.

133. Vale W, Rivier C, Hsueh A, et al. Chemical and biological characterization of the inhibin family of protein hormones. Rec Progress Horm Res 1988;44:1–34.

134. Groome N, O'Brian M. Immunoassays for inhibin and its subunits. J Immunol Meth 1993;165:167–176.

135. Groome NP, Illingworth PJ, O'Brien M, et al. Detection of dimeric inhibin throughout the human menstrual cycle by two-site enzyme immunoassay. Clin Endocrinol 1994;40:717–723.

136. Knight GJ, Palomaki GE, Neveux LM, Haddow JE, Lambert-Messerlian GM. Clinical validation of a new dimeric inhibin-A assay suitable for second trimester Down's syndrome screening. J Med Screen 2001;8:2–7.

137. MacRae AR, Allen LC, Lepage N, Tokmakjian S. Validation of an automated dimeric inhibin A assay for use in maternal serum screening for Down syndrome. Clin Chem 2001;47:A150.

138. Cuckle HS, Wald NJ, Densem JW, Canick J, Abell KB. Second trimester amniotic fluid oestriol, dehydroepiandrosterone sulphate, and human chorionic gonadotrophin levels in Down's syndrome. Br J Obstet Gynaecol 1991;98:1160–1162.

139. Wald NJ, Cheng R, Cuckle HS, et al. Maternal serum levels of the estriol precursor, 16αOH-DHEAS, are low in Down syndrome pregnancy. Am J Hum Genet 1992;51:A1046.

140. Kronquist KE, Dreazen E, Keener SL, Nicholas TW, Crandall BF. Reduced fetal hepatic alpha-fetoprotein levels in Downs syndrome. Prenat Diagn 1990;10:739–751.

141. Cuckle HS, Wald NJ, Lindenbaum RH, Jonasson J. Amniotic fluid AFP levels and Down syndrome. Lancet 1985;1:290–291.

142. Davis RO, Cosper P, Huddleston JF, et al. Decreased levels of amniotic fluid alpha-fetoprotein associated with Down syndrome. Am J Obstet Gynecol 1985;153:541–544.

143. MacRae AR, Heick HMC, Canick JA, Kellner LH. Does the mid-trimester rise in serum unconjugated estriol truly conform to a log-linear pattern? Am J Hum Genet 1998;63:A168.

144. Watt HC, Wald NJ, Huttly WJ. The pattern of maternal serum Inhibin-A concentrations in the second trimester of pregnancy. Prenat Diagn 1998;18:846–848.

145. Wald NJ, Watt HC, Haddow JE, Knight GJ. Screening for Down syndrome at 14 weeks of pregnancy. Prenat Diagn 1998;18:291–293.

146. Benn PA, Borgida A, Home D, Briganti S, Collins R, Rodis JF. Down syndrome and neural tube defect screening: the value of using gestational age by ultrasonography. Am J Obstet Gynecol 1997;176:1056–1061.

147. Haddow JE, Palomaki GE, Knight GJ, Canick JA. In: Prenatal Screening for Major Fetal Disorders, vol. II: Screening for Down Syndrome. Scarborough, ME: Foundation for Blood Research, 1998.

148. Jou H, Shyu M, Shih J, et al. Second trimester maternal serum hCG level in an Asian population: normal reference values by ultrasound dating. J Matern Fetal Med 2000;9:118–121.

149. Benn PA, Clive JM, Collins R. Medians for second-trimester maternal serum alpha-fetoprotein, human chorionic gonadotropin, and unconjugated estriol; differences between races or ethnic groups. Clin Chem 1997;43:333–337.

150. Wald NJ, Cuckle HS, Densem JW, Stone RB. Maternal serum unconjugated oestriol and human chorionic gonadotrophin levels in pregnancies with insulin-dependent diabetes: implications for screening for Down's syndrome. Br J Obstet Gynaecol 1992;99:51–53.

151. Wallace EM, Crossley JA, Ritoe SC, Groome NP, Aitken DA. Maternal serum inhibin-A in pregnancies complicated by insulin dependent diabetes mellitus. Br J Obstet Gynaecol 1997;104:946–948.

152. Wald NJ, Watt HC, George L. Maternal serum inhibin-A in pregnancies with insulin dependent diabetes: implications for screening for Down's syndrome. Prenat Diagn 1996;16:923–926.

153. Watt HC, Wald NJ, George L. Maternal serum inhibin-A levels in twin pregnancies: implications for screening for Down's syndrome. Prenat Diagn 1996;16:927–929.

154. Wald N, Cuckle H, Wu TS, George L. Maternal serum unconjugated oestriol and human chorionic gonadotrophin levels in twin pregnancies: implications for screening for Down's syndrome. Br J Obstet Gynaecol 1991;98:905–908.

155. Muller F, Dreux S, Dupoizat H, et al. Second-trimester Down syndrome maternal serum screening in twin pregnancies: impact of chorionicity. Prenat Diagn 2003;23:331–335.

156. Rudnicka AR, Wald NJ, Huttly W, Hackshaw AK. Influence of maternal smoking on the birth prevalence of Down syndrome and on second trimester screening performance. Prenat Diagn 2002;22:893–897.

157. Bernstein L, Pike MC, Lobo RA, Depue RH, Ross RK, Henderson BE. Cigarette smoking in pregnancy results in marked decrease in maternal hCG and oestradiol levels. Br J Obstet Gynaecol 1989;96:92–96.

158. Palomaki GE, Knight GJ, Haddow JE, Canick JA, Wald NJ, Kennard A. Cigarette smoking and levels of maternal serum alpha-fetoprotein, unconjugated estriol, and hCG: impact on Down syndrome screening. Obstet Gynecol 1993;81:675–678.

159. Benn PA. Advances in prenatal screening for Down syndrome: I. General principles and second trimester testing. Clin Chim Acta 2002;323:1–16.

160. Wald NJ, Watt HC. Serum markers for Down's syndrome in relation to number of previous births and maternal age. Prenat Diagn 1996;16:699–703.

161. Spong CY, Ghidini A, Stanley-Christian H, Meck JM, Seydel FD, Pezzullo JC. Risk of abnormal triple screen for Down syndrome is significantly higher in patients with female fetuses. Prenat Diagn 1999;19:337–339.

162. Sancken U, Bartels I. Preliminary data on an association between blood groups and serum markers used for the so-called "triple screening": free oestriol MoM values are decreased in rhesus-negative (Rh-) women. Prenat Diagn 2001;21:194–195.

163. Larsen SO, Christiansen M, Nergaard-Pedersen B. Inclusion of serum marker measurements from a previous pregnancy improves Down syndrome screening performance. Prenat Diagn 1998;18:706–712.

164. Wald NJ, White N, Morris JK, Huttly WJ, Canick JA. Serum markers for Down's syndrome in women who have had in vitro fertilisation: implications for antenatal screening. Br J Obstet Gynaecol 1999;106:1304–1306.

165. Hsu TY, Ou CY, Hsu JJ, Kung FT, Chang SY, Soong YK. Maternal serum screening for Down syndrome in pregnancies conceived by intra-uterine insemination. Prenat Diagn 1999;19:1012–1014.

166. Palomaki GE, Neveux LM, Haddow JE. Can reliable Down's syndrome detection rates be determined from prenatal screening intervention trials? J Med Screen 1996;3:12–17.

167. Haddow JF. Antenatal screening for Down's syndrome: where are we, where next? Commentary on Snijders et al.1998. Lancet 1998;351:336–337.

168. Wald NJ, Hackshaw AK, Huttly W, Kennard A. Empirical validation of risk screening for Down's syndrome. J Med Screen 1996;3:185–187.

169. Canick JA, Rish S. The accuracy of assigned risks in maternal serum screening. Prenat Diagn 1998;18:413–415.

170. Meier C, Huang T, Wyatt PR, Summers AM. Accuracy of expected risk of Down syndrome using the second-trimester triple test. Clin Chem 2002;48:653–655.

171. Spencer K. Accuracy of Down syndrome risks produced in a first-trimester screening programme incorporating fetal nuchal translucency thickness and maternal serum biochemistry. Prenat Diagn 2002;22:244–246.

172. Palomaki GE, Haddow JE, Beauregard LJ. Prenatal screening for Down's syndrome in Maine, 1980 to 1993. N Engl J Med 1996;334:1409–1410.

173. MacRae AR, Allen LC, Krishnan S, Lepage N, Quesnel R, Tokmakjian S. Maternal serum unconjugated estriol is cost-justified in screening for fetal trisomy. Clin Biochem 1999;32:308.

174. Carroll JC, Reid AJ, Woodward CA, et al. Ontario Maternal Serum Screening Program: practices, knowledge and opinions of health care providers. Can Med Assoc J 1997;156:775–784.

175. Allanson A, Michie S, Marteau TM. Presentation of screen negative results on serum screening for Down's syndrome: variations across Britain. J Med Screen 1997;4:21–22.

176. Marteau TM, Saidi G, Goodburn S, Lawton J, Michie S, Bobrow M. Numbers or words? a randomized controlled trial of presenting screen negative results to pregnant women. Prenat Diagn 2000;20:714–718.

177. Welkenhuysen M, Evers-Kiebooms G, d'Ydewalle G. The language of uncertainty in genetic risk communication: framing and verbal versus numerical information. Patient Educ Couns 2001;43:179–187.

178. Marteau TM, Cook R, Kidd J, et al. The psychological effects of false-positive results in prenatal screening for fetal abnormality: a prospective study. Prenat Diagn 1992;12:205–214.

179. Statham H, Green J. Serum screening for Down's syndrome: some women's experiences. Br Med J 1993;307:174–176.

180. Goel V, Glazier R, Summers A, Holzapfel S. Psychological outcomes following maternal serum screening: a cohort study. Can Med Assoc J 1998;159:651–656.

181. Kornman LH, Wortelboer MJ, Beekhuis JR, Morssink LP, Matingh A. Women's opinions and the implications of first versus second trimester screening for fetal Down's syndrome. Prenat Diagn 1997;17:1011–1018.

182. Canick JA, Kellner LH, Cole LA, Cuckle HS. Urinary analyte screening: a noninvasive detection method for Down syndrome? Mol Med Today 1999;5:68–73.

183. Cole LA, Cermik D, Bahado-Singh R. Oligosaccharide variants of hCG-related molecules: potential screening markers for Down syndrome. Prenat Diagn 1997;17:1187–1190.

184. Cole LA, Omrani A, Cermik D, Bahado-Singh RO, Mahoney MJ. Hyperglycosylated hCG: a potential alternative to hCG in Down syndrome screening. Prenat Diagn 1998;18:926–933.

185. Cole LA, Shahabi S, Oz UA, et al. Urinary screening tests for fetal Down syndrome: II. Hyperglycosylated hCG. Prenat Diagn 1999;19:351–359.

186. Vendely PM, Lu J, Plewnia J, et al. Measurement of second trimester maternal serum invasive trophoblast antigen (ITA) for Down syndrome (DS) screening. Clin Chem 2003;49:A132.

187. Cuckle HS, Shahabi S, Sehmi IK, Jones R, Cole LH. Maternal urine hyperglycosylated hCG in pregnancies with Down syndrome. Prenat Diagn 1999;19:918–920.

188. Simpson JL, Elias S. Isolating fetal cells from maternal blood: advances in prenatal diagnosis through molecular technology. JAMA 1993;270:2357–2361.

189. Bianchi DW. Current knowledge about fetal cells in the maternal circulation. J Perinat Med 1998;26:175–185.

190. Hahn S, Sant R, Holzgreve W. Fetal cells in maternal blood: current and future perspectives. Mol Hum Reprod 1998;4:515–521.

191. Bianchi DW, Williams JM, Sullivan LM, Hanson FW, Klinger KW, Shuber AP. PCR quantitation of fetal cells in maternal blood in normal and aneuploid pregnancies. Am J Hum Genet 1997;61:822–829.

192. Lo YMD, Corbetta N, Chamberlain PF, et al. Presence of fetal DNA in maternal plasma and serum. Lancet 1997;350:485–487.

193. Lo YMD, Tein MSC, Lau TK, et al. Quantitative analysis of fetal DNA in maternal plasma and serum: implications for noninvasive prenatal diagnosis. Am J Hum Genet 1998;62:768–775.

194. Lo YMD, Lau TK, Zhang J, et al. Increased fetal DNA concentrations in the plasma of pregnant women carrying fetuses with trisomy 21. Clin Chem 1999;45:1747–1751.

195. Lee T, LeShane ES, Messerlian GM, et al. Down syndrome and cell-free fetal DNA in archived maternal serum. Am J Obstet Gynecol 2002;187:1217–1221.

196. Xiao YZ, Burk MR, Troeger C, Jackson LR, Holzgreve W, Hahn S. Fetal DNA in maternal plasma is elevated in pregnancies with aneuploidy fetuses. Prenat Diagn 2000;20:795–798.

197. Benn PA. Advances in prenatal screening for Down syndrome: II. First trimester testing, integrated testing, and future directions. Clin Chim Acta 2002;324:1–11.

198. Bayes-Genis A, Conover CA, Overgaard MT, et al. Pregnancy-associated plasma protein A as a marker of acute coronary syndromes. N Engl J Med 2001;345:1022–1029.

199. Wald NJ, Stone R, Cuckle HS, et al. First trimester concentrations of pregnancy associated plasma protein A and placental protein 14 in Down's syndrome Br Med J. 1992;305:28.

200. Spencer K, Aitken DA, Crossley JA, et al. First trimester biochemical screening for trisomy 21: the role for free beta hCG, alpha fetoprotein and pregnancy associated plasma protein A. Ann Clin Biochem 1994;31:447–454.

201. Brambati B, Tului L, Bonacchi I, Shrimanker K, Suzuki Y, Grudzinskas JG. Serum PAPP-A, free β-hCG are first trimester screening markers for Down syndrome. Prenat Diagn 1994;14:1043–1047.

202. Wald NJ, George L, Smith D, Densem JW, Petterson K. Serum screening for Down's syndrome between 8 and 14 weeks of pregnancy. Br J Obstet Gynaecol 1996;103:407–412.

203. Brizot ML, Snijders RJ, Bersinger NA, Kuhn P, Nicolaides KH. Maternal serum pregnancy-associated plasma protein A and fetal nuchal translucency thickness for the prediction of fetal trisomies in early pregnancy. Obstet Gynecol 1994;84:918–922.

204. Haddow JE, Palomaki GE, Knight GJ, Williams J, Miller WA, Johnson A. Screening of maternal serum for fetal Down's syndrome in the first trimester. N Engl J Med 1998;338:955–961.

205. Cuckle HS, van Lith JM. Appropriate biochemical parameters in first-trimester screening for Down syndrome. Prenat Diagn, 1999;19:505–512.

206. Bersinger NA, Brizot ML, Johnson A, et al. First trimester maternal serum pregnancy-associated plasma protein A and pregnancy-specific beta 1-glycoprotein in fetal trisomies. Br J Obstet Gynaecol 1994;101:970–974.

207. Cuckle H, Arbuzova S. The efficiency and clinical practicality of multi-modality screening strategies. In: Macck M, Bianchi D, Cuckle H, eds. Early Prenatal Diagnosis, Fetal Cells and DNA in the mother: Proceedings of the 12th Fetal Cell Workshop. Prague: Charles University Press, 2002.

208. Hallahan T, Krantz D, Orlandi F, et al. First trimester biochemical screening for Down syndrome: free beta hCG versus intact hCG. Prenat Diagn, 2000;20:785–789.

209. Haddow JE, Palomaki GE, Knight GJ. Response to Hallahan et al. Prenat Diagn 2000;20:790–791.

210. Spencer K, Berry E, Crossley JA, Aitken DA, Nicolaides KH. Is maternal serum total hCG a marker of trisomy 21 in the first trimester of pregnancy? Prenat Diagn 2000;20:311–317.

211. Berry E, Aitken DA, Crossley JA, Macri JN, Conner JM. Screening for Down's syndrome: changes in marker levels and detection rates between first and second trimesters. Br J Obstet Gynaecol 1997;104:811–817.

212. de Graaf IM, Cuckle HS, Pajkrt E, Leschot NJ, Bleker OP, van Lith JM. Co-variables in first trimester maternal serum screening. Prenat Diagn 2000;20:186–189.

213. Spencer K, Ong CYT, Liao AWJ, Nicolaides KH. The influence of ethnic origin on first trimester biochemical markers of chromosomal abnormalities. Prenat Diagn 2000;20:491–494.

214. Spencer K. The influence of smoking on maternal serum PAPP-A and free beta hCG levels in the first trimester of pregnancy. Prenat Diagn 1999;19:1065–1066.

215. Spencer K, Ong CY, Liao AW, Papademetriou D, Nicolaides KH. First trimester markers of trisomy 21 and the influence of maternal cigarette smoking status. Prenat Diagn 2000;20:852–853.

216. Bronshtein M, Rottem S, Yoffe N, Blumenfeld Z. First-trimester and early second-trimester diagnosis of nuchal cystic hygroma by transvaginal sonography: diverse prognosis of the septated from the nonseptated lesion. Am J Obstet Gynecol 1989;161:78–82.

217. Cicero S, Curcio P, Papageorghiou A, Sonek J, Nicolaides K. Absence of nasal bone in fetuses with trisomy 21 at 11–14 weeks of gestation: an observational study. Lancet 2001;358:1665–1667.

218. Pandya PP, Snijders RJ, Johnson SP, De Lourdes Brizot M, Nicolaides KH. Screening for fetal trisomies by maternal age and fetal nuchal translucency thickness at 10 to 14 weeks of gestation. Br J Obstet Gynaecol 1995;102:957–962.

219. Chitty LS, Pandya PP. Ultrasound screening for fetal abnormalities in the first trimester. Prenat Diagn 1997;17:1269–1281.

220. Devine PC, Malone FD. First trimester screening for structural abnormalities: nuchal translucency sonography. Semin Perinatol 1999;23:382–392.

221. Pajkrt E, Mol BW, Bleker OP, Bilardo CM. Pregnancy outcome and nuchal translucency measurements in fetuses with a normal karyotype. Prenat Diagn 1999;19:1104–1108.

222. Pandya PP, Kondylios A, Hilbert KH. Abnormalities of the heart and great arteries in first trimester chromosomally abnormal fetuses. Am J Med Genet 1995;5:15–19.

223. Hyett JA, Perdu M, Shariand GK, Snijders RS, Nicolaides KH. Increased nuchal translucency at 10–14 weeks of gestation as a marker for major cardiac defects. Ultrasound Obstet Gynecol 1997;10:242–246.

224. Snijders R, Smith E. The role of fetal nuchal translucency in prenatal screening. Curr Opin Obstet Gynecol 2002;14:577–585.

225. Souka AP, Krampl E, Bakalis S, Heath V, Nicolaides KH. Outcome of pregnancy in chromosomally normal fetuses with increased nuchal translucency in the first trimester. Ultrasound Obstet Gynecol 2001;18:9–17.

226. Cullen MT, Gabrielli S, Green JJ, et al. Diagnosis and significance of cystic hygroma in the first trimester. Prenat Diagn 1990;10:643–651.

227. Nicolaides KH, Azar G, Byrne D, Mansur C, Marks K. Fetal nuchal translucency: ultrasound screening for chromosomal defects in first trimester of pregnancy. Br Med J 1992;304:867–869.

228. Pandya PP, Brizot ML, Kuhn P, Snijders RJ, Nicolaides KH. First-trimester fetal nuchal translucency thickness and risk for trisomies. Obstet Gynecol 1994;84:420–423.

229. Pandya PP, Kondylios A, Hilbert L, Snijders RJ, Nicolaides KH. Chromosomal defects and outcome in 1015 fetuses with increased nuchal translucency. Ultrasound Obstet Gynecol 1995;5:15–19.

230. Snijders RJM, Johnson S, Sebire NJ, Noble PL, Nicolaides KH. First trimester ultrasound screening for chromosomal defects. Ultrasound Obstet Gynaecol 1996;7:216–226.

231. Schuchter K, Wald N, Hackshaw AK, Hafner E, Liebhart E. The distribution of nuchal translucency at 10–13 weeks of pregnancy. Prenat Diagn 1998;18:281–286.

232. Faraut T, Cans C, Althuser M, Jouk PS. Combined use of nuchal translucency, gestational age and maternal age for evaluation of the risk of trisomy 21. [French] J Gynecol Obstet Biol Reprod (Paris) 1999;28:439–445.

233. Wald NJ, Hackshaw AK. Combining ultrasound and biochemistry in first-trimester screening for Down's syndrome. Prenat Diagn 1997;17:821–829.

234. Snijders RJM, Noble P, Sebire N, Souka A, Nicolaides KH. UK multicentre project on assessment of risk of trisomy 21 by maternal age and fetal nuchal-translucency thickness at 10–14 weeks of gestation. Lancet 1998;351:343–346.

235. Mol BW, Lijmer JG, van der Meulen J, Pajkrt E, Bilardo CM, Bossuyt PM. Effect of study design on the association between nuchal translucency measurement and Down syndrome. Obstet Gynecol 1999;94:864–869.

236. Chasen ST, Skupski DW, McCullough LB, Chervenak FA. Prenatal informed consent for sonogram: the time for first-trimester nuchal translucency has come. J Ultrasound Med 2001;20:1147–1152. Comments: J Ultrasound Med 2002;21:481–487.

237. Zoppi MA, Ibba RM, Floris M, Monni G. Fetal nuchal translucency screening in 12495 pregnancies in Sardinia. Ultrasound Obstet Gynecol 2001;18:649–651.

238. Crossley JA, Aitken DA, Cameron AD, McBride E, Connor JM. Combined ultrasound and biochemical screening for Down's syndrome in the first trimester: a Scottish multicentre study. Br J Obstet Gynaecol 2002;109:667–676.

239. Logghe H, Cuckle H, Sehmi I. Centre-specific ultrasound nuchal translucency medians needed for Down syndrome screening. Prenat Diagn 2003;23:389–392.

240. Edwards A, Mulvey S, Wallace EM. The effect of image size on nuchal translucency measurement. Prenat Diagn 2003;23:284–286.

241. Jou HJ, Wu SC, Li TC, Hsu HC, Tzeng CY, Hsieh FJ. Relationship between fetal nuchal translucency and crown–rump length in an Asian population. Ultraound Obstet Gynecol 2001;17:111–114.

242. Chen M, Lam YH, Tang MH, et al. The effect of ethnic origin on nuchal translucency at 10–14 weeks of gestation. Prenat Diagn 2002;22:576–578.

243. Maymon R, Padoa E, Dreazen E, Herman A. Nuchal translucency measurements in consecutive normal pregnancies: is there a predisposition to increased levels? Prenat Diagn 2002;22:759–762.

244. Spencer K, Ong CY, Liao AW, Nicolaides KH. The influence of parity and gravidity on first trimester markers of chromosomal abnormality. Prenat Diagn 2000;20:792–794.

245. Monni G, Zoppi MA, Ibba RM. Absence of nasal bone and detection of trisomy 21. Lancet 2002;359:1343.

246. Otano L, Aiello H, Igarzabal L, Matayoshi T, Gadow EC. Association between first trimester absence of fetal nasal bone on ultrasound and Down syndrome. Prenat Diagn 2002;22:930–932.

247. De Biasio P, Venturini PL. Absence of nasal bone and detection of trisomy 21. Lancet, 2002;359:1344.

248. Cicero S, Bindra R, Rembouskos G, Spencer K, Nicolaides KH. Integrated ultrasound and biochemical screening for trisomy 21 using fetal nuchal translucency, absent fetal nasal bone, free β-hCG and PAPP-A at 11 to 14 weeks. Prenat Diagn 2003;23:306–310.

249. Whittle M. Down's syndrome screening: where to now? Br J Obstet Gynaecol 2001;108:559–561.

250. Hackshaw AK, Wald NJ, Haddow JE. Down's syndrome screening with nuchal translucency. Lancet 1996;348:1740.

251. Cuckle HS. Growing complexity in the choice of Down's syndrome screening policy. Ultrasound Obstet Gynecol 2002;19:323–326.

252. Nicolaides KH, Snijders RJ, Cuckle HS. Correct estimation of parameters for ultrasound nuchal translucency screening. Prenat Diagn 1998;18:519–523.

253. Bewley S, Roberts LJ, Mackinson AM, Rodeck CH. First trimester fetal nuchal translucency: problems with screening the general population. Br J Obstet Gynaecol 1995;102:386–388.

254. Hyett JA, Sebire NJ, Snijders RJM, Nicolaides KH. Intrauterine lethality of trisomy 21 fetuses with increased nuchal translucency thickness. Ultrasound Obstet Gynecol 1996;7:101–103.

255. Wald NJ. First-trimester nuchal translucency screening. J Ultrasound Med 2002;21:481.

256. Noble PL, Abraha HD, Snijders RJ, Sherwood R, Nicolaides KH. Screening for fetal trisomy 21 in the first trimester of pregnancy: maternal serum free beta-hCG and fetal nuchal translucency thickness. Ultrasound Obstet Gynecol 1995;6:390–395.

257. Spencer K, Noble P, Snijders RJ, Nicolaides KH. First-trimester urine free beta hCG, beta core, and total oestriol in pregnancies affected by Down's syndrome: implications for first-trimester screening with nuchal translucency and serum free beta hCG. Prenat Diagn 1997;17:525–538.

258. Brizot ML, Snijders RJ, Butler J, Bersinger NA, Nicolaides KH. Maternal serum hCG and fetal nuchal translucency thickness for the prediction of fetal trisomies in the first trimester of pregnancy. Br J Obstet Gynaecol 1995;102:127–132.

259. Spencer K, Spencer CE, Power M, Moakes A, Nicolaides KH. One stop clinic for risk assessment for fetal anomalies: a report of the first year of prospective screening for chromosome anomalies in the first trimester. Br J Obstet Gynaecol 2000;107:1271–1275.

260. Wapner R, Thom E, Simpson JL, et al. First-trimester screening for trisomies 21 and 18. N Engl J Med 2003;349:1405–1413.

261. Hackshaw AK, Wald NJ. Estimation of risk in second trimester serum screening for Down syndrome among women who have already had first trimester screening. Prenat Diagn 2002;22:1051–1055.

262. Hackshaw AK, Wald NJ. Assessment of the value of reporting partial screening results in prenatal screening for Down syndrome. Prenat Diagn 2001;21:737–740.

263. Wald NJ, Watt HC, Hackshaw AK. Integrated screening for Down's syndrome on the basis of tests performed during the first and second trimesters. N Engl J Med 1999;341:461–467.

264. Hook EB, Cross PK, Schreinemachers DM. Chromosomal abnormality rates at amniocentesis and in live-born infants. JAMA 1983;249:2034–2038.

265. Hook EB, Topol BB, Cross PK. The natural history of cytogenetically abnormal fetuses detected at midtrimester amniocentesis which are not terminated electively: new data and estimates of the excess and relative risk of later fetal death associated with the 47,+21 and some other abnormal karyotypes. Am J Hum Genet 1989;45:855–861.

266. Carter PE, Pearn JH, Bell J, Martin N, Anderson NG. Survival in trisomy 18. Clin Genet 1985;27:59–61.

267. Schneider AS, Mennuti MT, Zackai EH. High cesarean section rate in trisomy 18 births: a potential indication for late prenatal diagnosis. Am J Obstet Gynecol 1981;140:367–370.

268. Canick JA, Palomaki GE, Osthanondh R. Prenatal screening for trisomy 18 in the second trimester. Prenat Diagn 1990;10:546–548.

269. Palomaki GE, Knight GJ, Haddow JE, Canick JA, Saller DN Jr, Panizza DS. Prospective intervention trial of a screening protocol to identify fetal trisomy 18 using maternal serum alpha-fetoprotein, unconjugated oestriol, and human chorionic gonadotropin. Prenat Diagn 1992;12:925–930.

270. Palomaki GE, Haddow JE, Knight GJ, et al. Risk-based prenatal screening for trisomy 18 using alpha-fetoprotein, unconjugated oestriol and human chorionic gonadotropin. Prenat Diagn 1995;15:713–723.

271. Benn PA, Leo MV, Rodis JF, Beazoglou T, Collins R, Horne D. Maternal serum screening for fetal trisomy 18: a comparison of fixed cutoff and patient-specific risk protocols. Obstet Gynecol 1999;93:707–711.

272. Hogge WA, Fraer L, Melegari T. Maternal serum screening for fetal trisomy 18: benefits of patient-specific risk protocol. Am J Obstet Gynecol 2001;185:289–293.

273. Aitken DA, Wallace EM, Crossley JA, et al. Dimeric inhibin-A as a marker for Down's syndrome in early pregnancy. N Engl J Med 1996;334:1231–1236.

274. Lambert-Messerlian GM, Saller DN Jr, Tumber MB, French CA, Peterson CJ, Canick JA. Second trimester maternal serum inhibin A levels in fetal trisomy 18 and Turner syndrome with and without hydrops. Prenat Diagn 1998;18:1061–1067.

275. Spencer K, Nicolaides KH. A first trimester trisomy 13/trisomy 18 risk algorithm combining fetal nuchal translucency thickness, maternal serum free beta-hCG and PAPP-A. Prenat Diagn 2002;22:877–879.

276. Sherod C, Sebire NJ, Soares W, Snijders RJM, Nicolaides KH. Prenatal diagnosis of trisomy 18 at the 10–14 week ultrasound scan. Ultrasound Obstet Gynecol 1997;10:387–390.

277. Tul N, Spencer K, Noble P, Chan C, Nicolaides K. Screening for trisomy 18 by fetal nuchal translucency and maternal serum free beta-hCG and PAPP-A at 10–14 weeks of gestation. Prenat Diagn 1999;19:1035–1042.

278. Palomaki GE, Neveux LM, Knight GJ, Haddow JE. Maternal serum-integrated screening for trisomy 18 using both first- and second-trimester markers. Prenat Diagn 2003;243–247.

279. Tint GS, Irons M, Elias ER, et al. Defective cholesterol biosynthesis associated with the Smith Lemli Opitz syndrome. N Engl J Med 1994;30:107–113.

280. Smith DW, Lemli L, Opitz JM. A newly recognized syndrome of multiple congential anomalies. J Pediatr 1964;64:210–217.

281. Bradley LA, Palomaki GE, Knight GJ, et al. Levels of unconjugated estriol and other maternal serum markers in pregnancies with Smith-Lemli-Opitz (RSH) syndrome fetuses. Am J Med Genet 1999;82:355–358.

282. Palomaki GE, Bradley LA, Knight GJ, Craig WY, Haddow JE. Assigning risk for Smith-Lemli-Opitz syndrome as part of 2nd trimester screening for Down's syndrome. J Med Screen 2002;9:43–44.

283. Saller DN Jr, Canick JA, Schwartz S, Blitzer MG. Multiple-marker screening in pregnancies with hydropic and nonhydropic Turner syndrome. Am J Obstet Gynecol 1992;167:1021–1024.

284. Laundon CH, Spencer K, Macri JN, Anderson RW, Buchanan PD. Free beta hCG screening of hydropic and non-hydropic Turner syndrome pregnancies. Prenat Diagn 1996;16:853–856.

285. Benn PA, Gainey A, Ingardia CJ, Rodis JF, Egan JFX. Second trimester maternal serum analytes in triploid pregnancies: correlation with phenotype and sex chromosome complement. Prenat Diagn 2001;21:680–686.

286. Oyer CE, Canick JA. Maternal serum hCG levels in triploidy: variability and need to consider molar tissue. Prenat Diagn 1992;12:627–629.

287. Saller DN Jr, Canick JA, Blitzer MG, et al. Second-trimester maternal serum analyte levels associated with fetal trisomy 13. Prenat Diagn 1999;19:813–816.

288. Caritis S, Sibai B, Hauth J, et al. Low-dose aspirin to prevent preeclampsia in women at high risk. N Engl J Med 1998;338:701–705.

289. Levine RJ, Hauth JC, Curet LB, et al. Trial of calcium to prevent preeclampsia. N Engl J Med 1997;337:69–76.

290. Cuckle H, Sehmi I, Jones R. Maternal serum inhibin A can predict preeclampsia. Br J Obstet Gynaecol 1998;105:1101–1103.

291. Aquilina J, Barnett A, Thompson O, Harrington K. Second-trimester maternal serum inhibin A concentrations as an early marker for preeclampsia. Am J Obstet Gynecol 1999;181:131–136.

292. Lambert-Messerlian GM, Silver HM, Petraglia F, et al. Second-trimester levels of maternal serum human chorionic gonadotropin and inhibin A as predictors of preeclampsia in the third trimester of pregnancy. J Soc Gynecol Invest 2000;7:170–174.

293. Wald NJ, Morris JK. Multiple marker second trimester serum screening for pre-eclampsia. J Med Screen 2001;8:65.

294. Gross SJ, Phillips OP, Shulman LP, et al. Adverse perinatal outcome in patients screen-positive for neural tube defects and fetal Down syndrome. Prenat Diagn 1994;14:609–613.

295. Pergament E, Stein AK, Fiddler M, Cho NH, Kupferminc MJ. Adverse pregnancy outcome after a false-positive screen for Down syndrome using multiple markers. Obstet Gynecol 1995;86:255–258.

296. Wilkins-Haug L. Unexplained elevated maternal serum alpha-fetoprotein: what is the appropriate follow-up? Curr Opin Obstet Gynecol 1998;10:469–474.

297. Huerta-Enochian G, Katz V, Erfurth S. The association of abnormal alpha-fetoprotein and adverse pregnancy outcome: does increased fetal surveillance affect pregnancy outcome? Am J Obstet Gynecol 2001; 184:1549–1553.

298. Balion CM, MacRae AR. Assay-dependent differences in the population distributions of five unconjugated estriol methods, and their effect on prenatal screening performance. Am J Human Genet 2000;67:A1344.

299. Sancken U, Bartels I, Louwen F, Eiben B. A retrospective evaluation of second-trimester serum screening for fetal trisomy 18: experience of two laboratories. Prenat Diagn 1999;19:947–954.

300. Sancken U, Bahner D. The effect of thermal instability of intact human chorionic gonadotropin (ihCG) on the application of its free beta-subunit (free beta hCG) as a serum marker in Down syndrome screening. Prenat Diagn 1995;15:731–738.

301. Tokmakejian SD, Haines MDS, Chan MK, MacRae AR. Development and validation of an extended-range hCG assay on the Technicon Immuno 1 analyser. In: proceedings of the 5th Technicon Immuno 1 International Symposium, Paris, France; 1996;86. Wilton, CT: Chase Medical Communications.

6 Chromosome Analysis in Prenatal Diagnosis

Syed M. Jalal, PhD, FACMG,
Adewale Adeyinka, MBBS, PhD,
and Alan Thornhill, PhD

CONTENTS

INTRODUCTION

Prenatal diagnosis for chromosome anomalies is an important aspect of preventive medicine. Historically, amniocentesis, a procedure to collect fetal amniotic fluid (AF) by transcervical or transabdominal puncture, has been practiced since the 1930s. It was demonstrated in the mid-1960s that human amniotic cells can be cultured and used for chromosome analysis and that the optimal timing for amniocentesis was around 16 wk gestation *(1,2)*. Amniocentesis is now common and is usually performed between 14 and 16 wk gestation, although early amniocentesis, around 12 wk gestation, or amniocentesis later than 16 wk are possible depending on the medical needs.

In addition to amniocentesis, another option for procurement of cells for cytogenetic studies is chorionic villus sampling (CVS) from the placenta by a catheter inserted transvaginally. The procedure has been in use in China since the 1970s. It has become an accepted prenatal procedure worldwide since the early 1980s *(3)*. The CVS procedure has the advantage compared to amniocentesis that it is performed earlier (9–12 wk gestation) but the risk for maternal cell contamination is higher.

Percutaneous umbilical cord blood sampling (PUBS) is another prenatal technique that is reserved for very critical clinical situations. It is a procedure to procure fetal blood from the umbilical cord by a needle guided by ultrasound images. The risk for spontaneous abortion or other complications is significantly more for PUBS compared to amniocentesis or CVS.

From: *Current Clinical Pathology: Handbook of Clinical Laboratory Testing During Pregnancy*
Edited by: A. M. Gronowski © Humana Press, Totowa, NJ

It is now possible to perform preimplantation genetic diagnosis (PGD) to test embryos for specific genetic disorders or chromosomal abnormalities before a pregnancy begins. Embryos derived from in vitro fertilization (IVF) techniques are tested for a specific genetic disorder or screened for chromosomal abnormalities by removing one or two cells for analysis. Embryos judged to be free of the disorder or chromosomal abnormality under test are transferred into the womb to initiate a pregnancy. PGD is an alternative to prenatal tests such as amniocentesis or CVS and because it is performed before a pregnancy has begun, it may be more acceptable to couples who have either had an affected child or a previous termination of pregnancy, or who have objections to termination of pregnancy.

Although PGD was developed initially for the prevention of specific single-gene defects, it is now used to identify common chromosome abnormalities in embryos. In this way, couples may have an increased chance of a healthy genetically related child by avoiding offspring with trisomies (such as Down syndrome) and recurrent miscarriages, many of which are caused by numeric chromosomal abnormalities (Tables 1 and 2).

In this chapter, we provide an overview of the techniques, results, and interpretation of amniocentesis, CVS, and PGD. Recent developments involving the use of fluorescent DNA probes and fluorescent *in situ* hybridization (FISH) for rapid results are highlighted.

OVERVIEW OF METHODS

Amniotic Fluid Cells

Amniocytes present in the AF are the most widely used tissue type for prenatal diagnosis. They can be grown in a fluid culture in flasks (T-type) or grown in monolayer attached to the glass surface of coverslips (*in situ* culture). The *in situ* culture has a faster turnaround time than the flask culture method, which is helpful in resolving the issue of mosaicism and is adaptable to a semiautomated harvesting system. However, when larger numbers of cells are needed, culture in flasks is necessary. Cell cultures are possible in appropriate combinations of a chemically defined medium (RPM1-1640, Chang medium, α MEM, etc.), biologically defined medium fetal bovine serum, L-glutamine, and antibiotics (penicillin and streptomycin).

An adequate sample size of AF is needed (optimally $\geq$20 mL) in sterile conditions for culture, although successful cultures can be established with 8–10 mL of fluid. The first 2 mL of AF that is obtained is contaminated up to 60% of the time (our experience) with maternal blood and is best discarded, especially for FISH analysis. Optimally, the sample is collected at 14–16 wk gestation, but smaller samples from 12 to 13 wk (proportion of living cells are more but fluid volume is less) or beyond 16 wk, including very late gestation (proportion of dead cells increases with increasing gestation), are possible.

Multiple cultures are set up in two separate incubators (with defined levels of nitrogen, oxygen, and carbon dioxide for optimum condition of cell growth) to ensure adequate and high quality of culture results and also ensure against incubator malfunction or single flask contamination. Many laboratories use automated robotic harvesting *(4)* systems and drying chambers *(5)* for harvesting the amniocytes in preparation of microscope analysis for increased efficiency and higher quality. In most cases, routine processing (guidelines set by accrediting agencies) is adequate. However, when mosaicism is suspected (e.g., more than two cells or two colonies have an extra chromosome or a structural abnormality, or three cells or three colonies have a missing chromosome), additional

Table 1
Incidence of Chromosome Abnormalities Among Newborns

Chromosome abnormalities	Incidence of abnormalities (rate/1000)			
	Norway[a] (1830 children)	Denmark[b] (34,910 children)	Japan[c] (14,835 children)	Pooled data (Canada, Europe, US, and USSR)[d] (54,749 children)
Numerical abnormalities				
Sex chromosomes	2.1	2.3	1.95	1.95
Autosomes	2.73	2.1	1.82	1.35
Structural balanced abnormalities				
Robertsonian translocations	2.19	1.23	0.74	0.95
Inversions	7.10	0.34	0.13	0.13
Inversion Y	3.14	0	0.13	0.26
Reciprocal translocations	2.73	1.4	0.74	0.84
Structural unbalanced abnormalities				
Robertsonian translocations	0	0	0.13	0.04
Reciprocal translocations	0	0.09	0.2	0.13
Deletions	0	0.11	0.06	0.09
Duplications	0	0.09	0	0
Others	2.19	0.8	0.4	0.35
Total Abnormalities	19.67	8.45	6.27	5.75

[a]Ref. 25, [b]Ref. 26, [c]Ref. 27, [d]Ref. 28.

quality control steps must be taken. Use of *in situ* culture is recommended and has the advantage that an average of 15 colonies (clone of cells arising from a single amniocyte results in a colony on a coverslip surface) are analyzed. If a single cell in a colony is abnormal, it is considered an artifact (it is common for such cultures and can be induced by the chemicals used for culturing and harvesting). If multiple cells of a colony and more than two or three colonies have the same abnormality, mosaicism is suspected. Usually, more colonies (e.g., 30 rather than the normal 15) are analyzed to establish the proportion of the mosaicism. For clinical diagnosis, establishment of the proportion of mosaicism is important. About 3% of Down syndrome patients may have mosaicism (47,XX or XY,+21/46,XX, or XY); up to 75% of Turner patients may have mosaicism (45,X/46,XX), especially when more than one tissue (blood and skin biopsy) is examined: and mosaicism is relatively common in spontaneous abortions especially early in gestation (Table 2).

Maternal cell contamination from blood is common (up to 60% in our experience), which does interfere with culturing success but is of no consequence in reporting results because the blood cells are eliminated in the processing. However, maternal cells from skin can culture with amniocytes (1 in about 118 specimens in our experience) and must be considered in interpreting results.

Table 2
Types and Frequency of Chromosome Abnormalities in Spontaneous Abortions

Chromosome constitution	Number of miscarriages				
	1000[a]	460[b]	571[c]	420[d]	Average/1000
Trisomy 1	0	0	0	0	0
Trisomy 2	5	5	7	4	8.57
Trisomy 3	1	3	2	0	2.45
Trisomy 4	8	4	1	1	5.71
Trisomy 5	1	0	0	1	0.82
Trisomy 6	3	1	1	3	3.26
Trisomy 7	8	3	7	3	8.57
Trisomy 8	7	3	6	4	8.16
Trisomy 9	1	3	1	4	3.67
Trisomy 10	1	3	1	1	2.45
Trisomy 11	1	2	1	1	2.04
Trisomy 12	2	0	1	1	1.63
Trisomy 13	10	15	10	11	18.77
Trisomy 14	5	7	5	11	11.42
Trisomy 15	14	9	11	22	22.85
Trisomy 16	51	32	42	19	58.75
Trisomy 17	2	0	0	2	1.63
Trisomy 18	5	4	7	4	8.16
Trisomy 19	0	1	0	0	0.41
Trisomy 20	7	1	3	2	5.30
Trisomy 21	26	9	7	12	22.03
Trisomy 22	29	28	14	16	35.50
Double trisomy	9	7	4	9	11.83
Mosaic trisomy	12	0	10	0	8.98
Autosomal trisomy (NOS)	9	0	0	0	3.67
Sex Trisomy	2	1	2	1	2.45
Monosomy X	112	42	22	18	79.15
Triploidy	70	59	39	27	79.56
Tetraploidy	33	6	10	10	24.07
Structural abnormalities	20	23	15	8	26.93
Other abnormalities	1	1	0	0	0.82

[a]Ref. 29, [b]Ref. 30, [c]Ref. 31, [d]Ref. 32.

The average turnaround time (time between the receipt of the specimen and reporting out of results) varies between 7 and 21 d, but the in situ method allows an average turnaround time of 7–10 d.

CVS

Prenatal analysis can also be performed from a biopsy of placental chorionic villi. A thin plastic catheter is used transvaginally to obtain samples of the villi. Generally, the risk for complications, including abortion, is quite low (about 1%). The procedure is most commonly performed between 9 and 12 wk gestation. Because of the physical nature of sampling, maternal cell contamination is quite common. An adequate sample of CVS is 15–20 mg and chances for adequate results are low if the sample is less than 5 mg.

Chorionic villi are cultured using either direct method or culture technique. In the direct method, dividing cells from the chorionic villi are used for analysis without culture or only a short-term culture (24–48 h). Because of high maternal cell contamination (decidua), direct culture is generally followed by a long-term culture technique. Long-term culture technique involves culturing cells obtained from villi that have been carefully cleaned and macerated, and the cells are isolated after enzymatic treatments (trypsin and collagenase). Once the cells are isolated, the culture technique is similar to that described for the amniocyte culture. The quality of metaphases (dividing cells for analysis) is generally superior from long-term culture, and maternal cell contamination is limited. For greater detail on culture, harvest, and analysis, other references are available *(6,7)*.

Preimplantation Genetic Diagnosis

The first laboratory component of PGD involves the collection of diagnostic material for testing (as would be required for amniocentesis or CVS). This is usually performed in a clinical IVF laboratory under sterile conditions. The second step involves the diagnostic test itself, which can be performed in an area adjacent to the IVF laboratory equipped to perform FISH analysis or in a completely separate dedicated cytogenetics laboratory with experience in processing single-cell samples.

A set of micromanipulators linked to an inverted microscope with phase contrast optics and facilities for extended embryo culture are the essential requirements to carry out diagnostic biopsy procedures. Theoretically, diagnostic material can be collected at any developmental stage between the mature oocyte (egg) and blastocyst (embryo with up to 200 cells). If PGD is performed using an egg, only maternal abnormalities can be identified whereas both maternal and paternal abnormalities can be diagnosed in the developing embryo. Irrespective of the stage at which diagnostic material is obtained, the biopsy method is a two-step procedure: the first step is to breach the zona pellucida (outer coat of the egg or embryo) and the second involves the removal of cellular material. Zona breaching can be achieved mechanically (by means of a sharp microneedle), chemically (using acidified Tyrode's solution, pH 2.2) or by thermal ablation (using a noncontact laser). Currently, the stage at which most centers obtain genetic material for PGD is on the third day following insemination when the embryo has between 6 and 10 cells. At this stage, embryonic cells are generally equivalent in size and developmental potential, and embryo survival and metabolism appears to be unaffected by the biopsy procedure *(8)*. Removal of cellular material is generally carried out using a glass micropipet attached to a pneumatic- or hydraulic-based suction system (Fig. 1).

While recent reports suggest that successful biopsy is achieved in 97% of cases *(9)*, two obstacles must be overcome once diagnostic material is obtained. First, the diagnostic procedure must be sensitive enough to be successful on only a single cell, and second, the interpretation of the result must consider the possibility that each of the embryonic cells is not genetically equivalent to the other cells. Indeed, the existence of mosaicism in human embryos has raised concerns about the diagnostic accuracy of PGD *(10,11)*.

The first successful clinical use of fluorescent labeled DNA and FISH on preimplantation embryos was embryonic sex determination to avoid X-linked disease *(12)*. In recent years, the use of FISH for PGD has flourished with the availability of commercial directly labeled probes with different fluorochromes. PGD is now possible for couples carrying reciprocal and Robertsonian translocations *(13)* and, more frequently, for chro-

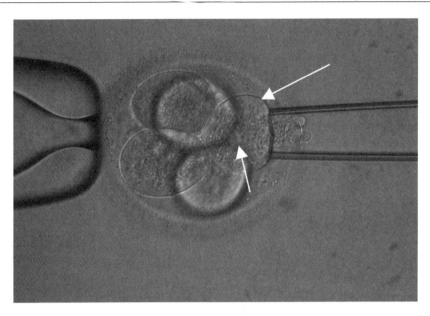

Fig. 1. Cleavage stage embryo biopsy. An eight-cell stage human embryo is held in place while a single embryonic cell is removed for diagnosis (large arrow). The nucleus is visible in this cell (small arrow).

mosomal aneuploidy screening in embryos from women of advanced maternal age or who have had recurrent miscarriage or repeated implantation failure following IVF treatment *(14–16)*.

Fluorescent Labeled DNA and FISH

It is now possible to determine numeric (loss or gain of whole chromosomes) chromosome abnormalities of chromosomes 13, 18, 21, X, and Y rapidly (24-h test) by use of fluorescently labeled DNA and FISH (a process of pairing between the probe DNA and chromosomal DNA). The numeric abnormalities of these five chromosomes cumulatively account for about 80% of cases at live birth of all major chromosomal anomalies. However, for numeric abnormalities of other chromosomes and structural anomalies of all chromosomes, standard karyotype analysis needs to be done as a follow-up to the FISH test.

FISH in a human was successfully performed in 1986 *(17)* both for dividing and undividing cells including amniocytes. Uncultured amniocytes were used in 1991 *(18)* with this method to detect aneuploidy (numeric chromosome anomaly) of 13, 18, and 21. By 1992 *(19–21)*, FISH techniques were in use to detect the numeric abnormality of chromosomes 13, 18, 21, X, and Y from nondividing AF cells. By 1998 *(22)*, these techniques were simplified for accuracy and efficiency, and the probes were commercially available. Prenatal aneuploidy detection by FISH is now widely available.

TECHNIQUE AND PRECAUTION
AF and Chorionic Villi

Direct-labeled DNA probes for 13, 18, 21, X, and Y in different colors are commercially available. The centromere-specific probes for each of the three chromosomes are aqua for 18, green for X, and orange for Y. The locus-specific probe for chromosome 13 based on 13q14 is green and for chromosome 21 based on 21q22.13–q22 is orange.

For each specimen, 2–4 mL of AF is used without culture for preparation of slides by standard harvesting procedure. Cells on the slide and probe DNA are denatured and allowed to hybridize for a minimum of 6 h. The analysis is done by fluorescence microscopy. An example of a normal female cell is shown in Fig. 2A with two green and two aqua signals for chromosomes X and 18, respectively. A normal male cell is shown in Fig. 2B. One green signal for X, one orange signal for Y, and two aqua signals for chromosome 18 are visible. A case of trisomy 18 (T18) (Edwards syndrome) is illustrated in Fig. 2C. Three aqua signals and two green signals are present in a female and three aqua signals are present with one green and one orange in a male (Fig. 2D). In Turner syndrome, only one green signal (single X) is present with two aqua signals for chromosome 18 (Fig. 2E). In a Klinefelter male, two green, one orange, and two aqua signals for chromosomes X, Y, and 18, respectively, are present (Fig. 2F). A normal pattern for chromosomes 13 and 21 are two green and two orange signals (Fig. 2G). Down syndrome (trisomy 21) will have three orange and two green signals (Fig. 2H). Patau syndrome (trisomy 13) will have three green signals and two orange signals (Fig. 2I). The loci for 13 and 21 are in the q (long) arms of the chromosomes, and the presence of three copies of the long arm (13q or 21q) results in the Patau or Down syndrome, respectively. Whole arm translocations that are phenotypically normal of these chromosomes (Robertsonian translocation) are common (1.2 per 1000). The FISH procedure provides counts of the long arms, so it is effective both for diagnosing trisomy as well as Robertsonian translocations involving these long arms.

The commercially available probes for the five chromosomes have a high rate of hybridization success and analytic sensitivity (detection rate of normal pattern) ranging from 89.1 to 98.7% (Table 3) based on the analysis of 30 AF specimens that were chromosomally normal. Because these probes are analyzed from nondividing (interphase) cells in two dimensions *(5)*, artifacts caused by overlapping signals are relatively common. Other artifacts are also possible because of inadequate hybridization or difficulty in interpretation of hybridization signals during the DNA duplication phase (S) or interphase. It is, therefore, important to establish normal cut off values (upper limits of normal) for each laboratory *(23)* for each of the chromosomes being analyzed. For us, this was determined for each of the five chromosomes (Table 4). For instance, for chromosome 21, the maximum number of abnormal signals observed in a normal cell was 9%; the 95% confidence interval (CI from a one-sided binomial distribution) was 13%. This means that unless the abnormal signals exceed 13%, they will be within the normal limit. Most of the abnormal signals were, however, monosomes (single rather than two or more signals). When only trisomics (three signals) are considered, only 1% was the maximum observed, and the normal cutoff value at 95% CI was 2%. This means that theoretically, trisomic signal patterns above 2% are real and abnormal. However, at levels below 10%,

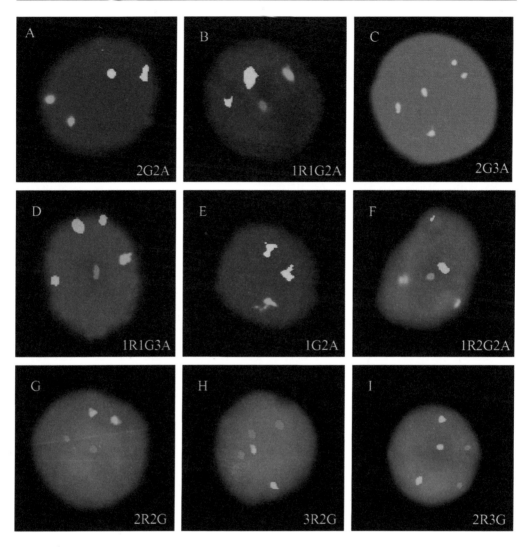

Fig. 2. Direct labeled, commercially available, fluorescent DNA probes were used for chromosomes 13, 18, 21, X, and Y to detect their numeric abnormalities by *in situ* hybridization to chromosome preparations of AF nondividing (interphase) cells without culture. The probes were used in two groups. Centromeric probes were used for chromosomes 18, X, and Y in aqua, green, and orange (red in figures), respectively. Locus-specific probes were used for chromosome 13 and 21 in green and orange, respectively. In a normal female cell, two green and two aqua signals for chromosomes 18 and X are seen (A) whereas in a normal male cell, one green, one orange, and two aqua signals occur for X, Y, and 18 (B). In the case of T18 (Edwards syndrome), three aqua signals are present with two green signals in a female (C), whereas three aqua signals are present with a green and an orange signal in a male Edwards syndrome (D). In Turner syndrome, only one green signal (single X) is present with two aqua signals for chromosome 18 (E). In a Klinefelter male (XXY), two green, one orange, and two aqua signals for chromosomes X, Y, and 18 are present (F). A normal pattern for chromosomes 13 and 21 are two green and two orange, respectively (G), whereas Down syndrome (trisomy 21 or three copies of 21 long arm) will result in three copies of the orange signal with two green (H) and Patau syndrome (trisomy 13) results in three green signals and two orange signals (I).

Table 3
Results of AF Analysis by Interphase FISH: Detection of Aneuploidy

Number of cases analyzed	Karyotype	Mean signal pattern (%)[a]					
		LSI-13	CEP-18	LSI-21	CEP-XX	CEP-XY	Other
6	Normal	97.6	91.5	94.5	95.8	99.0	—
2	Trisomy 13	94.2[b]	89.0	96.0	99.0	100.0	—
4	Trisomy 18	97.5	89.0[b]	96.2	95.7	99.0	—
4	Trisomy 21	97.0	92.7	92.9[b]	97.5	100.0	—
2	47,XXY	98.7	92.2	96.2	—	—	97.2[c]
1	45,X	98.5	91.5	96.0	—	—	99.5[c]
1	47,XXX	98.0	96.5	97.5	—	—	94.5[c]
1	47,XYY	100.0	97.0	96.5	—	7.0	92.5
1	47,XY,+22	98.0	98.0	95.0	15.5	84.0	—
1	mos45,X/46,XY	98.0	97.0	96.5	0.5	65.5	34.0[c]
1	mos46,XY/47,XYY	98.5	93.5	94.0	—	64.0	34.5[c]

[a]All signal patterns were disomic except b, which were trisomic, and c, which were consistent with abnormal karyotype or abnormal clone of the karyotype.
From ref. 22.

Table 4
Maximum Proportion of Abnormal Hybridization Signals
and Estimated Upper Bound Confidence Intervals[a]

Probe	Maximum abnormal signals (%)	[b]Upper bound confidence interval at 95%	Maximum abnormal trisomy (%)	[c]Upper bound confidence interval at 95%
LSI-13	8.5	13	1.5	4
CEP-18	14.5	19	1.0	2
LSI-21	9.0	13	1.0	2
CEP-XX	9.0	13	2.5	7
CEP-XY	4.5	8	.5	2

[a]CEP, chromosome enumeration probes; CI, confidence interval; LSI, locus-specific identifier.
[b]Based on the analysis of up to 200 interphase cells per specimen for each probe from 30 normal samples.
[c]95% upper bound values (rounded up) were calculated from one-sided binomial distribution.
From ref. 22.

a chromosome follow-up is necessary to confirm the low-level mosaic abnormality. For nonmosaic (pure) trisomy, the sensitivity (with three signals) is again high (92.9% for trisomy 21, Table 3). We have now studied more than 2000 of these cases, and the data are similar.

Preimplantation Genetic Diagnosis

The FISH technique, when applied to single cells, is essentially the same as that used for larger numbers of cells. Clearly, there is less tolerance for hybridization failure and technical artifact when only one or two cells are available for diagnosis. Moreover, the need to select unaffected embryos for uterine transfer in a timely fashion puts an additional constraint on the turnaround time for this diagnostic procedure. To meet these limitations, a number of considerations not necessary in conventional FISH diagnostic work must be used for single-cell FISH for PGD.

SELECTION OF THE SINGLE CELL(S)

Selection of each biopsied embryonic cell (blastomere) is critical owing to the relatively high incidence of nuclear and chromosomal abnormalities present in human embryos. Blastomeres should be checked for the presence of a single interphase nucleus because anucleate cellular fragments can be mistaken for blastomeres, and abnormal nucleation needs to be avoided as it is frequently associated with chromosomal abnormality.

AVOIDING CONTAMINATING CELLS

Because only a single cell is under investigation, the presence of an extraneous cell on the slide could be disastrous for PGD. All efforts must be made to ensure that no maternal cumulus cells (the cells that surround the egg during maturation) or other cells come into contact with the slide or reagents used for the diagnostic procedure.

NUMBER OF CELLS BIOPSIED

In deciding how many cells to biopsy from cleavage-stage embryos, it is necessary to balance diagnostic accuracy with potential of the embryo to implant and develop, which is progressively compromised as a greater proportion of the embryo is removed (24). At present, there is no consensus over whether to take one or two cells for analysis in clinical PGD (9).

NUCLEAR FIXATION

For conventional FISH applications, cells are generally prepared using a standard methanol:acetic acid fixative. In PGD, several methods have been successfully used to obtain high-quality single nuclei for FISH analysis, one of which involves methanol:acetic acid fixation, while the other employs a weak acid and detergent mixture to free the nucleus from the surrounding cytoplasm and fix the nucleus simultaneously. Each method gives a strikingly different preparation in terms of nuclear size after fixation (Fig. 3). Nevertheless, both methods are in widespread use, and both appear to provide high-quality FISH results.

REDUCED TIMES FOR HYBRIDIZATION

Owing to time constraints when dealing with human embryos growing in culture, the FISH test has been shortened considerably to allow biopsy, diagnostic testing, selection,

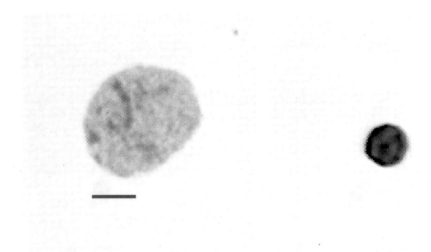

Fig. 3. Examples of Giemsa-stained blastomere nuclei using different fixation methods. Blastomere nuclei from eight-cell stage mouse embryos fixed in (**left**) methanol/acetic acid or (**right**) Tween/HCl. Bar = 10 μm.

and embryo transfer all on the same day if necessary. The hybridization step is generally shortened considerably for most probe combinations, and FISH can be successful with as little as 30 min hybridization time. With improvements in extended embryo culture, the requirement for rapid FISH testing is less acute, although rapid testing also allows multiple tests to be performed on the same cell or retesting when results are unclear.

Dedicated Slide-Washing Facilities

Because of the disastrous consequences of having even a few stray cells float from one slide to another, slides for single cell FISH analysis are washed in unused Coplin jars to minimize exposure to other clinical samples.

Locating the Nucleus

For PGD, the rapid location of the single fixed nucleus on the glass microscope slide is a crucial element in making an accurate and timely diagnosis. Clearly, this procedure becomes trivial when the slide is covered with thousands of cells available for analysis in conventional FISH applications. Locating the single nucleus can be achieved by carefully mapping the location of the fixed nucleus on the slide at the time of fixation, recording microscope stage coordinates, or by using an England finder.

FISH Errors

The FISH technique has been shown to work efficiently on single blastomeres using a variety of probes, but technical problems do arise for a variety of reasons. FISH errors including hybridization failure, signal overlap, and splitting of signals may be quantified when large numbers of cells of known genotype are analyzed. However, the margin for error when diagnosing a single cell is much smaller than for conventional diagnoses.

INTERPRETATION
AF and CVS

Chromosome abnormalities constitute a significant component of genetic disorders both prenatally and at birth. It is estimated, based on relatively large population studies, that chromosome anomalies occur with a frequency of 6–20 per 1000 live births (Tables 1 and 2) (25–28). Of these, balanced abnormalities (structural anomalies that result in no net gain or loss of genetic material and thus generally cause no phenotypic abnormality) range from 2 to 15 per 1000 live births. The unbalanced chromosome anomalies (numeric or structural) do cause dysmorphic features, reproductive problems, and abnormal development. Their rate of occurrence is 7–12 per 1000 live births. Of these, 80% or more result from numeric (gain or loss of whole chromosomes) abnormalities. The vast majority of the numeric chromosome disorders at birth involve chromosomes 13, 18, 21, X, and Y.

In the prenatal period, the rate of chromosome abnormalities is significantly higher than that reported at live births. It is estimated that more than 50% of spontaneously aborted fetuses have a chromosomal abnormality. The rate of such abnormality is higher the earlier the gestational age. Numeric chromosome abnormalities are the most common (Table 1) (29–32). Monosomy X resulting in Turner syndrome (45,X) and triploidy (69 chromosome count) are the most common anomalies, at 79 per 1000. Trisomies (presence of extra chromosome) involving autosomes (chromosomes 1–22 besides the sex chromosomes) are most frequent for chromosome 16 (59 per 1000), followed by chromosomes 22 (35 per 1000), 21 (22 per 1000), and 15 (22 per 1000). Although in these four studies, trisomy 1 was not detected, it has been reported by others. Because chromosome 1 is the largest chromosome, it is rarely encountered as a trisomy because when it does happen, fetal demise results very early in gestation. The level of structural abnormalities (deletion, duplication, inversion, and translocation) is relatively low at 27 per 1000. The reason is that only major structural abnormalities result in spontaneous abortion. Other structural abnormalities and some numeric disorders do not result in spontaneous abortions.

It is widely believed that the risk of chromosome nondisjunction (failure of chromosomes to normally segregate during cell division) resulting in numeric chromosome abnormalities increases with the increasing age of females. It is estimated that more than 90% of these result from maternal meiotic error (33). This is related to the long oocyte maturation process in human females when they may be exposed to environmental agents or a natural slowing down of physiological activities with age. During the third month of fetal development, oogonia enter meiosis (germinal cell division). These oocytes do not mature until puberty. Most of the oocytes out of almost 1 million degenerate by birth and only about 400 reach maturity between ages 12 to about 50 yr in conjunction with ovulation. When an ovum is released in the oviduct, the first half of meiosis is completed. It is only after fertilization of the ovum by a sperm that the rest of meiosis is completed. As oogenesis is completed, an egg with massive cytoplasm is produced along with three polar bodies that degenerate.

The point of increasing risk with age, especially beyond 35 yr, is well documented for Down syndrome with extra chromosome 21 (Table 5) (34–36). On the basis of several relatively large population surveys, risk for Down syndrome at age 24 is estimated to range from 1:1294 to 1:1877 compared to age 35, when it is 1:250 to 1:404. The risk rises to 1:24 to 1:44 at age 45, and it is dramatically higher at ages beyond 45. It is therefore a standard medical practice to offer amniocentesis for chromosome anomalies to females at age 35 or older even without any family history for genetic disorders. The rate of nondisjunction does increase somewhat in males with age, but it is insignificant because males complete the process of meiosis in 64 d, and they produce a large number of sperms throughout their life starting at puberty. Numeric chromosome problems involve all the chromosomes, but most of these abort spontaneously. Generally, the smaller the chromosome (21 is the smallest), the more the chances of its occurrence as a trisomy (extra copy) in a live birth.

Besides advanced maternal age, other significant reasons for offering amniocentesis for chromosome analysis to women include abnormal concentrations of hormones (such as human chorionic gonadotropin [hCG], α-fetoprotein [AFP], and estriol) in the blood during pregnancy, detection of fetal abnormalities at ultrasound examination, and a history of chromosome abnormality or birth defects in a previous pregnancy (Fig. 4). Advanced maternal age and the presence of abnormal concentrations of hormones in maternal blood account for a very small proportion of chromosomal anomalies in our referral pattern (Fig. 4).

Standard chromosome analysis from amniocentesis is based on eight primary cultures (cells grown on eight coverslips) of AF cells from in situ cultures or from multiple flasks grown in a fluid culture environment. Chorionic villi are analyzed from direct preparations or also cultured in multiple flasks. If 20 metaphase cells from 15 colonies (based on three or more primary cultures) have the same result (normal or abnormal), the result is reported. Similarly, from the flask system, if 20 metaphase cells from two or more flasks have the same result, it is reported.

Mosaicism (occurrence of both normal and abnormal cells) poses a particular problem of interpretation because low levels can be difficult to detect and interpret. About 3% of Down syndrome patients have mosaicism, and some can have very low levels of the extra 21 chromosome-containing cells mixed in with normal cells. Low levels of numeric (gain or loss) as well as structural abnormalities (translocation, inversion, deletion, and duplication) may also occur as artifacts from exposure to chemicals used for culturing. If one or more cells are abnormal but others are normal in a colony, it is considered to be an artifact (level I mosaicism) and disregarded. If a single colony has an abnormality involving every cell (level II mosaicism) but other colonies are normal, up to 15 more colonies (a total of 30) are analyzed. If a single colony remains abnormal, it is reported and follow-up chromosome study is advised after the birth of the baby, provided the numeric anomaly (gain or loss) involves well-established syndromes (sex chromosomes, and chromosomes 13, 18, 21, 8, and 9). If two colonies have identical numeric or structural abnormality, clonal abnormality is established and it is regarded as a true mosaic (level III). These results are reported regardless of the chromosomes involved. For the flask culture method, three or more flasks must be used for analysis to make these conclusions. Phenotypic dysmorphism can vary widely as a result of mosaicism. However, in general, the higher the level of mosaicism involving the proportion of abnormal clones, the more severe the dysmorphic features.

When the FISH test is used for rapid detection (24-h test) of numeric anomalies of chromosomes 13, 18, 21, X, and Y, nonmosaic results are easily interpreted (Table 1). However, mosaicism, especially at a low level (10% or lower) must be confirmed by the follow-up chromosome analysis, although higher levels can be reliably detected by the 24-h interphase FISH test (Table 3).

Table 5
Estimated Maternal Age-Specific Risk of Down Syndrome Live Birth

Maternal age (yr)	Asia[a] 1975–1995	Australia[b] 1960–1989	Pooled data (Australia, Canada, Europe, and US)[c] 1963–1991
16	n.c.	1:1748	1:1448
17	n.c.	1:1704	1:1442
18	1:7977	1:1661	1:1434
19	1:6682	1:1613	1:1423
20	1:5394	1:1577	1:1408
21	1:3992	1:1538	1:1389
22	1:3275	1:1499	1:1365
23	1:2403	1:1460	1:1333
24	1:1877	1:1425	1:1294
25	1:1377	1:1389	1:1244
26	1:993	1:1353	1:1184
27	1:735	1:1319	1:1111
28	1:583	1:1285	1:1027
29	1:504	1:1253	1:933
30	1:470	1:1221	1:831
31	1:408	1:978	1:725
32	1:357	1:789	1:620
33	1:346	1:629	1:519
34	1:315	1:504	1:426
35	1:250	1:404	1:344
36	1:207	1:324	1:273
37	1:183	1:259	1:215
38	1:175	1:208	1:167
39	1:166	1:167	1:128
40	1:135	1:133	1:98
41	1:112	1:107	1:75
42	1:106	1:86	1:57
43	n.c.	1:69	1:43
44	n.c.	1:55	1:32
45	n.c.	1:44	1:24
46	n.c.	1:35	1:18
47	n.c.	1:28	1:14
48	n.c.	1:23	1:10
49	n.c.	n.c.	1:8
50	n.c.	n.c.	1:6

n.c., Data not collected in this single age group.
[a]Ref. 34.
[b]Ref. 35.
[c]Ref. 36.

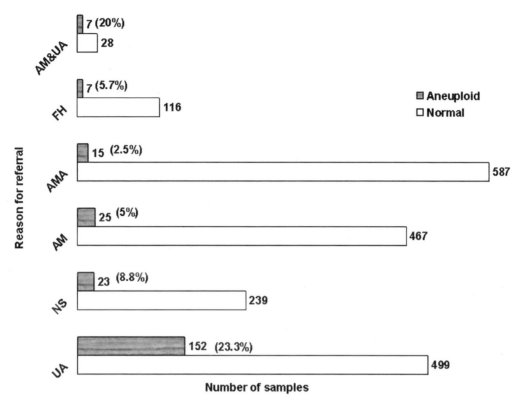

Fig. 4. Rate of aneuploidy detection by FISH in relation to reason for referral among 2165 informative samples analyzed at Mayo Clinic. AM, abnormal serum markers; AMA, advanced maternal age; FH, family history of chromosome abnormality or birth defects; NS, non specific; UA, ultrasound detected fetal anomalies.

What is the accuracy of the 24-h FISH test and how can the FISH results be used clinically? Eiben et al. *(37)* reported no false negatives (FISH results abnormal but chromosome analysis normal) or false positives (FISH results normal but chromosome analysis abnormal), based on 904 samples. Our own experience is similar, based on more than 2000 samples analyzed, although both groups experienced a few samples that were unsuccessful because of technical problems. Overall, we were able to obtain informative test results in 99.2% and detection of aneuploidy in 10.5% of 2182 samples analyzed. The results of FISH analysis can be provided to the patients with extensive counseling. These results may now be used for decision for elective abortion provided the abnormality detected by FISH is confirmed by anomalies detected by ultrasound examination of the fetus. Indeed, in our own experience, the highest rate of aneuploidy was among pregnancies in which fetal anomalies were detected at ultrasound examination (Fig. 4). When normal, FISH analysis results are also helpful to alleviate the anxiety of the mother, especially when there is a history or risk for trisomies (Fig. 4) involving the five (13, 18, 21, X, and Y) chromosomes. In the case of equivocal FISH results as well as mosaicism, chromosome follow-up studies must be done.

Signals from single cells are generally scored according to the same criteria as for conventional clinical samples. For example, probe signals are initially scored simultaneously and subsequently using individual filter sets by two independent observers. Same-color signals that touch, regardless of the size or length, that are joined by a signal strand of the same color, or that are less than one signal width apart are counted as one signal. Signal overlap is judged to occur when two different color signals have clearly merged (with a component of each remaining discrete) in the absence of any background within the nucleus.

Clearly, the more signals there are present within the same nucleus, the more cumulative opportunity for error. Currently, aneuploidy screening is undertaken with anywhere from 3 to 10 different chromosome-specific probes depending on the particular indication for testing. The identification of chromosomes X, Y, 13, 18, and 21 at preimplantation stages is considered useful for preventing the development of a trisomic or Turner syndrome pregnancy in women with a high risk or who are of advanced maternal age. The addition of chromosomes 16, 22, 14, and 15 is considered to be useful in reducing the potential for miscarriages (Table 2).

Preimplantation Genetic Diagnosis

The availability of only a single cell for analysis poses a significant diagnostic challenge in that commercially available chromosome-specific DNA probes are only available in a limited range of colors. In conventional FISH testing where abundant diagnostic material is present, this problem is resolved by performing multiple tests simultaneously using different probe combinations on different diagnostic sites of the same sample. With single cell analyses, one must determine the optimal probe combination to obtain the maximum amount of diagnostic information from the least number of consecutive hybridizations using the available probe combinations. Figure 5 demonstrates the use of the commercially available polar body testing probe set (containing probes specific for chromosomes 13, 16, 18, 21, and 22) followed by washing and rehybridization of the same blastomere nucleus with probes specific for chromosomes X, Y, 14, and 15. The combination should theoretically identify trisomies most likely to result in spontaneous abortions (Table 2) and is the most extensive FISH screen of human embryos to date *(16)*.

As probe combinations have become more difficult to configure and more chromosomes have become candidates for implantation failure of embryos, novel techniques have been devised to attempt greater diagnostic power within single nuclei. Such innovations include fusion of mouse *(38)* or bovine eggs *(14)* with human blastomeres to create an artificial metaphase (potentially allowing analysis of all chromosomes) and whole genome amplification followed by comparative genome hybridization to allow identification of gross chromosome aberrations or aneuploidies *(39,40)*. The initial step requires amplification of the DNA from the single cell, and this same process could also be followed in the future using an approach based on a DNA-chip.

SUMMARY

It is estimated that chromosome anomalies occur with a frequency of about 13 per 1000 live births. Nearly 80% of genetic disorders at birth from chromosomal abnormalities involve gain or loss (numeric) of chromosomes 13, 18, 21, X, and Y. The proportion of chromosomal abnormalities is considerably higher in the prenatal period. It is estimated

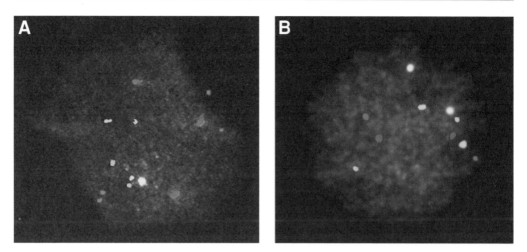

Fig. 5. Detection of common aneuploidies from a single blastomere nuclei from (A) an abnormal and (B) a normal human embryo using centromeric or locus-specific probes for the following chromosomes: 13 (red), 16 (aqua), 18 (blue), 21 (green), and 22 (gold). The abnormal blastomere (a) is trisomic for chromosomes 13 and 16, tetrasomic for chromosome 18, monosomic for chromosome 22, and disomic for chromosome 21. The normal blastomere (b) is disomic for all of these chromosomes.

that more than 50% of spontaneous abortions during early gestation have major chromosome abnormalities. It is also estimated that more than 90% of numeric chromosome abnormalities arise as maternal meiotic error. This is especially true for females beyond the age of 35. In addition to advancing age, other risks for prenatal chromosome anomalies are family history for chromosome abnormality, abnormal ultrasound results of the fetus, and abnormal maternal blood hormone concentrations during pregnancy.

Standard chromosome analyses are conducted by amniocentesis based on culture of cells from AF, generally during 14–16 wk gestation. Chromosome analysis can also be conducted at earlier gestation from samples of villi of the placenta. Both of these procedures are time tested and quite safe. For special medical needs, PUBS can be sampled, but that does have a significant risk for abortion.

A 24-h FISH test is available to rule out numeric abnormalities of chromosomes of 13, 18, 21, X, and Y. The test is approved by the Federal Drug Administration and is reliable. However, it is neither designed to detect numeric abnormalities of chromosomes other than the five listed above nor can it identify structural abnormalities of any chromosomes. In combination with ultrasound results, this FISH test can be helpful for rapid diagnosis of numeric anomalies of chromosomes 13, 18, 21, X, and Y. For a complete analysis of all structural and numeric anomalies of all chromosomes, however, a follow-up of standard chromosome analysis is essential.

It is now possible to have limited genetic testing of embryos prior to their implantation in the womb in cases of assisted reproduction of infertile couples or other special circumstances. A limited number of laboratories around the world provide PGD. The PGD test can involve detection of numeric anomalies of chromosomes 13, 16, 18, 21, 22, X, and Y by FISH or diagnosis of some single-gene disorders by molecular analysis. Embryos judged to be normal are then transferred into the womb to initiate pregnancy.

REFERENCES

1. Steele M, Berg W. Chromosome analysis of human amniotic-fluid cells. Lancet 1966;1:383–385.
2. Jacobson C, Barber R. Intrauterine diagnosis and management of genetic defects. Am J Obstet Gynecol 1967;99:796–806.
3. Kazy Z, Rozovsky L, Bakharev V. Chorion biopsy in early pregnancy: a method of early prenatal diagnosis for inherited disorders. Prenat Diagn 1982;2:39–45.
4. Spurbeck JL, Carlson RO, Allen JE, Dewald GW. Culturing and robotic harvesting of bone marrow, lymph nodes, peripheral blood, fibroblasts, and solid tumors with in situ techniques. Cancer Genet Cytogenet 1988;32:59–66.
5. Spurbeck J, Zinsmeister A, Meyer K, Jalal S. Dynamics of chromosome spreading. Am J Med Genet 1996;61:387–393.
6. Verma R, Babu A. Human chromosomes: principles and techniques New York: Pergamon Press, 1995, p. 419.
7. Gersen S, Keagle B. The principle of clinical cytogenetics: Totawa, NJ: Humana Press, 1999, p. 558.
8. Hardy K, Martin K, Leese II, Winston R, Handyside Λ. Human preimplantation development in vitro is not adversely affected by biopsy at the 8-cell stage. Hum Reprod 1990;5:708–714.
9. ESHRE preimplantation genetic diagnosis consortium: data collection III (May 2001). Hum Reprod 2002;17:233–246.
10. Delhanty J, Griffin D, Handyside A, et al. Detection of aneuploidy and chromosomal mosaicism in human embryos during preimplantation sex determination by fluorescent in situ hybridisation (FISH). Hum Mol Genet 1993;2:1183–1185.
11. Munne S, Weier H, Grifo J, Cohen J. Chromosome mosaicism in human embryos. Biol Reprod 1994;51:373–379.
12. Griffin D, Wilton L, Handyside A, Atkinson G, Winston R, Delhanty J. Diagnosis of sex in preimplantation embryos by fluorescent in situ hybridisation. Br Med J 1993;306:1382.
13. Munne S, Sandalinas M, Escudero T, Fung J, Gianaroli L, Cohen J. Outcome of preimplantation genetic diagnosis of translocations. Fertil Steril 2000;73:1209–1218.
14. Verlinsky Y, Cieslak J, Freidine M, et al. Pregnancies following pre-conception diagnosis of common aneuploidies by fluorescent in-situ hybridization. Hum Reprod 1995;10:1923–1927.
15. Gianaroli L, Magli M, Ferraretti A, Fiorentino A, Garrisi J, Munne S. Preimplantation genetic diagnosis increases the implantation rate in human in vitro fertilization by avoiding the transfer of chromosomally abnormal embryos. Fertil Steril 1997;68:1128–1231.
16. Munne S, Magli C, Bahce M, et al. Preimplantation diagnosis of the aneuploidies most commonly found in spontaneous abortions and live births: XY, 13, 14, 15, 16, 18, 21, 22. Prenat Diagn 1998;18:1459–1466.
17. Pinkel D, Straume T, Gray J. Cytogenetic analysis using quantitative, high-sensitivity fluorescence hybridization. Proc Natl Acad Sci USA 1986;83:2934–2938.
18. Kuo WL, Tenjin H, Segraves R, Pinkel D, Golbus MS, Gray J. Detection of aneuploidy involving chromosomes 13, 18, or 21, by fluorescence in situ hybridization (FISH) to interphase and metaphase amniocytes. Am J Hum Genet 1991;49:112–119.
19. Klinger K, Landes G, Shook D, et al. Rapid detection of chromosome aneuploidies in uncultured amniocytes by using fluorescence in situ hybridization (FISH). Am J Hum Genet 1992;51:55–65.
20. Ward BE, Gersen SL, Carelli MP, et al. Rapid prenatal diagnosis of chromosomal aneuploidies by fluorescence in situ hybridization: clinical experience with 4,500 specimens. Am J Hum Genet 1993;52:854–865.
21. Philip J, Bryndorf T, Christensen B. Prenatal aneuploidy detection in interphase cells by fluorescence in situ hybridization (FISH). Prenat Diagn 1994;14:1203–1215.
22. Jalal S, Law M, Carlson R, Dewald G. Prenatal detection of aneuploidy by directly labeled multicolor probes and interphase fluorescence in situ hybridization. Mayo Clinic Proc 1998;73:132.
23. American College of Medical Genetics. Prenatal interphase fluorescence in situ hybridization (FISH) policy statement. Am J Hum Genet 1993;53:526–527.
24. Liu J, Van den Abbeel E, Van Steirteghem A. The in-vitro and in-vivo developmental potential of frozen and non-frozen biopsied 8-cell mouse embryos. Hum Reprod 1993;8:1481–1486.
25. Hansteen IL, Varslot K, Steen-Johnsen J, Langard S. Cytogenetic screening of a new-born population. Clin Genet 1982;21:309–314.
26. Nielsen J, Wohlert M. Chromosome abnormalities found among 34,910 newborn children: results from a 13-year incidence study in Arhus, Denmark. Hum Genet 1991;87:81–83.

27. Maeda T, Ohno M, Matsunobu A, Yoshihara K, Yabe N. A cytogenetic survey of 14,835 consecutive liveborns. Jpn J Human Genet 1991;36:117–129.
28. Nielsen J, Sillesen I. Incidence of chromosome aberrations among 11,148 newborn children. Humangenetik 1975;30:1–12.
29. Hassold T, Chen N, Funkhouser J, et al. A cytogenetic study of 1000 spontaneous abortions. Ann Hum Genet 1980;44:151–178.
30. Kalousek D. Anatomic and chromosome anomalies in specimens of early spontaneous abortion: seven-year experience. Birth Defects Orig Artic Ser 1987;23:153–168.
31. Griffin DK, Millie EA, Redline RW, Hassold TJ, Zaragoza MV. Cytogenetic analysis of spontaneous abortions: comparison of techniques and assessment of the incidence of confined placental mosaicism. Am J Med Genet 1997;72:297–301.
32. Stephenson MD, Awartani KA, Robinson WP. Cytogenetic analysis of miscarriages from couples with recurrent miscarriage: a case-control study. Hum Reprod 2002;17:446–451.
33. Warburton D. Human female meiosis: new insights into an error-prone process. Am J Hum Genet 1997;61:1–4.
34. Sheu BC, Shyu MK, Lee CN, Kuo BJ, Tseng YY, Hsieh FJ. Maternal age-specific risk of Down syndrome in an Asian population: a report of the Taiwan Down Syndrome Screening Group. Prenat Diagn 1998;18:675–682.
35. Staples AJ, Sutherland GR, Haan EA, Clisby S. Epidemiology of Down syndrome in South Australia, 1960–1989. Am J Hum Genet 1991;49:1014–1024.
36. Bray I, Wright DE, Davies C, Hook EB. Joint estimation of Down syndrome risk and ascertainment rates: a meta-analysis of nine published data sets. Prenat Diagn 1998;18:9–20.
37. Eiben B, Trawicki W, Hammans W, Goebel R, Epplen JT. A prospective comparative study on fluorescence in situ hybridization (FISH) of uncultured amniocytes and standard karyotype analysis. Prenat Diagn 1998;18:901–906.
38. Willadsen L, Munne S, Schimmel T, Marquez C, Scott R, Cohen J. Rapid visualization of metaphase chromosomes in single human blastomeres after fusion with in-vitro matured bovine eggs. Hum Reprod 1999;14:470–475.
39. Wilton L, Williamson R, McBain J, Edgar D, Voullaire L. Birth of a healthy infant after preimplantation confirmation of euploidy by comparative genomic hybridization. N Engl J Med 2001;345:1537–1541.
40. Wilton L. Preimplantation genetic diagnosis for aneuploidy screening in early human embryos: a review. Prenat Diagn 2002;22:512–518.

7

Diagnosis and Monitoring of Ectopic and Abnormal Pregnancies

Gary Lipscomb, MD

CONTENTS

INTRODUCTION
LABORATORY TESTING
OTHER TESTING
SUMMARY
REFERENCES

INTRODUCTION

Vaginal bleeding during the first half of pregnancy is considered a threatened abortion. This occurs in 30–40% of all pregnancies with approx 50% of these pregnancies eventually progressing to spontaneous abortion. If sensitive assays for human chorionic gonadotropin (hCG) are used, more than half of all pregnancies have been shown to end in abortion. Most of these abortions will not be recognized as they occur before or at the time of the next expected menses. Of clinically recognized pregnancies, only 15–20% will end as a spontaneous abortion, 80% of which will be in the first trimester *(1)*. The differential diagnosis of first-trimester bleeding includes vaginitis, trauma, gestational trophoblastic disease, and ectopic pregnancy. Evaluation of a threatened abortion should include serial hCG measurements unless an intrauterine pregnancy (IUP) has been documented. The consideration of ectopic pregnancy is of special concern because of its increasing incidence.

In the United States, the incidence of ectopic pregnancy has increased from 0.37% in 1948 to 1.97% in 1992 *(2)*. Despite the continued increase in the rate of ectopic pregnancy, the maternal death rate associated with this condition has declined 10-fold from 1979 to 1992 *(3)*. This decrease in death rate is primarily the result of earlier diagnosis prior to tubal rupture made possible by more sensitive and specific immunoassays for hCG, serum progesterone screening, high-resolution transvaginal sonography, and the widespread availability of laparoscopy. The earlier diagnosis of unruptured ectopic pregnancies also allows for the use of more conservative tubal-preserving treatment options. In fact, in selected patients, surgery may be avoided entirely and replaced with medical management.

This chapter attempts to elaborate on the proper use of laboratory testing, particularly hCG and progesterone, to make the diagnosis of ectopic pregnancy as well as failed IUP.

From: *Current Clinical Pathology: Handbook of Clinical Laboratory Testing During Pregnancy*
Edited by: A. M. Gronowski © Humana Press, Totowa, NJ

LABORATORY TESTING

Ideally, because of their life-threatening nature, ectopic pregnancies would be diagnosed as rapidly as possible. However, since the protocols for diagnosing ectopic pregnancies can be cumbersome and complex, the orderly and logical use of diagnostic tests can be difficult, particularly for individuals who do not use these protocols on a regular basis. As such, diagnostic algorithms have been developed to simplify the management of suspected ectopic pregnancies. Initially, these algorithms relied on quantitative hCG concentrations and transabdominal ultrasound followed by diagnostic laparoscopy to confirm the diagnosis of ectopic pregnancy. As the sensitivity and specificity of the diagnostic tests increased, the need for laparoscopy to confirm the diagnosis decreased. Subsequently, an algorithm developed by Stovall and others to diagnose ectopic pregnancy without the use of laparoscopy proved 100% accurate in a randomized clinical trial *(4)*. This algorithm was an extension of the ectopic screening algorithm then in use at the University of Tennessee, Memphis. The current version of this nonlaparoscopic algorithm now in use at this institution is presented in Fig. 1. The use of each of the diagnostic modalities used in this algorithm is discussed in detail in the following section.

Serum Progesterone

Historically, serum progesterone has been proposed as both a screening tool to identify patients with failed pregnancies or potential ectopic pregnancies and to determine candidates for dilation and curettage (D&C) to rule out ectopic pregnancy. Because progesterone concentrations associated with ectopic pregnancy are generally lower than those associated with IUPs, serum progesterone would appear to be a logical diagnostic tool for ectopic pregnancies. Unfortunately, although preliminary studies suggested that all ectopic pregnancies were associated with serum progesterone concentrations below certain thresholds, later studies have shown considerable overlap in progesterone concentrations for viable IUPs, failed IUPs, and ectopic pregnancies (Table 1) *(5–7)*. Although this data invalidated serum progesterone concentrations for the definitive diagnosis of an ectopic pregnancy, the authors of these studies suggested certain thresholds for serum progesterone that could be used as part of a screening program for ectopic pregnancies.

Because only 1–2% of abnormal pregnancies (abortions or ectopic pregnancies) in the previously mentioned studies were associated with progesterone of 25 ng/mL or more, patients with concentrations of 25 mg/mL or more generally do not require further evaluation for ectopic pregnancy. Exceptions would be patients at extremely high risk for ectopic pregnancy such as those with a previous ectopic pregnancy or prior tubal ligation. Serum progesterone concentrations of 25 ng/mL or more that were associated with an ectopic pregnancy generally indicated an ongoing and viable pregnancy that frequently exhibited cardiac activity on transvaginal ultrasound.

In these studies, a serum progesterone concentration less than 6.5 ng/mL was always associated with a nonviable pregnancy. However, a low serum progesterone did not indicate whether the failed pregnancy was intrauterine or ectopic. Because this progesterone concentration was considered indicative of a failed pregnancy, D&C to document a failed IUP could then be performed without fear of interrupting a viable pregnancy. This threshold for pregnancy viability was subsequently lowered to 5 ng/mL and recently two viable pregnancies with serum progesterones of 3.9 ng/mL have been reported from the same database *(8)*. Thus, although a serum progesterone of 5 ng/mL or less is highly

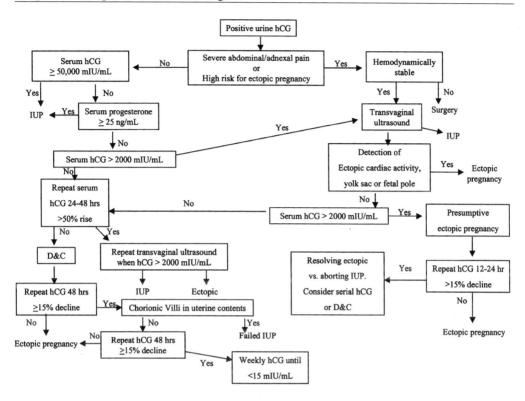

Fig. 1. University of Tennessee, Memphis, Diagnostic Algorithm for Ectopic Pregnancy. D&C, dilation and curettage; IUP, intrauterine pregnancy.

Table 1
Status of Pregnancies Presenting to an Emergency Room
by Progesterone Concentration

Final diagnosis N = 1994	Progesterone ≥25 ng/mL N = 1136	Progesterone < 25 ng/mL N = 858
Viable IUP n = 1476 (74%)	1129 (76.5%)	347 (23.5%)
Ectopic pregnancy n = 161 (8.1%)	5 (3.1%)	156 (96.9%)
Incomplete abortion n = 154 (7.7%)	0 (0%)	154 (100%)
Complete abortion n = 174 (8.7%)	0 (0%)	174 (100%)
Fetal demise n = 29 (1.5%)	2 (7.1%)	27 (92.9%)

Modified from ref. 6.

suggestive of an abnormal pregnancy, be it intra- or extrauterine, it can no longer be considered definitive and should not be used as the sole criteria to determine candidates for D&C.

Serum progesterone is not commonly used to diagnose fetal demise (impending miscarriage) in known IUPs. Serum progesterone only provides a snapshot of fetal condition at the time of the assay and is not predictive of continued viability. Therefore, a high serum progesterone in a known IUP is encouraging but it does not rule out the possibility of a later miscarriage. Alternatively, extremely low progesterone concentrations are almost invariably associated with a failed pregnancy. Generally, such a diagnosis is confirmed with the use of transvaginal ultrasound.

Although, serum progesterone concentrations have not proved as valuable a diagnostic tool as previously thought, they still remain a useful screening tool for the diagnosis of ectopic pregnancies if readily available. Currently, the use of serum progesterone concentrations as a screening tool for ectopic pregnancy is limited by the lack of universal availability of the test itself. Many smaller laboratories do not perform the assay, and even large laboratories often perform progesterone assays only a few times a week. In these circumstances, other screening and diagnostic tools must be used to diagnose the early unruptured ectopic pregnancy.

hCG

hCG concentrations are standardized against one of three reference preparations that are not completely interchangeable. Unfortunately, the exact reference preparation used for standardization is frequently not stated even in journal articles. The First International Standard (1st IS) was introduced by the World Health Organization in the 1930s. It is no longer used and is of historical interest only. The Second International Standard (2nd IS) was adopted in 1964 and is still used in some laboratories to report hCG concentrations. The material used to standardize the 2nd IS was relatively impure and contained large amounts of both the α and β subunits of hCG in addition to the intact hormone. Because many of the various immunoassays developed shortly after the adoption of the 2nd IS also had varying sensitivities to the α and β subunits, considerable differences in hCG concentrations were obtained on the same specimen by the different assays. This made correlation between the different assays difficult (see Chapter 2).

The First International Reference Preparation (1st IRP) was subsequently developed using a highly purified form of intact hCG. The 1st IRP, also known as the 3rd International Standard, was authorized in 1975 and should be used when reporting hCG concentrations. One nanogram of purified hCG is equivalent to 5.0 mIU of the 2nd IS or 9.3 mIU of the 1st IRP *(9)*. Thus, an hCG concentration referenced to the 1st IRP is roughly twice that of the same concentration referenced to the 2nd IS. All hCG concentrations in this article are referenced to the 1st IRP unless otherwise stated.

In the past, the sensitivity of available pregnancy tests was such that only a positive test was useful. Biologic and immunologic tests in the mid-1970s frequently were not readily available, could require 24 h or more to perform, and could detect hCG only at concentrations of 1500 mIU/mL or greater. Using these tests, only 50% of ectopic pregnancies had a positive pregnancy test *(10)*.

The development of rapid, extremely sensitive enzyme-linked immunosorbent assay (ELISA) pregnancy tests has simplified the diagnosis of ectopic pregnancy. Currently available qualitative assays can be performed in minutes and will detect hCG at concentrations of 20–50 mIU/mL. Using these ELISA tests, hCG can sometimes be detected in first-voided maternal urine by day 21 of the menstrual cycle *(11)*. Prior to the development of ELISA pregnancy tests, the low sensitivity of available urine pregnancy tests made them unreliable with dilute urine specimens. However, the increased sensitivity of the ELISA urine pregnancy test should detect all but the earliest pregnancy without the need for a first-voided concentrated urine specimen. Likewise, these tests can be used as an initial screening test for pregnancy in patients presenting with symptoms consistent with ectopic pregnancy because all symptomatic ectopic pregnancies should have sufficiently high hCG concentrations to produce a positive urine test.

Serum concentrations of hCG can be quantified down to 2 mIU/mL using automated immunoassay methods. The use of monoclonal antibodies has also markedly reduced cross-reactivity to luteinizing hormone, follicle-stimulating hormone, and thyroid-stimulating hormone. Using these assays, hCG can reliably be detected in maternal serum as early as 8 d after the LH surge (day 22 of menstrual cycle). Quantitative hCG plays a pivotal role in diagnosing the suspected ectopic pregnancy and allows for proper interpretation of the other diagnostic modalities. In IUPs, hCG concentrations rise in a curvilinear fashion until they plateau at approx 100,000 mIU/mL. However, the rise in hCG concentrations is essentially linear prior to 41 d gestation *(12)*. Because of this linearity, the rate of hCG doubling can be used to assess viability of a pregnancy.

The mean doubling time for serum hCG in a normal IUP has been reported to be 1.4 to 2.1 d *(13–16)*. However, in patients with an ectopic pregnancy, hCG will typically rise at a much slower rate. Based on studies of doubling times, serum hCG concentrations will rise by at least 66% in 48 h in 85% of normal pregnancies (1 standard deviation [SD] from the mean) *(13,14,16)*. Thus, 15% of normal IUPs will rise less than this in 48 h. However, a rise of less than 50% is more than 3 SDs from the mean and would be associated with an abnormal pregnancy 99.9% of the time. Because the interassay variability of hCG is 10–15%, a change of less than this amount is considered to be a plateau. Plateaued hCG concentrations are the most predictive of ectopic pregnancy.

These doubling times apply only to early IUPs. Research by Daya has identified three gestational age ranges within which the hCG rise is linear (0–41 d, 41–57 d and 57–65 d) *(12)*. Although the rise in hCG remains linear within each group, the rate of rise is less for each successive group, with normal 48-h rises in hCG being 103, 33, and 5%, respectively for each group. Fortunately, all normal IUPs should reach the discriminatory zone for both transvaginal and transabdominal ultrasound prior to 41 d gestation.

hCG concentrations of 50,000 or more are rarely (<0.1%) associated with an ectopic pregnancy. At hCG concentrations of 2000 mIU/mL or more, transvaginal ultrasound should visualize an intrauterine sac in all normal IUPs *(17)*. Patients with an abnormal rise in hCG (<50% in 48 h) or plateaued concentrations (±15%) may undergo D&C without fear of interrupting an ongoing viable intrauterine pregnancy. A plateaued or rising concentration after D&C indicates the presence of persistent trophoblastic tissue, usually an ectopic pregnancy.

Caution should be used when interpretating hCG concentrations from different institutions. More than 50 different quantitative hCG assays are sold in the United States. There are numerous different antibody binding sites on the hCG molecule. Each commercial test uses a different combination of capture and tracer antibodies. This is compounded by the heterogeneity of the hCG molecule and its degradation products that exist in the body. hCG exists as the intact molecule, nicked hCG, free β subunit, and several other forms. Two different assays can, in certain circumstances, give greatly varying hCG results (see Chapter 2).

Quantitative serum hCG assays can also be falsely elevated when no real hCG exists in the serum. This recently noted phenomenon is known as phantom hCG *(18,19)*. Most cases of phantom hCG are caused by heterophilic antibodies that bind to the animal antibodies used in the assay. Such falsely positive hCG concentrations are usually in the range of 10–600 mIU/mL. Phantom hCG can be ruled out with a positive urine pregnancy test, because the antibodies are not secreted into the urine, or with special dilutional techniques on the serum specimen. It is our practice to use a positive urine pregnancy test as the initial step in our ectopic algorithm. Likewise, a test for urine hCG should be considered when hCG concentrations do not respond appropriately to treatment or there is doubt of the diagnosis (see Chapter 2).

OTHER TESTING

The sonographic identification of an intrauterine gestational sac essentially excludes an ectopic pregnancy. The earliest sonographic finding of an IUP is a gestational sac. However, intrauterine fluid accumulations may produce a pseudosac that may be falsely interpreted as a true gestational sac. Failing IUPs may also appear sonographically as a pseudosac. Prior to development of a yolk sac, verifying the double decidual sac sign (two concentric echogenic rings separated by a hypoechoic space) is the best method to differentiate a true intrauterine sac from a pseudosac.

Vaginal ultrasound permits visualization of a gestational sac at much lower hCG concentrations than with transabdominal scanning. While an IUP will be apparent at hCG concentrations of 6000–6500 mIU/mL with transabdominal ultrasound scanning, an experienced transvaginal sonographer should be able to visualize a viable IUP at an hCG titer of 2000 mIU/mL *(15,17)*. However, the minimal hCG titer at which an intrauterine gestational sac should always be seen is not known, and thus each institution must develop its own lower limits for transvaginal detection of an IUP.

The addition of color doppler transvaginal sonography can help differentiate among a completed abortion, incomplete abortion, and early IUP before visualization of a gestational sac. Vaginal ultrasound can also accurately image oviducts and ovaries such that ectopic pregnancies and their dimensions can be defined.

An ectopic pregnancy more than 4 cm in greatest dimension, or the presence of adnexal cardiac activity in ectopics larger than 3.5 cm, are both relative contraindications to methotrexate therapy. When determining candidates for methotrexate therapy, the protocol at the University of Tennessee considers only the gestational mass or sac size and not the overall size of the hematosalpinx or hematoma. If the gestational mass cannot be distinguished from the surrounding hematoma, then the size of the entire mass must be used. Because ectopic pregnancies are generally associated with lower hCG concentrations than IUPs of similar gestational age, they can often be visualized by transvaginal ultrasound at far lower hCG concentrations than an IUP. However, the finding of an adnexal mass in a patient with a presumed ectopic pregnancy and hCG concentrations less than 2000 mIU/mL should not automatically be assumed to be an ectopic pregnancy without the presence of a yolk sac, fetal pole, or cardiac activity. Frequently, such masses are, in reality, corpus luteum cysts associated with an early IUP.

D&C

Traditionally, D&C has played an important role in the diagnosis of ectopic pregnancy. Now, technical advances, particularly in ultrasound, frequently allow the differentiation of ectopic or failed IUPs at increasingly earlier gestations and often eliminate the need for D&C. Nevertheless, D&C still plays an important role in the diagnosis of ectopic pregnancies with hCG concentrations below the ultrasound discriminatory zone. Except in the rare case of heterotopic pregnancy, the identification of chorionic villi in uterine contents obtained by curettage or from spontaneous passage essentially eliminates the diagnosis of ectopic pregnancy. The use of D&C also prevents giving methotrexate unnecessarily to a patient with a failed IUP.

D&C is particularly important in those patients with hCG concentrations below the discriminatory zone of ultrasound. In these patients, the appropriate use of hCG doubling times and serum progesterone concentrations is necessary to avoid the possibility of interrupting a viable IUP. Patients with plateauing hCG concentrations (<15% change) or an hCG rise of less than 50% in 48 h should undergo D&C to differentiate between a failed IUP and an ectopic pregnancy. Because the diagnosis of an ectopic pregnancy can be delayed by several days while awaiting final histologic pathology, hCG concentrations are followed postoperatively. As noted in the ectopic algorithm (Fig. 1), a serum hCG collected at the time of D&C is followed by repeat testing in 12–24 h. Rising or inappropriately falling concentrations after D&C are considered diagnostic of an ectopic pregnancy.

In patients with appropriately falling hCG concentrations, D&C and its potential surgical morbidity and cost can be usually be avoided. Most patients with falling hCG concentrations will represent a resolving failed IUP, although a small number will represent a spontaneously resolving ectopic pregnancy. Because our treatment protocol is essentially the same for spontaneously resolving ectopics as for resolving failed IUPs, D&C serves little purpose in these patients. However, since the actual success rate for expectant management is less certain than with other treatment options, many clinicians still prefer to perform a D&C to verify a failed IUP in these situations. Unfortunately, villi will be absent on final histology in up to 50% of these cases *(20)*. Because only the presence of villi is diagnostic, those without villi will still require serial hCG concentrations.

Laparoscopy

Laparoscopy remains the gold standard for the diagnosis of ectopic pregnancy. However, with the recent development of diagnostic algorithms that do not require the use of laparoscopy, we are rapidly moving toward a point where laparoscopy is a surgical modality rather than a diagnostic tool. As one eliminates laparoscopy, the risks, costs, and morbidity associated with diagnosis and treatment of the ectopic pregnancy are decreased.

SUMMARY

It is the intention of this chapter to simplify the use of common laboratory tests used to diagnose and monitor both ectopic and abnormal pregnancies. The appropriate use of these tests should allow the clinician to manage these conditions efficiently and accurately.

REFERENCES

1. Poland BJ, Miller JR, Jones DC, Trimble BK. Reproductive counseling in patients who have had a spontaneous abortion. Am J Obstet Gynecol 1977;127:685–691.
2. DeVoe R, Pratt JH. Simultaneous intrauterine and extrauterine pregnancy. Am J Obstet Gynecol 1948;56:1119.
3. Centers for Disease Control. Ectopic pregnancy—United States, 1990–1992. Morb Mortal Wkly Rep 1995;44:46–48.
4. Stovall TG, Ling FW, Carson SA, Buster JE. Nonsurgical diagnosis and treatment of tubal pregnancy. Fertil Steril 1990;54:537–538.
5. Stovall TG, Ling FW, Cope BJ, Buster JE. Preventing ruptured ectopic pregnancy with a single serum progesterone. Am J Obstet Gynecol 1989;160:1425–1428; discussion 28–31.
6. Stovall TG, Kellerman AL, Ling FW, Buster JE. Emergency department diagnosis of ectopic pregnancy. Ann Emerg Med 1990;19:1098–1103.
7. Stovall TG, Ling FW, Andersen RN, Buster JE. Improved sensitivity and specificity of a single measurement of serum progesterone over serial quantitative beta-human chorionic gonadotrophin in screening for ectopic pregnancy. Hum Reprod 1992;7:723–725.
8. McCord ML, Muram D, Buster JE, Arheart KL, Stovall TG, Carson SA. Single serum progesterone as a screen for ectopic pregnancy: exchanging specificity and sensitivity to obtain optimal test performance. Fertil Steril 1996;66:513–516.
9. Storring PL, Gaines-Das RE, Bangham DR. International reference preparation of human chorionic gonadotrophin for immunoassay: potency estimates in various bioassay and protein binding assay systems; and International reference preparations of the alpha and beta subunits of human chorionic gonadotrophin for immunoassay. J Endocrinol 1980;84:295–310.
10. Hallatt JG. Repeat ectopic pregnancy: a study of 123 consecutive cases. Am J Obstet Gynecol 1975;122:520–524.
11. Lipscomb GH, Spellman JR, Ling FW. The effect of same-day pregnancy testing on the incidence of luteal phase pregnancy. Obstet Gynecol 1993;82:411–413.
12. Daya S. Human chorionic gonadotropin increase in normal early pregnancy. Am J Obstet Gynecol 1987;156:286–290.
13. Kadar N, Caldwell BV, Romero R. A method of screening for ectopic pregnancy and its indications. Obstet Gynecol 1981;58:162–166.
14. Kadar N, DeCherney AH, Romero R. Receiver operating characteristic (ROC) curve analysis of the relative efficacy of single and serial chorionic gonadotropin determinations in the early diagnosis of ectopic pregnancy. Fertil Steril 1982;37:542–547.
15. Kadar N, DeVore G, Romero R. Discriminatory hCG zone: its use in the sonographic evaluation for ectopic pregnancy. Obstet Gynecol 1981;58:156–161.
16. Pittaway DE, Reish RL, Wentz AC. Doubling times of human chorionic gonadotropin increase in early viable intrauterine pregnancies. Am J Obstet Gynecol 1985;152:299–302.
17. Bernaschek G, Rudelstorfer R, Csaicsich P. Vaginal sonography versus serum human chorionic gonadotropin in early detection of pregnancy. Am J Obstet Gynecol 1988;158:608–612.
18. Rotmensch S, Cole LA. False diagnosis and needless therapy of presumed malignant disease in women with false-positive human chorionic gonadotropin concentrations. Lancet 2000;355:712–715.
19. Cole LA. Phantom hCG and phantom choriocarcinoma. Gynecol Oncol 1998;71:325–329.
20. Lindahl B, Ahlgren M. Identification of chorion villi in abortion specimens. Obstet Gynecol 1986;67:79–81.

8 Thyroid Disease During Pregnancy
Assessment of the Mother

Corinne R. Fantz, PhD
and Ann M. Gronowski, PhD, DABCC

CONTENTS

Because of the normal physiologic changes associated with pregnancy, maternal thyroid status is often difficult to assess. This chapter focuses on the evaluation of the mother and examines changes that occur both in normal pregnancy and thyroid disease states during pregnancy. A careful clinical review of the patient's history, symptoms, and laboratory measurements will aid the physician in an accurate assessment of maternal thyroid status to avoid inappropriate management of the patient.

THYROID FUNCTION IN NORMAL PREGNANCY

Increase in Circulating Concentrations of Thyroxine-Binding Globulin

Circulating thyroid hormones are bound to three serum proteins: thyroxine-binding globulin (TBG), transthyretin (prealbumin), and albumin. Despite the low concentrations of TBG in serum, TBG has a high affinity for thyroid hormones and thus is responsible for the majority of thyroxine (T_4) and tri-iodothyronine (T_3) transport [1]. During pregnancy, the binding affinities of the three transport proteins are not significantly altered. However, the circulating concentration of TBG more than doubles while the concentrations of the other transport proteins remain relatively constant [2-4]. Elevations in serum concentrations of TBG are observed beginning around 8 wk postfertilization, increase rapidly during the first trimester, reach a plateau around midgestation, and remain high until parturition (Fig. 1). The observed elevation of serum TBG concentrations during normal pregnancy is a result of estrogenic-induced hepatic synthesis of TBG and sialylation of TBG [2,4,5]. Modification of TBG sialic acid content is associated with a reduced hepatic clearance and thus an extended half-life.

From: *Current Clinical Pathology: Handbook of Clinical Laboratory Testing During Pregnancy*
Edited by: A. M. Gronowski © Humana Press, Totowa, NJ

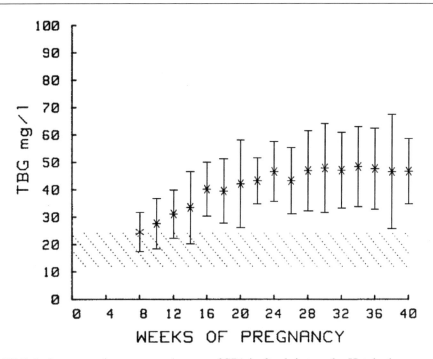

Fig. 1. TBG during normal pregnancy (mean ± 2SD) in 2-wk intervals. Hatched area: normal nonpregnant range of fertile women (n = 290). (Reprinted with permission from ref. *3*.)

Regulation of Thyroid Hormones

Paralleling the increase in TBG, the concentrations of both total thyroxine (TT_4) and total tri-iodothyronine (TT_3) rise substantially in the first trimester, reach a plateau around midgestation, and remain stable throughout the remainder of the pregnancy *(4)*. Despite the body's ability to maintain a euthyroid condition, circulating concentrations of total thyroid hormones, TT_4 and TT_3, often exceed the normal reference intervals. In addition to the influences of TBG on the circulating concentrations of total thyroid hormones, increases in maternal plasma volume may also contribute to the increased demand for the total hormone pools *(6)*. It has also been suggested that increases in total thyroid hormones is caused by placental type III deiodinase *(6)*. Placental type III deiodinase has extremely high activity during pregnancy and has been shown to convert maternal hormones that cross the placenta from T_4 and T_3 to rT_3 and T_2, respectively *(7)*. It has been proposed that this rapid turnover rate generates an increased demand for total thyroid hormones during pregnancy *(8,9)*.

There is typically a slight transient increase in the concentration of biologically active, free T_4 hormone during the first trimester of pregnancy paralleling the increase in human chorionic gonadotropin (hCG) and the decrease in thyroid-stimulating hormone (TSH) *(10)*. Progression into the second and third trimesters, however, may yield significant decreases (20–40% below the normal mean) in the concentration of serum free T_3 and free T_4 *(11)*, and it is important to mention that this phenomenon is exacerbated among women in iodine-deficient areas *(12)*. In fact, two recent reports suggest a need for gestation-dependent reference ranges for pregnant women to avoid unnecessary referrals or misdiagnosis of thyroid dysfunction in normal pregnancies *(13,14)*. Currently, measurement of free T_4 concentrations (together with TSH) is recommended for the evaluation of thyroid status during each trimester of pregnancy *(11)*. Measurement of free T_3 hormone concentrations is usually reserved for cases of thyrotoxicosis with normal free T_4 concentrations and suppressed concentrations of TSH *(10)*.

Increase in Thyroglobulin

Thyroid hormones are synthesized and stored in the colloid matrix of the thyroid follicles in the form of thyroglobulin (TG) *(1)*. Despite having no known hormonal function, serum concentrations of TG can indicate the physiologic activity and volume status of the thyroid gland *(15)*. Thyroidal stimulation during the second and third trimesters of pregnancy often results in an elevation of serum TG concentration, though an increase in TG may be apparent as early as the first trimester *(4)*. The increase in TG concentrations correlates with increased thyroid volume *(4)*. Although goiter is observed in only a small percent of pregnant women (<15%) in the United States, women in iodine-deficient areas have significant increases in thyroid volume and, consequently, elevation in circulating concentrations of TG *(16,17)*.

Plasma Iodine Concentrations

The circulating concentrations of iodine are regulated by an established equilibrium between the stores of iodine present in the thyroid and kidneys with the iodine present in the plasma *(4)*. In pregnancy, the glomerular filtration rate is considerably increased over the nonpregnant state, which results in lower concentrations of plasma iodine *(18)*. Renal losses produce a compensatory increase in thyroidal iodine clearance, often more than two times over that observed in nonpregnant patients *(19)*. In areas of inadequate dietary supplies, renal loss of iodine can rapidly induce overt hypothyroidism and goiter especially following the first trimester of pregnancy when maternal iodine crosses the placenta in response to fetal demands *(20)*. In contrast, in Western civilizations and other areas of the world where iodine intake is adequate, the iodine losses in the urine are not clinically relevant.

Thyroidal Stimulation by Human Chorionic Gonadotropin

Pituitary hormones including hCG, TSH, lutenizing hormone (LH), and follicle-stimulating hormone (FSH) belong to a family of heterodimeric glycoproteins that share a common α-subunit and differ only by a hormone-specific β-subunit *(1)*. Extensive homology exists between TSH and hCG in the β-subunit and several conserved cysteine residues strongly suggest similar tertiary structures *(21)*. In addition, the LH/hCG and TSH receptors also share structural homology *(21)*. Kosugi et al. demonstrated cross-reactivity of hCG to TSH receptors that induces cellular responses leading to TSH suppression *(22)*. Various reports indicate that the hCG in blood is a heterogenous mixture, and certain oligosaccharide side chain modifications can affect the thyrotropic effect of hCG. For instance, removal of the sialic acid residues on hCG can increase its thyrotropic activity *(23,24)*.

Approaching the end of the first trimester, when hCG concentrations are highest, hCG stimulates the thyroid to release thyroid hormones, resulting in a transient suppression of TSH (Fig. 2) *(17)*. This inverse relationship of hCG and TSH is recognized as some of the most convincing evidence of the thyrotropic activity of hCG. Numerous studies have

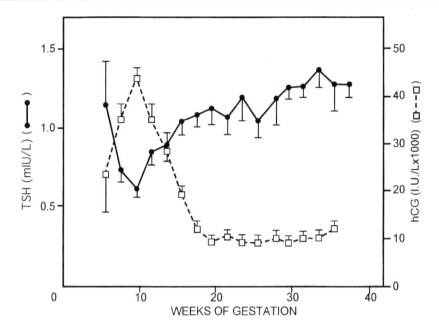

Fig. 2. Serum TSH and hCG as a function of gestational age. Serum hCG determined at initial evaluation; TSH was determined at initial evaluation and during late gestation. The data points represent the mean values (± SE) for samples pooled for 2 wk of gestation. Each point corresponds to the mean of 33 determinations for hCG and 49 for TSH. (Reprinted with permission from ref. 7.)

documented the thyrotropic effect of hCG (21,25–31), including a study demonstrating thryotropic activity on FRTL-5 rat thyroid cells by placing sera on them from women in their first trimester of pregnancy. The effect was confirmed when the sera was treated with an anti-hCG antibody that immunoprecipitated hCG and resulted in a loss of thyrotropic activity (26). In normal pregnancy, TSH suppression is a transient phenomenon that remains within normal reference intervals; however, in approx 18% of otherwise euthyroid women, TSH may be lowered below the normal reference range (32). Abnormal TSH values are usually observed only in cases when the hCG concentration exceeds 50,000 IU/L (4,25). In certain pathological conditions such as molar pregnancies and trophoblastic disease, circulating concentrations of hCG are extremely elevated for extended periods of time, and the thyroid stimulatory effects of hCG are more severe, often inducing thyroid hyperfunction (4). In these cases, thyrotropic stimulation is relieved with complete removal of the placenta and products of conception (33).

HYPERTHYROIDISM IN PREGNANCY

Etiology

Graves' disease, toxic multinodular goiter, subacute thyroiditis, toxic adenoma, TSH hypersecretion, and hormone overreplacement may cause thyroid hyperfunction in the general population. Any of these conditions may be observed during pregnancy as well (34). Estimates of the incidence of hyperthyroidism complicating pregnancy range from 0.1 to 0.4% and have been presumed to be increasing (34–36). This rise has in part been attributed to greater physician awareness and increased sensitivity of assays in detecting mild forms of the disease. Graves' disease is by far the most common etiology of hyper-thyroidism occurring in pregnancy *(37)*. Hyperemesis gravidarum and hydatiform mole are pregnancy-specific associations that can induce hyperthyroidism and are discussed below.

Inadequate control of hyperthyroidism in pregnancy can lead to deleterious side effects for both the mother and fetus *(4)*. Although most pregnancies can tolerate mild hyperthyroidism, it is crucial to monitor hyperthyroid patients. Some maternal compli-cations include congestive heart failure, thyroid storm, infection, spontaneous abortions, increased rate of stillbirths, low birth weights, preterm delivery, severe preeclampsia, fetal or neonatal hyperthyroidism, and intrauterine growth retardation *(10,37–39)*. Euthyroid pregnant women may exhibit tachycardia, insomnia, wide pulse pressures, hypertension, and mild heat intolerance that may make differentiating hyperthyroidism from normal pregnancy-related symptoms more difficult *(37,40)*. However, a careful clinical interpretation of observed symptoms, medical history, and laboratory thyroid function tests should lead to the appropriate assessment of thyroid status.

Diagnosis and Laboratory Assessment

Distinguishing between symptoms of hyperthyroidism and the hypermetabolic state of pregnancy can be particularly challenging. The clinical suspicion of hyperthyroidism should be explored if symptoms such as weight loss or inappropriate weight gain, the presence of goiter, lid lag, fatigue, heart rate greater than 100 bpm, onycholysis, and opthalmopathy are present in the pregnant patient *(16)*. Laboratory testing is similar to that in nonpregnant patients; however, measurements of thyroid function should include TSH and free, not total, hormone concentrations. As discussed earlier, total T_4 and T_3 measurements are influenced by fluctuations in serum TBG concentrations during preg-nancy and therefore should not be used *(2,4,40)*. Concentrations of the free hormones can be determined either directly or by a calculated index. Calculated indices are useful in determining free hormone concentrations, despite the elevation of TBG during preg-nancy *(10)*. Additionally, hyperthyroid patients may exhibit mild increases in certain routine laboratory tests including white blood count, calcium, bone alkaline phosphatase, and liver enzymes *(41)*. Table 1 summarizes thyroid-related changes that occur during pregnancy *(5,6)*.

Graves' Disease and Pregnancy

Graves' disease is by far the most common cause of hyperthyroidism in pregnancy, accounting for more than 85% of all cases *(16,42,43)*. Typically, there is a history of Graves disease or at least thyrotoxic symptoms that predate the pregnancy. It is important to obtain a complete medical history and carefully evaluate clinical symptoms because a missed diagnosis can pose serious threats to the mother and fetus. In properly managed cases of Graves' disease during pregnancy, the prognosis for both the mother and child is excellent *(44)*. Graves' disease is characterized by the presence of goiter; tachycardia; warm, moist skin; and mild heat intolerance *(1)*. Ophthalmic findings suggestive of Graves' disease include proptosis and diplopia resulting from eye muscle dysfunction *(39)*. In most cases, exophthalmos is absent or mild, with one eye appearing slightly more prominent than the other. Pretibial myxedema is rare, where as edema of the conjunctiva and stare are both relatively common *(34)*. When clinical symptoms are inconclusive on routine examination, swollen eye muscles of Graves' ophthalmopathy may be detected

Table 1
Effects of Pregnancy on Thyroid Function Tests

Physiologic change	Thyroid-related consequences
↑ serum estrogens	↑ serum TBG
↑ serum TBG	↑ demand for T_4 and T_3 h in total T_4 and T_3
↑ hCG	↓ TSH (in reference range unless hCG >50,000 IU/L) transient ↑ in free T_4 (1st trimester, in reference range unless hCG >50,000 IU/L)
↑ renal iodine clearance	↑ dietary requirement for I⁻ ↑ 24-hour RAIU ↓ in hormone production in I⁻ deficient areas
↑ type III deiodinase	↑ in T_4 and T_3 degradation and production ↑ demand for T_4 and T_3
↑ demand for TT_4 and TT_3	↑ serum thyroglobulin ↑ thyroid volum ↑ goiter in I⁻ deficient areas
↑ plasma volume	↑ in T_4 and T_3 pool size

Modified from refs. 5,6.

by ultrasonography (39). However, treatment and intervention for endocrine orbitopathy during pregnancy have not been well described in the literature. Retrobulbar irradiation and surgical decompression are both contraindicated in pregnancies; therefore, most clinicians rely on the administration of high-dose glucocorticoids for the medical management of pregnant patients (45).

Pregnancy alters the natural course of Graves' disease. Because of increased thyroid activity in the first trimester, there is initially an observed aggravation followed by an amelioration of symptoms in the second and third trimesters of pregnancy. This transient relief of symptoms has been attributed to immunosuppression associated with pregnancy. However, as the immune system rebounds, there is typically an exacerbation of symptoms during the postpartum period (46). Although immunosuppression is largely recognized as a major contributing factor in changing the course of disease in pregnancy, several other factors are currently being investigated to determine their role in the temporary diminution of clinical symptoms during the second and third trimesters of pregnancy. For example, some have suggested that the renal iodine losses during pregnancy may be ironically beneficial for women with Graves' disease (6). Recent studies examining the changes in cytokine production during pregnancy may also provide additional clues to the pregnancy-induced change of the course of Graves' disease (47).

Thyroid Antibodies

Autoimmune thyroid disease alters thyroid function by humoral and cellular mechanisms. Currently, there are no laboratory tests available to detect cell-mediated processes, but most clinical laboratories provide thyroid antibody testing for the assessment of the humoral response (11). Thyroid peroxidase (TPO), TG, and the TSH receptor are recognized as the three principal thyroid autoantigens. The clinical significance and diagnostic/prognostic utility of each thyroid autoantibody is discussed below.

TPO antibodies are most notably associated with autoimmune tissue destruction. TPO antibody testing is the most sensitive test for detecting autoimmune thyroiditis, and TPO antibodies are often present before the development of thyroid dysfunction (48). There are several methods currently available for detecting TPO antibodies including older antimicrosomal antibody immunofluorescence assays and passive tanned red cell agglutination tests, as well as both competitive and noncompetitive immunoassays (11). For this reason, sensitivity is method dependent, with the more current immunoassays achieving higher sensitivities. One should also be aware of the wide reference intervals for normal patients reported among different manufacturers. Patients with TPO antibodies detected in early pregnancy are at risk for developing postpartum thyroiditis (49). In addition, newly published guidelines recommending that TSH and TPO antibody concentrations be measured in the first trimester of pregnancy are based on recent reports that demonstrate lower IQs among children born to mothers with elevations in TSH and/or TPO antibodies (11,50,51).

TG antibodies are also associated with autoimmune thyroiditis. Because of the complex nature of the immunologic structure of TG, these assays are extremely difficult to standardize (11). As with TPO antibody testing, are a number of different methods of detecting TG antibodies are currently available, including older immunofluoresence assays to competitive and noncompetitive immunoassays. For these reasons, sensitivity and specificity depends on the method employed. TG antibodies are detectable without TPO antibodies in less than 3% of individuals with no risk factors for thyroid dysfunction (52). Therefore, in iodine-sufficient areas, TPO antibodies alone are sufficient for confirmation of autoimmune thyroid disease (53). However, serum TG antibody measurement may be useful for detecting autoimmune thyroid disease in patients with nodular goiter in iodine-deficient areas (11).

Thyrotropin receptor antibodies (TRAbs) are most often measured to investigate the etiology of hyperthyroidism when the diagnosis is not clinically apparent. The presence of TPO antibodies suggests an autoimmune etiology, and TRAbs are more specific for Graves' disease (54). TRAbs are heterogenous and may stimulate the thyroid, causing hyperthyroidism, or alternatively, block the action of the TSH receptor and result in hypothyroidism. Heterogeneity can exist even in an individual patient, and the ratio of the antibodies may change over time (55,56). There are bioassays commercially available to measure the ability of TRAbs to stimulate or inhibit TSH activity and receptor assays that measure the ability of the antibody in serum to block the action of TSH. Bioassays, including thyroid-stimulating antibody (TSAb) assays and TSH receptor blocking antibody (TBAb/TSBAb) assays, measure biological activity based on the production of cyclic adenosine monophosphate from the stimulation or inhibition of the TSH receptor in cultured cells. There are also receptor assays, including thyroid binding inhibiting immunoglobulin assays, that quantify the inhibition of the binding of ^{125}I-labeled TSH to a TSH receptor (57). TRAbs have prognostic implications for fetal and neonatal hyperthyroidism (37,38,55,58). TRAbs have been shown to cross the placenta and, at high concentrations, bind to TSH receptors and stimulate the fetal thyroid (59). There is a strong correlation between high titers of TRAbs (>500% over normal) in maternal serum and fetal or neonatal dysfunction (16). The fetus of expectant mothers with a previous history of Graves' disease should be closely monitored for signs of TRAb stimulating activity (even if the mother is clinically euthyroid during pregnancy) because 2–10% of mothers with high concentrations of TRAbs will deliver babies with hyperthyroidism (60,61).

Women should have their hyperthyroidism under control prior to conception; however, if it becomes necessary to clinically manage the symptoms in the pregnant patient, antithyroid drugs (ATDs) are the treatment of choice *(38)*. The dosage should be adjusted to achieve the minimum amount of drug required to maintain the free thyroid hormone concentrations in the upper third of the normal range *(35,62)*. ATDs can cross the placenta and suppress thyroid function in the fetus; therefore, administration of ATDs should be reduced or stopped when the symptoms of Graves' disease begin to diminish in the second and third trimesters *(37,63)*. Subtotal thyroidectomy should be performed only if there is an allergic reaction to ATDs or if there is sufficient evidence for drug resistance *(16)*. If surgery is deemed necessary, it should be delayed until the second trimester *(35)*. ^{131}I treatment is contraindicated in pregnancy *(63)*.

Nonimmune Causes of Transient Hyperthyroidism

Gestational transient thyrotoxicosis is a broad term encompassing a collection of nonautoimmune causes for transient hyperthyroidism associated with pregnancy *(4)*. Although the majority of cases of transient hyperthyroidism in pregnancy can be associated with hyperemesis gravidarum, other obstetrical conditions such as multiple gestation and hydatidiform mole can also result in transient hyperthyroidism with or without symptoms of hyperemesis. Therefore, another term, transient hyperthyroidism of hyperemesis gravidarum (THHG), has been adopted to describe the syndrome of transient hyperthyroidism in pregnancy associated with severe vomiting *(64)*. One interesting, yet extremely rare, cause of THHG was recently published in the *New England Journal of Medicine (65)*. This report describes a case of familial gestational hyperthyroidism where a mother and daughter were both found to have a mutation in the TSH receptor. The mutant receptor functioned normally in the absence of hCG. However, despite maintaining normal pregnant concentrations of hCG, this mutant receptor was discovered to be more sensitive to hCG, resulting in a recurrence of hyperthyroidal symptoms during pregnancy *(65)*.

Hyperemesis gravidarum is known to occur in approx 0.2% of all pregnancies, with more than half of those patients manifesting symptoms of hyperthyroidism *(64,66)*. These patients typically have no previous history of thyroid illness prior to pregnancy, and goiter is usually absent, as are thyroid antibodies *(4,67)*. Free T_4 concentrations are often found to be elevated over free T_3 concentrations *(5)*. Several studies suggest hyperemesis gravidarum is most often associated with extremely elevated concentrations of hCG in early pregnancy, although there is not always a correlation *(16,26,68)*. Additionally, variants of hCG including desialylated forms have been isolated from the serum of patients experiencing hyperemesis gravidarum and, therefore, a prolonged half-life may in part explain increased thyroid stimulating activity *(16)*. Further, a recent study demonstrated that maternal age, free T_4, and TSH were all independent variables for hyperemesis gravidarum *(69)*. Although the complete mechanism of hyperemesis gravidarum remains elusive, published reports include theories that suggest a combination of estradiol produced by sustained concentrations of hCG in combination with elevated free T_4 concentrations may play a role in promoting hyperemesis *(26,68,70)*. Fortunately, the symptoms associated with THHG typically do not require treatment and disappear on resolution of the hyperemesis *(10,67)*.

Gestational trophoblastic disease (GTD) is another nonautoimmune condition associated with transient hyperthyroidism of pregnancy *(71,72)*. GTD is a general designation

that includes both benign and malignant conditions of hydatidiform mole and choriocar-
cinomas. Goiter is rarely identified in patients with GTD *(42)*. Hyperthyroidism is attributed to substantial and persistent elevations in serum hCG concentrations, which in some
cases may exceed the upper limit of normal by 1000-fold. Laboratory evaluation finds
increases in free hormone concentrations and marked elevation in serum hCG *(4)*. As is
the case with hCG-induced stimulation, the T_4 to T_3 ratio is commonly increased over
ratios observed in Graves' disease patients *(21)*. Complete removal of the GTD rapidly
cures the hyperthyroidism.

THYROID HYPOFUNCTION DURING PREGNANCY

Etiology

The incidence of hypothyroidism among pregnant women has been estimated to be
0.3–0.7%, which is considerably lower than the frequency of hypothyroidism in the
general population, 0.6–1.4% *(4)*. This discordance has been attributed to the known
association between hypothyroidism and infertility *(73–75)*. Iodine deficiency,
Hashimoto's disease, thyroidectomy, radioactive iodine treatment, and subacute thyroiditis are all known to cause hypofunction of the thyroid during and after pregnancy.
In developed countries, the most common etiology of hypothyroidism in pregnancy is
Hashimoto's disease and is characterized by the production of antithyroid antibodies.
This is in contrast to iodine deficiency, which accounts for the most common etiology
worldwide *(70)*. The American College of Obstetricians and Gynecologists suggests that
even certain poorly nourished and immigrant subpopulations located within developed
countries may benefit from iodine treatment *(10)*. Inadequate treatment of hypothyroidism can have serious consequences for both the mother and fetus. Hypothyroidism during
pregnancy has been associated with pregnancy-induced hypertension, placental
abruption, postpartum hemorrhage, an increase in the frequency of low birth weight
infants, and possibly a decrease in the IQ of children *(16,51)*.

Diagnosis and Laboratory Assessment

It should be noted that is it extremely rare for advanced hypothyroidism to present
during pregnancy *(10)*. The classic signs of hypothyroidism are essentially the same in
the pregnant and nonpregnant individual. Patients may present with fatigue, constipation,
cold intolerance, muscle cramps, hair loss, dry skin, and carpal tunnel syndrome. These
symptoms, many nonspecific in nature, may be difficult to separate from symptoms
commonly associated with pregnancy *(1,10)*. The diagnosis of hypothyroidism in pregnancy can be established using TSH and an assessment of free hormone values, measured
either directly or via a calculated index. As with the assessment of hyperthyroidism,
measurement of total T_4 and T_3 should be considered unreliable due to the increase in
TBG concentrations during pregnancy.

Because of the autoimmune nature of Hashimoto thyroiditis, anti-TPO antibodies and
anti-TG antibodies are increased in most patients with Hashimoto thyroiditis and therefore may be useful in establishing a diagnosis. Immunosuppression associated with the
second and third trimesters of pregnancy alters the natural course of this disease by
providing transient relief of hypothyroid symptoms in the second half of pregnancy,
followed by an aggravation in the postpartum period *(46)*. In addition, pregnant patients
who are on thyroid replacement therapy require, on average, 45% more TT_4 compared

with nonpregnant patients. This increased requirement is a direct result of the pregnancy-associated changes in TBG concentration, volume of distribution, and placental action of type III deiodinase *(4,16)*. Women on thyroid replacement therapy should have their TSH monitored closely, and the dose should be titrated to maintain the concentration of TSH within the reference interval.

POSTPARTUM THYROID DISEASE

Although this chapter focuses on thyroid function during pregnancy, the assessment of the mother imparts an extension of this topic to the postpartum period. Postpartum thyroid disease (PPTD) is recognized as an autoimmune destruction of thyroid follicles leading to transient hyperthyroidism (1–3 mo postpartum) followed by hypothyroidism (3–8 mo postpartum) *(76,77)*. PPTD occurs in approx 5–9% of unselected postpartum women *(77–79)*. More than 80% of women who suffer from PPTD are euthyroid within 12 mo of delivery *(80)*. The release of preformed T_4 and T_3 from the damaged thyroid makes this condition characteristically distinct from Graves' disease *(81)*. Graves' disease can be differentiated from PPTD on the basis of low radioactive iodine or technetium uptake in the thyroid during the thyrotoxic phase. Serum TSH is a good screening test, and if it is abnormal, a free T_4 (either direct or calculated) should be performed. Fifty percent of women with anti-TPO positivity do not develop PPTD despite the strong association of TPO antibodies with PPTD *(77,78)*. Occasionally, anti-TG antibodies are present and, in rare cases, anti-TG antibodies are the only antithyroid antibodies found *(82)*. Although PPTD is a transient state of thyroid dysfunction, there is an increased risk for permanent hypothyroidism *(83)*. Treatment is usually not required because symptoms of PPTD generally are mild and nonspecific. In fact, PPTD is often underdiagnosed. Overt symptoms should be treated and thyroid function should be monitored yearly to assess thyroid status for subsequent pregnancies and for the development of permanent thyroid dysfunction.

SUMMARY

Correct assessment of thyroid function during pregnancy is critical to avoid both maternal and fetal complications. It is important to recognize that thyroid function and regulation is altered during normal pregnancy by (1) significant increases in serum TBG, TG, total T_4 and total T_3; (2) an increase in renal iodine clearance; and (3) hCG stimulation. Whereas determination of the above parameters is not useful in the investigation of thyroid disease during pregnancy, assessment of both hyper- and hypothyroidism should be performed with a careful clinical review of the patient's symptoms as well as laboratory evaluation of TSH and free thyroid hormones. Measurement of thyroid autoantibodies may also be useful to diagnose maternal Graves' disease, Hashimoto thyroiditis, and postpartum disease. The physician can properly determine thyroid status by knowing the patient's history and clinical symptoms, and, moreover, realizing the changes associated with thyroid function in pregnancy.

REFERENCES

1. Larsen PR, Davies TF, Hay ID. The thyroid gland. In: Wilson JD, Foster DW, Kronenberg HM, Larsen PR, eds. Williams Textbook of Endocrinology. Philadelphia: W.B. Saunders, 1998:389–515.

2. Ain KB, Mori Y, Refetoff S. Reduced clearance rate of thyroxine-binding glogulin (TBG) with increased sialylation: a mechanism for estrogen-induced elevation of serum TBG concentration. J Clin Endocrinol Metab 1987;65:689–696.

3. Skjoldebrand L, Brundin J, Carlstrom A, Pettersson T. Thyroid associated components in serum during normal pregnancy. Acta Endocrinol (Copenh) 1982;100:504–511.

4. Glinoer D. The regulation of thyroid function in pregnancy: pathways of endocrine adaptation from physiology to pathology. Endocr Rev 1997;18:404–433.

5. Brent GA. Maternal thyroid function: interpretation of thyroid function tests in pregnancy. Clin Obstet Gynecol 1997;40:3–15.

6. Glinoer D. Thyroid regulation and dysfunction in the pregnant patient. In: www.thyroidmanager.org/ thyroidbook.htm, eds. The Thyroid and Its Diseases. Endocrine Education, Inc., 2001, pp. 1–14.

7. Roti E, Fang SL, Green K, Emerson CH, Braverman LE. Human placenta is an active site of thyroxine and 3,3',5-triiodothyronine tyrosyl ring deiodination. J Clin Endocrinol Metab 1981;53:498-501.

8. Burrow GN, Fisher DA, Larsen PR. Maternal and fetal thyroid function. N Engl J Med 1994;331: 1072–1078.

9. Fisher DA, Polk DH, Wu SY. Fetal thyroid metabolism: a pluralistic system. Thyroid 1994;4:367–371.

10. ACOG Practice Bulletin No. 37. Thyroid disease in pregnancy. Am Fam Physician 2002;100(2): 387–396.

11. Demers LM, Spencer CA. Laboratory medicine practice guidelines: laboratory support for the diagnosis and monitoring of thyroid disease. National Academy of Clinical Biochemistry, 2002.

12. Glinoer D. Maternal and fetal impact of chronic iodine deficiency. Clin Obstet Gynecol 1997;40: 102–116.

13. McElduff A. Measurement of free thyroxine (T4) levels in pregnancy. Austr NZ Obstet Gynecol 1999;39:158–161.

14. Pansesar NS, Li CY, Rogers MS. Reference intervals for thyroid hormones in pregnant Chinese women. Ann Clin Biochem 2001;38:329–332.

15. Spencer CA, Wang C-C. Thyroglobulin measurement: techniques, clinical benefits, and pitfalls. Endocrinol Metab Clin North Am 1995;24:841–863.

16. Mestman J, Goodwin TM, Montoro MM. Thyroid disorders of pregnancy. Endocrinol Metab Clin North Am 1995;24:41–71.

17. Glinoer D, DeNayer P, Bourdoux P, et al. Regulation of maternal thyroid during pregnancy. J Clin Endocrinol Metab 1990;71:276–287.

18. Dafnis E, Sabatini S. The effect of pregnancy on renal function: physiology and pathophysiology. Am J Med Sci 1992;303:184–205.

19. Pochin EE. The iodine uptake of the human thyroid throughout the menstrual cycle and in pregnancy. Clin Sci 1952;11:441–445.

20. Thilly CH, Vanderpas JB, Bebe N, et al. Iodine deficiency, other trace elements, and goitrogenic factors in the etiopathogeny of iodine deficiency disorders (IDD). Biol Trace Elem Res 1992;32:229–243.

21. Goodwin TM, Hershman JM. Hyperthyroidism due to inappropriate production of human chorionic gonadotropin. Clin Obstet Gynecol 1997;40:32–44.

22. Kosugi S, Mori T. TSH receptor and LH receptor. Endocrinol J 1995;45:587–606.

23. Yoshimura M, Pekary AE, Pang XP, Berg L, Goodwin TM, Hershman JM. Thyrotropic activity of basic isoelectric forms of human chorionic gonadotropin extracted from hydatidiform mole tissues. J Clin Endocrinol Metab 1994;78:862–866.

24. Mann K, Schneider N, Hoermann R. Thyrotropic activity of acidic isolectric varients of human chorionic gonadotropin from trophoblastic tumors. Endocrinol 1986;118:1558–1566.

25. Guillaume J, Schussler GC, Goldman J, Wassel P, Bach L. Components of the total serum thyroid hormone concentrations during pregnancy: high free thyroxine and blunted thyrotropin (TSH) response to TSH-releasing hormone in the first trimester. J Clin Endocrinol Metab 1985; 0:678–684.

26. Yoshimura M, Hershman JM. Thyrotropic action of human chorionic gonadotropin. Thyroid 1995;5:425–434.

27. Yoshikowa N, Nishikawa M, Horimoto M, et al. Thyroid-stimulating activity in sera of normal pregnant women. J Clin Endocrinol Metab 1989;69:891–895.

28. Yoshimura M, Hershman JM, Pang XP, Berg L, Pekary AE. Activation of the thyrotropin (TSH) receptor by human chorionic gonadotropin and leutinizing hormone in Chinese hamster ovary cells expressing functional human TSH receptors. J Clin Endocrinol Metab 1993;77:1009–1013.

29. Ball R, Freedman DB, Holmes JC, Midgley JEM, Sheehan CP. Low-normal concentrations of free thyroxin in serum in late pregnancy: physiological fact, not detected artifact. Clin Chem 1989;35: 1891–1896.

30. Tomer Y, Huber GK, Davies TF. Human chorionic gonadotropin (hCG) interacts directly with recombinant human TSH receptors. J Clin Endocrinol Metab 1992;74:1477–1479.

31. Davies TF, Platzer M. hCG-induced TSH receptor activation and growth acceleration in FRTL-5 thyroid cells. Endocrinol 1986;118:2149–2151.

32. Glinoer D, DeNayer P, Robyn C, Lejeune B, Kinthaert J, Meuris S. Serum levels of intact human chorionic gonadotropin (hCG) and its free alpha and beta subunits, in relation to maternal thyroid stimulation during normal pregnancy. J Endocrinol Invest 1993;16:881–888.

33. Norman RJ, Green-Thompson RW, Jialal I, Soutter WP, Pillay NL, Joubert SM. Hyperthyroidism in gestational trophoblastic neoplasia. Clin Endocrinol 1981;15:395–401.

34. Mestman J. Perinatal thyroid dysfunction: prenatal diagnosis and treatment. Medscape Women's Health 1997;2:1–11.

35. Glinoer D. Thyroid hyperfunction during pregnancy. Thyroid 1998;8:859–864.

36. Wang C, Crapo LM. The epidemiology of thyroid disease and implications for screening. Endocrinol Metab Clin North Am 1997;26:189–218.

37. Masiukiewicz US, Burrow GN. Hyperthyroidism in pregnancy: diagnosis and treatment. Thyroid 1999;9:647–652.

38. Mestman JH. Hyperthyroidism in pregnancy. Endocrinol Metab Clin North Am 1998;27:127–149.

39. Hamburger JH. Diagnosis and management of Graves' disease in pregnancy. Thyroid 1992;2:219–224.

40. Lazarus JH. Treatment of hyper- and hypothyroidism in pregnancy. J Endocrinol Invest 1993;16:391–396.

41. Mestman JH. Hyperthyroidism in pregnancy. Clin Obstet Gynecol 1997;40:45–64.

42. Bishnoi A, Sachmechi I. Thyroid disease in pregnancy. Am Fam Physician 1996;53:215–220.

43. Lazarus JH. Thyroid disease in relation to pregnancy: a decade of change. Clin Endocrinol 2000;53: 265–278.

44. Mitsuda N, Tamaki H, Amino N, Hosono T, Miyai K, Tanizawa O. Risk factors for developmental disorders in infants born to women with Graves' disease. Obstet Gynecol 1992;80:359–364.

45. Nüßgens Z, Roggenkämper P, Schweikert HU. Entwicklung einer endokrinen orbitopathie während einer schwangerschaft. Klin Monatsbl Augenheilkd 1993;202:130–133.

46. Amino N, Tada H, Hidaka Y. Autoimmune thyroid disease in pregnancy. J Endocrinol Invest 1996;19:59–69.

47. Jones BM, Kwok JSY, Kung AWC. Changes in cytokine production during pregnancy in patients with Graves' disease. Thyroid 2000;10:701–707.

48. Mariotti S, Caturegli P, Piccolo P, Barbesino G, Pinchera A. Antithyroid peroxidase autoantibodies in thyroid diseases. J Clin Endocrinol Metab 1990;71:661–669.

49. Nohr SB, Jorgenson A, Pederson KM, Laurberg P. Postpartum thyroid dysfunction in pregnant thyroid peroxidase antibody positive women living in an area with mild to moderate iodine deficiency: is iodine supplementation safe? J Clin Endocrinol Metab 2000;85:3191–3198.

50. Pop VJ, DeVries E, van Baar AL, et al. Maternal thyroid peroxidase antibodies during pregnancy: a marker for impaired child development? J Clin Endocrinol Metab 1995;80:3561–3566.

51. Haddow JE, Palomaki GE, Allan WC, et al. Maternal thyroid deficiency during pregnancy and subsequent neuropsychological development of the child. N Engl J Med 1999;341:549–555.

52. Hollowell JG, Staehling NW, Hannon WH, Gunter EW, Spencer CA, Braverman LE. Serum thyrotropin, thyroxine, and thyroid antibodies in the United States population (1988–1994): national health and nutrition examination survey (NHAANES III). J Clin Endocrinol Metab 2002;87:489–499.

53. Nordyke RA, Gilbert FI, Miyamoto LA, Fleury KA. The superiority of antimicrosomal over antithyroglobulin antibodies for detecting Hashimoto's thyroiditis. Arch Intern Med 1993;153: 862–865.

54. Cove DH, Johnston P. Fetal hyperthyroidism: experience of treatment in four siblings. Lancet 1985;1:430–432.

55. Ueta Y, Fukui H, Murakami M, et al. Development of primary hypothyroidism with the appearance of blocking-type antibody to thyrotropin receptor in Grave's disease in late pregnancy. Thyroid 1999;9: 179–182.

56. Gupa MK. Thyrotropin-receptor antibodies in thyroid diseases: advances in detection techniques and clinical application. Clin Chem Acta 2000;293:1–29.

57. Costaglioa S, Morganthaler NG, Hoermann R, et al. Second generation assay for thyrotropin receptor antibodies has superior diagnostic sensitivity for Graves' disease. J Clin Endocrinol Metab 1999;84: 90–97.
58. Skuza KA, Sills IN, Stene M, Rapaport R. Prediction of neonatal hyperthyroidism in infants born to mothers with Graves disease. J Pediatr 1996;128:264–268.
59. Wallace C, Couch R, Ginsberg J. Fetal thyrotoxicosis: a case report and recommendations for prediction, diagnosis and treatment. Thyroid 1995;5:125–128.
60. Polk DH. Diagnosis and management of altered fetal thyroid status. Fetal Drug Ther 2002;21:647–662.
61. Fantz CR, Dagogo-Jack S, Ladenson JH, Gronowski AM. Thyroid function during pregnancy. Clin Chem 1999;45:2250–2258.
62. Gardner DF, Cruikshank DP, Hayes PM, Cooper DS. Pharmacology of propylthiourcil (PTU) in pregnant hyperthyroid women: correlation of maternal PTU concentrations with cord serum thyroid function tests. J Clin Endocrinol Metab 1986;62:217–220.
63. Mulder JE. Thyroid disease in women. Med Clin North Am 1998;82:103–125.
64. Goodwin TM, Montoro M, Mestman JH. Transient hyperthyroidism and hyperemesis gravidarum: clinical aspects. Am J Obstet Gynecol 1992;167:648–652.
65. Rodien P, Bremont C, Sanson M-LR, et al. Familial gestational hyperthyroidism caused by a mutant thyrotropin receptor hypersensitive to human chorionic gonadotropin. N Engl J Med 1998;339: 1823–1826.
66. Mazzaferri EL. Evaluation and management of common thyroid disorders in women. Am J Obstet Gynecol 1997;176:507–514.
67. Caffrey TJ. Transient hyperthyroidism of hyperemesis gravidarum: a sheep in wolf's clothing. J Am Board Fam Pract 2000;13:35–38.
68. Goodwin TM, Montoro M, Mestman JH, Pekary AE, Hershman JM. The role of chorionic gonadotropin in transient hyperthyroidism of hyperemesis gravidarum. J Clin Endocrinol Metab 1992;75:1333–1337.
69. Volumenie JL, Polak M, Guibourdenche J, et al. Management of fetal thyroid goiters: a report of 11 cases in a single perinatal unit. Prenat Diag 2000;20:799–806.
70. Ecker JL, Musci TJ. Treatment of thyroid disease in pregnancy. Obstet Gynecol Clin North Am 1997;24:575–589.
71. Hershman JM. Hyperthyroidsim induced by trophoblastic thyrotropin. Mayo Clinic Proc 1972;47: 913–918.
72. Mizouchi T, Nishimura R, Derappes C, et al. Structures of the asparagine-linked sugar chains of human chorionic gonadotropin produced in choriocarcinoma. J Biol Chem 1983;258:14126–14129.
73. Grodstein F, Goldman MB, Ryan L, Cramer DW. Self reported use of pharmaceuticals and primary ovulatory infertility. Epidemiology 1993;4:151–156.
74. Aldersberg MA, Burrow GN. Focus on primary care: thyroid function and dysfunction in women. Obstet Gynecol Surv 2002;57:S1–S7.
75. Reindollar RH, Novak M, Tho SPT, McDonough PG. Adult-onset amenorrhea: a study of 262 patients. Am J Obstet Gynecol 1986;155:531–543.
76. Amino N, Miyai KJ, Onishi T, Hashimoto T, Arai K. Transient hypothyroidism after delivery in autoimmune thyroiditis. J Clin Endocrinol Metab 1976;42:296–301.
77. Kuijpens JL, Haan-Meulman MD, Vader HL, Pop VJ, Wiersinga WM, Drexhage HA. Cell-mediated immunity and postpartum thyroid dysfunction: a possibility for the prediction of disease. J Clin Endocrinol Metab 1998;83:1959–1966.
78. Gerstein HC. How common is postpartum thyroiditis? a methodologic overview of the literature. Arch Intern Med 1990;150:1397–1400.
79. Amino N, Mori T, Iwantani Y, et al. High prevalence of transient postpartum thyrotoxicosis and hypothyroidism. N Engl J Med 1982;306:849–852.
80. Lervang HH, Pryds O, Kristensen HP. Thyroid dysfunction after delivery: incidence and clinical course. Acta Med Scand 1987;222:369–374.
81. Emerson CH. Thyroid disease during and after pregnancy. In: Weiner JA, Ingbar SH, eds. The Thyroid. Philadelphia: Lippincott, 1991: 1263–1279.
82. Lazarus JH. Clinical manifestations of postpartum thyroid disease. Thyroid 2001;9:685–689.
83. Othman S, Phillips DW, Parkes AB, et al. A long term follow-up of postpartum thyroiditis. Clin Endocrinol 1990;32:559–564.

9

Thyroid Disease During Pregnancy
Assessment of the Fetus

Pratima K. Singh, MD
and Ann M. Gronowski, PhD, DABCC

INTRODUCTION

Fetal thyroid metabolism depends on normal fetal thyroid development and hormonogenesis as well as normal maternal thyroid physiology. Thyroid hormone production has been detected in the fetus as early as 10 wk gestation, and thyroid follicles have been identified histologically by 12 wk *(1,2)*. From the 13th wk of gestation until the third trimester, there are increases in fetal serum concentrations of thyroxine (T_4), thyroxine-binding globulin (TBG), and thyroid-stimulating hormone (TSH), independent of maternal serum concentrations *(3,4)*, indicating maturation of the fetal thyroid gland. Tri-iodothyroinine (T_3) does not rise significantly until the third trimester *(3)*, a finding that is explained by the late appearance of type I deiodinase, which catalyses the synthesis of T_3 from T_4.

Placental Transport

The interpretation of fetal thyroid hormone status requires an understanding of maternal–fetal interaction via the placenta. Early in fetal development, maternal iodothyronines such as T_3 and T_4 appear to cross the placental barrier, although this permeability significantly decreases during gestation as the fetus begins to synthesize thyroid hormones. The fetus is capable of independent thyroid hormone production by the end of the first trimester, although some maternal hormones, such as T_4, still undergo a degree of transplacental passage (Fig. 1) *(1)*. For example, fetuses with thyroid gland agenesis or iodination defects have detectable, albeit low, concentrations of T_4 in cord serum *(5)*. However, significant fetal hypothyroidism still occurs, even when maternal serum thyroid hormone concentrations are normal *(6)*, indicating insufficient contribution of maternal T_4 to compensate for fetal thyroid hormone deficiencies. During the second and third trimes-

From: *Current Clinical Pathology: Handbook of Clinical Laboratory Testing During Pregnancy*
Edited by: A. M. Gronowski © Humana Press, Totowa, NJ

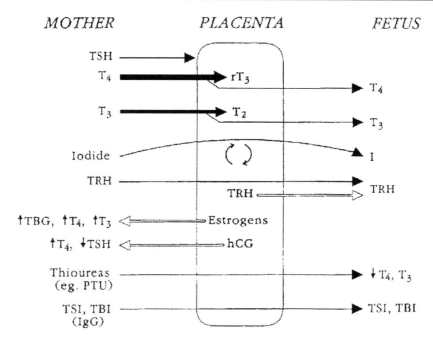

Fig. 1. Placental permeability to various thyroid system-related substances. (From ref. 9, with permission from Elsevier Science.)

ters of normal pregnancies, comparison of cord serum to maternal serum indicates that there are significant T_4 and T_3 concentration gradients, with higher concentrations present in the maternal serum (1,7,8). These data support the concept that there is an extremely limited physiological role for maternally derived iodothyronines in the second and third trimesters.

TSH does not appear to cross the placenta (9). It can be detected in fetal serum as early as 12 wk of gestation (10,11), and, throughout gestation, fetal serum TSH concentrations are actually higher than maternal serum concentrations (10). Thyrotropin-releasing hormone (TRH) does cross the placenta, and some authors have reported an increased fetal TSH response to maternal administration of TRH (9,12).

FETAL THYROID DISORDERS

Fetal Hypothyroidism

The most common thyroid disorder to affect the developing fetus is congenital hypothyroidism, which occurs in 1 per 4000 births (9). It is most often caused by dysgenesis or agenesis of the thyroid gland (9,13). Other, less common etiologies of congenital hypothyroidism include altered thyroid hormonogenesis caused by defects in iodide transport or thyroglobulin abnormalities, maternal antithyroidal medication, and immune-mediated thyroiditis (Table 1) (13).

Although congenital hypothyroidism is the most frequent fetal thyroid disease, these cases are usually not clinically evident during the perinatal period. Neonatal screening for congenital hypothyroidism has been instituted in many states, resulting in early diagnosis of affected individuals. Adequate treatment for these patients should be initiated as soon as possible in order to avoid sequelae such as mental retardation and hearing loss

Table 1
Causes of Congenital Hypothyroidism With Approximate Incidence

Thyroid dysgenesis	1:4000
Agenesis	
Dysgenesis	
Ectopia	
Thyroid dyshormonogenesis	1:30,000
TSH receptor defect	
Iodide trapping defect	
Organification defect	
Iodotyrosine deiodinase deficiency	
Thyroglobulin defect	
Transient hypothyroidism	1:40,000
Drug-induced	
Maternal antibody-induced	
Idiopathic	
Hypothalamic–pituitary hypothyroidism	1:100,000
Hypothalamic–pituitary anomaly	
Panhypopituitarism	
Isolated TSH deficiency	
TSH structural defect	

From ref. *9*, with permission from Elsevier Science.

(14,15). Fetal hypothyroidism can have adverse consequences in the prenatal period, such as fetal bradycardia, intrauterine growth retardation, and delayed ossification *(16)*. If a prenatal diagnosis is made, fetal hypothyroidism can be treated by *in utero* administration of T_4.

Fetal hypothyroidism can also be a result of maternal hypothyroidism caused by etiologies such as iodine deficiency or antibody-mediated hypothyroidism *(9)*. The fetus depends on maternal iodine for thyroid hormone production; therefore, maternal iodine deficiency can cause fetal hypothyroidism. Throughout the world, iodine deficiency is the most common cause of fetal hypothyroidism, although these cases are usually restricted to endemic iodine-deficient areas *(17)*. In the setting of immune-mediated maternal hypothyroidism, transplacental passage of immunoglobulins can occur, inducing hypothyroidism in the fetus *(9,18)*. Predictive antibody testing in pregnant women with immune-mediated hypothyroidism has not been extensively studied. However, one group has reported transient neonatal hypothyroidism when maternal thyrotropin-binding inhibitor immuoglobulin (TBII) concentrations were above 300 U/mL *(18)*.

Another significant cause of fetal hypothyroidism in developed countries is iatrogenic, caused by the administration of antithyroidal medication for maternal hyperthyroidism. The commonly used antithyroidal agents propylthiouracil and methimazole have been shown to cross the placenta and cause fetal hypothyroidism *(19–21)*; however, conservative dosing of these agents helps to prevent adverse fetal effects *(9,22)*.

Fetal Hyperthyroidism

Fetal hyperthyroidism is much less common than hypothyroidism and is extremely rare in the absence of maternal thyroid disease. Affected fetuses can manifest signs of hyperthyroidism such as tachycardia and advanced bone maturation *(6,23)*. In the neonatal period, hyperthyroidism can lead to tachycardia, hyperactivity, growth retardation, sweating, irritability, exophthalmos, and increased morbidity and mortality *(24,25)*. The fetal thyroid is responsive to stimulation by approx 25–28 wk and hyperthyroidism should be suspected if the fetal heart rate in the third trimester is greater than 160 beats/min *(25,26)*.

The most common cause of fetal hyperthyroidism is transplacental passage of thyroid stimulating and/or TSH-binding inhibitory antibodies, collectively known as TSH-receptor antibodies (TRAbs) *(25,27)*. Indeed, fetal hyperthyroidism appears to be restricted to mothers with elevated TRAb concentrations. In the evaluation of Graves' disease, two assays are primarily used to assess TRAb status. The first method detects the presence of thyroid-stimulating antibodies (TSAbs). It is an in vitro bioassay that measures cyclic adenosine monophosphate (cAMP) production when a thyroid cell culture is exposed to patient IgG in comparison to pooled normal immunoglobulin G (IgG) *(26)*. Although the nomenclature for this technique varies, it is most commonly known as either thyroid stimulating immunoglobulin or TSAb, and today results are usually reported as a percent of basal activity. The normal reference intervals provided for this test are variable and depend on the individual assay, but are generally less than 130% of basal activity (or less than 1.3-fold over basal). The second method is a radioreceptor assay that detects the presence of TSH-binding inhibitory antibodies. This assay measures the specific binding of ^{125}I-labeled TSH in the presence of patient IgG vs normal pooled IgG *(26)*. This test is commonly referred to as TBII and is reported as a percent inhibition. As would be expected, normal mean should be approx 0% inhibition, with reference intervals often quoted as –15 to +15% *(24,28)*.

The utility of these two tests rests primarily in their ability to predict neonatal outcome. The literature, however, does not provide a uniform set of guidelines in approaching test results. Some authors report a high likelihood of fetal involvement if both assays show elevation *(24,29)*. Mortimer et al. reported that TBII inhibition of more than 70% was associated with neonatal hyperthroidism, either at birth or shortly after *(28)*. TSI stimulating activity of 350–500% above basal has been associated with intrauterine hyperthyroidism *(30,31)*. Overall, the data suggest that even mild elevation of TRAbs, regardless of methodology, warrant careful follow-up of the fetus and neonate for any signs of involvement.

Diagnosing fetal thyroid disorders in the setting of maternal Graves' disease should be done with caution, because the fetus is at risk for hyperthyroidism from transplacental passage of TSAbs as well as iatrogenic hypothyroidism caused by any antithyroidal treatment that is initiated. For example, Ochoa-Maya et al. reported a case where a woman being treated for Graves' disease had one pregnancy affected by fetal hypothyroidism and then a subsequent pregnancy affected by fetal hyperthyroidism *(32)*.

DIAGNOSIS OF FETAL THYROID DISEASE

Ultrasound Findings in Fetal Dysthyroid States

Approximately 3% of fetal thyroid diseases will be associated with an enlarged fetal thyroid gland, or goiter *(33)*. The presence of a fetal goiter itself confers additional risks on the fetus such as neck dystocia and respiratory compromise caused by compression by the thyroid gland, which can complicate delivery *(33,34)*. Polyhydramnios is a particularly concerning finding in the setting of fetal goiter, because it can imply significant obstruction of the esophagus and possible upper airway obstruction as well.

A goiter can result from fetal hypo- or hyperthyroidism, and specific *in utero* treatments are available for fetal thyroid disorders. Therefore, the ability to differentiate between separate dysthyroid states is critical. For example, several case reports have demonstrated rapid resolution of hypothyroid fetal goiters using intrauterine T_4 administration or, in cases of fetal hypothyroidism caused by maternal antithyroidal medication, withdrawal (or dosage reduction) of the offending agent *(32,33,35–42)*. Conversely, cases of fetal hyperthyroid goiters in the setting of maternal Graves' disease have been treated successfully *in utero* by the administration of appropriate doses of oral antithyroidal medication such as propylthiovracil and methimazole to the mother *(33,43,44)*. Obviously, appropriate *in utero* treatments require definitive understanding of fetal thyroid pathophysiology.

Normal size ranges for fetal thyroid glands have been reported in the literature *(45,46)*. Figures 2 and 3 illustrate expected fetal thyroid measurements at different gestational ages. The presence of a goiter correlates well with abnormal fetal thyroid function *(46)*. Again, it should be noted that only a minority of fetal thyroid diseases present with a goiter *(33)*, stressing the continued need for widespread neonatal testing.

There are certain findings on ultrasound examination, apart from goiter, that can help support a particular dysthyroid state. For example, delayed bone maturation and reduced fetal movements are associated with fetal hypothyroidism, whereas fetal hyperthyroidism can cause tachycardia and advanced bone maturation *(33,47)*. When correlated with a suggestive clinical history, these ultrasound features can support a particular thyroid disease, but they cannot render a definitive diagnosis by themselves. The presence of fetal tachycardia should be interpreted with particular caution, because other factors, such as maternal bleeding, can cause fetal tachycardia in an otherwise hypothyroid fetus *(33)*.

All ultrasound findings should be considered in the context of the clinical presentation. If a fetal goiter is present in the setting of untreated maternal Graves' hyperthyroidism, then there is no reason to suspect fetal hypothyroidism. In fact, fetal goiter in this setting has been interpreted as hyperthyroidism and successfully treated by antithyroidal medication with no corroborative AF or cord serum evaluation *(33)*. It may be prudent, however, to have a low threshold for further fetal testing. AF and/or umbilical cord serum can provide a more specific assessment of fetal thyroid function for both diagnostic and therapeutic purposes.

AF Testing

The use of AF thyroid hormone measurements in diagnosing fetal dysthyroid states has been controversial. There has been much discussion about whether thyroid hormones in AF are of fetal or maternal origin. As previously discussed, the iodothyronines have a complex maternal–fetal physiology; therefore, the utility of measuring these hormones in AF is unclear. However, it is generally accepted that TSH does not cross the placenta *(48–50)*, so that AF TSH originates solely from the fetus.

Prior reports have discussed the futility of using AF to diagnose fetal thyroid disorders. In a widely cited study by Hollingsworth and Alexander *(51)*, the authors were unable to correlate AF concentrations of TSH, T_4, and T_3 to clinical outcome. However, there are numerous shortcomings to this paper. First, the reference intervals for AF TSH that this study provided are considerably wider than the reference intervals that have been reported in the literature since that time (Table 2). Therefore, cases that may otherwise have been

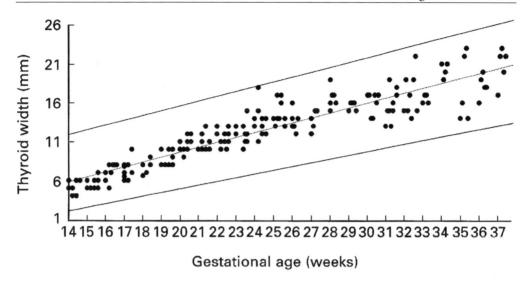

Fig. 2. Individual scatter plot showing the relationship between the thyroid width and gestational age of 193 normal fetuses (mean and 95% confidence limits) ($r = 0.911$). (From ref. *45*, with permission from Blackwell Science.)

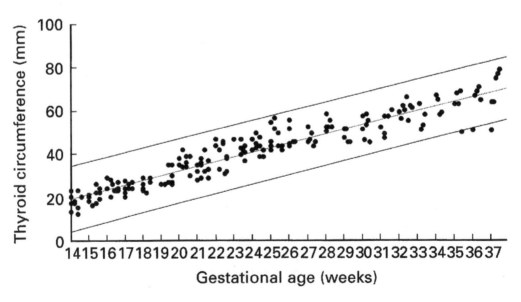

Fig. 3. Individual scatter plot showing the relationship between the thyroid circumference and gestational age of 193 normal fetuses (mean and 95% confidence limits) ($r = 0.931$). (From ref. *45*, with permission from Blackwell Science.)

diagnosed as fetal hypothyroidism using narrower reference intervals may have been missed. Second, the authors report that their TSH assay had cross-reactivity with human chorionic gonadotropin (hCG) and the AF matrix contributed a positive bias for TSH, making their TSH results unreliable. They further state that their AF TSH results "should not be taken as absolute values." Therefore, their assay should not have been used to define a reference interval. Finally, several of the case reports in Hollingsworth's paper do not confirm AF thyroid hormone concentrations with neonatal serum, which may

Other published reports have provided reference intervals for thyroid hormones in AF (Table 2). These reference intervals have been used to diagnose and manage fetal goiters by measuring AF TSH and in some cases, AF T_4 (35–39,52). There are six case reports of fetal hypothyroidism in which AF TSH was measured. In these cases, the AF TSH concentrations ranged from 1.1 to 28.9 µIU/mL, all of which are well outside the published reference intervals, with the exception of Hollingsworth and Alexander's study (Table 2). These high AF TSH concentrations allowed the investigators to make an *in utero* diagnosis of primary fetal hypothyroidism, supporting a diagnostic role for AF thyroid hormones, and AF TSH in particular. The utility of AF T_4 measurement is not clear, and some researchers have found AF total T_4 concentrations to be less reliable than AF TSH (39).

Based on knowledge of fetal thyroid physiology and published reports, TSH appears to be the single best marker to use for diagnosing fetal hypothyroidism in AF. However, there are some issues one should bear in mind when using AF TSH. First, in the case of hypothalamic or pituitary dysfunction, hypothyroidism is associated with decreased TSH concentrations (in contrast to the elevated concentrations expected in primary thyroid dysfunction). It should be noted that the incidence of fetal hypothyroidism as a result of dysfunction of the hypothalamic–pituitary system is exceedingly rare, with a prevalence of 1 per 100,000 per live births (48), whereas primary hypothyroidism is far more frequent (Table 1). Therefore, in the vast majority of cases of suspected fetal hypothyroidism, the presence of an elevated AF TSH concentration is sufficient for the diagnosis.

Second, AF concentrations of TSH are very low in normal pregnancies. Many normal AF specimens have TSH concentrations below the analytical sensitivity of second-generation immunoassays (53). This relative lack of sensitivity is significant, because the expected decrease in AF TSH in the setting of secondary hypothyroidism or primary fetal hyperthyroidism would not be detectable using this method. A more definitive lower reference range may be possible using third-generation TSH assays, but these studies have not yet been conducted.

The utility of AF thyroid hormone concentrations for diagnosing fetal hyperthyroidism is unclear. We know of no published case reports of fetal hyperthyroidism where AF thyroid tests were performed. It is not possible to know whether such testing is of use until AF thyroid hormone concentrations from several cases of fetal hyperthyroidism are reported in the literature. Although it may be predicted that the currently available reference intervals for AF TSH lack the sensitivity to be of clinical use in these cases, it is possible that reference intervals for total and free T_4 will aid in the diagnosis.

AF thyroid hormone measurements can be used not only for diagnosis but also for management. Many authors have reported cases of fetal hypothyroid goiter successfully treated with intrauterine T_4. These cases were followed with ultrasound examination to show regression of fetal goiter and AF testing to show decreases in AF TSH and/or increases in AF T_4 (35,37–39). Application of amniotic fluid reference intervals may

Table 2

Amniotic Fluid Thyroid Hormone Reference Intervals Published in the Literature

Reference	n	Gestational age in weeks	TSH method	TSH ($\mu IU/mL$)	Total T_4 method	Total T_4 ($\mu g/dL$)
Chopra, 1975 (67)	a) 26 b) 7	a) 36–42 b) 31–35	RIA	not detectable	RIA	a) mean 0.44 b) mean 0.31
Klein, 1980 (68)	138	10–42	n/d[a]	n/d	RIA	range ~0.08 to ~2.5
Kourides, 1982 (69)	a) 201 b) 21	a) 16–19 b) 3rd trimester	RIA	a) mean 0.4 range < 0.15–1.7 b) mean 0.25 range < 0.15–0.55	n/d	n/d n/d
Hollingsworth, 1983 (51)	a) 41 b) 28	a) 15–28 b) 36–42	Beckman solid-phase hTSH kit (Beckman, Fullerton, CA)	a) mean ± SD[c] 1.9 ± 0.6 range < 0.4–2.9 b) mean ± SD 0.7 ± 0.4 range 0.4 ± 1.7	RIA	a) mean ± SD 0.182 ± 0.176 range 0–0.675 b) mean ± SD 0.318 ± 0.153 range 0.108–0.728
Yoshida, 1986 (70)	21	38–41	IRMA (Riabead II, Dainabbot Co., Japan)	mean ± SD 0.129 ± 0.069	n/d	n/d
Singh, 2003 (53)	TSH-127 tT$_4$-129 fT$_4$-119	26–39	Abbott AxSym (Abbott Laboratories, Abbott Park, IL)	95% reference interval: < 0.1–0.4	Abbott AxSym (Abbott Laboratories, Abbott Park, IL)	2.3–3.9 free T$_4$ < 0.4–0.7 ng/dL

provide a more relevant endpoint for therapy than ultrasound monitoring, because the regression of goiter does not necessarily confer a euthyroid state. In addition, if intrauterine T_4 injections are being performed for treatment purposes, AF is a readily accessible sample.

AF thyroid hormone reference intervals (especially TSH) can be of significant use in the diagnosis and management of fetal hypothyroidism, potentially reducing the need for umbilical blood sampling in these patients.

Cord Serum Testing

The use of umbilical cord serum has been considered to be the gold standard for the diagnosis of fetal thyroid disease. In fact, most of our understanding of fetal thyroid physiology comes from studies of cord serum *(54–60)*. Many authors have successfully utilized cord serum to render diagnoses of particular fetal thyroid disorders *(35–37,39–44,61,62)*, using a variety of sources for reference intervals *(56–60)*. Although analysis of cord serum would appear to be the most definitive way to assess fetal dysthyroid states, there are some flaws with this approach. First of all, most studies examining normal concentrations of thyroid hormones in cord serum lack a suitably sized study population to establish proper reference intervals. Second, and even more important, almost all studies utilizing cord serum obtained samples from aborted fetuses or prematurely delivered neonates. This approach may not provide accurate reference intervals for thyroid hormones in cord serum, because parturitional stress contributes significantly to artificial elevation of cord serum TSH *(63)*.

Reference intervals for cord serum thyroid hormone values are provided in Table 3. The two studies utilized in this table are those of Radunovic et al. *(59)* and Santini et al. *(64)*. These studies were included in part because they utilized cordocentesis samples from living fetuses for analysis as opposed to aborted or newborn cord serum samples. Additionally, the study by Santini et al. had a larger sample size than many other studies of cord serum thyroid hormone concentrations. Although the purpose of Santini et al. was to examine fetal thyroid physiology and not to establish reference intervals, the results may still be used for such purposes. The study by Radunovic et al. was intended to provide reference intervals, but the number of samples utilized was small ($n = 12$ for gestational weeks 19–27, $n = 6$ for weeks 28–35, and $n = 3$ for weeks 36–42). The lack of a large study population in these articles also prevents the investigators from determining whether cord concentrations change significantly with gestational age. These data are needed to determine whether separate weekly or monthly reference intervals are necessary.

One of the major drawbacks in using cordocentesis is the potential risk to the fetus and mother during the procedure. Bleeding from the site of funipuncture is the most common complication, occurring in approx 40–50% of cordocentesis procedures *(65)*; however, the bleeding is usually transient and mild. Rarely, fetal exsanguination has been reported in cases of fetal platelet disorders. Other complications associated with cordocentesis are fetal bradycardia, chorioamnionitis, and fetomaternal hemorrhage. Infection is an important cause of morbidity and mortality, occurring in approx 1% of procedures. The rate of fetal loss caused by cordocentesis is low, cited at 1.4% by Ghidini et al. *(65)*; however, the mortality rate is extremely variable and appears highly dependent on the expertise of the physicians performing the procedure.

As stated earlier, the use of cord serum for the evaluation of fetal dysthyroid states has been considered the gold standard. This is despite the absence of well-established reference intervals for fetal serum thyroid hormone concentrations because of small sample

Table 3
Cord Serum Thyroid Hormone Reference Intervals

Analyte	Units	Weeks	Range	n	Weeks	Range	n	Weeks	Range	n	Reference
TSH	mU/L	19–27	4.1 ± 1.4[a]	76	28–35	6.9 ± 2.4	7	36–42	4.2 ± 1.5	37	64
Total T_4	µg/mL	19–21	7.79 ± 2.02	12	28–30	9.28 ± 2.13	6	34–35	11.03 ± 1.4	3	59
Total T_3	ng/mL	19–21	<10	12	28–30	18.5 ± 10.7	6	34–35	22.1 ± 15.8	3	59
Free T_4	pmol/L	19–27	7.4 ± 5.5	50	28–35	15 ± 2.1	7	36–42	17 ± 5.2	33	64
Free T_3	pmol/L	19–27	1.8 ± 0.66	25	28–35	2.1 ± 0.41	5	36–42	2.6 ± 0.67	6	64
TBG	µg/mL	19–21	8.13 ± 5.54	12	28–30	14.37 ± 2.58	6	34–35	17.1 ± 5.51	3	59

[a]Values represent the mean ± standard deviation.

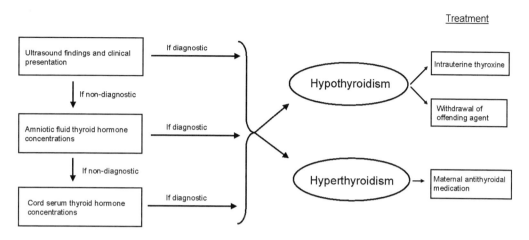

Fig. 4. Algorithm for diagnostic approach to fetal dysthyroid states.

sizes and the use of cord serum obtained from aborted fetuses or premature infants. In the literature, there is no significant clinical outcome data addressing AF versus cord serum thyroid hormone evaluation in terms of diagnostic or therapeutic superiority. Because of the higher complication rate, cordocentesis for fetal serum testing may be ideally left for those cases where the clinical setting, ultrasound findings, and AF thyroid hormone values fail to provide the diagnosis (Fig. 4).

SUMMARY

Fetal dysthyroid states are rare and may exist either with or without predisposing maternal thyroid disease. The importance in determining fetal thyroid function lies in the fact that *in utero* treatment is available, which can prevent complications of fetal goiter and neonatal thyroid problems.

As seen in Fig. 4, there are many ways that fetal thyroid disorders can be diagnosed. The first, and most important, is the clinical presentation. Some cases can be diagnosed solely on the basis of the clinical setting, such as diagnosing a fetal goiter as hyperthyroidism in the setting of untreated maternal Graves' hyperthyroidism. Ultrasound findings can provide a great deal of information as well. Apart from fetal thyroid size, evaluation of bone development and heart rate can provide support for a particular thyroid state, although these findings should be interpreted with caution.

AF or cord serum thyroid hormone concentrations provide a more definitive assessment of fetal thyroid status. There are reasons why either approach may be appropriate, depending on the clinical situation. The relative ease of obtaining AF gives it an advantage over cord serum in most cases, not only for diagnosis, but also in monitoring response to therapy. AF has more precisely defined reference intervals, which may be important in less severe thyroid disease or for therapy endpoints. Cord serum may be the method of choice if fetal hyperthyroidism is suspected, because AF thyroid hormone concentrations in fetal hyperthyroidism have not been studied. Cord serum may also be helpful in cases where other diagnostic modalities fail to yield the diagnosis.

The use of perinatal testing for fetal thyroid disorders is not currently recommended for screening an asymptomatic population. Rather, fetal testing should be reserved for those cases with high clinical suspicion because of either maternal thyroid disease or an incidentally discovered fetal goiter on ultrasound examination. Fetuses that have thyroid diseases in these clinical circumstances tend to have severe disease, and if the diagnosis is delayed until the neonatal period, they may have IQ deficits even with treatment *(66)*. For this reason, there may be significant advantages to diagnosing and treating affected cases *in utero*. Certainly, there are tremendous benefits to the fetus in the reversal of goiter prior to delivery.

REFERENCES

1. Burrow GN, Fisher DA, Larsen PR. Maternal and fetal thyroid function. N Engl J Med 1994;331: 1072–1078.
2. Rosen F, Ezrin C. Embryology of the thyrotroph. J Clin Endocrinol 1966;26:1343–1345.
3. Fisher DA, Dussault JH, Hobel CJ, Lam R. Serum and thyroid gland triiodothyronine in the human fetus. J Clin Endocrinol Metab 1973;36:397–400.
4. Klein AH, Oddie TH, Parslow M, Foley TP Jr, Fisher DA. Developmental changes in pituitary–thyroid function in the human fetus and newborn. Early Hum Dev 1982;6:321–330.
5. Vulsma T, Gons MH, de Vijlder JJM. Maternal–fetal transfer of thyroxine in congenital hypothyroidism due to a total organification defect or thyroid agenesis. N Engl J Med 1989;321:13–16.
6. Volumenie JL, Polak M, Guibourdenche J, et al. Management of fetal thyroid goiters: a report of 11 cases in a single perinatal unit. Prenat Diag 2000;20:799–806.
7. Ballabio M, Nicolini U, Jowett T, DeElvira MCR, Ekins RP, Rodeck CH. Maturation of thyroid function in normal human foetuses. Clin Endocrinol 1989;31:565–571.
8. Daffos F. Fetal blood sampling. Annu Rev Med 1989;40:319–329.
9. Polk DH. Diagnosis and management of altered fetal thyroid status. Fetal Drug Ther 2002;21:647–662.
10. Thorpe-Beeston JG, Nicolaides KH, McGregor AM. Fetal thyroid function. Thyroid 1992;2(3): 207–217.
11. Thorpe-Beeston JG, Nicolaides KH, Felton CV, Butler J, McGregor AM. Maturation of the secretion of thyroid hormone and thyroid-stimulating hormone in the fetus. N Engl J Med 1991;3243(8):532–536.
12. Thorpe-Beeston JG, Nicolaides KH, Snijders RJM, Butler J, McGregor AM. Fetal thyroid-stimulating hormone response to maternal administration of thyrotropin-releasing hormone. Am J Obstet Gynecol 1991;164:1244–1245.
13. Abuhamad AZ, Fisher DA, Warsof SF, et al. Antenatal diagnosis and treatment of fetal goitrous hypothyroidism: case report and review of the literature. Ultrasound Obstet Gynecol 1995;6:368–371.
14. Knipper M, Zinn C, Maier H, et al. Thyroid hormone deficiency before the onset of hearing causes irreversible damage to peripheral and central auditory systems. J Neurophysiol 2000;83(5):3101–3112.
15. Rovet J, Ehrlich R, Sorbara D. Intellectual outcome in children with fetal hypothyroidism. J Pediat 1987;110:700–704.
16. Utiger RD. Recognition of thyroid disease in the fetus. N Engl J Med 1991;324(8):559–561.
17. Fisher DA. Fetal thyroid function: diagnosis and management of fetal thyroid disorders. Clin Obstet Gynecol 1997;40(1):16–31.
18. Tamaki H, Amino N, Aozasa M, et al. Effective method for predication of transient hypothyroidism in neonates born to mothers with chronic thyroiditis. Am J Perinatol 1989;6(3):296–303.
19. Hamburger JH. Diagnosis and management of Graves' disease in pregnancy. Thyroid 1992;2:219–224.
20. Mestman J. Perinatal thyroid dysfunction: prenatal diagnosis and treatment. Medscape Women's Health 1997;2:1–11.
21. Momotani N, Noh JY, Ishikawa N, Ito K. Effects of propothiouracil and methimazole on fetal thyroid status in mothers with Graves' hyperthyroidism. J Clin Endocrinol Metab 1997;82:3633–3636.
22. Emerson CH. Thyroid disease during and after pregnancy. In: Weiner JA, Ingbar SH, eds. The Thyroid. Philadelphia: Lippincott, 1991, pp. 1263–1279.
23. Sagot P, David A, Yvinec M, et al. Intrauterine treatment of fetal goiters. Fetal Diagn Ther 1991;6:28–33.

24. Matsuura N, Konishi J, Fujieda K, et al. TSH-receptor antibodies in mothers with Graves' disease and outcome in their offspring. Lancet 1988;1(8575–6):14–17.
25. McKenzie JM, Zakarija M. Fetal and neonatal hyperthyroidism and hypothyroidism due to maternal TSH receptor antibodies. Thyroid 1992;2:155–159.
26. McKenzie JM, Zakarija M. The clinical use of thyrotropin receptor antibody measurements. J Clin Endocrinol Metab 1989;69:1093–1096.
27. Mestman J, Goodwin TM, Montoro MM. Thyroid disorders of pregnancy. Endocrinol Metab Clin North Am 1995;24:41–71.
28 Mortimer RH, Tyack SA, Galligan JP, Perry-Keene DA, Tan YM. Graves' disease in pregnancy: TSH receptor binding inhibiting immunoglobulins and maternal and neonatal thyroid function. Clin Endocrinol 1990;32:141–152.
29. Tamaki H, Amino N, Aozasa M, et al. Universal predictive criteria for neonatal overt thyrotoxicosis requiring treatment. Am J Perinatol 1988;5(2):152–158.
30. Clavel S, Madec AM, Bornet H, Deviller P, Stefanutti A, Orgiazzi J. Anti TSH-receptor antibodies in pregnant patients with autoimmune thyroid disorder. Br J Obstet Gynaecol 1990;97:1003–1008.
31. Zakarija M, McKenzie JM. Pregnancy-associated changes in the thyroid-stimulating antibody of Graves' disease and the relationship to neonatal hyperthyroidism. J Clin Endocrinol Metab 1983;57:1036–1040.
32. Ochoa-Maya MR, Frates MC, Lee-Parritz A, Seely EW. Resolution of fetal goiter after discontinuation of propylthiouracil in a pregnant woman with Graves' hyperthyroidism. Thyroid 1999;9(11):1111–1114.
33. Volumenie JL, Polak M, Guibourdenche J, et al. Management of fetal thyroid goiters: a report of 11 cases in a single perinatal unit. Prenat Diag 2000;20:799–806.
34. Utiger RD. Recognition of thyroid disease in the fetus. N Engl J Med 1991;324(8):559–561.
35. Bruner JP, Dellinger EH. Antenatal diagnosis and treatment of fetal hypothyroidism: a report of two cases. Fetal Diagn Ther 1997;12:200–204.
36. Nicolini U, Venegoni E, Acaia B, Cortelazzi D, Beck-Peccoz P. Prenatal treatment of fetal hypothyroidism: is there more than one option? Prenat Diag 1996;16:443–448.
37. Perelman AH, Johnson RL, Clemons RD, Finberg HJ, Clewell WH, Trujillo L. Intrauterine diagnosis and treatment of fetal goitrous hypothyroidism. J Clin Endocrinol Metab 1990;71:618–621.
38. Perrotin F, Sembely-Taveau C, Haddad G, Lyonnais C, Lansac J, Body G. Prenatal diagnosis and early in utero management of fetal dyshormonogenic goiter. Eur J Obstet Gynecol Reprod Biol 2001;94: 309–314.
39. Abuhamad AZ, Fisher DA, Warsof SF, et al. Antenatal diagnosis and treatment of fetal goitrous hypothyroidism: case report and review of the literature. Ultrasound Obstet Gynecol 1995;6:368–371.
40. Gruner C, Kollert A, Wildt L, Dorr HG, Beinder E, Lang N. Intrauterine treatment of fetal goitrous hypothyroidism controlled by determination of thyroid-stimulating hormone in fetal serum. Fetal Diagnosis and Therapy 2001;16:47–51.
41. Noia G, DeSantis M, Tocci A, et al. Early prenatal diagnosis and therapy of fetal hypothyroid goiter. Fetal Diagn Ther 1992;7:138–143.
42. Davidson KM, Richards DS, Schatz DA, Fisher DA. Successful in utero treatment of fetal goiter and hypothyroidism. N Engl J Med 1991;324(8):543–546.
43. Hadi HA, Strickland D. In utero treatment of fetal goitrous hypothyroidism caused by maternal Graves' disease. Am J Perinat 1995;12:455–458.
44. Friedland DR, Rothschild MA. Rapid resolution of fetal goiter associated with maternal Graves' disease: a case report. Int J Pediatr Otorhinolaryngol 2000;54:59–62.
45. Achiron R, Rotstein Z, Lipitz S, Karasik A, Seidman DS. The development of the foetal thyroid: in utero ultrasonographic measurements. Clin Endocrinol 1998;48:259–264.
46. Bromley B, Frigoletto FD, Cramer D, Osathanondh R, Benacerraf BR. The fetal thyroid: normal and abnormal sonographic measurements. J Ultrasound Med 1992;11:25–28.
47. Sagot P, David A, Yvinec M, et al. Intrauterine treatment of fetal goiters. Fetal Diagn Ther 1991;6:28–33.
48. Polk DH. Diagnosis and management of altered fetal thyroid status. Fetal Drug Ther 2002;21:647–662.
49. Ecker JL, Musci TJ. Treatment of thyroid disease in pregnancy. Obstet Gynecol Clin North Am 1997;24:575–589.
50. Emerson CH. Thyroid disease during and after pregnancy. In: Weiner JA, Ingbar SH, eds. The Thyroid. Philadelphia: Lippincott, 1991, pp. 1263–1279.
51. Hollingsworth DR, Alexander NM. Amniotic fluid concentrations of iodothyronines and thyrotropin do not reliably predict fetal thyroid status in pregnancies complicated by maternal thyroid disorders or anencephaly. Clin Endocronol Metab 1983;57:349–355.

52. Kourides IA, Berkowitz RL, Pang S, Van Natta FC, Barone CM, Ginsberg-Fellner F. Antepartum diagnosis of goitrous hypothyroidism by fetal ultrasonography and amniotic fluid thyrotropin concentration. J Clin Endocrinol Metab 1984;59:1016–1018.

53. Singh PK, Parvin CA, Gronowski AM. Establishment of reference intervals for markers of fetal thyroid status in amniotic fluid. J Clin Endocrinol Metab 2003;88:4175–4179.

54. Ballabio M, Nicolini U, Jowett T, DeElvira MCR, Ekins RP, Rodeck CH. Maturation of thyroid function in normal human foetuses. Clin Endocrinol 1989;31:565–571.

55. Daffos F. Fetal blood sampling. Annu Rev Med 1989;40:319–329.

56. Klein AH, Oddie TH, Parslow M, Foley TP Jr, Fisher DA. Developmental changes in pituitary–thyroid function in the human fetus and newborn. Early Hum Dev 1982;6:321–330.

57. Thorpe-Beeston JG, Nicolaides KH, McGregor AM. Fetal thyroid function. Thyroid 1992;2(3):207–217.

58. Fisher DA, Dussault JH, Hobel CJ, Lam R. Serum and thyroid gland triiodothyronine in the human fetus. J Clin Endocrinol Metab 1973;36:397–400.

59. Radunovic N, Dumez Y, Nastic D, Mandelbrot L, Dommergues M. Thyroid function in fetus and mother during the second half of pregnancy. Biol Neonate 1991;59:139–148.

60. Thorpe-Beeston JG, Nicolaides KH, Felton CV, Butler J, McGregor AM. Maturation of the secretion of thyroid hormone and thyroid-stimulating hormone in the fetus. N Engl J Med 1991;3243(8):532–536.

61. Wenstrom KD, Weiner CP, Williamson RA, Grant SS. Prenatal diagnosis of fetal hyperthyroidism using funipuncture. Obstet Gynecol 1990;76(3):513–517.

62. Van Loon AJ, Derksen JTM, Bos AF, Rouwe CW. In utero diagnosis and treatment of fetal goitrous hypothyroidism, caused by maternal use of propylthiouracil. Prenat Diagn 1995;15:599–604.

63. Chan LY, Leung TN, Lau TK. Influences of perinatal factors on cord blood thyroid-stimulating hormone level. Acta Obstet Gynecol Scand 2001;80:1014–1018.

64. Santini F, Cortelazzi D, Baggiani AM, Marconi AM, Beck-Peccoz P, Chopra IJ. A study of the serum 3,5,3'-triiodothyronine sulfate concentration in normal and hypothyroid fetuses at various gestational stages. J Clin Endocrinol Metab 1993;76:1583–1587.

65. Ghidini A, Sepulveda W, Lockwood CJ, Romero R. Complications of fetal blood sampling. Am J Obstet Gynecol 1993;168:1339–1344.

66. Rovet J, Ehrlich R, Sorbara D. Intellectual outcome in children with fetal hypothyroidism. J Pediat 1987;110:700–704.

67. Chopra IJ, Crandall BF. Thyroid hormones and thyrotropin in amniotic fluid. N Engl J Med 1975;293:740–743.

68. Klein AH, Murphy BEP, Artal R, Oddie TH, Fisher DA. Amniotic fluid thyroid hormone concentrations during human gestation. Am J Obstet Gynecol 1980;136:626–629.

69. Kourides IA, Heath CV, Ginsberg-Fellner F. Measurement of thyroid-stimulating hormone in human amniotic fluid. J Clin Endocrinol Metab 1982;54:635–637.

70. Yoshida K, Sakurada T, Takakashi T, Furruhashi N, Kaise K, Yoshinaga K. Measurement of TSH in human amniotic fluid: diagnosis of fetal thyroid abnormality in utero. Clin Endocrinol 1986;25:313–318.

10 Hematology and Hemostasis During Pregnancy

Charles S. Eby, MD

CONTENTS

INTRODUCTION

Numerous hematologic and hemostatic changes occur during an uncomplicated pregnancy. Presumably, these alterations have been selected for because they are beneficial to both the mother and the fetus. Plasma expansion in excess of increased red cell production leads to the anemia of pregnancy, and fetal and placental demands tax a mother's iron and folate stores. Hemostatic changes are associated with an increased risk of maternal morbidity and mortality caused by thrombotic complications, but theoretically may improve maternal and fetal viability by reducing blood loss during parturition. In order to accurately interpret changes in hematologic and hemostatic laboratory measurements when complications arise, it is necessary to first appreciate the physiologic adaptations that occur during normal pregnancies.

HEMATOLOGY

Changes in Plasma, Red Cell, and Blood Volumes

Plasma volume begins to expand at about the sixth week of pregnancy and rises steadily, until weeks 28–30, when the rate of increase diminishes or plateaus, typically increasing a total of about 1250 mL at term *(1)*. Plasma volume expansion varies considerably in normal pregnancies, ranging from 25 to 50% over baseline *(2)* (Fig. 1), and is positively correlated with birth weight and multiple pregnancies rather than maternal nonpregnant weight *(3)*. Gestational complications that produce small or nonsurviving fetuses are associated with small increases in plasma volume *(4)*. Although the physiologic mechanisms involved in the maternal plasma volume expansion remain unknown, it is considered to be important for fetal well-being.

From: *Current Clinical Pathology: Handbook of Clinical Laboratory Testing During Pregnancy*
Edited by: A. M. Gronowski © Humana Press, Totowa, NJ

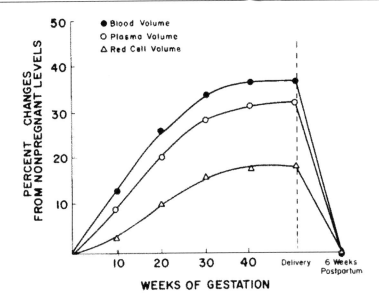

Fig. 1. Changes in blood, plasma, and red cell volumes during pregnancy and postpartum. (Reprinted with permission from ref. 2.)

Red cell mass may decrease slightly during the first trimester and then begins to increase until term, totaling about 180 mL in iron-unsupplemented women, and 350 mL in iron supplemented women (5), for an 18–30% increase compared to the nonpregnant state (3) (Fig. 1). Red cell survival is normal during uncomplicated pregnancies (6). Red cell expansion is also positively correlated with fetal birth weight and multiple births, and, like plasma expansion, the physiologic regulation is not completely understood (3).

During the first trimester, erythropoietin (EPO) (7), soluble transferrin receptor concentrations (7,8) and reticulocyte counts (9) are lower than predicted based on the degree of anemia, consistent with a blunted erythropoietic response. A possible explanation for these observations is a diminished hypoxic stimulus for EPO production because of a temporary increase in renal blood flow during the first trimester (3). EPO concentrations rise steadily during the second and third trimesters, increasing by 25% (10) to 75% (11) over first trimester concentrations, and reticulocyte counts trend slightly upward (11). Peak EPO concentrations are significantly higher in women whose hematocrit is less than 30% (11) or not taking iron supplements (10,12).

Estimates of the increase in oxygen demand in late pregnancy are similar to the measured increase in oxygen-carrying capacity of the expanded red cell mass. The arterio-venous oxygen difference is lower throughout pregnancy compared to nonpregnant women, indicating adequate delivery of oxygen to maternal and fetal tissue beds (3). These observations are consistent with an adequate expansion of red cell mass at least partly mediated through unknown, nonhypoxia-stimulated mechanisms that increase EPO production, as well as secondary, hypoxia-mediated increased EPO production in women who develop iron deficiency anemia (10).

The combined plasma and red cell expansion increases maternal blood volume by about 40% at term, preparing the mother for potential blood loss during delivery (Fig. 1). Because red cell volume increases less than plasma volume during pregnancy, the ratio of red cell to plasma volume decreases and is reflected in a decline in venous blood hematocrit and hemoglobin, frequently referred to as the anemia of pregnancy. Within six wk postpartum, plasma and red cell volumes return to nonpregnant values (Fig. 1).

Iron Reserves and Demands

Iron stores in most healthy nulliparous women are tenuous, averaging 200 mg (13), with no stainable iron on bone marrow examination in 24% (14) because of increased iron loss with menses. There are four major sources of increased iron utilization during an uncomplicated, singleton pregnancy: (1) the fetus, (2) the placenta, (3) the expanded maternal erythroid mass, and (4) the peripartum blood loss, totaling about 1100 mg of iron, of which about 600 mg is permanently lost and 500 mg is recovered as the expanded red cell mass is resorbed postpartum (Table 1). Gastrointestinal absorption of iron increases from the nonpregnant rate of about 2 mg/d in the first trimester to 5 mg/d in the third trimester (15). However, the dietary iron intake necessary to obtain maximal absorption is 10 mg/d (16), and this may be the limiting factor in many women, leading to depletion of iron stores. Puolakka et al. (17) performed sternal bone marrow aspirates at 16 and 32 wk gestation in 32 Finish pregnant women; 16 received iron supplements and 16 did not. In the supplemented group, no stainable iron was detected in 35% at 16 wk when iron treatment began, compared to 43% at 32 wk. In the nonsupplemented group, no stainable iron was detected in 20% at 16 wk, increasing to 80% at 32 wk. The National Academy of Science recommends 30 mg of elemental iron supplementation during pregnancy (18).

However, many aspects of maternal and fetal health, as they relate to iron metabolism, remain controversial after decades of investigation. Despite a high prevalence of borderline or depleted iron stores, the occurrence of microcytic, hypochromic anemia during pregnancy is rare in western societies, and the impact of exhausted maternal iron stores on fetal and neonatal heath is unclear (19) because the placenta is capable of transporting iron to the fetus against a high concentration gradient (20), and maternal iron stores improve postpartum when the expanded red cell mass is recycled (5).

Hemoglobin Nadir During Normal Pregnancy

The changes in hemoglobin, red cell indices, iron, and iron transport proteins that occur during gestation and postpartum with and without iron supplementation are shown in Fig. 2. Multiple longitudinal studies have been performed in developed countries randomizing healthy pregnant women to either placebo or iron supplementation. For iron-supplemented women, the mean hemoglobin nadir at 23–26 wk gestation ranges from 11.5 to 12.0 g/dL (21) with central 90% lower limits of 10–10.5 g/dL (22). Typically, hemoglobin concentration increases during the third trimester, approaching or surpassing first trimester concentrations (22,23). The hemoglobin nadir in women who do not take iron supplements ranges from 10.9 to 11.4 g/dL (21), with central 90% lower limits of 10 g/dL (22), and hemoglobin concentration may remain stable, decline, or increase slightly during the third trimester (22). Postpartum, hemoglobin concentrations rise in both groups, although improvement may be blunted in women who do not receive iron supplements (24).

Guidelines have been derived from the results of these investigations to assist clinicians in determining when other causes for anemia should be considered in addition to dilution because of increased plasma volume. The Centers for Disease Control published

Table 1
Estimated Iron Utilization During Pregnancy and Delivery

Baseline requirements:	
Fe loss in secretions and shed epithelial cells	200 mg
Increased requirements:	
Fetus	300 mg
Placenta	50 mg
Maternal red cell expansion[a]	500 mg
Blood loss with vaginal delivery[b]	250 mg
Decreased requirements:	
Cessation of menses × 9 mo	135 mg
Net iron demand during uncomplicated single-term pregnancy	1165 mg

[a]Portion not lost during delivery returned to iron stores postpartum as red cell mass declines to nonpregnant state.
[b]May be doubled for ceasarian section.
Derived from refs. *2,16,27,126*.

gestational age-specific anemia cutoffs for iron-supplemented pregnancies (Table 2), while the World Health Organization defined nonphysiologic anemia as a hemoglobin less than 11.0 g/dL anytime during pregnancy *(25)*.

Red Cell Indices During Pregnancy

Red cell mean cellular volume (MCV) increases slightly during pregnancy (Fig. 2). This appears to be a physiologic macrocytosis associated with pregnancy, but the mechanism is unknown, and folate supplementation has no impact on the MCV *(24)*. The average MCV typically increases 3–5 fL during gestation *(26)*, rarely exceeding the upper limit of the nonpregnant MCV reference interval, and rapidly declines postpartum *(22,24)*. In women not taking iron supplements, the increase in MCV is smaller and not sustained during the third trimester, but does not decline into the microcytic range *(24,26)*. Accompanying the increase in MCV, there is a trivial increase of red cell mean cell hemoglobin (MCH) and no change in mean cell hemoglobin concentration (MCHC) in iron-supplemented pregnancies *(22)*. However, by late third trimester, MCH and MCHC are abnormally low, compared to nonpregnant reference intervals, in 9.3 and 1.9%, respectively, of women not taking iron supplements, and may indicate iron deficiency erythropoiesis *(22)*.

Laboratory Evaluation of Iron Deficiency During Pregnancy

In men and nonpregnant women subjected to progressive iron depletion because of phlebotomy or pathologic blood loss, several stages of iron deficiency are identified based on measurements of serum iron; proteins involved in storage, transport, and uptake of iron; hemoglobin; and red cell indices *(27)* (Table 3). Typical cutoffs for iron defi-

Fig. 2. (*opposite page*) Changes (mean ± SD) in hemoglobin, red cell mean cell volume (MCV), serum iron, transferrin, transferrin saturation, and ferritin during and after pregnancy in women taking (■__■) and not taking (△__△) supplemental iron. Reference ranges provided for nonpregnant women with adequate (●) or absent (○) bone marrow iron stores. (Reprinted with permission from ref. *17*.)

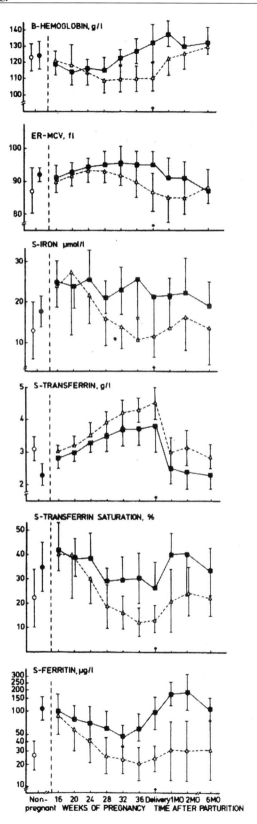

Table 2
Pregnancy Month-Specific and Trimester-Specific Hemoglobin (Hb) Cutoffs

Gestation (wk)	12	16	20	24	28	32	36	40
Mean Hb (g/dL) 5th percentile	12.2	11.8	11.6	11.6	11.8	12.1	12.5	12.9
Hb values (g/dL) Equivalent 5th percentile	11.0	10.6	10.5	10.5	10.7	11.0	11.4	11.9
Hematocrit values (%)	33.0	32.0	32.0	32.0	32.0	33.0	34.0	36.0

From: Morbidity Morality Weekly Report 1988;38:400–404.

Table 3
Stages of Iron Deficiency

	Depleted iron stores	Iron-restricted erythropoiesis	Iron deficiency anemia
Marrow iron stores	Absent	Absent	Absent
Ferritin	↓	↓	↓
Serum iron	nl	↓	↓
Transferrin	nl	↑	↑
Transferrin saturation	nl	↓	↓
Soluble transferrin receptor	nl	↑	↑
Reticulocyte count	nl	↓	↓
Hemoglobin	nl	nl	↓
Mean cell volume	nl	nl	↓

Adapted from ref. 27.

ciency and iron-restricted erythropoiesis in nonpregnant women are ferritin less than 10 μg/L (28) and transferrin saturation less than 16% (27), respectively. Iron deficiency anemia in nonpregnant women is usually defined as hemoglobin less than 12 g/dL (27). However, during pregnancy, serum iron and transferrin saturation are altered, independent of iron status, making low transferrin saturation nonspecific for iron-restricted erythropoiesis (Fig. 2). Increases in plasma volume and red cell mass cannot be accurately quantitated, reducing the reliability of hemoglobin and hematocrit measurements for diagnosing causes of anemia other than dilution. Decreased serum ferritin appears to be a reliable marker of depleted iron stores when compared to bone marrow iron staining (17) but is not specific for iron deficiency anemia (29).

Elevated serum transferrin receptor (sTFR) is a sensitive marker of iron-restricted erythropoiesis but is also elevated during increased erythropoietic activity in congenital and acquired hemolytic anemias. Investigations of sTFR in pregnancy have produced inconsistent findings. Carriaga et al. measured sTFR in 176 iron-supplemented women during the third trimester. Mean sTFR concentration did not differ significantly from a non-pregnant reference group. Fifteen of 18 women with ferritins less than 12 ng/mL had elevated sTFR, and 11 of 13 women with hemoglobin less than 11 g/dL had elevated sTFR. The authors concluded that sTFR was a sensitive marker of iron-restricted erythropoiesis, and other investigators support their findings *(30)*. However, another study of sTFR concentrations in pregnancy found a progressive increase in sTFR during gestation that was independent of storage iron or anemia status, and correlated with another measurement of increased erythropoietic activity: reticulocyte immaturity *(31)*. Therefore, the utility of measuring sTFR concentration in anemic, pregnant women is currently unclear and is not recommended.

Folate and Vitamin B_{12} Changes During Pregnancy

Folic acids are water-soluble vitamins involved in many one-carbon transfer reactions required for nucleic acid synthesis and amino acid metabolism. Like iron deficiency, pregnant women are at increased risk for folate deficiency because of inadequate tissue stores; increased maternal, fetal, and lactation demands on folate stores; and inadequate dietary sources. Nonpregnant folate stores approx 5 mg *(32)*. The daily folate requirements of 100–150 µg increase by 100–300 µg during pregnancy *(13)*. During pregnancy, serum folate concentration declines from approx 6.5 ng/mL to 4.0 ng/mL, probably because of plasma volume expansion, but red cell folate concentration is unchanged *(13)*. The first hematologic sign of folate deficiency is hypersegmented neutrophils on a peripheral smear. Progression to anemia, macro-ovalocyte red cells, and leukopenia and thrombocytopenia occurs after several months of exhausted folate stores. Typically, severe macrocytic anemia does not occur until the late stages of pregnancy or postpartum. A serum folate less than 3.0 ng/mL or red cell folate less than 20 ng/mL is considered evidence of folate deficiency during pregnancy *(33)*. Plasma homocysteine concentrations will also be elevated. As with iron, the fetal–placental unit is able to extract folate from the maternal circulation despite depleted reserves *(33)*. Prophylactic folic acid supplementation (0.4–1.0 mg/d) is recommended during pregnancy, even in women at low risk for inadequate dietary folate *(34)*.

Although folate deficiency is the most common cause of macrocytic anemia during pregnancy, the differential also includes vitamin B_{12} deficiency, hypothyroidism, reticulocytosis caused by hemolytic anemia, liver disease, excessive alcohol, and certain chemotherapy, antiviral, and anticonvulsant medications *(32)*. Pregnant women are at risk for combined iron and folate deficiency anemia, which can present as a normocytic anemia and normal ferritin or transferrin saturation because of ineffective erythropoiesis caused by folate deficiency *(32)*.

An increased risk of neural tube defects (NTDs) is associated with maternal folate deficiency and elevated homocysteine concentration *(35)*, and folate supplementation from preconception through the first trimester is associated with a decreased risk of NTDs *(36)*. In order to reduce the incidence of NTDs, grains and breads have been fortified with folate (0.14 mg/100g) since 1996 in the United States, leading to an improvement in population folate status *(37)*.

Vitamin B_{12} is a water-soluble vitamin synthesized by microorganisms and almost exclusively ingested by eating meat. B_{12} concentrations also decrease during pregnancy, from a nonpregnant range of 205–1025 pg/mL to 20–510 pg/mL at term *(13)*. Despite lower B_{12} concentrations, pregnant women do not have biochemical evidence of B_{12} deficiency based on methylmalonic acid and homocysteine concentrations *(38,39)*. B_{12}

deficiency is uncommon during pregnancy because maternal stores are adequate to meet fetal and maternal requirements, even in most vegetarians. Neonatal B_{12} deficiency caused by maternal pernicious anemia has been reported rarely because this disease is uncommon in women under 40 years old and usually causes infertility *(13)*.

Changes in Leukocytes and Platelets During Pregnancy

Longitudinal studies have consistently shown an increase in peripheral white blood cell count (WBC) during normal, term pregnancies *(40–42)*. WBC begins to rise during the first trimester, plateaus during the second and third trimesters, and returns to baseline by 6 wk postpartum (Table 4). Leukocyte counts as high as 12,200 may occur during pregnancy without signs or symptoms of an infection *(42)*. During spontaneous labor, there is a further, temporary increase in WBC (mean 20,000, ± SD 6,000) *(43)*. Women who smoke during pregnancy have higher WBC than nonsmokers, and the leukocytosis increases with the number of cigarettes smoked per day *(44)*. The WBC increase is primarily caused by an increase in mature neutrophils *(42)*. An increase in neutrophil count is also observed during the ovulatory phase of the menstrual cycle. Granulocyte-colony stimulating factor concentrations peak during ovulation and are elevated throughout pregnancy, suggesting a hormonal–cytokine interaction *(45)*. A mild monocytosis is also common during pregnancy and is also associated with an increase in macrophage-colony stimulating factor *(46)*. Absolute eosinophil and basophil counts typically decrease slightly, as does the total lymphocyte count *(40,42)*. In general, the relative numbers of T and B cells do not change significantly *(40)*. Inconsistent results have been reported for changes in lymphocyte subsets during pregnancy *(40)*. Interactions between the maternal immune system and the placenta and fetus, and their impact on maternal–fetal health, are areas of active investigation.

Most longitudinal studies have demonstrated that normal gestation has a minimal affect on maternal platelet counts *(41,47,48)* (Table 5). While some longitudinal *(42)* and cross-sectional *(49–51)*, studies have identified a downward trend for platelet counts during pregnancy, the changes are not clinically meaningful, and platelet counts remain above the lower limit of the nonpregnant reference interval. Possible causes for a lower platelet count during pregnancy include dilution from plasma volume expansion, decreased production, and shortened survival because of activation by prothrombotic forces. Mean platelet volume increases during pregnancy and is cited as evidence of increased platelet consumption with compensatory increased production of larger, young platelets *(47,49)*. However, this model is not supported by studies of platelet survival *(52)* and reticulated platelets, young platelets with detectable RNA, showing no evidence of decreased survival or increased production *(53)*. In one longitudinal study, smoking did not affect median platelet counts during pregnancy *(54)*.

There are multiple causes of thrombocytopenia during pregnancy, defined as a platelet count below the lower limit of the nonpregnant reference interval and typically less than 150,000/μL (Table 6). Several large population surveys have published incidences for different causes of maternal thrombocytopenia in late pregnancy (Table 7). Most often, thrombocytopenia associated with gestation is mild (≥70,000) and is an incidental finding in asymptomatic women with no other risk factors *(55–57)*. Preconception platelet counts are normal, the platelet count normalizes by 6 wk postpartum, and thrombocytopenia is likely to recur with subsequent pregnancies. Although the mechanisms

Table 4
Changes in Mean Leukocyte Counts During Normal Pregnancy

	WBC ($\times 10^3/\mu L$)		Granulocytes ($\times 10^3/\mu L$)		Lymphocytes ($\times 10^3/\mu L$)		Monocytes ($\times 10^3/\mu L$)	
	A	B	A	B	A	B	A	B
Nonpregnant controls	6.7	nd	4.6	nd	1.8	nd	.3	nd
First trimester	9.5	6.88	6.9	nd	2.0	1.65	.4	nd
Second trimester	10.5	8.12	8.2	nd	1.8	1.65	.5	nd
Third trimester	10.8	8.71	8.6	nd	1.7	1.78	.5	nd
1 wk postpartum	9.7	nd	7.2	nd	2.0	nd	.5	nd

nd, not done; WBC, white blood cell count.
A, ref. *40*
B, ref. *41*

Table 5
Changes in Platelet Counts During Normal Pregnancy
Mean Platelet Count ($\times 10^3/\mu L$)

	A	B
First trimester	262	205
Second trimester	269	197
Third trimester	268	211

A, ref. *41*.
B, ref. *48*.

Table 6
Causes of Thrombocypenia[a] During Pregnancy

Incidental, (gestational)
Hypertensive disorders of pregnancy
Immune thrombocytopenia purpura
Autoimmune disorders
Thrombotic thrombocytopenia purpura
Human immunodeficiency virus
Aplastic anemia
Folate, B_{12} deficiencies
Hematologic malignancies
Disseminated intravascular coagulopathy
Acute hemorrhage
Inherited thrombocytopenia
Type 2B von Willebrand disease
Drug-induced
Pseudothrombocytopenia

[a]Defined as platelet count less than 150,000/μL.

Table 7
Frequency of Maternal and Neonatal Thrombocytopenia

References	(56)	(57)	(55)
Maternal thrombocytopenia[a]	6.6%	7.3%	11.6%
Incidental	73.6%	81.0%	94.0%
Hypertensive disorders of pregnancy	21.0%	16.0%	4.5%
ITP & SLE	3.8%	3.0%	0.5%
Other	2.6%	1.0%	
Neonatal thrombocytopenia[b]	0.12%		
Incidental	0.13%		
Hypertensive disorders of pregnancy	1.8%		
ITP & SLE	6.4%		
High-risk for neonatal alloimmune thrombocytopenia	50.0%		

[a]Platelets count less than 150,000/μL.
[b]Umbilical cord platelet count less than 50,000/μL.

involved in incidental thrombocytopenia of pregnancy are unknown, infants born to these mothers are not at higher risk for significant thrombocytopenia or bleeding complications (56,57).

Immune thrombocytopenia purpura (ITP) is an autoimmune disorder that infrequently causes thrombocytopenia during pregnancy (Table 7). Platelet counts range from less than 10,000/μL, to slightly less than 100,000/μL, precede conception, and do not recover postpartum. Diagnosis of ITP is typically based on exclusion of other causes of thrombocytopenia (Table 6); however, some experts recommend laboratory evaluation for platelet-specific antibodies and other autoimmune serologies (58). It can be difficult to distinguish mild ITP from incidental thrombocytopenia of pregnancy in primigravida women with no previous platelet counts. Fortunately, the maternal and fetal outcomes are excellent in both situations, and no specific interventions during pregnancy or delivery are recommended (58).

Preeclampsia is the most common cause of thrombocytopenia in women with hypertensive disorders of pregnancy. Thrombocytopenia may precede the onset of hypertension or develop during its course. Typically, platelet decrements are mild, and recovery is rapid after delivery (see Chapter 18).

Thrombocytosis (platelet count >600,000/μL) during pregnancy is extremely uncommon and is typically caused by an underlying myeloproliferative disorder, most often essential thrombocytosis (ET). There is a higher rate of spontaneous abortion in women with ET, but late gestational complications appear to be less frequent (59). Management of ET is controversial, ranging from no intervention to daily aspirin, or α-interferon to inhibit platelet aggregation and lower the platelet count, respectively (60).

A reactive thrombocytosis is seen commonly postpartum, usually returning to prepregnancy concentrations within a month. Women who are preeclamptic (61) or undergo cesarean section (62) have higher mean postpartum platelet counts compared to women who are normotensive or undergo a vaginal delivery. These investigators have speculated that postpartum thrombocytosis is a risk factor for thrombotic complications (62), but outcome data are lacking.

HEMOSTASIS

Pregnancy-Associated Thromboembolic Complications

Pregnancy and the puerperium are recognized as temporary prothrombotic conditions on the basis of clinical and laboratory observations. However, the reduction in uteroplacental hemorrhagic complications during gestation and delivery may more than compensate for the increased morbidity and mortality caused by thrombotic events *(63,64)*. The leading cause of maternal mortality in developed countries is pulmonary embolism (PE) (2.1/100,000 pregnancies), 2.5 and 5 times more common than death from hypertension and hemorrhage, respectively *(65)*. The incidence of venous thromboembolic events (VTE) during pregnancy ranges from 0.55 to 0.86/1000 deliveries *(66,67)*. Although it is widely accepted that VTEs are more common during pregnancy than in comparable nonpregnant women, an accurate estimate of the increased risk associated with pregnancy is lacking. The incidence of deep vein thromboses (DVT) compared to PE is about 2:1 *(66,67)*. DVT are more common antepartum and are distributed fairly equally among all trimesters *(68)*. DVT usually arise in the proximal iliofemoral veins and approx 90% involve the left leg *(68)*. A reasonable explanation for the left-side bias is the anatomic relation between the iliac veins and arteries: the right iliac artery crosses over the left iliac vein, and there is no vascular compression of the right iliac vein. PEs are fairly equally distributed between antepartum and postpartum periods, and are more common after delivery by cesarean section. Arterial thromboembolic events are uncommon during pregnancy and postpartum *(69,70)*. Atherosclerotic risk factors are frequently present in women who suffer myocardial infarctions *(70)*, and strokes are associated with hypertensive complications of pregnancy and cesarean sections *(69)*.

Physiology and Laboratory Monitoring of Hemostasis

Rapid formation of an occlusive plug at the site of vascular injury while maintaining patency and blood flow involves many complicated interactions between blood procoagulant, anticoagulant, and fibrinolytic proteins; circulating blood cells; and vessel components *(71)*. Analysis of changes in the viscoelasticity of whole blood as it first clots and then lysis ex vivo has led to the development of instruments for the global assessment of hemostasis. Primarily used to monitor hemostasis during liver transplantation and cardiothoracic surgery, limited studies performed on pregnant subjects demonstrate hypercoaguable behavior throughout pregnancy *(72–74)*.

Laboratory tests to assess primary hemostasis include von Willebrand factor (vWF) antigen and activity, the platelet count, bleeding time, an in vivo measurement of the time it takes for a forearm incision to stop bleeding, in vitro platelet aggregation studies, and PFA-100® (Dade-Bohring) closure time, an instrument that measures the rate of platelet aggregation in anticoagulated whole blood when exposed to collagen and adenosine diphosphate (ADP), or collagen and epinephrine under high shear stress conditions *(75)*.

The standard screening tests for secondary hemostasis are the prothrombin time (PT) and activated partial thromboplastin time (aPTT). Both tests monitor the time to form a fibrin clot following the addition of reagents to activate the coagulation factor pathway (Fig. 3). The PT test adds tissue factor to activate factor VII (extrinsic pathway), and the aPTT test adds phospholipid and a negatively charged material to activate factor XII (intrinsic pathway). Coagulation factors, and proteins that regulate them, are measured with either functional or antigenic assays.

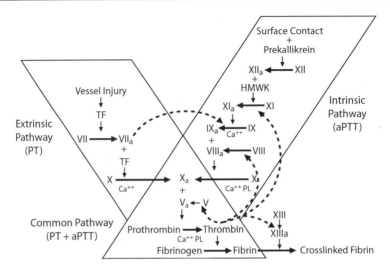

Fig. 3. In vivo, the coagulation cascade is initiated by exposure of blood to tissue factor (TF) at the site of vascular injury, leading to activation of factor VII (extrinsic pathway). Factor VII$_a$ activates factors X and IX, and activated factor X (X$_a$) activates prothrombin to thrombin (common pathway). Thrombin acts on many substrates. It converts fibrinogen to fibrin, activates cofactors VIII and V, and activates factor XI to XI$_a$ to sustain and accelerate thrombin generation. Thrombin also activates factor XIII to XIII$_a$, which covalently cross-links fibrin monomers to form a durable clot. In vitro, the coagulation cascade can be initiated by exposure of plasma to negatively charged surfaces (intrinsic pathway). However, the factors involved in surface activation (factor XII, prekallikrein, and high-molecular-weight kininogen) are not required for in vivo hemostasis. The Prothombin Time (PT) monitors extrinsic and common pathways and the activated partial thromboplastin time (aPTT) monitors the intrinsic and common pathways.

Plasmin-mediated clot lysis releases fibrin degradation products (FDP) into blood (Fig. 4) *(76)*. The D-dimer is an FDP that contains covalently cross-linked D-domains from two fibrin molecules. Immunoassays using polyclonal antibodies to detect FDP or monoclonal antibodies specific for D-dimer are used to monitor in vivo fibrinolytic activity. In vitro tests to assess global fibrinolytic activity and quantitate tissue plasminogen activator, plasminogen, and their inhibitors are not routinely performed in clinical laboratories.

Primary Hemostasis Changes During Pregnancy

Platelet counts do not change significantly during normal pregnancy *(41)*. Investigations into platelet function have produced inconsistent results. Bleeding times are shortened *(77)* or unchanged *(78)* during pregnancy compared to nonpregnant controls. PFA-100 ADP closure times in 110 late third-trimester uncomplicated pregnancies were all within the normal limits, and only 6 of 110 epinepherine closure times were minimally prolonged *(79)*. Investigations of platelet aggregation in normal, hypertensive, and preclamptic pregnancies have produce varied and inconsistent results. Whigham et al. reported no difference between platelets from women with uncomplicated pregnancies and platelets from nonpregnant controls when aggregation was induced with collagen, ADP, arachadonic acid, and adrenaline *(80)*. However, platelets from patients with severe

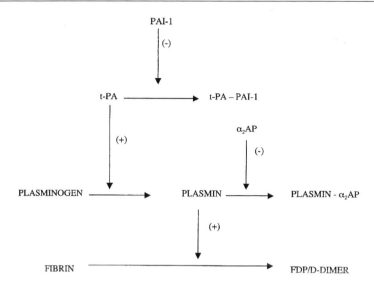

Fig. 4. Fibrinolytic system. Tissue-type plasminogen activator (t-PA) converts plasminogen to plasmin, and plasmin degrades fibrin into soluble fragments (fibrin degradation products [FDP] including D-dimer). Two proteins regulate fibrinolysis; plasminogen activator inhibitor-1 (PAI-1), which binds to t-PA, and α_2-antiplasmin (α_2-AP), which binds to plasmin.

preeclampsia were less responsive to the agonists, suggesting that circulating platelets were "exhausted" because of partial platelet activation while flowing through a perturbed microcirculation. Using the same agonists, O'Brien et al. observed a similar reduction in platelet aggregation with platelets from normal as well as mild and severe pregnancy-induced hypertensive pregnant patients when compared to nonpregnant controls (81). Other investigators have reported increased platelet activity during normal pregnancies based on in vitro aggregation studies (82,83). Overall, there is no convincing evidence for platelet hyperactivity being a major component of the hypercoaguable state during pregnancy (77).

Secondary Hemostasis Changes During Pregnancy

PT and partial thromboplastin time (PTT) tend to shorten during pregnancy (84), but the changes are not clinically significant. Evidence for a prothrombotic hemostatic physiology during pregnancy is derived primarily from changes in concentrations of coagulation, fibrinolytic, and anticoagulant proteins. Results from both longitudinal (85,86) and cross-sectional (87,88) surveys are summarized in Table 8. Fibrinogen rises steadily during pregnancy, increasing by 20–50% at term. The vitamin K-dependent serine protease factors X, IX, VII, and II (prothrombin) all increase during pregnancy, although reported magnitudes vary. vWF antigen increases 200–300%, and factor VIII, which circulates noncovalently bound to vWF, increases 50–100% by the end of the third trimester. Factor V, a cofactor for activation of prothrombin to thrombin, is unchanged or increases slightly, and factor XI decreases as gestation progresses. Factor XIII, a transglutaminase enzyme that covalently crosslinks fibrin monomers, decreases throughout pregnancy, but it is not clinically significant (89).

Table 8
Changes in Hemostasis Factors During Pregnancy

Protein (references)	Decrease	No Change	Increase
Factor XII *(86,87)*			▬ (No Change–Increase)
Prekallikrein *(86)*		▬	
Factor XI *(86,87)*	▬ (Decrease–No Change)		
Factor IX *(87)*		▬	
Factor VIII *(85–87)*			▬
vWF: Ag *(85–87)*			▬
Factor VII *(85)*			▬ (No Change–Increase)
Factor X *(85–87)*			▬ (No Change–Increase)
Factor V *(85,87)*			▬ (No Change–Increase)
Prothrombin *(85,87)*			▬ (No Change–Increase)
Fibrinogen *(85–87)*			▬ (No Change–Increase)
Factor XIII *(89)*	▬ (Decrease–No Change)		
Antithrombin *(85–87)*		▬	
Protein C *(87,88)*		▬	
Total Protein S *(87,88,90)*	▬ (Decrease–No Change)		
Free Protein S *(87,88,90)*	▬		
Plasminogen *(86,127)*			▬ (No Change–Increase)
PAI-1 *(127)*			▬
A2-antiplasmin			▬ (No Change–Increase)
t-PA	▬ (Decrease–No Change)		

Of the three proteins that regulate thrombin generation, two (protein C and antithrombin) do not change significantly during pregnancy *(88)*. However, the functional state of protein S (free protein S, unbound to Complement 4b binding protein) decreases steadily beginning in the second trimester *(88,90)*. A consistent finding has been an increase of coagulation factor activation markers during gestation. Concentrations of thrombi–antithrombin complexes *(91,92)*, as well as the prothrombin peptide fragment F^{1+2} *(76,92)* that is released during activation to thrombin, rise steadily as gestation progresses. However, there is no evidence that the concentrations of coagulation activation markers are predictive of thrombotic complications for individual pregnancies *(91,92)*.

The changes in coagulation protein concentrations during pregnancy are similar to the alterations that occur in women taking oral contraception pills (OCPs) *(93)*, confirming the link between sex hormones and hemostasis. OCP use is also associated with a fourfold increased risk of VTE compared to age-matched women who are not taking them *(94)*. In addition, elevated factor IX *(95)*, factor VIII *(96)*, and prothrombin *(96)* are associated with an increased risk of VTE among nonpregnant women and men.

Fibrinolytic Pathway Changes During Pregnancy

Dramatic and complex changes occur to the components of the fibrinolytic system (Fig. 4) during pregnancy, yet their physiologic significance remains incompletely understood *(97)*. It is generally accepted that fibrinolytic activity is inhibited during pregnancy, thus promoting uteroplacental vascular integrity *(98)*. This model is supported by histologic evidence of replacement of the smooth muscle and elastic lamina of dilated uterine spiral arteries by trophoblasts and fibrin *(98)*, and decreased systemic fibrinolytic activity *(77,85)*. Plasma concentrations of plasminogen parallel increases in fibrinogen during pregnancy *(98)*. Wright et al. observed a progessive decrease in tissue-type plasminogen activator (t-PA) and increase in plasminogen activator inhibitor-1 (PAI-1) activities during uncomplicated pregnancies, consistent with the observed decreased fibrinolytic activity using the euglobulin lysis method *(99)*. In addition to PAI-1, the placenta produces an antigenically and functionally distinct t-PA inhibitor, plasminogen activator inhibitor-2 (PAI-2), and circulating concentrations of PAI-2 change from undetectable to higher than PAI-1 concentrations toward the end of gestation *(98)*. However, using different methods to measure in vitro fibrinolytic activity, other investigators have reported no change *(97)* or increased *(100)* fibrinolytic activity during pregnancy.

A progessive rise in FDP and D-dimer concentrations during uncomplicated pregnancies is a consistent finding *(85,101)* (Fig. 5). These findings may represent ongoing localized deposition and remodeling of fibrin within the uteroplacental unit during normal gestation rather than a state of systemic low-grade disseminated intravascular coagulation (DIC).

Peripartum and Postpartum Hemostatic Changes

Mechanical (uterine contractions) and hemostatic forces combine to minimize blood loss following separation of the placenta from the uterine wall. During and shortly after labor, changes in hemostasis parameters are consistent with activation of the intrinsic coagulation pathway (factor XII) *(89)*, contributing to increased generation of thrombin and fibrin *(86)*; a mild, temporary drop in platelet count *(86)*; and increased fibrin proteolysis *(85)*. PAI-1 falls to a nonpregnant concentration within hours of placental sepa-

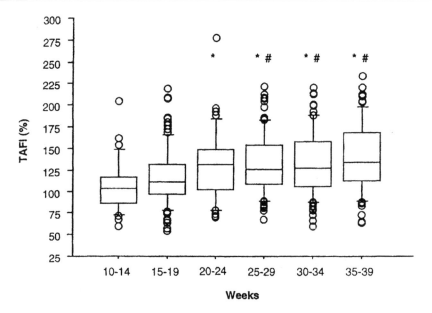

Fig. 5. Box plots of D-dimer values as a function of pregnancy periods. Boxes represent 50% of the values, the horizontal bar inside the median, and the lower and the upper bars the 10th and 90th percentiles, respectively. (Reprinted with permission from ref. *101*.)

ration, while PAI-2 concentrations remain elevated for several days *(97)*. Factor VIII and vWF antigen concentrations gradually return to baseline, and by 6–8 wk postpartum, coagulation and fibrinolytic systems have returned to nonpregnant baseline status *(86,97)*.

Hemostatic Consequences of Pregnancy Complications

Fetal and placental tissues and amniotic fluid (AF) are rich sources of tissue factor. Sudden disruptions of the fetal–maternal barrier can precipitate acute DIC, because of tissue factor-mediated systemic activation of the extrinsic coagulation pathway, excessive thrombin generation, and subsequent platelet activation and secondary fibrinolysis. Clinical consequences include consumption of clotting factors and platelets, hyperfibrinolysis, and life-threatening hemorrhage. Typical laboratory findings would include prolonged PT and aPTT, hypofibrinogenemia (<100 mg/dL), markedly elevated D-dimer, and thrombocytopenia *(102)*. Examples of gestational emergencies that can lead to severe DIC are AF embolism, abruptio placentae, and abortion complications. A more chronic and usually less severe form of DIC occurs when fetal death *in utero* is not recognized and tissue factor from fetal tissue slowly enters the maternal bloodstream. Changes in hemostatic parameters consistent with DIC can also develop during hypertensive disorders of pregnancy (see Chapter 18).

Management of pregnancy-associated DIC depends on the clinical impact and underlying cause. Debridement and curretage (D&C), leads to prompt hemostatic recovery in most cases of retained placental or fetal tissue. Delivery of the fetus and placenta resolves the coagulopathy associated with preeclampsia, abruptio placentae, and dead fetus. If cardiopulmonary complications of AF embolism are not fatal, the coagulopathy is typically self-limited. Blood component support may be indicated for severe coagulopathy or thrombocytopenia to prevent or treat active bleeding *(103)*.

Inherited Hemostatic Defects and Pregnancy

vWF is a large, multimeric plasma glycoprotein and has an important role in both primary hemostasis, facilitating platelet adhesion at sites of endothelial injury, and secondary hemostasis, binding factor VIII and protecting it from rapid degradation (104). von Willebrand disease (vWD) is the most common inherited bleeding disorder, with an estimated symptomatic prevalence of 0.01% (104). Bleeding complications in patients with vWD, caused by quantitative (type 1,3) or qualitative (type 2) abnormalities of vWF, depend on the severity of the defect (105). Approximately 80% of patients diagnosed with vWD are type 1, which is characterized by autosomal inheritance of a partial deficiency of vWF. Typical bleeding complications of type 1 vWD include excessive bruising, bleeding from mucous membranes, and mennorrhagia (105). During pregnancy in women with vWD type 1, vWF antigen and factor VIII activity progressively rise, possibly achieving concentrations found in nonpregnant women, and bleeding complications typically diminish. However, postpartum, vWF and factor VIII concentrations can rapidly return to baseline, and delayed uterine bleeding may occur (106). Women with type 2 (qualitative vWF defects) and type 3 (severe quantitative deficiency of vWF) remain at risk for major bleeding complications during gestation and postpartum. Infusions of blood components containing vWF are indicated to prevent bleeding during labor and postpartum and to manage antepartum bleeding complications (107).

Inherited Risk Factors for VTEs and Pregnancy

Women who inherit risk factors associated with an increased risk of VTEs are at increased risk for both maternal and fetal complications during pregnancy. Factor V Leiden (FVL) is a common genetic polymorphism (G1691A) and is a risk factor for VTEs (108). Among Caucasians, the incidence of heterozygosity is approx 5%. The mutation eliminates a site where activated protein C cleaves factor Va, leading to prolonged thrombin generation (109). Most people who inherit FVL will not have a VTE. However, when FVL is combined with acquired risk factors, the incidence of VTE increases. The frequency of FVL genotype in women with pregnancy-associated VTEs ranges from 8% (67) to 46% (110). Although the relative risk for VTE during pregnancy in FVL carriers is increased (111), an estimate of the absolute risk (based on an incidence of VTE in 1 of 1500 pregnancies) is 0.2% (112). A polymorphism in the prothrombin gene (G20210A) is associated with elevated plasma prothrombin concentrations and increased risk for VTE, and is found in approx 2% of Caucasians (113). The incidence of the G20210A prothrombin gene mutation in women whose pregnancies are complicated by VTE ranges from 9 (114) to 17% (112), and the reported ranges for relative and absolute VTE risk are similar to those for FVL (111,112). Homozygosity for a common polymorphism in the gene encoding 5,10,-methylenetetrahydrofolate reductase (MTHFR C667T) is associated with elevations in plasma homocysteine, but its role as an independent risk factor for venous and arterial thromboembolic events is controversial (115,116). Current data do not support a convincing association between MTHFR C677T and VTE (111,112,114). The prevalences of congenital partial deficiencies of the coagulation regulating proteins, antithrombin, protein C, and protein S, are lower than FVL, and the relative risks for VTEs during pregnancy associated with them are difficult to accurately quantify because of the low frequency of deficiencies in cases and controls. However, the clinical impression is that congenital antithrombin deficiency is the most potent inherited risk factor for VTE complications during pregnancy (117).

Inherited VTE risk factors have also been associated with other obstetrical complications including preeclampsia, abruptio placentae, stillbirth, and intrauterine growth retardation *(118)*. Kupferminc et al. identified FVL, G20210A prothrombin gene mutation, or MTHFR C677T in 52% of 110 women who had one of these pregnancy complications compared to 17% in 110 women with histories of uncomplicated pregnancies. Other investigators have confirmed an association between FVL *(111,119)* and G20210A prothrombin gene mutation *(111)* and late unexplained fetal loss. A recent meta-analysis of studies investigating inherited thrombophilia and fetal loss identified an association for FVL, G20210A prothrombin gene mutation, and protein S deficiency with early and late recurrent fetal loss and as well as late nonrecurrent fetal loss *(120)*. There was no association between fetal loss and MTHFR C677T, protein C, or antithrombin deficiency.

Thrombophilic risk factors have not been associated with an increased risk of intrauterine growth retardation in the absence of hypertensive complications of pregnancy *(121–124)*. While hypertensive complications during pregnancy can lead to prothrombotic hemostatic alterations, the results of investigations into whether FVL, MTHFR C677T, and G20210A prothrombin gene mutation are associated with an increased risk for development of preeclampsia are inconsistent *(106,124,125)*. Furthermore, studies to test the hypothesis that inherited risk factors for VTE increase the risk for placental vascular insufficiency, placental infarction, and maternal–fetal complications are limited and inconclusive *(121)*.

Although the cumulative evidence linking some thrombophilic risk factors to an increased risk of VTEs, and some maternal–fetal complications is convincing, it is not appropriate to screen asymptomatic women for their presence *(106,124)*. The predictive values of a positive or negative result for these risk factors in regard to pregnancy-associated complications are unknown, as is the effectiveness of possible therapeutic interventions.

SUMMARY

Maternal and fetal well-being during pregnancy depends on increases of maternal plasma and red cell volumes. Since plasma expansion is proportionately greater than red cell expansion, the hematocrit declines during the second trimester and early third trimesters. Maternal iron stores, often minimal before conception, are frequently depleted during gestation because of fetal demands and increased maternal hemoglobin synthesis. Distinguishing between physiologic anemia of pregnancy with depleted iron stores and physiologic anemia of pregnancy plus early iron-restricted erythropoiesis for individual patients is often difficult with currently available laboratory tests. Therefore, it is appropriate to provide iron supplementation to all pregnant women.

Maternal hematologic complications of folate deficiency occur late in pregnancy; whereas the risk for fetal NTDs can be reduced with folate supplementation during the first month of gestation. Therefore, it is appropriate to provide folate supplementation prior to conception and throughout pregnancy.

Gestation and delivery are associated with hemorrhagic risk. Changes in maternal hemostatic functions appear to tilt the balance toward thrombus formation. This is supported by the increased incidence of VTEs during pregnancy and in the immediate postpartum period, and a decrease in blood loss during delivery in women with FVL, an inherited thrombophilic risk factor *(64)*.

Some inherited thrombophilic risk factors are also associated with early and late fetal loss. Investigators continue to search for pathophysiologic explanations to link maternal–fetal complications with thrombophilic risk factors and to evaluate the utility of prophylaxis strategies in women who inherit them.

REFERENCES

1. Koller O, Haram K, Sagen N. Maternal hemoglobin concentration and fetal health. In: Bern MM, Frigoletto FDJ, eds. Hematologic Disorders in Maternal–Fetal Medicine. New York: Wiley-Liss, 1990, pp. 31–46.
2. Hiss RG. Evaluation of the anemic patient. In: Laros RK, ed. Blood Disorders in Pregnancy. Philadelphia: Lea & Febiger, 1986, pp. 1–18.
3. Hytten F. Blood volume changes in normal pregnancy. Clin Haematol 1985;14:601–612.
4. Gibson HM. Plasma volume and glomerular filtration rate in pregnancy and their relation to differences in fetal growth. J Obstect Gyneacol Br Commonwealth 1973;80:1067–1074.
5. Taylor DJ, Lind T. Red cell mass during and after normal pregnancy. Br J Obstet Gynaecol 1979;86: 364–370.
6. Cabaniss CD, Cabaniss ML. Physiologic hematology of pregnancy. In: Kitay DZ, ed. Hematologic Problems in Pregnancy. ORadell, N.J.: Medical Economics Books, 1987, pp. 3–14.
7. Bequin Y, Lipscei G, Thoumsin H, Fillet G. Blunted erythropoietin production and decreased erythropoiesis in early pregnancy. Blood 1991;78:89–93.
8. Bianco I, Mastropietro F, D'Asero C, et al. Serum levels of erythropoietin and soluble transferrin receptor during pregnancy in non-B-thalassemic and B-thalassemic women. Haematologia 2000; 85:902–907.
9. Mercelina-Roumans PE, Ubachs JM, van Wersch JW. The reticulocyte count and its subfractions in smoking and non-smoking pregnant women. Eur J Clin Chem Clin Biochem 1995;33:263–265.
10. Milman N, Graudal N, Nielsen OJ, Agger AO. Serum erythropoietin during normal pregnancy: relationship to hemoglobin and iron status markers and impact of iron supplementation in a longitudinal, placebo-controlled study on 118 women. Int J Hematol 1997;66:159–168.
11. Harstad TW, Mason RA, Cox SM. Serum erythropoietin quantitation in pregnancy using an enzyme-linked immunoassay. Am J Perinatol 1992;9:233–235.
12. Barton PJD, Joy MT, Lappin TR, et al. Maternal erythropoietin in singleton pregnancies: a randomized trial on the effect of oral hematinic supplementation. Am J Obstet Gynecol 1994;170:896–901.
13. Taylor DJ. Pregnancy haemopoiesis. In: Turner T, ed. Perinatal Haematological Problems. Hoboken, NJ, John Wiley & Sons, 1991, pp. 1–22.
14. Scott DE, Pritchard JA. Iron deficiency in healthy young college women. JAMA 1967;147:147–150.
15. Hallberg L, Hulten L. Iron requirements, iron balance, and iron deficiency in menstruating and pregnant women. In: Halberg L, Asp NG, eds. Iron Nutrition in Health and Disease. London: George Libbey, 1996, pp. 165–182.
16. Graves BW, Barger MK. A conservative approach to iron supplementation during pregnancy. J Midwifery Womens Health 2001;46:159–166.
17. Puolakka J, Janne O, Jarvinen PA, Vihko R. Serum ferritin as a measure of iron stores during and after normal pregnancy with and without iron supplements. Acta Obstet Gynecol Scand 1980;95(suppl):43–51.
18. Johnson TRB, Niebyl JR. Preconception and prenatal care: part of a continuum. In: Gabbe SG, Niebly JR, Simpson JL, eds. Obstetrics: Normal and Problem Pregnancies; London: Churchill Livingstone, 2002, pp. 139–160.
19. US Preventive Services Task Force. Routine iron supplementation during pregnancy: policy statement and review article. JAMA 1993;270:2846–2854.
20. Gordon MC. Maternal physiology in pregnancy. In: Gabbe SG, Niebly JR, Simpson JL, eds. Obstetrics: Normal and Problem Pregnancies. London: Churchill Livingstone, 2002, pp. 63–91.
21. Milman N, Bergholt T, Byg KE, Eriksen L. Iron status and iron balance during pregnancy: a critical reappraisal of iron supplementation. Acta Anaesthesiol Scand 1999;78:749–757.
22. Milman N, Byg KE, Agger AO. Hemoglobin and erythrocyte indices during normal pregnancy and postpartum in 206 women with and without iron supplementation. Acta Anaesthesiol Scand 2000;79:89–98.

23. Taylor DJ, Mallen C, McDougall N, Lind T. Effect of iron supplementation on serum ferritin levels during and after pregnancy. Br J Obstet Gynaecol 1982;89:1011–1017.

24. Chanarin I, McFadyen IR, Kyle R. The physiological macrocytosis of pregnancy. Br J Obstet Gynaecol 1977;84:504–508.

25. Nutritional anemias: report of a WHO scientific group. World Health Organization Technical Report Service 1968;405:5–37.

26. Taylor DJ, Lind T. Haematological changes during normal pregnancy: iron induced macrocytosis. Br J Obstet Gynaecol 1976;83:760–767.

27. Puolakka J. Serum ferritin as a measure of iron stores during pregnancy. Acta Obstet Gynecol Scand 1980;95(suppl):8–31.

28. Blinder M. Anemia and transfusion therapy. In: Ahya SN, Flood K, Paranjothi S, eds. The Washington Manual of Medical Therapeutics. Lippincott Williams & Wilkins, Philadelphia, PA, 2001, pp. 413–428.

29. Carriaga MT, Skikne BS, Finley B, Cutler B. Serum transferrin receptor for the detection of iron deficiency in pregnancy. Am J Clin Nutr 1991;54:1077–1081.

30. Akesson A, Bjellerup P, Berglund M, Bremme K. Serum transferrin receptor: a specific marker of iron deficiency in pregnancy. Am J Clin Nutr 1998;68:1241–1246.

31. Choi JY, Pai SH. Change in erythropoiesis with gestational age during pregnancy. Ann Hematol 2001;80:26–31.

32. Frenkel EP, Yardley DA. Clinical and laboratory features and sequelae of deficiency of folic acid and vitamin B_{12} in pregnancy and gynecology. Hematol Oncol Clin North Am 2000;14:1079–1100.

33. Pryor JA, Morrison JC. Nutritional anemias. In: Bern MM, Frigoletto FD, eds. Hematologic Disorders in Maternal–Fetal Medicine. New York: Wiley-Liss, 1990, pp. 93–1121.

34. Beisher NA, Mackay EV, Colditz P. Obstetrics and the New Born. London: W. B. Saunders, 1997, pp. 86–89.

35. Mills JL, McPartin JM, Kirke PN. Homocysteine metabolism in pregnancies complicated by neural tube defects. Lancet 1995;345:149–151.

36. Czeizel AE, Dudas I. Prevention of the first occurrence of neural tube defects by periconceptional vitamin supplementation. N Engl J Med. 1992;327:1442–1446.

37. Rader JI, Yetley EA. Nationwide folate fortification has complex ramifications and requires careful monitoring over time. Arch Intern Med 2002;162(letter):608–609.

38. Pardo J, Peled Y, Bar J, Hod M. Evaluation of low serum vitamin B_{12} in the non-anaemic pregnant patient. Hum Reprod 2000;15:224–226.

39. Metz J, McGrath K, Bennett M, Hyland K. Biochemical indices of vitamin B_{12} nutrition in pregnant patients with subnormal serum vitamin B_{12} levels. Am J Hematol 1995;48:251–255.

40. Kuhnert M, Strohmeier R, Stegmuller M, Halberstadt E. Changes in lymphocyte subsets during normal pregnancy. Eur J Obstet Gynecol Reprod Biol 1998;76:147–151.

41. Sill PR, Lind T, Walker W. Platelet values during normal pregnancy. Br J Obstet Gynaecol 1985;92: 480–483.

42. Pitkin RM, Witte DL. Platelet and leukocyte counts in pregnancy. JAMA 1979;242:2696–2698.

43. Delgado I, Reinhard N, Dudenhausen JW. Changes in white blood cells during parturition in mothers and newborn. Gynecol Obstet Investi 1994;38:227–235.

44. Mercelina-Roumans PE, Ubachs JM, van Wersch JW. Leucocyte count and leucocyte differential in smoking and non-smoking females during pregnancy. Eur J Obstet Gynecol Reprod Biol 1994;55: 169–173.

45. Makinoda S, Mikuni M, Furuta I, Okuyama K. Serum concentration of endogenous G-CSF in women during the menstrual cycle and pregnancy. Eur J Clin Invest 1995;25:877–879.

46. Tsakonas DP, Nicolaides KH, Tsakona CP, Worman CP. Changes in maternal plasma macrophage-colony stimulating factor levels during normal pregnancy. Clin Lab Haemat 1995;17:57–59.

47. Tygart SG, McRoyan DK, Spinnato JA, McRoyan CJ. Longitudinal study of platelet indices during normal pregnancy. Am J Obstet Gynecol 1986;154:883–887.

48. Fenton V, Saunders K, Cavill I. The platelet count in pregnancy. J Clin Path 1977;30:68–69.

49. Fay RA, Hughes AO, Farron NT. Platelets in pregnancy: hyperdestruction in pregnancy. Obstet Gynecol 1983;61:238–240.

50. Verdy E, Bessous V, Dreyfus M, Kaplan C, Tchernia G, Uzan S. Longitudinal analysis of platelet count and volume in normal pregnancy. Thromb Haemost 1997;77:806–807.

51. O'Brian JR. Platelet counts in normal pregnancy. J Clin Path 1976;29:174.

52. Wallenburg HC, Van Kessel PH. Platelet lifespan in normal pregnancy as determined by a nonradioisotopic technique. Br J Obstet Gynaecol 1978;85:33–36.

53. Rinder HM, Bonan JL, Anandan S, Rinder CS. Noninvasive measurement of platelet kinetics in normal and hypertensive pregnancies. Am J Obstet Gynecol 1994;170:117–122.
54. Mercelina-Roumans PE, Ubachs JM, van Wersch JW. Platelet count and platelet indices at various stages of normal pregnancy in smoking and non-smoking women. Eur J Clin Chem Clin Biochem 1995;33:267–269.
55. Boehlen F, Hohlfeld P, Extermann P, Perneger TV, de Moerloose P. Platelet count at term pregnancy: a reappraisal of the threshold. Obstet Gynecol 2000;95:29–33.
56. Burrows RF, Kelton JG. Fetal thrombocytopenia and its relation to maternal thrombocytopenia. N Engl J Med 1993;329:1463–1466.
57. Saino S, Kekomaki R, Riikonen S, Teramo K. Maternal thrombocytopenia at term: a population-based study. Acta Obstet Gynecol Scand 2000;79:744–749.
58. Gill KK, Kelton JG. Management of idiopathic thrombocytopenic purpura in pregnancy. Sem Hematol 2000;37:275–289.
59. Tefferi A, Silverstein MN, Petitt RM, Hoagland HC. Outcome analysis of 34 pregnancies in women with essential thrombocythemia. Arch Intern Med 1995;155:1217–1222.
60. Vantroyen B, Vanstraelen D. Management of essential thrombocythemia during pregnancy with aspirin, interferon alpha-2a and no treatment: a comparative analysis of the literature. Acta Haematol. 2002;107:158–169.
61. Aune B, Gjesdal K, Oian P. Late onset postpartum thrombocytosis in preeclampsia. Acta Anaesthesiol Scand 1999;78:866–870.
62. Atalla RK, Thompson JR, Oppenheimer CA. Reactive thrombocytosis after ceasarean section and vaginal delivery: implications for maternal thromboembolism and its prevention. Br J Obstet Gynaecol 2000;107:411–414.
63. Hathaway WE, Bonnar J. Hemostatic disorders of the pregnant woman and newborn infant. New York: Elsevier, 1987, pp. 39–56.
64. Lindqvist PG, Svensson PF, Dahback B, Marsal K. Factor V Q506 mutation (activated protein C resistance), associated with reduced intrapartum blood loss: a possible evolutionary selection mechanism. Thromb Haemost 1998;79:69–73.
65. de Swiet M. Maternal mortality: confidential enquiries into maternal deaths in the United Kingdom. Am J Obstet Gynecol 2000;182:760–766.
66. Rutherford S, Montoro M, McGhee W, Strong T. Thromboembolic disease associated with pregnancy: an 11 year review. Am J Obstet Gynecol 1991;164(suppl).
67. McColl MD, Ramsay JE, Tait RC, et al. Risk factors for pregnancy associated venous thromboembolism. Thromb Haemost 1997;78:1183–1188.
68. Ginsberg JS, Brill-Edwards P, Burrows RF. DVT during pregnancy: leg and trimester of presentation. Thromb Haemost 1992;67:519–520.
69. Lanska DJ, Kryscio RJ. Risk factors for peripartum and postpartum stroke and intracranial venous thrombosis. Stroke 2000;31:1274–1282.
70. Roth A, Elkayam U. Acute myocardial infarction associated with pregnancy. Ann Intern Med 1996;125:751–762.
71. Rosenberg RD, Aird WC. Vascular-bed specific hemostasis and hypercoaguable states. N Engl J Med 1999;340:1555–1564.
72. Sharma SK, Philip J, Whitten CW. Thromboelastography in preeclamptic patients. Reg Anesth Pain Med 1996;21:493–495.
73. Kjellberg U, Hellgren M. Sonoclot signature during normal pregnancy. Intensive Care Med 2000;26:206–211.
74. Steer PL, Krantz HB. Thromboelastography and sonoclot analysis in the healthy parturients. J Clin Anesth 1993;5:419–424.
75. Kundu SK, Heilmann EJ, Sio R, Garcia C, Davidson RM, Ostgaard RA. Description of an in vitro platelt function analyzer: PFA-100. Sem Thromb Hemost 1995;21(suppl 2):106–112.
76. Kjellberg U, Andersson NE, Rosen S, Tengborn L, Hellgren M. APC resistance and other haemostatic variables during pregnancy and puerperium. Thromb Haemost 1999;81:527–531.
77. Beller FK, Ebert C. The coagulation and fibrinolytic enzyme system in pregnancy and in the puerperium. Eur J Obstet Gynecol Reprod Bio 1982;13:177–197.
78. Reid DE, Frigoletto FD, Tullis JL, Hinman J. Hypercoagulable states in pregnancy. Am J Obst Gynecol 1971;111:493–504.
79. Vincelot A, Nathan N, Collet D, Mehaddi Y, Grandchamp P, Julia A. Platelet function during pregnancy: an evaluation using the PFA-100 analyser. Br J Anaesth 2001;87:890–893.

80. Whigham KAE, Howie PW, Drummond AH, Prentice CRM. Abnormal platelet function in preeclampsia. Br J Obstet Gynaecol 1978;85:28–32.

81. O'Brien WF, Saba HI, Knuppel RA, Scerbo JC, Cohen GR. Alterations in platelet concentration and aggregation in normal pregnancy and preeclampsia. Am J Obstet Gynecol 1986;155:486–490.

82. Norris LA, Sheppard BL, Bonnar J. Increased whole blood platelet aggregation in normal pregnancy can be prevented in vitro by aspirin and dazmegrel. Br J Obstet Gynaecol 1992;99:253–257.

83. Lewis PJ, Boylan P, Friedman LA, Hensbey CN, Downing I. Prostacyclin in pregnancy. Br Med J 1980;282:1581–1582.

84. Frigoletto FD, Tullis JL, Reid DE, Hinman J. Hypercoagulability in the dysmature syndrome. Am J Obstet Gynecol 1971;111:867–873.

85. Stirling Y, Woolf L, Norht WRS, Seghatchian MJ, Meade TW. Haemostasis in normal pregnancy. Thromb Haemost 1984;52:176–182.

86. Hellgren M, Blomback M. Studies on blood coagulation and fibrinolysis in pregnancy, during delivery, and in the puerperium. Gynecol & Obstetric Investigation. 1981;12:141–154.

87. Clark P, Brennand J, Conkie JA, McCall F, Greer IA, Walker ID. Activated protein C sensitivity, protein C, protein S and coagulation in normal pregnancy. Thromb Haemost 1998;79:1166–1170.

88. Faught W, Garner P, Jones G, Ivey B. Changes in protein C and protein S levels in normal pregnancy. Am J Obstet Gynecol 1995;172:147–150.

89. Suzuki S, Sakamoto W. The kinetics of blood coagulability: fibrinolytic and kallikrein-kinin system at the onset and during labor. Eur J Obstet Gynecol Reprod Biol 1984;17:209–218.

90. Comp PC, Thurnas GR, Welsh J, Esmon CT. Functional and immunolgic protein S levels are decreased during pregnancy. Blood 1986;68:881–885.

91. Bombeli T, Raddatz-Mueller P, Fehr J. Coagulation activation markers do not correlate with the clinical risk of thrombosis in pregnant women. Am J Obstet Gynecol 2001;184:382–389.

92. Eichinger S, Weltermann A, Philipp K, et al. Prospective evaluation of hemostatic system and thrombin potential in healthy pregnant women with and without factor V Leiden. Thromb Haemost 1999;82:1232–1236.

93. Kluft C, Lansink M. Effect of oral contraceptives on haemostasis variables. Thromb Haemost 1997;78:315–326.

94. Vanderbroucke JP, Koster T, Briet E, Reitsman PH, Bertina RM, Rosendaal FR. Increased risk of venous thrombosis in oral-contraceptive users who are carriers of factor V Leiden mutation. Lancet 1994;344:1453–1457.

95. van Hylckama A, van der Linden IK, Bertina RM, Rosendaal FR. High levels of factor IX increase the risk of venous thrombosis. Blood 2000;95:3678–3682.

96. van der Meer FJM, Koster T, Vanderbroucke JP, Briet E, Rosendaal FR. The Leiden Thrombophilia Study (LETS). Thromb Haemost 1997;78:631–635.

97. Kruithof EKO, Tran-Thang C, Gudinchet AH, et al. Fibrinolysis in pregnancy: a study of plasminogen activator inhibitors. Blood 1987;69:460–466.

98. Bonnar J, Daley L, Sheppard B. Changes in the fibrinolytic system during pregnancy. Sem Thromb Hemost 1990;16:221–229.

99. Wright JG, Cooper P, Astedt B, et al. Fibrinolysis during normal human pregnancy: complex inter-relationships between plasma levels of tissue plasminogen activator and inhibitors and the euglobulin lysis clot lysis time. Br J Haematol 1988;69:253–258.

100. Arias F, Andrinopoulos G, Zamora J. Whole blood fibrinolytic activity in normal and hypertensive pregnancies and its relation to the placental concentration of urokinase inhibitor. Am J Obstet Gynecol 1979;133:624–629.

101. Chabloz P, Reber G, Boehlen F, Hohfeld P, de Moerloose P. TAFI antigen and D-dimer levels during normal pregnancy and at delivery. Br J Haematol 2001;115:150–152.

102. Williams E. Disseminated intravascular coagulation. In: Loscalzo J, Schafer AI, eds. Thrombosis and Hemorrhage. Baltimore: Williams & Wilkins, 1998, pp. 963–985.

103. Oshiro BT, Branch DW. Maternal hemostasis: coagulation problems of pregnancy. In: Loscalzo J, Schafer AI, eds. Thrombosis and Hemorrhage. Baltimore: Williams & Wilkins, 1998, pp. 1005–1026.

104. Sadler JE. Biochemistry and genetics of von Willebrand factor. Annu Rev Biochem 1998;67:395–424.

105. Nichols WC, Cooney KA, Ginsberg D, Ruggeri ZM. von Willebrand disease. In: Loscalzo J, Schafer AI, eds. Thrombosis and Hemorrhage. Baltimore: Williams & Wilkins, 1998, pp. 729–755.

106. Greer IA. Thrombosis in pregnancy: maternal and fetal issues. Lancet 1999;353:1258–1265.

107. Greer IA, Lowe GDO, Walker JJ, Forbes CD. Haemorrhagic problems in obstetrics and gynaecology in patients with congenital coagulopathies. Br J Obstet Gynaecol 1991;98:909–918.

108. Ridker PM, Miletich JP, Hennekens CH, Buring JE. Ethnic distribution of factor V Leiden in 4047 men and women: implications for venous thromboembolism screening. JAMA 1997;277:1305–1307.

109. Bertina RM, Koelman PC, Koster T, Rosendaal FR. Mutation in blood coagulation factor V associated with resistance to activated protein C. Nature 1994;369:64–67.

110. Bokarewa MI, Bremme K, Blomback M. Arg 506-Gln mutation in factor V and risk of thrombosis during pregnancy. Br J Haematol 1996;92:473–478.

111. Martineli IM, De Stevano V, Taioli E, Paciaroni K, Rossi E, Mannucci PM. Inherited thrombophilia and first venous thromboembolism during pregnancy and puerperium. Thromb Haemost 2002;87:791–795.

112. Gerhardt A, Scharf RE, Beckmann MW, et al. Prothrombin and factor V mutations in women with a history of thrombosis during pregnancy and the puerperium. N Engl J Med 2000;342:374–380.

113. Poort SR, Rosendaal FR, Koelman PC, Koster T. A common genetic variation in the 3'-untranslated region of the prothrombin gene is associated with elevated plasma prothrombin levels and an increase in venous thrombosis. Blood 1996;88:3698–3703.

114. McColl MD, Reid DE, Tait RC, Walker ID, Greer IA. Prothrombin G20210A, MTHFR C677T mutations in women with venous thromboembolism associated with prengnancy. Br J Obstet Gynaecol 2000;107:565–569.

115. Ray JG, Shmorgun D, Chan WS. Common C6778T polymorphism of the methylenetetrahydrofolate reductase gene and the risk of venous thromboembolism: meta-analysis of 31 studies. Pathophysiol Haemost Thromb 2002;32:51–58.

116. Kelly PJ, Rosand J, Kistler JP, Shih VE, Silveira S. Homocysteine, MTHFR C677T polymorphism and risk of ischemic strokes: results of a meta-analysis. Neurology 2002;59:529–536.

117. Ginsberg JS, Greer IA, Hirsh J. Use of antithrombotic agents during pregnancy. Chest 2001; 119(suppl):122S–131S.

118. Alfirevic Z, Roberts D, Martlew V. How strong is the association between maternal throbophilia and adverse pregnancy outcome? a systematic review. Eur J Obstet Gynecol 2002;101:6–14.

119. Meinardi JR, Middeldorp S, de Kam P, et al. Increased risk for fetal loss in carriers of the factor V Leiden mutation. Ann Intern Med 1999;130:736–739.

120. Rey E, Kahn SR, Shrier I. Thrombophilic disorders and fetal loss: a meta-analysis. Lancet 2003;361:901–908.

121. McCowan LME, Craigie S, Taylor RS, Ward C, McLintock C, North RA. Inherited thrombophilias are not increased in "idiopathic" small-for-gestational-age pregnancies. Am J Obstet Gynecol 2003; 188:981–985.

122. Infante-Reivard C, Rivard G, Yotov WV, Genin E, Gurigeut M, Weinbert C. Absence of association of thrombophilia polymorphisms with intrauterine growth restriction. N Engl J Med 2002;347:19–25.

123. Verspyck E, Le Cam-Duchez V, Goffinet F, Tron F, Marpeau L, Borg JY. Thrombophilia and immunological disorders in pregnancies as risk factors for small for gestational age infants. Br J Obstet Gynaecol 2002;109:28–33.

124. Morrison ER, Meidzbrodzka H, Campbell DM, et al. Prothrombotic genotypes are not associated with pre-eclampsia and gestational hypertension: results from a large population-based study and systematic review. Thromb Haemost 2002;87:779–785.

125. Benedetto CM, Salton L, Maula V, Chieppa G, Massobrio M. Factor V Leiden and factor II G20210A in preeclampsia and HELLP syndrome. Acta Obstet Gynecol Scand 2002;81:1095–1100.

126. Meeks GR, Gookin K, Morrison JC. Iron deficiency anemia in pregnancy. In: Kitay DZ, ed. Hematologic Problems in Pregnancy. Oradell, NJ: Medical Economics Books, 1987.

127. van Wersch JW, Ubachs JM. Blood coagulation and fibrinolysis during normal pregnancy. Eur J Clin Chem Clin Biochem 1991;29:45–50.

11 Hemolytic Disease of the Newborn

David G. Grenache, PhD

Contents

INTRODUCTION

Hemolytic disease of the newborn (HDN) is characterized by the destruction of fetal red blood cells by maternal immunoglobulin G (IgG) directed against antigens present on fetal erythrocytes. These paternally inherited antigens are not present on maternal cells and can stimulate the maternal immune system to produce antibodies when antepartum or intrapartum fetomaternal hemorrhage occurs. Maternal sensitization often occurs during the first pregnancy with a fetus that expresses the erythrocyte antigens and although this fetus is at low risk of HDN, future antigen-positive fetuses are at substantial risk of developing the disease. Transplacental passage of the resulting antibodies into the fetal circulation often leads to hemolysis that can range from mild to extreme depending on several factors including, among others, the antibody concentration, the transfer rate of immunoglobulin from the maternal to the fetal circulation, the antibody specificity, the functional maturity of the fetal spleen, and the IgG subclass (Fig. 1) *(1)*.

The lysis of red cells in HDN does not occur through complement activation but rather through interactions between the Fc portion of the IgG molecules on the sensitized erythrocyte and effector cells present in the fetal spleen *(2)*. Splenic macrophages are believed to be the principal effector cells responsible for the red cell destruction, which occurs via erythrophagocytosis.

Clinical Manifestations

Clinical manifestations of HDN depend on the nature of the immune response, and disease severity can range from mild hemolysis to severe anemia. When anemia is severe, the erythrocyte production in the bone marrow cannot match the red blood cell destruction, and extramedullary sites of hematopoiesis are stimulated, leading to hepatosplenomegaly and the appearance of erythroblasts in the fetal circulation. Indeed, the term erythroblastosis fetalis, often used to describe HDN, is derived from this clinical finding.

From: *Current Clinical Pathology: Handbook of Clinical Laboratory Testing During Pregnancy*
Edited by: A. M. Gronowski © Humana Press, Totowa, NJ

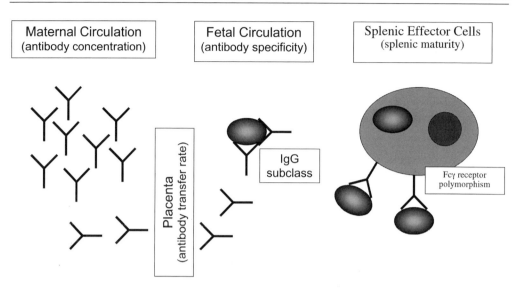

Fig. 1. Various factors that can influence the severity of hemolytic disease of the newborn. (Adapted from ref. *1*.)

Severe anemia can also result in hypoxic injury to the liver and heart. Impaired hepatic synthesis of plasma proteins results in a decrease in plasma oncotic pressure that, in conjunction with heart failure, causes generalized edema termed hydrops fetalis. This finding carries grave prognostic implications and frequently results in death *in utero* or shortly after birth *(3)*. After birth, when the placenta is no longer able to remove the excess bilirubin from the fetal blood, unconjugated bilirubin can pass through the blood–brain barrier, leading to bilirubin encephalopathy (kernicterus), which that can impair neurodevelopment, produce nerve deafness, spastic cerebral palsy, or even death *(4)*.

Etiology

Numerous alloantibodies have been cited as a cause of HDN. These include antibodies with specificity toward the antigens of the rhesus (Rh) blood group system (c, C, D, e, and E), and those of the Kell (K and k); Duffy (Fy^a); Kidd (Jk^a and Jk^b); and MNSs (M, N, S, and s) systems *(4)*. Anti-D is the most common cause of HDN in the Western world, followed by anti-c, anti-K, and anti-E *(1,4–6)*. Despite the availability since 1968 of effective prophylaxis with anti-D immune globulin, the Centers for Disease Control reported in 1991 that the incidence of Rh hemolytic disease in the United States was 1 per 1000 total births *(7)*. Failure to receive anti-D prophylaxis and sensitization to antigens other than D has been sited as the likely causes of maternal alloimmunization *(5)*.

Prophylaxis

Anti-D immune globulin (RhoGAM®, Ortho Clinical Diagnostics, Raritan, NJ) is manufactured from human plasma containing anti-D and is used to prevent maternal alloimmunization to the RhD antigen by antibody-mediated immune suppression. The exact mechanism by which anti-D immune globulin works remains unclear. Suppression may result from clearance of RhD-positive fetal cells from the maternal circulation, antigen blocking, or central inhibition *(2)*. The latter hypothesis is perhaps the most plausible and is likely to involve the sequestration of anti-D-coated fetal erythrocytes in the maternal spleen. The accumulation of anti-D complexes may suppress the primary immune response by interrupting the T-cell mediated clonal expansion of RhD-specific B-cells *(2)*.

A single dose of RhoGAM contains 300 μg (1500 IU) of anti-D and is sufficient to suppress the immune response of 15 mL or less of RhD-positive red blood cells *(8)*. It is recommended that RhoGAM be administered to RhD-negative women between 28 and 32 wk of gestation and again postpartum if the infant is RhD-positive *(8)*.

Clinical Management and Treatment

Clinical management of potential HDN is aimed at the early detection of maternal alloantibodies associated with HDN and early detection of fetal hemolytic anemia when it occurs. If alloantibodies are detected, then the genotype of the fetus's father can be determined to assess the risk of HDN to the fetus. If the father of the fetus does not possess the antigen, then the fetus is not at risk and continued monitoring for fetal anemia is not required. If the father possesses the antigen, then the fetus is potentially at risk for developing HDN and further follow-up studies are performed. In cases where the father is heterozygous, polymerase chain reaction can be used to determine the fetal Rh genotype from DNA obtained from cells collected by amniocentesis or chorionic villus sampling *(9)* (Fig. 2).

When hemolytic anemia is identified, treatment with blood transfusions (peritoneal or direct intravascular) and/or early delivery with appropriate neonatal care can be initiated. Unfortunately, invasive therapeutic procedures have associated risks such as fetomaternal hemorrhage that can worsen maternal alloimmunization and exacerbate fetal anemia. Fetal loss rates in groups that require intrauterine transfusion are still 4 to 15%, with the highest mortality associated with severely anemic fetuses that are already hydropic when the diagnosis is made *(10)*. Clearly, detecting fetal anemia prior to the onset of hydrops is the main goal in the management of these complicated pregnancies. Perhaps even more desirable is the availability of noninvasive tests that could reliably predict the severity of HDN earlier in gestation and would allow optimal and judicious use of invasive clinical procedures.

Clinical Laboratory Tests

The focus of this chapter is on in vitro assays that have been advocated or investigated as indicators of HDN severity. These include tests to detect and quantify alloantibodies in the maternal serum, functional or cellular assays that measure the ability of maternal antibodies to modulate cellular interactions that lead to the hemolysis of fetal erythrocytes, and tests performed on amniotic fluid (AF) to predict and/or monitor the severity of fetal red blood cell hemolysis.

The gold standard test for assessing fetal anemia is the hematologic analysis of fetal blood collected via fetal blood sampling, also known as cordocentesis or percutaneous umbilical cord blood sampling (PUBS). It is performed for both diagnostic and therapeutic purposes and has an approx 2% risk of a serious complication *(11)*. Table 1 summarizes fetal hematologic measurements according to gestational age *(11a)*.

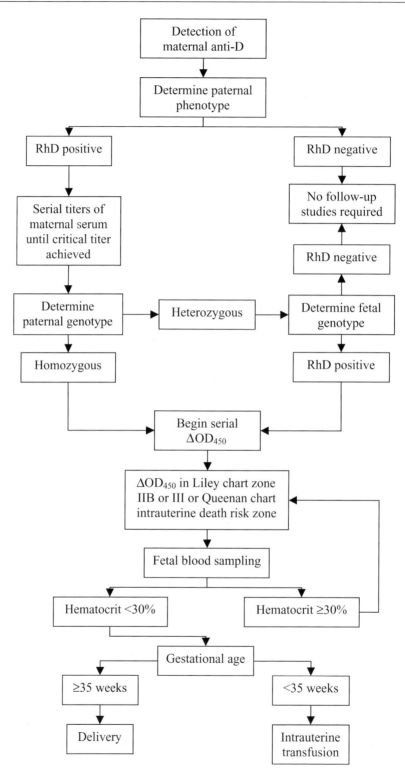

Fig. 2. Algorithm for the clinical management of maternal alloimmunization during pregnancy. (Adapted from ref. 60.)

Table 1
Evolution of Hematologic Values of 2860 Normal Fetuses During Pregnancy (mean ± SD)

Week of gestation	WBC[a] (× 10^9/L)	Total WBC counts (× 10^9/L)	PLT (× 10^9/L)	RBC (× 10^12/L)	Hb (g/dL)	Ht (%)	MCV (fL)
18–21 (n = 760)	4.68 ± 2.96	2.57 ± 0.42	234 ± 57	2.85 ± 0.36	11.69 ± 1.27	37.3 ± 4.32	131.11 ± 10.97
22–25 (n = 1200)	4.72 ± 2.82	3.73 ± 2.17	247 ± 59	3.09 ± 0.34	12.2 ± 1.6	38.59 ± 3.94	125.1 ± 7.84
26–29 (n = 460)	5.16 ± 2.53	4.08 ± 0.84	242 ± 69	3.46 ± 0.41	12.91 ± 1.38	40.88 ± 4.4	118.5 ± 7.96
>30 (n = 440)	7.71 ± 4.99	6.40 ± 2.99	232 ± 87	3.82 ± 0.64	13.64 ± 2.21	43.55 ± 7.2	114.38 ± 9.34

[a]Including normoblasts. (From ref. *11a*. Copyright American Society of Hematology, used with permission.)

SEROLOGICAL ASSAYS

Although a variety of techniques have been utilized for detecting IgG antibodies to red blood cells *(12)*, the indirect antiglobulin test (IAT), also known as the indirect Coomb's test, is considered to be the best serological test to identify them *(13)*. In conjunction with ABO and RhD typing of maternal red blood cells as part of the initial tests performed on an obstetrical patient at her first prenatal visit, the IAT is also performed to identify antibodies, such as anti-D, that have the potential to cause HDN.

Semiquantitative Techniques

In the United States, semiquantitative assessment of the maternal alloantibody is accomplished by titration performed by preparing twofold serial dilutions of serum that are then tested for antibody activity by IAT. The titer is recorded as the reciprocal of the highest dilution that gives a 1+ agglutination reaction (i.e., a 1 in 64 dilution produces a reaction at a titer of 64) *(14)*. It is recommended that titers be determined when potentially hemolyzing antibodies are first identified and then repeated at 20 wk gestation and approximately every 4 wk thereafter *(6)*. The purpose of performing the titer is to determine when to initiate other types of fetal monitoring such as fetal blood sampling to determine fetal hemoglobin/hematocrit or amniocentesis to evaluate the severity of fetal hemolysis by measuring the deviation in optical density at 450 nm (ΔOD_{450}). Titrations performed in the first trimester can provide baseline values for comparison with titers performed later in gestation. Patients with rising titers or titers above a "critical titer" (the titer below which fetal hydrops is not anticipated and additional fetal monitoring is unnecessary), require subsequent monitoring.

Antibody titration methods are inherently imprecise, and the correlation between titer and HDN severity is generally regarded as poor. Several studies that have investigated their use in the prediction of HDN severity have produced mixed results. A summary of some studies that have investigated the use of titration in estimating HDN severity is shown in Table 2. There is wide variability in the predictive values of titration, which is likely caused by the inherent variation that is observed between laboratories performing the test. The variation in the critical titers utilized by individual studies is also a contributing factor.

The limitations of titration in assessing HDN severity were made apparent in a retro-spective analysis of RhD-sensitized pregnancies in which 24% (12 of 49) of mothers with a titer of 16 or less had infants with mild to severe HDN *(15)*. This finding prompted the authors to recommend that the concept of the critical titer be abandoned entirely and suggested that all women with a positive IAT be managed by serial evaluations of AF, irrespective of the titer. Others, however, have argued against that recommendation, pointing out that amniocentesis is an invasive procedure and one that may result in additional maternal alloimmunization *(16)*.

The largest shortcoming of antibody titration in predicting HDN severity appears to be its poor specificity (Table 2), which puts fetuses unaffected by HDN at risk for invasive investigative procedures. One multicenter study reported an increase in titration specific-ity from 18 to 64% with no decrease in the sensitivity when the critical titer was increased to 128 from 16 *(17)*. However, the authors urged that laboratories and physicians use their own clinical experience to determine critical titers. As a guideline, the American College of Obstetricians and Gynecologists (ACOG) has recommended a critical titer between 16 and 32 *(6)*.

Quantitative Techniques

Although this test is not available in the United States, the concentration of maternal anti-D is quantitated in the United Kingdom and other European countries using a Technicon AutoAnalyzer. Originally described in 1969, the AutoAnalyzer quantitates anti-D by diluting serum that is subsequently incubated with an excess of RhD-positive red blood cells *(18)*. After any resulting agglutinates are removed, the remaining cells are lysed and the optical density of the lysate is measured spectrophotometrically. Sera with either high or low titers of anti-D produce low or high optical densities, respectively, and are compared against a reference standard to produce results of anti-D in IU/mL (5 IU = 1 μg) *(2)*. As is the case with titration, quantitation by AutoAnalyzer is used to make decisions regarding clinical interventions and, for this purpose, a cutoff value of 15 IU/mL has been recommended *(19)*. Advantages of the AutoAnalyzer include its ability to process a large number of samples, quantify antibody concentration against a standard preparation of anti-D, and generate results with greater precision than is achievable by titration *(1)*.

It is generally accepted that quantitative results have greater predictive values than titration, although there are few published comparisons between the two methods. Like those observed with titration, the predictive values of quantitative anti-D measurements are broad (Table 2). However, data from some studies suggest that it is possible to define a concentration of anti-D below which severe HDN is not likely to occur *(19–21)*. One of these studies identified an anti-D concentration of 4 IU/mL as a concentration at or below which no infant had a cord blood hemoglobin less than 10 g/dL ($n = 78$, 100% NPV) *(20)*. Unfortunately, there is no cutoff above which anti-D concentrations are reliably predictive of HDN, and numerous women with high concentrations of anti-D deliver unaffected infants.

Summary

Overall, these two serological measurements of anti-D appear to behave similarly and are of limited value in the assessment of the severity of HDN. At best, they both do a fair job of identifying infants that are least likely to be affected by HDN (Table 2, NPV).

Table 2

Studies Investigating the Clinical Performance of Serological Tests in the Prediction of HDN Severity, the Need for Neonatal Treatment, or Fetal Anemia

Reference	Test type	n	Critical titer or anti-D cutoff concentration	Outcome measured	Sensitivity (%)	Specificity (%)	PPV (%)	NPV (%)	Accuracy (%)
Gall and Miller (15)	Titration	49	> 16	HDN severity	71	71	94	29	71
Moise et al. (17)	Titration	47	≥ 16	HDN severity	100	18	45	100	51
Gottvall et al. (57)	Titration	222	≥ 64	Neonatal treatment	86	73	62	91	77
Filbey et al. (34)	Titration	42	> 32	HDN severity	87	47	67	75	69
Oepkes et al. (28)	Titration	172	≥ 32	Neonatal treatment	100	40	52	100	63
Zupanska et al. (30)	Titration	72	≥ 32	HDN severity	74	80	96	33	75
Sacks et al. (31)	Titration	33	≥ 16	Neonatal treatment	100	39	42	100	56
Bowell et al. (20)	AutoAnalyzer	184	> 4 IU/mL	Neonatal anemia	100	48	22	100	55
Nicolaides and Rodeck (19)	AutoAnalyzer	237	> 15 IU/mL	Fetal anemia	ND	ND	ND	100	ND
Gottvall et al. (57)	AutoAnalyzer	54	≥ 3.5 IU/mL	Neonatal treatment	80	79	83	76	80
Filbey et al. (34)	AutoAnalyzer	42	> 4 IU/mL	HDN severity	74	58	68	65	67
Hadley et al. (26)	AutoAnalyzer	27	≥ 5 IU/mL	HDN severity	95	25	75	67	74
Garner et al. (27)	AutoAnalyzer	44	>11 IU/mL	HDN severity	74	92	96	60	80
Buggins et al. (21)	AutoAnalyzer	20	≥ 15 IU/mL	Fetal anemia	100	30	59	100	65
Hadley et al. (58)	AutoAnalyzer	132	> 15 IU/mL	HDN severity	70	74	88	46	71

ND, not done; NPV, negative predictive value; PPV, positive predictive value.

Clearly, their largest failure is in accurately predicting which infants are likely to suffer from the disorder because it is not possible to identify a threshold above which HDN can be reliably predicted (Table 2, PPV). Despite their performance characteristics, both tests continue to be widely used in the management of HDN to determine which patients should undergo fetal blood sampling or amniocentesis.

FUNCTIONAL/CELLULAR ASSAYS

As mentioned previously, a variety of factors influence the severity of HDN, and serologic methods assess only the antibody concentration. Functional or cellular assays have been developed that measure the ability of maternal antibodies bound to erythrocytes to interact with the Fc receptors on effector cells such as monocytes or lymphocytes. The resulting effects of that interaction are then quantitated. These types of tests include the antibody-dependent cell-mediated cytotoxicity (ADCC) assay, the monocyte monolayer assay (MMA), and the chemiluminescence (CL) assay.

ADCC Assay

The ADCC assay measures the lysis of sensitized red blood cells by effector cells. Chromium-51 (^{51}CR)-labeled RhD-positive erythrocytes are incubated with maternal serum and either monocytes (M-ADCC) or killer cells (K-ADCC) and percent lysis is measured by the release of ^{51}Cr from the red cells into the supernatant (22). Table 3 summarizes the data from some of the studies investigating the use of this assay in predicting HDN severity or the need for neonatal treatment for HDN.

Despite it being the first cellular assay investigated for predicting HDN severity, reports using the K-ADCC assay are few. The first report of this assay demonstrated that it was able to differentiate infants with no or mild HDN from severely affected infants. This was true despite all patients having concentrations of anti-D that were greater than 19 IU/mL (23). In contrast, a study by Hadley et al. reported no correlation between the percent lysis of K-ADCC and HDN severity (24).

Studies using the M-ADCC assay are more numerous, and most seem to suggest that M-ADCC results are more accurate than either antibody titration or anti-D quantitation, although some conclude that it may be only slightly more useful than anti-D quantitation in predicting the severity of fetal anemia (25–27).

A recent retrospective study investigated the use of the M-ADCC assay and antibody titer in the management of 172 RhD-sensitized pregnancies with RhD-positive fetuses (28). Fetal blood sampling and intrauterine transfusion were performed on 30 infants with severe HDN diagnosed by ultrasonographic scans, Doppler examinations, or ΔOD_{450} analysis. Of the remaining 142 infants, 105 were unaffected by HDN and required no neonatal therapy, whereas 37 received either top-up or exchange transfusions after birth. A cutoff of more than 50% lysis by the M-ADCC assay correctly identified 64 out of 84 (positive predictive value [PPV], 75%) infants who required any type of treatment for HDN and 100% of infants who required intrauterine transfusion therapy (28). The same cutoff correctly predicted 84 out of 87 (negative predictive value [NPV], 97%) infants who did not require therapy. By comparison, use of a critical anti-D titer of 32 or more produced many more false-positives and correctly identified only 67 out of 130 (PPV, 52%) infants who required therapy. Similar to the findings discussed earlier by Moise et al. (17), the authors of this study reported that the critical titer could safely be increased to 128 or more with only a 1% decrease in sensitivity (to 99%) but with an increase in specificity from 40 to 70%.

Table 3

Studies Investigating the Clinical Performance of Functional Assays in the Prediction of HDN Severity or Need for Neonatal Treatment

Reference	Test type	n	Cutoff	Outcome measured	Sensitivity (%)	Specificity (%)	PPV (%)	NPV (%)	Accuracy (%)
Engelfriet and Ouwehand (22)	M-ADCC	62	> 3 SD[a]	HDN severity	79	90	94	67	82
Urbaniak et al. (23)	K-ADCC	11	< 30%[b]	HDN severity	100	75	88	100	91
Hadley et al. (26)	M-ADCC	27	> 25%	HDN severity	89	75	89	75	85
Garner et al. (27)	M-ADCC	44	> 28%	HDN severity	84	100	100	72	89
Oepkes et al. (28)	M-ADCC	172	> 50%	Neonatal treatment	96	80	75	97	86
Nance et al. (29)	MMA	16	≥ 20%	HDN severity	100	83	91	100	94
Zupanska et al. (30)	MMA	72	≥ 20%	HDN severity	68	100	100	33	72
Sacks et al. (31)	MMA	33	≥ 20%	Neonatal treatment	100	43	43	100	61
Garner et al. (27)	MMA	44	≥ 22%	HDN severity	61	100	100	52	73
Lucas et al. (32)	MMA	22	≥ 20%	HDN severity	75	43	43	75	55
Lucas et al. (32)	CL	22	≥ 10%[c]	HDN severity	88	71	64	91	77
Buggins et al. (21)	CL	20	≥ 7	Fetal anemia	100	80	83	100	90
Filbey et al. (34)	CL	42	> 30%	HDN severity	65	79	79	65	71
Hadley et al. (58)	CL	132	> 30%	HDN severity	82	94	98	64	85

CL, chemiluminescence assay; K-ADCC, K-cell antibody-dependent cell-mediated cytotoxicity assay; M-ADCC, monocyte antibody-dependent cell-mediated cytotoxicity assay; MMA, monocyte monolayer assay; NPD, negative predictive value; PPD, positive predictive value.

[a]>3 standard deviations above results from unaffected infants.

[b]Although the authors did not report the use of this cutoff specifically, visual interpretation of their data as well as their conclusions would support the use of this value.

[c]CL assay cutoffs are expressed as either a percent of the response obtained from a positive control or as an index (no units) obtained from the response of a negative control.

MMA

The MMA, also known as the phagocytosis assay, involves adherence of monocytes to a chamber slide to create a cell monolayer. Erythrocytes sensitized with alloantibodies from maternal serum are added to the chamber slide and incubated with the monocytes for 1 h. After rinsing away nonadherent cells, the slide is stained and examined under light microscopy to determine the percentage of monocytes that have adhered to and/or phagocytized erythrocytes. Unlike the ADCC assays, there is no need for the use of radioactive isotope; however, the results are more subjective. A summary of performance data using the MMA is given in Table 3.

Initial reports of the MMA indicated that it produced very good predictive values and suggested a correlation with disease severity that was better than antibody titration *(29,30)*. This was true primarily when the assay was used to differentiate unaffected from severely affected fetuses rather than moderately affected ones. Several other studies, however, have reported that the MMA correlated poorly with HDN severity and offered no benefit over antibody titration *(31,32)*.

One study examined the correlation between results from the MMA and M-ADCC tests and antibody subclass and reported that although the number of cell-bound IgG1 antibodies correlated poorly with the MMA ($r = 0.33$), it was highly correlated with the M-ADCC assay ($r = 0.76$) *(27)*. The authors concluded that the M-ADCC assay was superior to that of the MMA because HDN severity was also more closely correlated to IgG1 ($r = 0.58$) than to IgG3 ($r = 0.16$). They suggest that the poorer predictive value of the MMA, relative to that of the M-ADCC, was a function of its apparent dependence on an antibody subclass that was less likely to be implicated in HDN *(27)*.

CL Assay

The CL assay measures the metabolic response of monocytes that occurs during phagocytosis of sensitized erythrocytes *(33)*. Red blood cells that are sensitized with maternal serum are added together with luminol to a cuvette containing monocytes pooled from six donors (multiple donors are used to decrease interassay variation), and the cuvette is incubated at 37°C. During this incubation, oxygen radicals released from the monocytes during erythrophagocytosis react with the luminol, producing luminescence that can be monitored with a luminometer. Results are expressed either as a percentage of the response obtained from monoclonal anti-D-sensitized (positive) control cells or as an index calculated from the response obtained from unsensitized (negative) control cells. Like the MMA, this test does not require the use of radioisotopes, yet it has the benefit of being a more objective test similar to the ADCC assay.

Several studies suggest that the ability of the CL test to predict HDN severity is better than that of the MMA (Table 3). Others, showing it to be a better predictor of fetal anemia, have proposed that its use in managing alloimmunized pregnancies could decrease the need for fetal blood sampling if the CL test result was negative *(21)*.

One study suggested the use of the CL test in a stepwise approach in conjunction with serological assays beginning with titration to identify patients with quantities of anti-D above a critical titer (32 in their study) *(34)*. Specimens exceeding that cutoff would receive quantitation by AutoAnalyzer, and those in excess of 4 IU/mL would then be analyzed by the CL test. It was speculated that this approach would reduce AutoAnalyzer quantitation of low titer antibodies that rarely cause HDN but would identify high concentrations of low functional antibodies that are also less likely to be associated with HDN. Although such an idea is intriguing, it has yet to be investigated and reported.

Summary

Functional assays like the ones discussed here would appear to have some clinical utility in the prediction and management of HDN. However, to ensure assay performance, these technically difficult tests need to be carefully validated, performed frequently, and observed closely. As such, they are best suited to be performed by reference laboratories. From the evidence available in the literature, it would seem that among the functional tests, the ADCC and CL assays have better predictive values than the MMA (Table 3), which may be because of the more objective nature of their results.

Functional tests do not have to have the same performance characteristics in all spectrums of HDN severity. When appropriately utilized, these tests are most likely to be of benefit in identifying nonaffected or severely affected fetuses and may help in clinical decision making regarding the use of invasive procedures such as amniocentesis or fetal blood sampling. In contrast, their ability to identify mildly affected fetuses is poor, but this shortcoming can be overlooked because these mildly affected fetuses rarely require *in utero* transfusion therapy.

In a recent review of in vitro tests for predicting HDN severity, Hadley proposes a structured approach to using serological and functional antibody assays so that the more technically demanding functional assays are used only in pregnancies that are likely to have the highest risk of HDN *(1)*. His approach takes the form of a pyramid whose base consists of all pregnant women who undergo serological tests to screen for red cell alloantibodies associated with HDN. In the pyramid's center are those women with positive screening tests who then receive antibody titration or anti-D quantitation. Women with antibody concentrations that exceed a specified cutoff and undergo testing with a functional assay by a reference laboratory make up the top of the pyramid.

Although various functional assays are used selectively in the United Kingdom and other European countries, they are not used in the United States or they are used only rarely *(35)*. As mentioned earlier, in the United States, in vitro serological tests are performed to determine when to initiate invasive tests such as amniocentesis or PUBS, not to predict HDN severity. To accomplish the latter, spectrophotometric analysis of AF has been the accepted method for over 40 yr for determining the severity of fetal erythrocyte hemolysis.

AF SPECTROPHOTOMETRY

During normal pregnancy, AF bilirubin peaks at approx 19–22 wk at concentrations of 1.6 to 1.8 mg/L *(36)*. Intrauterine hemolysis severe enough to cause erythroblastosis fetalis can increase the bilirubin concentration of AF to approx 10 mg/L *(37,38)*. Because the concentration of AF bilirubin is often too low to be measured by standard chemical techniques, an alternative method using scanning spectrophotometry has been devised. The principal of this approach is based on the fact that the deviation in AF optical density at 450 nm is caused by the presence of bilirubin. As bilirubin absorbs light maximally at 450 nm, the extent to which the curve deviates from a baseline (drawn between the optical

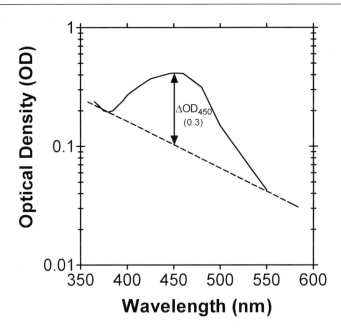

Fig. 3. Graph of the spectrophotometric analysis of AF taken from an Rh-sensitized pregnancy. The solid line is the plot of the optical density of the bilirubin-containing fluid versus wavelengths scanned. The dashed line represents the baseline (drawn between the optical density readings at 350 and 550 nm) expected from AF that does not contain bilirubin). The difference between the optical density of the solid line and the dashed line at 450 nm is the ΔOD_{450} value (0.3 in this example).

density readings at 350 and 550 nm) at this wavelength is proportional to the concentration of bilirubin in the AF, and it is this change in absorbance that is known as the ΔOD_{450} *(39)* (Fig. 3).

The Liley Chart

First introduced into clinical practice in 1961 by Liley *(40)*, the ΔOD_{450} has become the most widely used test to predict the severity of HDN *(10)*. Liley measured the ΔOD_{450} in 101 sensitized pregnancies beginning at 27 wk gestation and correlated the results to clinical outcome. From these data he constructed a graph, referred to as the Liley chart (Fig. 4), which is now well known and is used to predict the severity of HDN. Liley created his chart by plotting the ΔOD_{450} value on the *y*-axis relative to the gestational age (in wk) on the *x*-axis and then divided the chart into three zones. Results falling within zone I (low zone) were associated with unaffected or very mildly affected infants, results in zone II (mid zone) included infants with mild to severe anemia, and results within zone III (high zone) represented the most severely affected infants, most of whom died *in utero* *(40)*. Liley later advocated dividing zones II and III into two equal subzones *(41)*.

The importance of serial amniocentesis and measurement of the ΔOD_{450} in evaluating fetal anemia was also made clear by Liley because decreasing values in his studies were associated with mild disease, and stable or rising values were associated with severe anemia *(40,41)*. Others have supported the value of this trend analysis. Queenan analyzed serial ΔOD_{450} results in 223 women who delivered unaffected to either mildly, moder-

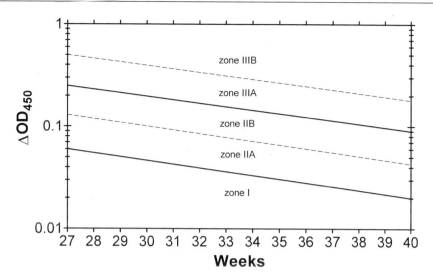

Fig. 4. The Liley chart. (Adapted from ref. *40*.)

ately, or severely affected infants and reported a downward trend in ΔOD_{450} results in all but the severely affected infants *(42)*. Results from these severely affected fetuses showed higher values with mixed trends, and results from 13 infants who died *in utero* demonstrated upward trends in all cases with the exception of one downward trend. That single case was complicated by polyhydramnios that produced a dilutional influence on the AF bilirubin concentration and the subsequent lowering of the ΔOD_{450} *(42)*. A horizontal or rising trend is an ominous sign and indicates the need for clinical intervention either by transfusion or early delivery. Although there are no reliable data concerning the frequency of testing, the ACOG recommends repeating amniocentesis every 1 to 4 wk if results are in zone II and every 3 to 4 wk if results drop into zone I *(6)*.

An evaluation of Liley's chart with 36 RhD-sensitized women in whom both ΔOD_{450} and fetal hematocrit were measured on 63 occasions between 17 wk gestation and term reported incorrect predictions of HDN severity in 21% (13 of 63) of instances *(43)*. Seven (54%) of these incorrect predictions occurred in samples collected at less than 27 wk gestation with the use of a Liley chart in which the zones had been extrapolated backward. This is notable because Liley's chart was originally developed with specimens collected at no less than 27 wk gestation and the authors of the current study did not validate the utility of extrapolated zones.

The use of the Liley chart with zones that were linearly extrapolated behind the chart's original 27 wk was widely adopted (without appropriate validation) when the need to diagnose fetal anemia in the second trimester became necessary because of advances in fetal blood sampling and transfusion therapy. Studies that have investigated the clinical usefulness of the extrapolated Liley chart have reported conflicting results and recommendations. Nicolaides et al. reported that ΔOD_{450} values plotted on the extrapolated Liley chart did not accurately predict fetal anemia and pointed out that results within zones I and II (suggesting mild to moderate anemia) were observed for 68% (21 of 31) of severely affected fetuses (sensitivity, 32%) *(44)*. However, the sensitivity for predicting hemoglobin concentrations less than 6.0 g/dL increased to 84% (26 of 31) when a cutoff based on the subdivided zone II (greater than or equal to zone IIB) was utilized (Table 4). The poor performance of the Liley chart prompted the authors to conclude that fetal blood sampling was the only accurate method to assess fetal anemia in the second trimester *(44)*. It is worth noting that 14 fetuses with hydrops fetalis were included in the analysis. As was previously mentioned, polyhydroaminos in these infants exerts a dilution effect on the AF bilirubin concentration and, importantly, ΔOD_{450} analysis is superfluous for these infants because they are clearly severely affected by HDN. From the data provided in the study, and after excluding the hydropic fetuses, the sensitivity for predicting severe HDN increased to 94% when using zone IIB or greater as the cutoff with no decrease in the specificity (Table 4).

Similarly, fetal blood sampling was also recommended by the authors of a 10-year retrospective study of 111 pregnancies that compared the last ΔOD_{450} result to the first neonatal hemoglobin concentration *(45)*. They reported excellent neonatal outcome when results were in zones I or IIA but that one death and seven cases of neonatal morbidity were the direct result of clinical action based on false-positive information obtained from results falling into zones IIB or III. The lack of absolute correlation between ΔOD_{450} and neonatal hemoglobin results prompted the conclusion that the ΔOD_{450} could at best be regarded as an indirect evaluation of fetal anemia and that fetal blood sampling should be considered when ΔOD_{450} values fall in zones IIB or III *(45)*.

In recent years, the use of Doppler ultrasonography to measure blood flow through the middle cerebral artery has been investigated as a noninvasive method that could potentially replace amniocentesis in the assessment of fetal anemia *(17)*. Although the data supporting its use are encouraging, additional studies are required before its use is widely adopted *(10)*. Because this approach may one day be used as the principal diagnostic test in the assessment of HDN, Sikkel et al. revisited the use of the ΔOD_{450} and the extrapolated Liley chart in the second and third trimesters to predict severe fetal anemia *(46)*. The study utilized data from AF and fetal blood specimens that had been analyzed at a single center over a 13-yr period. Samples were included if they were collected from RhD-sensitized singleton pregnancies with nonhydropic fetuses that had not been transfused and if AF specimens had been collected less than 4 d before fetal blood sampling. Samples from 79 fetuses collected between 20 and 35 wk gestation met the inclusion criteria. Of these, one was unaffected (hemoglobin concentration within the reference range), 11 had moderate anemia (hemoglobin concentration between 2 and 5 SD below the reference range), and 67 had severe anemia (hemoglobin concentration >5 SD below the reference range). Overall, the extrapolated Liley chart correctly identified 97% (65 of 67) of severely anemic fetuses from unaffected or moderately affected ones when using ΔOD_{450} results that fell within or above the upper third of zone II (zone IIC) (Table 4) *(46)*. Similar sensitivities were obtained at gestational ages of 20 to 27 wk (95%) and 27 to 35 wk (98%). A high number of false-positive results were observed at the same cutoffs that produced low specificities (Table 4). One unaffected fetus and eight moderately anemic fetuses were in or above zone IIC (specificity, 25%) and although the specificity for fetuses at less than 27 wk gestation increased to 60%, it fell to 0% when fetuses at greater than or equal to 27 wk were examined *(46)*. The authors concluded that the high sensitivity of the ΔOD_{450} allowed it to remain a useful diagnostic test, despite the specificity, especially in light of the comparative risk of fetal loss between amniocentesis (0.25–1%) and the gold standard method for diagnosing fetal anemia, fetal blood sampling (1–3%) *(46)*.

Table 4
Studies Investigating the Clinical Performance of the ΔOD_{450} in the Prediction of Fetal Anemia

Reference	n	Cutoff	Outcome measured	Gestational age range (wk)	Sensitivity (%)	Specificity (%)	PPV (%)	NPV (%)	Accuracy (%)
Nicolaides et al. (44)	59	≥ Liley zone IIB	Fetal hemoglobin	18–25	84	43	62	71	64
	45[a]	≥ Liley zone IIB	Fetal hemoglobin	18–25	94	43	50	92	62
Ananth and Queenan (59)	41	≥ 0.09 ΔOD_{450}	Fetal outcome	16–20	100	37	65	100	71
Sikkel et al. (46)	79	≥ Liley zone IIC	Fetal hemoglobin	20–35	97	25	88	60	86
	24	≥ Liley zone IIC	Fetal hemoglobin	< 27	95	60	90	75	88
	55	≥ Liley zone IIC	Fetal hemoglobin	≥ 27	98	0	87	0	85
Scott and Chan (52)	72	Queenan's intrauterine death risk zone	Fetal hemoglobin	16–38	100	79	22	100	81

NVP, negative predictive value; PPV, positive predictive value.
[a]Hydropic fetuses excluded.

Chloroform Extraction

The ΔOD_{450} is subject to various sources of analytical error. Several of these, including the use of AF contaminated with blood, were addressed by Liley himself (41). While the presence of oxyhemoglobin can alter the spectrophotometric analysis at 450 nm and lead to incorrect interpretations, this interference can be removed by chloroform extraction of AF. Using this approach, equal volumes of chloroform and AF are combined, shaken for 30 s, and then centrifuged for 5 min (47). Theoretically, any bilirubin present in the AF will be extracted into the chloroform layer, which is then subjected to scanning spectrophotometry using a chloroform blank.

A study that utilized AF specimens contaminated with exogenous bilirubin demonstrated that all of the bilirubin was successfully extracted by chloroform and that the ΔOD_{450} values from these specimens were the same as those obtained from unextracted samples (47). The same was true when these specimens were also contaminated with exogenously added maternal red blood cells. However, in 52% (11 of 21) of visibly bloody AF specimens obtained by amniocentesis, chloroform extraction resulted in a significant change (defined as a variation >0.01 nm at 450 nm) in ΔOD_{450} results when compared to unextracted aliquots (the ΔOD_{450} was decreased in eight and increased in three specimens). When pre- and postextraction ΔOD_{450} results were plotted on a Liley chart, there were major zone changes in 55% (6 of 11) of these bloody specimens (two higher and four lower), all of which were correctly correlated with clinical outcome (47). The reason that chloroform extraction produced variable results was not discussed, but the authors did recommend chloroform extraction on all AF specimens that produce absorbance peaks between 410 and 420 nm—wavelengths at which oxyhemoglobin demonstrates maximum absorbance.

In a separate study, chloroform extraction was also shown to produce variable ΔOD_{450} values from AF specimens with both endogenous and exogenous bilirubin sources *(48)*. For specimens with exogenously added bilirubin, postextraction ΔOD_{450} results were lower than those obtained from unextracted specimens in 83% (10 of 12) of specimens. This included specimens that were also adulterated with exogenously added hemoglobin. Similarly, ΔOD_{450} results were lower in 90% (9 of 10) of specimens that did not contain exogenous bilirubin. The authors reported that during the chloroform extraction procedure a precipitate often formed within the organic layer, and they hypothesized that this material trapped some of the bilirubin, thereby producing ΔOD_{450} values that were lower than baseline *(48)*.

Spinnato et al. also utilized the extrapolated Liley chart and reported accurate predictions of fetal status when AF specimens were chloroform extracted *(49)*. Like other reports utilizing chloroform extraction, the procedure resulted in a significant decrease in the mean ΔOD_{450} in 90% (93 of 103) of specimens when compared to unextracted values (0.086 vs 0.108, $p < 0.05$) *(49)*. Patient management was based on the chloroform-extracted ΔOD_{450} values. Although the authors reported that no patients were categorized inaccurately ($n = 28$ patients with known clinical outcomes data), one of only five fetuses that underwent blood sampling because of ΔOD_{450} values in zone III or the upper third of zone II had a normal hematocrit. Trend analysis performed on seven patients correctly revealed a reassuring (downward) trend in all cases. The authors suggested that the use of chloroform extraction in AF bilirubin analysis permitted accurate assessment of fetal status, and they argued that its use avoids unnecessary fetal blood sampling *(49)*.

Several studies have reported a significant decrease in ΔOD_{450} results following extraction of AF specimens (including those without visible blood contamination) with chloroform. Therefore, if individual laboratories wish to utilize this method for the removal of heme pigments, then it would seem pertinent to perform the extraction on all specimens rather than reserving this treatment for those contaminated with blood.

The Queenan Chart

In 1993, Queenan et al. reported an alternative to the extrapolated Liley chart for the clinical management of Rh-immunized pregnancies *(50)*. They established a reference AF ΔOD_{450} pattern using 682 specimens collected between 14 and 40 wk gestation from 464 Rh-immunized women who delivered unaffected Rh-negative fetuses and 56 women who underwent amniocentesis for genetic purposes and were without blood group incompatibilities. When ΔOD_{450} results were plotted on a linear scale relative to gestational age, ΔOD_{450} values showed a slight increasing trend from 14 to 22 wk, leveled off until 24 wk, and then declined to term (Fig. 5). ΔOD_{450} results were also obtained from 107 AF specimens collected between 14 and 40 wk gestation from 74 Rh-immunized women who delivered Rh-positive infants. The clinical outcomes of these pregnancies were used to categorize the fetuses as either affected with HDN but surviving or affected with HDN but with the potential for fetal death (likely or actual). The authors then developed their own chart with zones demarcated by the ΔOD_{450} data from pregnancies unaffected and affected by HDN (Fig. 6). The lowest zone, the "unaffected" zone, was established as the area below the mean ΔOD_{450} for the unaffected population. Fetuses within this zone were either unaffected or had mild HDN. The authors recommended that one additional amniocentesis be performed as clinically indicated on infants who fall in this zone to ensure that the ΔOD_{450} stayed within that zone and indicated that a term delivery was

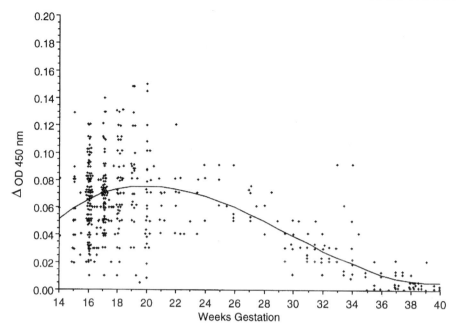

Fig. 5. AF ΔOD_{450} values from pregnancies unaffected by HDN plotted from 14 to 40 wk gestation. Mean values are shown as a polynomial fitted regression line. (Reprinted from rcf. *50*.)

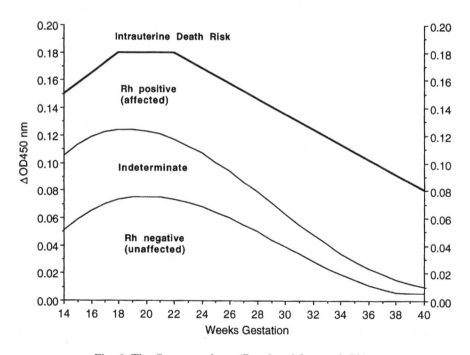

Fig. 6. The Queenan chart. (Reprinted from ref. *50*.)

appropriate *(50)*. The highest zone was defined from potentially fatal cases of HDN and was labeled the "intrauterine death risk" zone. Most fetuses in this zone were born alive because of intrauterine transfusion therapy although some did die from severe HDN. Clinical management of fetuses within this zone (or with serially obtained results that suggested that this zone would be entered) included intrauterine transfusion and/or early delivery *(50)*. Between these two extreme zones was an area that included many fetuses representing all possible clinical outcomes (unaffected to severe HDN) although the fetuses in this zone were not in immediate danger of intrauterine death. The authors divided this area in half by creating a zone of +2 SD above the mean ΔOD_{450} for the unaffected population and labeled it the "indeterminate" zone. They noted that 50% of the unaffected fetuses were in this zone but that it also included some mildly and moderately affected fetuses, all of which survived. It was recommended that fetuses in this zone be monitored by ΔOD_{450} analysis every 2 to 4 wk *(50)*. The last zone is the area between the indeterminate and the death risk zones and was labeled the "Rh-positive, affected" zone. This zone rarely included unaffected fetuses and those affected fetuses survived when appropriately managed. The authors recommended serial AF ΔOD_{450} measurements every 1 to 2 wk for these fetuses *(50)*.

When the performance of the Queenan chart was compared to that of the Liley chart, the authors noted that the while the Queenan chart correctly categorized all 18 fetuses with potentially fatal HDN, 15 of these fell into Liley's zone III and 3 fell into zone II *(50)*. No additional comparisons with the Liley chart were reported. The excellent performance of the Queenan chart in this study is not surprising considering that it was constructed from the same population that it then used to evaluate clinical management.

A direct comparison between the Queenan and Liley charts has been reported by two different groups of investigators. Consistent with their previous recommendation regarding the use of chloroform, Spinnato et al. compared the accuracy of both charts using 231 chloroform-extracted AF specimens collected from 73 alloimmunized pregnancies between 20 and 39 wk gestation *(51)*. When the ΔOD_{450} results were plotted on both charts, the Queenan chart generated more false positive results than the extrapolated Liley chart. Overall, the Queenan chart significantly overestimated risk in 19% (13 of 67) of fetuses compared to the 10% (7 of 67) estimated by the Liley chart ($p = 0.031$) *(51)*. Similarly, the Queenan chart also overestimated fetal risk when used at or before 28 wk gestation (20 vs 8%, $p = 0.031$, $n = 49$) *(51)*. Fetal blood sampling or transfusions were required in 16% (12 of 73) of patients and both charts performed equivalently on 10 of these occasions, although only the Liley chart was used for clinical management. Underestimations of fetal risk were not significantly different between the two charts, leading the investigators to conclude that the performance of the extrapolated Liley chart was superior to that of the Queenan chart because it did not overestimate fetal risk as frequently *(51)*.

The other study compared the clinical usefulness of both charts by examining ΔOD_{450} results from 72 amniocenteses, half of which were performed before 27 wk gestation *(52)*. AF specimens were labeled with fetal condition at the time of collection. All specimens from infants found to be RhD-negative were labeled unaffected. Specimens from RhD-positive babies were labeled affected and the severity of HDN was defined by the hemoglobin concentration determined at birth or from a fetal blood sample. Infants with a hemoglobin deficit less than 2 g/dL were considered mildly affected, moderately affected fetuses were those with a deficit of 2 to 7 g/dL, and those with a deficit greater than 7 g/dL were considered to be severely affected. There were instances (n = not reported) where fetuses received intrauterine transfusions, yet no pretransfusion hemoglobin concentration was available. The authors labeled these fetuses as moderately affected if hydrops was not present, despite this apparent subjective approach being a potential source of bias. Similarly, the clinical status of those fetuses for which hemoglobin concentrations were not available within a week of amniocentesis (n = not reported) was determined using criteria that lacked accuracy. ΔOD_{450} results were labeled mildly affected if they were obtained from AF specimens that had been collected more than 1 wk before a fetus was found to be moderately affected or more than 2 wk before a fetus was found to be severely affected. Similarly, specimens obtained 8 to 13 d before the fetus was found to have severe HDN were labeled moderately affected (52).

ΔOD_{450} results from unaffected fetuses were scattered over Liley zones I and II and Queenan's lower three zones, whereas mildly affected fetuses were scattered over all zones on both charts. Six percent (4 of 72) of fetuses were severely affected and all received transfusions before 25 wk gestation. All of these ΔOD_{450} results fell in Queenan's intrauterine death risk zone but the authors' use of Liley's original chart and not an extrapolated one prevented a direct comparison of the two charts. Also in Queenan's intrauterine death risk zone were 11 moderately affected fetuses and 3 mildly affected ones. Therefore, although Queenan's chart correctly identified all severely affected fetuses (sensitivity, 100%), it produced a specificity of 79% (54 of 68) (Table 4) (52). The authors commented that the usefulness of the Liley chart is now limited given the technological advances made in perinatal medicine since the chart's inception. Like Spinnato et al. the authors acknowledged that the Queenan chart, with its lower cutoff levels, is more conservative than the Liley chart and may overestimate fetal risk. Still, they considered the use of the Queenan chart as an appropriate tool to manage alloimmunized pregnancies in the second and third trimesters (52).

The Ovenstone Factor

A standardized approach to the ΔOD_{450} was proposed in 1968 by Ovenstone and Connon (53). Rather than plotting the optical density of AF against wavelength, the authors plotted the derivative of the fluid's spectral curve. The primary analytical advantage of this method was the minimization of variation in the ΔOD_{450} from differences among spectrophotometers and within specimens themselves. For example, the presence of heme pigments can introduce significant error into ΔOD_{450} measurements. Central to their approach is the fact that at 490 nm, the slope of the bilirubin absorbance curve is at its maximum decrease, whereas other pigments that may be present in AF demonstrate relatively small changes in optical density. In contrast, the rate of optical density increase for bilirubin at 430 nm is slight compared to the large decreasing rates for the heme pigments (Fig. 7). Therefore, the rate of change in optical density with respect to wavelength is capable of revealing the presence or absence of pigments (bilirubin) within a sample even when they might otherwise be influenced by other factors (heme pigments). When the derivatives of the slope of the AF spectral curve are plotted against wavelength, two distinct peaks are revealed from specimens that contained both bilirubin and blood (Fig. 8).

Connon reported that the Ovenstone factor (OF) was easily calculated by subtracting the optical density of AF at 500 nm from the optical density at 480 nm and multiplying

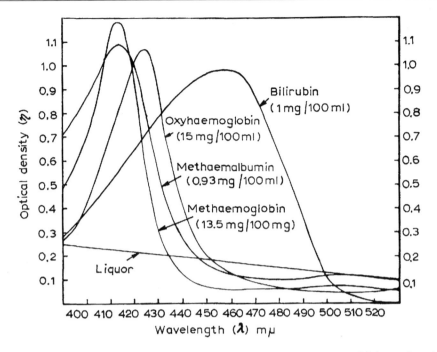

Fig. 7. Optical densities of "pure" AF, bilirubin, oxyhemoglobin, methemoglobin, and methemal-bumin. (Reprinted from ref. *53*)

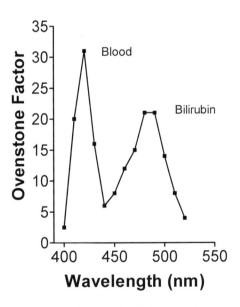

Fig. 8. A plot of the first derivative of the optical densities between a bloody amniotic fluid specimen containing bilirubin between 400 and 540 nm. The peak of the curve at 490 nm (21 in this example) is the Ovenstone factor caused by the presence of bilirubin. (Adapted from ref. *54*.)

Table 5
Correlation of the Ovenstone Factor and Its Interpretation
With Specific Zones of the Liley Chart

Ovenstone factor	Ovenstone interpretation	Liley zone
0–10	Unaffected/Mild	I
10–20	Mild/Moderate	IIA
20–30	Moderate/Severe	IIB
30–40	Severe	IIIA
> 40	Very severe	IIIB

the product by 230 [OF = 230 × (OD 480 – OD 500)][1] *(54)*. Also reported were five different OF cutoffs that were correlated to the five grades of HDN severity on the Liley chart (Table 5). To investigate the performance of the Liley chart and the OF in predicting HDN severity, AF specimens from 106 Rh-sensitized pregnancies were evaluated by both methods and compared to fetal outcome. Infants were classified as unaffected (Rh-negative) or affected with HDN, and disease severity was evaluated according to the degree of anemia and jaundice, the number of transfusions received, or the occurrence of death. For each of the two prediction methods, results were considered accurate if the prediction and outcome were identical. Results were considered equivocal if there was one grade difference in either direction and were called inaccurate when there were two or more grades of difference. The OF correctly predicted fetal outcome in 72% (76 of 106) of infants compared to 47% (50 of 106) by the Liley chart *(54)*. There were also fewer incorrect predictions according to the OF than by the Liley chart (3% vs 15%). Similar results were observed when the 20 infants found at birth to be Rh-negative were excluded from the analysis. There were no incorrect predictions by the OF in these unaffected infants compared to the 30% incorrectly predicted by the Liley chart. The author concluded that the OF offers clear advantages over the Liley chart for predicting outcome and points out that, unlike the Liley chart, the OF can be interpreted without regard to gestational age *(54)*.

Another study that investigated the use of the OF and the Liley chart reached similar conclusions *(55)*. This study included 324 AF specimens collected between 18 and 40 wk gestation from 90 Rh-sensitized pregnancies. The authors found that an OF of 30 or more at any time during gestation indicated a very poor outcome, as did a greater than 10 OF unit increase obtained from serially collected samples *(55)*. The OF correctly predicted 10 babies as significantly affected that were called unaffected by the Liley chart. Specimens from three infants affected by HDN gave negative results for both the OF and the Liley chart. Although the Liley chart produced more false-negative results, the authors recommended that both analyses be performed and interpreted together rather than relying on a single method.

The superior performance of the OF in predicting HDN severity was also reported in a study of 78 AF specimens collected from 46 patients between 24 and 40 wk *(56)*. Using a scheme similar to that of Connon *(54)* for correlating prediction to infant outcome, the

---

[1] This formula is corrected from the one originally published by Connon as 2.30 × (OD 480 – OD 500).

OF correctly predicted outcome more often than did the Liley chart (80 vs 67%) and produced fewer inaccurate predictions (7 vs 13%) *(56)*. The OF also performed better than the Liley chart when only Rh-negative infants were considered (93 vs 71% correct). Like Connon, the authors concluded that the higher accuracy of the OF made its use preferable to that of the Liley chart.

A more recent study suggested that OF interference from heme pigments is possible. When the OF was calculated from spectrophotometric data obtained from AF specimens with exogenously added bilirubin and hemoglobin, positive interference in the OF was observed (range: 35–119% compared to baseline specimens without added hemoglobin) *(48)*.

Summary

The use of the Liley chart for predicting the severity of HDN in the third trimester is effective and it remains in widespread use. Advances in maternal–fetal medicine, however, have prompted the use of the Liley chart with zones linearly extrapolated backward into the second trimester. The clinical utility of this modified Liley chart is clearly controversial and there is published evidence that both supports and discourages its use. It should be recognized that the use of serial amniocentesis to identify trends in the ΔOD_{450} are more informative than single determinations. The efforts by Queenan et al. to develop a method for the clinical management of HDN in the second and third trimesters were helpful, especially their data regarding second-trimester ΔOD_{450} results in pregnancies unaffected by HDN. Almost all the published data regarding the use of Liley's and Queenan's charts were obtained from relatively small numbers of patients in retrospective analyses. A large prospective study of both methods is required to effectively determine the efficacy of these prediction methods. It is difficult to imagine how such a study could be conducted considering the low incidence of HDN. The lack of published data after 1977 regarding the utility of the OF is curious. Other investigators confirmed initial reports demonstrating its enhanced performance over the Liley chart, yet its use has never gathered widespread attention.

Despite the availability of fetal blood sampling as the gold-standard method for diagnosing fetal anemia, determining the ΔOD_{450} remains a valuable diagnostic test in the management of alloimmunized pregnancies. This is in part because of the higher fetal loss rate associated with fetal blood sampling techniques and the risk of fetomaternal hemorrhage and subsequent exacerbation of HDN caused by a maternal anamnestic immune response. The use of ultrasonography in predicting HDN has been (and continues to be) explored. As a completely noninvasive technique, this approach has obvious advantages, but until additional data are available, it is unlikely to replace the ΔOD_{450}.

CONCLUSIONS

Despite a substantial reduction in its incidence, hemolytic disease of the newborn continues to be a clinical problem. The successful management of pregnancies complicated by red blood cell alloimmunization involves a multidisciplinary approach that includes an evaluation of obstetrical history, careful and frequent clinical assessment of the fetus, and the appropriate utilization of laboratory tests.

Laboratory testing is involved in the entire spectrum of HDN. Serological techniques such as the IAT are used to identify maternal alloantibodies associated with the disease, whereas titration and quantitation have been used to predict severity or, in the United

States, to determine when to initiate invasive methods of fetal monitoring. Overall, serological methods perform poorly as predictors of severity, which is not surprising because antibody concentration is only one variable involved in the pathogenesis of HDN.

As tests that quantitate interactions between sensitized erythrocytes and effector cells, functional assays would be expected to be better predictors of severity. Among the ones discussed here, the ADCC and CL assays have the highest accuracies, yet all available functional tests produce potentially misleading results, especially when fetuses are mildly to moderately affected. It has been recommended that the use of functional assays be limited to those pregnancies that have antibody concentrations above a given threshold and that these tests be performed by reference laboratories (1). Because none of these types of tests are 100% predictive, it is difficult to see how they can be used to safely manage sensitized pregnancies without the need for performing invasive tests to assess the extent of fetal anemia.

The spectrophotometric analysis of AF and the determination of the ΔOD_{450} are widely used in the assessment of fetal anemia, and different methods for interpreting the value have been described. Irrespective of the approach adopted by a laboratory, the trend of ΔOD_{450} values obtained from serial amniocenteses should be emphasized rather than reliance on a single result.

It is important to realize that HDN is not managed solely on the basis of test results. Although laboratory data can be of great benefit to the physician who encounters HDN, it provides insight into only part of what is a much broader picture of a rarely encountered fetal condition.

REFERENCES

1. Hadley AG. A comparison of in vitro tests for predicting the severity of haemolytic disease of the fetus and newborn. Vox Sang 1998;74(suppl 2):375–383.
2. Urbaniak SJ, Greiss MA. RhD haemolytic disease of the fetus and the newborn. Blood Rev 2000;14(1):44–61.
3. Kliegman RM, Stoll BJ. Blood disorders. In: Behrman RE, Kliegman RM, Jenson HB, eds. Nelson Textbook of Pediatrics. Philadelphia: W.B. Saunders, 2000, pp. 520–527.
4. Luban NL. Hemolytic disease of the newborn: progenitor cells and late effects. N Engl J Med 1998;338(12):830–831.
5. Hadley AG. In vitro assays to predict the severity of hemolytic disease of the newborn. Transfus Med Rev 1995;9:302–313.
6. ACOG Educational Bulletin. Management of isoimmunization in pregnancy. Int J Gynecol Obstet 1996;55:183–190.
7. Chavez GF, Mulinare J, Edmonds LD. Epidemiology of Rh hemolytic disease of the newborn in the United States. JAMA 1991;265(24):3270–3274.
8. Ortho Clinical Diagnostics. Rho(D) Immune Globulin (Human) RhoGAM, Package Insert. 2001. Raritan, NJ: Ortho Clinical Diagnostics.
9. Bennett PR, Le Van KC, Colin Y, et al. Prenatal determination of fetal RhD type by DNA amplification. N Engl J Med 1993;329(9):607–610.
10. Oepkes D. Invasive versus non-invasive testing in red-cell alloimmunized pregnancies. Eur J Obstet Gynecol Reprod Biol 2000;92(1):83–89.
11. Harman CR. Percutaneous fetal blood sampling. In: Creasy RK, Resnik R, eds. Maternal–fetal Medicine. Philadelphia: W.B. Saunders, 1999, pp. 341–363.
11a. Forestier F, Daffos F, Catherine N, et al. Developmental hematopoiesis in normal human fetal blood. Blood 1991,77:2360–2362.
12. Engelfriet CP, Reesink HW, Arbolla L, et al. What is the best technique for the detection of red cell antibodies? Vox Sang 1995;69:292–300.
13. Contreras M, Garner SF, de Silva M. Prenatal testing to predict the severity of hemolytic disease of the fetus and newborn. Curr Opin Hematol 1996;3(6):480–484.

14. Technical Manual of the American Association of Blood Banks, 14th ed. Bethesda: American Association of Blood Banks, 2002.

15. Gall SA, Miller JM Jr. Rh isoimmunization: a 24 year experience at Duke University Medical Center. Am J Obstet Gynecol 1981;140(8):902–908.

16. Judd WJ, Luban NL, Ness PM, Silberstein LE, Stroup M, Widmann FK. Prenatal and perinatal immunohematology: recommendations for serologic management of the fetus, newborn infant, and obstetric patient. Transfusion 1990;30(2):175–183.

17. Moise KJ, Jr., Perkins JT, Sosler SD, et al. The predictive value of maternal serum testing for detection of fetal anemia in red blood cell alloimmunization. Am J Obstet Gynecol 1995;172(3):1003–1009.

18. Moore BP. Automation in the blood transfusion laboratory. I. Antibody dectection and quantitation in the technicon autoanalyzer. Can Med Assoc J 1969;100(8):381–387.

19. Nicolaides KH, Rodeck CH. Maternal serum anti-D antibody concentration and assessment of rhesus isoimmunisation. Br Med J 1992;304(6835):1155–1156.

20. Bowell P, Wainscoat JS, Peto TE, Gunson HH. Maternal anti-D concentrations and outcome in rhesus haemolytic disease of the newborn. Br Med J (Clin Res Ed) 1982;285(6338):327–329.

21. Buggins AG, Thilaganathan B, Hambley H, Nicolaides KH. Predicting the severity of rhesus alloimmunization: monocyte-mediated chemiluminescence versus maternal anti-D antibody estimation. Br J Haematol 1994;88(1):199–200.

22. Engelfriet CP, Ouwehand WH. ADCC and other cellular bioassays for predicting the clinical significance of red cell alloantibodies. Baillieres Clin Haematol 1990;3(2):321–337.

23. Urbaniak SJ, Greiss MA, Crawford RJ, Fergusson MJ. Prediction of the outcome of rhesus haemolytic disease of the newborn: additional information using an ADCC assay. Vox Sang 1984;46(5):323–329.

24. Hadley AG, Kumpel BM, Leader KA, Poole GD, Fraser ID. Correlation of serological, quantitative and cell-mediated functional assays of maternal alloantibodies with the severity of haemolytic disease of the newborn. Br J Haematol 1991;77(2):221–228.

25. Garner SF, Wiener E, Contreras M, et al. Mononuclear phagocyte assays, autoanalyzer quantitation and IgG subclasses of maternal anti-RhD in the prediction of the severity of haemolytic disease in the fetus before 32 weeks gestation. Br J Haematol 1992;80(1):97–101.

26. Hadley AG, Garner SF, Taverner JM. AutoAnalyzer quantification, monocyte-mediated cytotoxicity and chemiluminescence assays for predicting the severity of haemolytic disease of the newborn. Transfus Med 1993;3:195–200.

27. Garner SF, Gorick BD, Lai WY, et al. Prediction of the severity of haemolytic disease of the newborn: quantitative IgG anti-D subclass determinations explain the correlation with functional assay results. Vox Sang 1995;68(3):169–176.

28. Oepkes D, van Kamp IL, Simon MJ, Mesman J, Overbeeke MA, Kanhai HH. Clinical value of an antibody-dependent cell-mediated cytotoxicity assay in the management of Rh D alloimmunization. Am J Obstet Gynecol 2001;184(5):1015–1020.

29. Nance SJ, Nelson JM, Horenstein J, Arndt PA, Platt LD, Garratty G. Monocyte monolayer assay: an efficient noninvasive technique for predicting the severity of hemolytic disease of the newborn. Am J Clin Pathol 1989;92(1):89–92.

30. Zupanska B, Brojer E, Richards Y, Lenkiewicz B, Seyfried H, Howell P. Serological and immunological characteristics of maternal anti-Rh(D) antibodies in predicting the severity of haemolytic disease of the newborn. Vox Sang 1989;56(4):247–253.

31. Sacks DA, Nance SJ, Garratty G, Petrucha RA, Horenstein J, Fotheringham N. Monocyte monolayer assay as a predictor of severity of hemolytic disease of the fetus and newborn. Am J Perinatol 1993;10(6):428–431.

32. Lucas GF, Hadley AG, Nance SJ, Garratty G. Predicting hemolytic disease of the newborn: a comparison of the monocyte monolayer assay and the chemiluminescence test. Transfusion 1993;33:484–487.

33. Hadley AG, Kumpel BM, Merry AH. The chemiluminescent response of human monocytes to red cells sensitized with monoclonal anti-Rh(D) antibodies. Clin Lab Haematol 1988;10(4):377–384.

34. Filbey D, Garner SF, Hadley AG, Shepard SL. Quantitative and functional assessment of anti-RhD: a comparative study of non-invasive methods in antenatal prediction of Rh hemolytic disease. Acta Obstet Gynecol Scand 1996;75(2):102–107.

35. Engelfriet CP, Reesink HW. Laboratory procedures for the prediction of the severity of haemolytic disease of the newborn. Vox Sang 1995;69(1):61–69.

36. Benzie RJ, Doran TA, Harkins JL, Owen VM, Porter CJ. Composition of the amniotic fluid and maternal serum in pregnancy. Am J Obstet Gynecol 1974;119(6):798–810.

37. Rosenthal P, Blanckaert N, Kabra PM, Thaler MM. Liquid-chromatographic determination of bilirubin and its conjugates in rat serum and human amniotic fluid. Clin Chem 1981;27(10):1704–1707.
38. The Merck Manual of Diagnosis and Therapy. 17th ed. Whitehouse Station, NJ: Merck, 1999.
39. Ashwood ER. Clinical chemistry of pregnancy. In: Burtis CA, Ashwood ER, eds. Tietz Textbook of Clinical Chemistry. Philadelphia: W.B. Saunders, 1999, pp. 1736–1775.
40. Liley AW. Liquor amnii analysis in the management of the pregnancy complicated by rhesus sensitization. Am J Obstet Gynecol 1963;82:1359–1370.
41. Liley AW. Errors in the assessment of hemolytic disease from amniotic fluid. Am J Obstet Gynecol 1963;86:485–494.
42. Queenan JT. Current management of the Rh-sensitized patient. Clin Obstet Gynecol 1982;25(2):293–301.
43. MacKenzie IZ, Bowell PJ, Castle BM, Selinger M, Ferguson JF. Serial fetal blood sampling for the management of pregnancies complicated by severe rhesus (D) isoimmunization. Br J Obstet Gynaecol 1988;95(8):753–758.
44. Nicolaides KH, Rodeck CH, Mibashan RS, Kemp JR. Have Liley charts outlived their usefulness? Am J Obstet Gynecol 1986;155(1):90–94.
45. Steyn DW, Pattinson RC, Odendaal HJ. Amniocentesis: still important in the management of severe rhesus incompatibility. S Afr Med J 1992;82(5):321–324.
46. Sikkel E, Vandenbussche FP, Oepkes D, Meerman RH, Le Cessie S, Kanhai HH. Amniotic fluid delta OD 450 values accurately predict severe fetal anemia in D-alloimmunization. Obstet Gynecol 2002;100(1):51–57.
47. Hochberg CJ, Witheiler AP, Cook H. Accurate amniotic fluid bilirubin analysis from the "bloody tap:" a preliminary report. Am J Obstet Gynecol 1976;126(5):531–534.
48. Foster K, Hankins K, Gronowski AM. The effect of blood contamination on delta 450 bilirubin measurement: a comparison of different corrective methods. 2003. Unpublished work.
49. Spinnato JA, Ralston KK, Greenwell ER, Marcell CA, Spinnato JA III. Amniotic fluid bilirubin and fetal hemolytic disease. Am J Obstet Gynecol 1991;165(4 Pt1):1030–1035.
50. Queenan JT, Tomai TP, Ural SH, King JC. Deviation in amniotic fluid optical density at a wavelength of 450 nm in Rh-immunized pregnancies from 14 to 40 weeks' gestation: a proposal for clinical management. Am J Obstet Gynecol 1993;168(5):1370–1376.
51. Spinnato JA, Clark AL, Ralston KK, Greenwell ER, Goldsmith LJ. Hemolytic disease of the fetus: a comparison of the Queenan and extended Liley methods. Obstet Gynecol 1998;92(3):441–445.
52. Scott F, Chan FY. Assessment of the clinical usefulness of the "Queenan" chart versus the "Liley" chart in predicting severity of rhesus iso-immunization. Prenat Diagn 1998;18(11):1143–1148.
53. Ovenstone JA, Connon AF. Optical density differencing: a new method for the direct measurement of bilirubin in liquor amnii. Clin Chim Acta 1968;20:397–406.
54. Connon AF. Improved accuracy of prediction of severity of hemolytic disease of the newborn. Obstet Gynecol 1969;33:72–78.
55. Amstey MS, Hochberg CJ, Choate JW, Wax SH, Lund CJ. Comparative analysis of amniotic fluid bilirubin. Obstet Gynecol 1972;39:407–410.
56. Moore GI, Hochberg CJ. Ovenstone factor in the management of Rh sensitization. South Med J 1977;70:1093–1095.
57. Gottvall T, Hilden JO, Selbing A. Evaluation of standard parameters to predict exchange transfusions in the erythroblastotic newborn. Acta Obstet Gynecol Scand 1994;73(4):300–306.
58. Hadley AG, Wilkes A, Goodrick J, Penman D, Soothill P, Lucas G. The ability of the chemiluminescence test to predict clinical outcome and the necessity for amniocenteses in pregnancies at risk of haemolytic disease of the newborn. Br J Obstet Gynaecol 1998;105(2):231–234.
59. Ananth U, Queenan JT. Does midtrimester delta OD450 of amniotic fluid reflect severity of Rh disease? Am J Obstet Gynecol 1989;161(1):47–49.
60. Moise KJ Jr. Management of rhesus alloimmunization in pregnancy. Obstet Gynecol 2002;100(3):600–611.

12 Prenatal Screening and Diagnosis of Congenital Infections

Lynn Bry, MD, PhD

INTRODUCTION

Infections acquired prior to or during pregnancy can profoundly impact fetal and postnatal development. Most infections acquired during pregnancy affect the maternal upper respiratory or gastrointestinal tract, and resolve without adverse impact on the mother or fetus. Of concern are infections with pathogens that enter the circulation and have the capacity to actively or passively traverse the placenta to infect the fetus. *In utero*, these infections may have teratogenic effects or otherwise adversely impact fetal development.

Screening for congenital infections has the following aims: (1) assess maternal immunity to a specific pathogen, and (2) detect the presence of an active or underlying infection for diseases with potentially severe sequelae for the fetus or adversely impacting maternal health. Follow-up testing may then be performed to specifically diagnose infection in the mother or fetus.

The World Health Organization has provided the following guidelines for instituting population-based screening programs *(1)*:

1. The target condition should be common, or a serious though less common problem.
2. Screening should be able to lead to a clear diagnosis in the majority of cases.
3. The natural history of the condition should be well enough understood to permit prediction of outcomes.
4. There should be an effective and acceptable management strategy (treatment and/or prevention).
5. The program should be cost effective.

Routine screening of pregnant women for underlying infectious diseases or immunity is consistently performed to identify (1) chronic carriers of hepatitis B virus, (2) human immunodeficiency virus (HIV) infection, (3) group B streptococcal colonization, (4) immu-

From: *Current Clinical Pathology: Handbook of Clinical Laboratory Testing During Pregnancy*
Edited by: A. M. Gronowski © Humana Press, Totowa, NJ

nity to rubella virus, and (5) syphilis. In addition, women receive purified protein derivative (PPD) placement for detection of tuberculosis. The American Association of Obstetricians and Gynecologists and other organizations in the United States and abroad recommend that all pregnant women receive testing for these agents.

Though originally described as "TORCHES" for <u>to</u>xoplasmosis, <u>r</u>ubella, <u>c</u>ytomegalovirus (CMV), <u>her</u>pes virus, and <u>s</u>yphilis, screening for agents such as toxoplasmosis, CMV, herpes simplex virus (HSV), and others including *Chlamydia trachomatis*, gonorrhea, and hepatitis C is more commonly targeted toward high-risk groups, or women from high prevalence areas. In these situations, the screening serves to identify women with underlying infection, or sero-negative women, who may be vaccinated or more specifically counseled to limit risks of exposure.

Other agents, including enteroviruses *(2)* and spirochetal infections other than syphilis *(3,4)* can rarely cause congenital infection, but are not discussed in this chapter. The impact of other infectious agents including West Nile virus *(5)* and bunyaviruses *(6)* on development of congenital infection in women infected during pregnancy remain to be determined.

Sensitivity, Specificity of Screening Tests, and Prevalence of Disease

No test perfectly distinguishes all disease-free individuals from those with a given condition. The limitations of the testing technologies and the diversity of human populations and pathogenic organisms lead to the inevitable situation that some individuals with a particular disease will not give a positive result when tested, while some disease-free individuals will test positive even though they do not have the disease. Table 1 defines positive and negative predictive values relative to prevalence within a population, as well as calculations for determining the ratio of individuals likely to give positive or negative results for a test with a given sensitivity and specificity. Each concept may be defined succinctly as:

- Sensitivity: ability to predict disease
- Specificity: ability to predict health
- Positive predictive value (PPV): likelihood that a positive test means that the patient has the disease
- Negative predictive value (NPV): likelihood that a negative test means the patient does not have the disease

The predictive values of test results are thus directly related to the prevalence of the disease in the population tested. Mittendorf *et al.* have written an excellent review concerning impact of test sensitivity, specificity, and disease prevalence on screening of maternal infections that provides additional in-depth discussion of the topic *(7)*.

Test sensitivity and specificity may also be defined on the basis of analytical and biological factors. Analytic specificity refers to the lack of reaction with other components in the assay besides the analyte under investigation, whereas analytical sensitivity refers to the lowest concentration of the analyte that can be reliably detected over background. In contrast, biological sensitivity refers to the lowest biological concentration, or point in a disease process, at which a test can report clinically useful results. Biological specificity refers to the ability of a test to reliably diagnose a specific condition.

Diagnosis of a disease is thus ideally based on multiple factors including subjective components of a patient's history and physical exam and objective markers that include laboratory test results. This combination of factors results in defining the prevalence of

Table 1
Calculations for Determining Predictive Values of Testing Relative
to Disease Prevalence in a Population

Value	Calculation
True Positives (TP)	$= \text{Prevalence} \times \text{Sensitivity}$
True Negatives (TN)	$= (1 - \text{Prevalence}) \times \text{Specificity}$
False Positives (FP)	$= (1 - \text{Prevalence}) \times (1 - \text{Specificity})$
False Negatives (FN)	$= \text{Prevalence} \times (1 - \text{Sensitivity})$
Positive Predictive Value (PPV)	$= \dfrac{\text{Prevalence} \times \text{Sensitivity}}{(\text{Prevalence} \times \text{Sensitivity}) + [(1 - \text{Prevalence}) \times (1 - \text{Specificity})]}$ $= \dfrac{\text{TP}}{\text{TP} + \text{FP}}$
Negative Predictive Value (NPV)	$= \dfrac{(1 - \text{Prevalence}) \times \text{Specificity}}{[(1 - \text{Prevalence}) \times \text{Specificity}] + [\text{Prevalence} \times (1 - \text{Sensitivity})]}$ $= \dfrac{\text{TN}}{\text{TN} + \text{FN}}$

a disease in a given population. Prevalence of each disease in individual populations greatly impacts the utility of implementing screening measures in pregnant women from particular geographic regions. An understanding of the impact of disease prevalence on the PPVs and NPVs of tests proves critical when interpreting results that could have profound impact on further maternal and fetal care.

Figure 1 calculates the PPVs and NPVs of a hypothetical test for toxoplasmosis in three populations with different sero-prevalences. The hypothetical test has a sensitivity of 98%: 98 out of every 100 people with the disease will test positive, whereas two positive individuals will test negative; and a specificity of 99%: 99 out of every 100 negative individuals tested will return a negative result, whereas one truly negative person will give a falsely positive result.

Although the PPV and NPV of this test remain above 95% in high-prevalence populations, as encountered in France and other parts of western Europe, the PPV in a low prevalence population is poor and drops even further in populations with disease prevalences less than 1.0%. Thus, even a test with good sensitivity and specificity has low PPV in populations with low disease prevalence. For this reason, screening tests used in low-prevalence populations should have high sensitivity and should always be followed with further confirmatory testing with high specificity to provide a high PPV associated with the results. Given the impact of positive results in maternal screening, further testing procedures, including confirmatory testing and ultrasound, are warranted to fully determine the extent of disease and potential impact on the fetus before making clinical decisions or undertaking invasive procedures.

LABORATORY METHODS

Maternal–fetal testing for infectious diseases employs a variety of laboratory methods. An understanding of the assay techniques and their limitations can help with the selection of tests for particular situations and with the interpretation of results.

Impact of disease prevalence on predictive values of testing.

Example: Toxoplasmosis IgG assay with sensitivity = 98%, specificity = 99%, applied to a population of 10,000.

Prevalence:	1%	10%	60%
Disease Positive:	100	1,000	6,000
Disease Negative:	9,900	9,000	4,000

True Positives = Prevalence X Sensitvity X 10,000

	= 0.01 X .98 X 10,000	= 0.1 X .98 X 10,000	= 0.6 X .98 X 10,000
	= 98	= 980	= 5880

True Negatives = (1-Prevalence) X Specificity X 10,000

	= 0.99 X 0.99 X 10,000	= 0.9 X 0.99 X 10,000	= 0.4 X 0.99 X 10,000
	= 9,801	= 8,910	= 3,960

False Positives = (1- Prevalence) X (1-Specificity) X 10,000

	= 0.99 X 0.01 X 10,000	= 0.9 X 0.01 X 10,000	= 0.4 X 0.01 X 10,000
	= 99	= 90	= 40

False Negatives = (Prevalence) X (1-Sensitivity) X 10,000

	= 0.01 X 0.02 X 10,000	= 0.1 X 0.02X 10,000	= 0.6 X 0.02 X 10,000
	= 2	= 20	= 120

PPV = TP / (TP + FP) X 100

	= 98 / (98+99) X 100	= 980 / (980+90) X 100	= 5880 / (5880+40) X 100
	= 49.75%	= 91.59%	= 99.32%

NPV = TN / (TN + FN) X 100

	= 9,801 / (9,801 + 2) X 100	= 8,910 / (8,910+20) X 100	= 3,960 / (3,960+120) X 100
	= 99.97%	= 99.78%	=98.51%

Fig. 1. Calculations that illustrate the effect of prevalence on the positive and negative predictive value of a test.

Serological Testing

Serologies measure the host's antibody response. Tests commonly assay pathogen-specific serum immunoglobulin G (IgG) or immunoglobulin M (IgM) as a means for determining immune status to a particular pathogen or assisting with the diagnosis of a primary infection. Interpreting the results of serological testing requires an understanding of the evolving humoral immune response during primary infection and during secondary challenge or reactivation.

Primary infections have a window period during which time the pathogen is present in the body, but the host has not yet mounted a specific, adaptive immune response. This period may last from days to weeks after initial exposure. Reactive B cells first produce IgM, a pentameric immunoglobulin with low affinity but high avidity for the antigen. Further stimulation of antigen-specific B cells leads to isotype switching to other heavy-chain classes such as IgG, the primary isotype found in blood, and immunoglobulin A (IgA), the primary isotype found in mucosal secretions. Reactive IgM thus appears earliest during a primary infection. Over the subsequent weeks, IgM concentrations commonly peak and fall, to be replaced by rising titers of serum IgG. Somatic hypermutation and gene conversion that occur during subsequent class switching events can improve the affinity of individual antibodies from clonal B cell populations, resulting in increased avidity of the total population of reactive antibodies with the infectious agent *(8,9)*.

The timing of testing is critical for measuring the antibody response to infection. Fourfold increases in IgG titers from acute and convalescent samples collected 14–21 d apart indicate recent infection or reactivation. However, the time needed for these analyses makes them unacceptable for rapid diagnosis. Comparison of IgG and IgM titers can assist with the identification of primary infection but must be used with caution, given the decreased specificity of many IgM assays. When screening or testing for congenital infection *in utero* or in the neonate, maternal immune status must be considered when interpreting results, as maternally transferred IgG commonly persists in the infant for 6–18 mo after birth.

A variety of patient, disease, and laboratory factors impact the presence of false-positive and false-negative results. Laboratory errors in labeling of specimens, sample preparation, and performance of assays can also impact the results obtained. False-negative serologic results commonly occur in the early stages of disease when the infected person has not yet developed an antibody response, or in individuals with underlying defects in antibody production. Of importance to testing for infectious disease is the fact that severely immunocompromised women, particularly HIV-positive women with chronically low CD4+ T-cell counts, may fail to mount robust antibody responses during infection. In such cases, direct assay for potential pathogens, using culture or molecular methods, should be considered to obtain a diagnosis.

Conversely, false-positive results may occur when an individual has antibody that reacts with components of the assay aside from the antigen, or if the antigen used cross-reacts with antibodies against epitopes on other pathogens. Rheumatologic or underlying infectious diseases may produce falsely positive results with cross-reactive antibodies or excessively high total Ig concentrations that impact the formation of detectable antigen/antibody complexes. Significant derangements in total Ig concentration will also adversely impact results of serological testing because they skew the antibody to antigen ratio in the assay.

METHODOLOGIES

A variety of techniques are employed to assay antibody titers against specific pathogens. Older methods using complement fixation or hemagglutination assays have largely been replaced by enzyme immunoassays and solution-based agglutination assays. These two latter formats have been adopted to permit testing on high throughput analyzers used in many clinical laboratories.

IMMUNOASSAY

The immunoassay format commonly uses a capture antigen to bind reactive antibody from patient samples. After washing, a secondary anti-human immunoglobulin specific for human IgG, IgM, or other isotype allows detection of the bound Patient Ig. Secondary reagents are commonly conjugated to fluorescent tags (fluorescent immunoassay [FIA]), radioisotopes (radioimmunoassay [RIA]), or an enzyme with readily detected biochemical amplification signal (enzyme immunoassay [EIA]). Immobilization of the capture antigen on 96-well plates forms the basis for many enzyme-linked immunosorbent assays

(ELISAs) that may be manual or semi- or fully automated. Commercial assays also commonly include reagents to selectively remove rheumatoid factor or serum IgG from patient serum to improve the specificity of the tests for IgM and other isotypes. Automated plate readers determine mean fluorescence intensity or optical density for colorimetric enzymatic reactions to determine quantity of captured antibody. Dilutions of the patient sera allow quantitative titering of reactive antibody species. Results may be correlated with known standards to provide a concentration per mL. More commonly, laboratories report values in ELISA units (EU)/mL that correlate with optical density or fluorescence readings. Laboratories may validate manufacturers' recommended cutoffs to determine positive, negative, or indeterminate results, or assign specific cutoff values to obtain particular sensitivities and specificities for assays.

The source of the capture antigen impacts the specificity of many assays used in infectious disease testing. First-generation assays commonly use crude preparations of the organism or cell lysates from viral cultures. These assays often have lower specificities because they may detect antibody directed against the cell or media in which the pathogens were cultured. As understanding of the disease progresses, including the identification of immunodominant epitopes shared by all or most pathogenic strains, assays improve by using purified, recombinant, or synthetic antigens. Purified recombinant antigens may be more sensitive and specific for detecting reactive antibody than synthetic antigens, which may not fold properly and bind nonspecifically with reactive antibody in patient samples, or may lack a potentially immunodominant epitope that is present in the native molecule.

Variations of the typical "sandwich ELISA" include competitive inhibition EIAs where patient antibody is added to a solution containing labeled antibody with specificity for the antigen analyzed. Reactive patient antibody from the patient sample competes with the labeled antibody for binding sites. Increased binding from the patient sample reduces detection of the label and can be correlated with a concentration or titer. Many competitive EIAs have been developed for testing on random-access, high-throughput analyzers, allowing more rapid and high volume testing.

Methods specifically used for IgM detection include double-sandwich and immunosorbent agglutination assays (ISAGA). Both methods have higher specificities than routine EIAs because they allow for purification of IgM, or removal of IgG, from patient sera to limit false-positive results caused by rheumatoid factor or high concentrations of IgG. The double-sandwich assay uses an IgM capture antibody to bind human IgM. Added antigen then binds reactive, captured antibody. Detection is provided by a labeled secondary antibody that recognizes bound antigen. The ISAGA captures IgM onto a solid substrate and then assess agglutination after addition of particulate material containing reactive antigen. The assay is used in many countries for identifying toxoplasmosis-specific IgM that reacts with heat or formalin-fixed parasites to promote agglutination.

INDIRECT IMMUNOFLUORESCENCE (IFA)

Titered patient serum may be applied to prepared slides of the organism or virally infected cell lines. Bound antibody is then detected with a fluorescently conjugated secondary immunoglobulin, and the pattern of binding is determined by analyzing the slides by fluorescence microscopy. IFA assays are more time consuming and require expensive equipment, compared with EIA and other formats. Furthermore, patients with anti-DNA antibodies may give false-positive results for many assays.

AGGLUTINATION ASSAYS

Agglutination assays commonly use latex particles coated with purified antigen. Addition of patient sera may agglutinate the beads directly, or agglutination may be detected after addition of an antihuman Ig that promotes cross-linking among beads with antibody–antigen complexes. The limitations of agglutination assay follow those for EIAs, including antigen source and purity, and Ig concentration in patient samples.

WESTERN BLOTS/IMMUNOBLOTS

Western blots/immunoblots detect antibody that reacts with defined protein antigens. Antigen samples are subjected to polyacrylamide gel electrophoresis (PAGE) to separate proteins based on size and charge, depending on the conditions used. The proteins are then transferred to a membrane and probed with patient sera. Antibodies bind transferred proteins and may subsequently be detected with tagged antihuman immunoglobulin reagents. The end result produces a discrete band on the membrane or on autoradiograph film with fluorescent amplification or radioisotopes. Because the procedure is time consuming and highly labor intensive, it is not routinely used for screening purposes or to titer patient sera.

Interpretation of the blots may be hindered by the integrity and purity of the antigens, following appropriate blocking and washing procedures during incubation of the membranes, and the skill of the individuals performing and interpreting the blots. Many commercial confirmatory western blot assays for hepatitis C, Lyme disease, and HIV provide pretransferred membranes that have undergone stringent quality control measures to limit errors that may be made during electrophoresis and transfer.

AVIDITY ASSAYS

Avidity assays are gaining acceptance for use in clinical testing under particular circumstances. Avidity is defined as the overall binding strength of a given population of antibodies, as opposed to affinity, which defines the binding strength between an antigen and antibody. The technique associates an avid, or mature and strongly binding, Ig response with past infections, whereas recent infections have less avid responses that are more easily dissociated with denaturation agents. Modifications of standard sandwich ELISAs assay the avidity of IgG for antigen. After primary incubation of patient sample with the capture reagents, methods incubate samples in 6–8M urea to disrupt weakly bound IgG. Ratios of treated to untreated wells generate an aviditiy index (AI) with cutoffs to indicate strong or weak IgG avidity. Infection in the previous 3–5 mo commonly results in a low AI, whereas a high AI indicates infection prior to that time period. The method has an advantage in that recent versus past infection can potentially be determined with a single patient sample. However, the accuracy of the test is very much operator dependent and subject to significant fluctuation in values if the incubation, denaturation, and washing steps are not followed appropriately. In-house assays may also be limited by the extent of validation used to define cutoffs and by use of cutoffs defined for one disease entity to define results for another.

DIPSTICK/IMMUNOCHROMATOGRAPHIC LATERAL FLOW ASSAYS

Lateral flow assays have provided many highly sensitive and specific rapid diagnostic tests for infectious diseases that may be performed in a clinical laboratory or ambulatory setting or at home.

The assays use an Ig binding protein, commonly protein A, conjugated to a dye or other readily detected compound. A loop provided with the assay kit is used to transfer a small amount of patient blood, serum, or saliva to a solution containing the reagent. The mixed solution flows through a nitrocellulose membrane encased in a dipstick by capillary action. Areas of the membrane are impregnated with purified antigen (test band) or with a control reagent (control band) that reacts with added patient sample. If the patient has antibody that reacts with the antigen, the antibody-protein A-dye conjugates bind to the antigen on the dipstick, producing a visible test band. The same happens for the control band. Presence of the control band indicates only a negative result, whereas presence of both the control and test band are interpreted as positive. Bands appearing outside of the specified areas or appearance of test bands, with no control bands, are reported as indeterminate results and require further testing *(10)*.

Antigen Assays

Antigen assays commonly detect protein or carbohydrate epitopes specific for the infecting agent by using a capture reagent, frequently a monoclonal antibody with known specificity for the antigen. Sensitivity of these assays may be limited by the affinity of the capture reagent for the antigen and by the frequency at which pathogenic strains express the antigen. Assay factors impacting the specificity of the testing include the purity of the capture reagent and uniqueness of the antigen for the particular pathogen of interest.

Nucleic Acid Detection

Direct testing for DNA or RNA produced by a pathogen has revolutionized testing for infectious agents. As opposed to serological methods, nucleic acid appears well before the generation of the antibody response and often before the onset of symptomatic illness.

In addition to polymerase chain reaction (PCR), other amplification schemes including ligase chain reaction (LCR), transcription-mediated amplification (TMA), nucleic acid sequence-based amplification, and branched-DNA detection (B-DNA) have been developed to detect low quantities of organisms present in patient samples. Amplification of a particular nucleic acid target is generally more sensitive than methods such as strand displacement or direct hybridization that probe without an amplification step. Most amplified assays attain high specificity by having sequence-specific primers that amplify a unique sequence that is subsequently confirmed as originating from the target by a variety of techniques, including restriction fragment digestion of amplified products, internal amplification of target sequences with a separate primer set, or hybridization with one or more tagged molecular beacon probes that permit fluorescent detection of the target. Furthermore, it is critical that laboratories run appropriate positive and negative controls. Positive controls are necessary to assess whether the amplification reaction was successful given the potential for inhibitors to be present in patient samples. Negative controls ensure that common buffers and materials used in preparing reactions have not been contaminated with amplified products from other samples. The checklist from the College of American Pathologists (CAP) for molecular pathology provides detailed guidelines concerning performance of molecular assays for patient testing *(11)*.

Culture Methods

Prior to the advent of molecular testing in infectious disease, culture methods remained the gold standard for diagnosing many bacterial and viral infections. In many cases, culture still plays a vital role for providing a specific diagnosis. Bacterial culture in particular includes the benefit of providing antibiotic susceptibility data for common pathogens.

BACTERIAL CULTURE

Samples from specific anatomical locations are commonly plated on selective and nonselective solid media and/or broth to enrich for growth of pathogens. Subsequent biochemical and susceptibility tests help speciate organisms and determine their susceptibility to antibiotics. Most common bacterial pathogens, culturable under routine conditions, can be identified within 24–72 h.

VIRAL CULTURE

Viral culture is performed by culturing patient material with cell lines that support the growth of the viruses of interest. Detection of some viruses may be improved by centrifuging the patient sample onto plated cell lines, as is performed with shell vial cultures for CMV, or through direct detection of virally induced reporter genes in genetically modified cell lines *(12)*. Appropriate samples include body fluids, tissue samples, and swabs of vesicular fluid or ulcerated lesions. Because many viruses are temperature labile and sensitive to drying, samples should be placed in viral transport media and transported to the laboratory within a reasonable time frame. Swabs used to collect samples for culture should have Dacron or rayon tips and plastic or metal shafts because compounds in wood or treated cotton may be toxic to cell lines and inhibit the growth of any virus.

Staining Methods

HISTOCHEMICAL STAINS

Stains can be rapidly performed and have good sensitivity and specificity if performed and interpreted by trained personnel. Although more than 100 yr old, the Gram stain remains the initial decision point in the routine identification and speciation of most bacterial pathogens. Direct staining of amniotic fluid (AF) may occasionally assist in identifying bacterial causes of chorioamnionitis, and the stain permits detection of protozoal parasites if present. Wright-Giemsa staining of peripheral blood smears forms the basis for diagnosing blood-borne infections including malaria and trypanosomiases. However, detection is limited by the pathogen burden in the patient sample, the volume subjected to staining, and the expertise of the individuals performing and interpreting the slides.

IMMUNOFLUORESCENCE

Fluorescent dyes or antibodies against specific infectious agents are used in many situations to identify pathogens in body fluids or tissues, or to confirm positive viral cultures. Interpretation requires a fluorescent microscope with appropriate objectives and filters, and interpretation by qualified personnel.

ELECTRON MICROSCOPY

In the past, electron microscopy (EM) provided a common means of diagnosing congenitally acquired viral infections by analyzing viral morphology from AF or tissues. EM still plays a role in identifying pathogens for which few other diagnostic modalities exist or in identifying newly emerging pathogens for which tests have not yet been developed. However, the time-consuming nature of EM, expensive equipment required, and extensive expertise needed to prepare, process, and interpret samples limit its use in most settings for routine diagnosis of infectious diseases.

Pathological Tissue Analysis

Gross and microscopic analysis of placenta, fetal, or neonatal samples can assist with diagnosis of infections contracted *in utero*. Histological staining of placenta, in particular, can be instrumental in identifying protozoal and viral pathogens.

INFECTIONS

Viral Infections

Cytomegalovirus

Cytomegalovirus (CMV) is a double-stranded herpesvirus and a common viral cause of congenital infection. The virus may be transmitted by oral and respiratory secretions, breast milk, blood transfusion, sexual contact, and vertically. Primary infection produces nonspecific symptoms of heterophile-negative mononucleosis in young adults, including fatigue and malaise, athough many individuals and older adults manifest no overt symptoms. As with other herpesviruses, CMV establishes latent infection after primary disease and can be reactivated during pregnancy and with immunosuppression *(13)*.

Rates of sero-positivity increase with age but do so more rapidly in urban areas and developing countries *(14)*. The sero-prevalence in industrialized countries approaches 25% in young adults, but 80% or more in urban areas and in many developing countries. In the United States, 2% of sero-negative women acquire primary CMV infection during pregnancy. Most of these women demonstrate no signs of infection, although 40% of primary maternal infections result in vertical transmission to the fetus. Maternal immunity to CMV lowers the rate of vertical transmission significantly among different populations, resulting in congenital infection in 0.4–1.9% of pregnancies *(15,16)*.

Of congenital infections resulting in live births, 7–10% of these infants have discernable defects or indications of congenital infection while the remainder appear normal at birth. Vertical transmission during the first half of pregnancy is thought to produce worse outcomes including low birth weight, hepatitis, deafness, microcephaly, and other findings *(16,17)*. Many studies have also indicated that maternal immune status cannot necessarily predict the presence or absence of congenital defects once infection has occurred in the fetus. Among congenitally infected infants with no signs or symptoms at birth, 85–95% develop normally, but the remainder develop adverse sequelae in infancy and childhood including hearing and vision loss, and other neurological deficits *(16,18)*.

Screening. Routine serological screening for CMV immune status is not recommended except for women with high risk of exposure, including health care and child-care workers and HIV-positive women. Baseline serologies serve to identify sero-negative individuals and allow specific education of these women concerning exposure risks and measures for limiting risks for infection.

Immune status can be determined with CMV IgG serology. Available commercial assays include EIA kits produced by Diamedix, Wampole Laboratories, Abbott Laboratories, BioMérieux, and Diagnostic Products Corporation. Assays have sensitivities of 91–99% and specificities of 93–100% *(19)*.

Maternal Diagnosis. Diagnosis of primary maternal infection commonly uses IgG and IgM serologies to ascertain the evolving immune response to CMV infection. A fourfold increase in IgG titers from paired acute and convalescent sera, drawn 14–21 d apart, indicates either primary infection or reactivation. IgM serologies are frequently employed to distinguish primary infection from reactivation or reinfection. However, maternal serologies cannot predict the likelihood of *in utero* infection. Likewise, although PCR, CMV pp65 antigenemia, and viral load assays can assist in diagnosis of CMV-related disease in transplant, HIV-positive, and other immunocompromised women, their use in immunocompetent pregnant women cannot predict or detect vertical transmission of the virus to the fetus.

Fetal Diagnosis. PCR or CMV culture on AF can be used to detect fetal infection after 21 wk gestation. Sensitivity of PCR detection prior to 21 wk has been reported to be 45% with specificity of 100% *(20)*. Other assays have reported sensitivities of 80–100% and specificities of 100% when using CMV-specific primers with internal confirmation of amplified sequences on samples obtained after 21 wk gestation *(21,22)*. In contrast, viral culture has reported sensitivity of 50–70% and specificity of 100% with most culture and confirmation systems *(23,24)*. Small numbers of case reports have described use of serial viral load determinations in AF to predict presence of fetal infection and fetal disease *(25,26)*. Although promising, further studies are warranted to determine the predictive values of serial testing and defined viral load cutoffs that can predict disease and outcomes.

Neonatal Diagnosis. Diagnosis of congenital infection in the neonate commonly uses shell vial viral culture on human fibroblast lines or PCR performed on urine or saliva. Samples collected for viral culture should be stored at 4°C until transported to the laboratory. Culture from neonatal urine or saliva has reported sensitivity of 94–95% and specificity of 100% *(27)*. PCR amplification strategies have sensitivities and specificities approaching 100% in congenitally infected infants *(28)*.

HEPATITIS B

Hepatitis B is a double-stranded DNA hepadnavirus. Transmission occurs through exposure to blood and body fluids, and less commonly via sexual contact or congenital infection. Countries with successful vaccination programs for hepatitis B have prevalences of 0.6% or less in the general population *(29,30)*. Worldwide, the highest prevalence of infection occurs in sub-Saharan Africa, parts of South America, southeast Asia, and in certain populations such as the Inuit and Australian aborigines, where documented infections may occur in more than 40% of the population, with chronic carriage present in 7–10% of adults *(31,32)*.

The prevalence of hepatitis B infection among pregnant women in North America and Europe ranges from 0.6 to 0.9% but has been reported to be 5.79% among some Asian populations *(33)*. Vertical transmission occurs in more than 90% of chronically infected women and in 60% of women acquiring primary infection during pregnancy *(34)*. Conflicting reports have indicated no association, or potential association, of maternal infection with stillbirths, prematurity, or congenital defects *(34,35)*, although more recent reports suggest no association between maternal infection and adverse perinatal outcomes *(36)*. Higher rates of vertical transmission have been found in Taiwan and other regions in Asia than in other parts of the world, suggesting that differences in viral strains or genetic makeup of infected populations may predispose to *in utero* infection. However, congenital infection clearly predisposes to chronic carriage of hepatitis B virus and early development of liver cirrhosis and hepatocellular carcinoma *(37,38)*.

Table 2
Interpretation of Test Results for Hepatitis B

HBs Ag	HBe Ag	Anti-HBsAg	Anti-HBc	HBV-DNA	Interpretation
−	−	+	−	−	Consistent with prior vaccination for hepatitis B
−	−	−	−	+	Very early infection. Repeat testing in patient.
±	±	−	−	+	Early infection
+	+	−	±	+	Consistent with symptomatic primary infection
+	−	+	+	−	Consistent with recent infection
−	−	+	+	−	Past infection
+	±	+	+	+	Chronic infection

Adapted from refs. *39,51,54.*

Table 2 describes typical profiles seen for hepatitis B antigens and serologies for primary and chronic infection. Symptoms of primary maternal infection may appear 5 wk to 6 mo after initial exposure and include malaise, fatigue, jaundice, and sometimes urticaria, other rashes, and arthritis, and less commonly with symptoms of glomerulone-phritis and vasculitis. Sensitive assays detect hepatitis B surface antigen (HBsAg) and viral DNA (HBV-DNA) 1–11 wk postexposure. The hepatitis B early antigen (HbeAg) commonly appears within days of HBsAg and persists through symptomatic disease. Individuals developing acute disease usually manifest symptoms within 4 weeks of detection of HBsAg. Symptoms last for 1–2 wk, after which HBsAg and HbeAg fall in individuals clearing the infection. Early IgM responses develop against core antigen (anti-HBc) 8–12 wk postexposure and may persist for several months to 1 yr. Specific IgG against HBc appears earliest at 12 wk postexposure, with specific IgG against HBe and HBsAg arising over the next 2 mo, as individuals resolve disease and clear the virus. Individuals resolving the virus clear it from the blood within weeks of the first appearance of symptoms *(39)*.

Subclinical disease is most commonly detected with anti-HBc antibody in the face of other negative serological or antigen tests. Many individuals manifest either transient or absent HBsAg. Chronic carriers of hepatitis B virus represent up to 10% of all infected individuals and are diagnosed by the presence of persistently positive HBsAg and viral DNA in blood.

Screening. Routine screening commonly uses HBsAg to identify newly infected or chronic carriers of the virus. Abbott Laboratories, Roche Diagnostics, Murex, Diasorin, Diagnostic Products Corporation, and Ortho-Clinical Diagnostics produce commercial kits for measuring HBsAg. Sensitivites of these assays range from 96 to 100% and have specificities of 97.6–100% in most populations *(40,41)*. Highly sensitive HBsAg assays detect tens of pg/mL amounts of the antigen, which has a half-life of 1–2 wk in serum *(42)*. Detection of primary infection can thus potentially be determined for a few months after resolution of symptomatic disease in individuals clearing the virus.

HBsAg is a viral coat protein that contains five major epitopes, including the immunodominant "a" epitope that forms the basis of detection for many commercial assays, as well as surface antigen vaccines *(43–45)*. Three overlapping reading frames in the virus produce the glycoproteins S1, S2, and S, all of which contain the "S" segment. Prior to 1990, the majority of characterized strains contained the HBsAg a epitope. However, pre-S mutant strains of hepatitis B, particularly ones with the G->A mutation at nucleotide 587 that substitutes an arginine for glycine at position 145, lack this immunodominant epitope and may not be detected by assays for HBsAg *(46,47)*. Presence of pre-S mutations capable of infecting vaccinated individuals has also raised issues concerning the long-term use of current vaccines for hepatitis B *(46,48)*. In some areas of North America, Asia, and Europe, these strains may comprise 10–40% of isolates infecting patients *(46,49)*. If suspected, detection of HBc antibody should be used to screen with follow-up measurement of hepatitis B DNA levels. This testing should also be performed if acute or underlying infection is suspected in individuals negative for HBsAg and markers for other hepatitis viruses.

Diagnosis. Women testing positive for HBsAg require further diagnostic evaluation. Full serologies, including HBc and surface IgG and IgM, HbeAg, and viral DNA load should be performed. Table 2 lists common diagnostic patterns for HBsAg, HbeAg, HBV-DNA, and serologies against HBsAg. Vaccinated women should have anti-HBsAg antibody but no reactivity with HBc or other viral components. Of available assays for hepatitis B virus, viral load of hepatitis B DNA has become the best predictor of infectivity *(50)*, particularly for women near delivery *(51)*. Other studies have indicated that HBV-DNA, HBsAg load, and HbeAg can predict potential for vertical transmission *(52,53)*.

Neonatal Diagnosis. Diagnosis in the neonate and infant is best made with detection of HBsAg *(54)* or detection of HBV-DNA in blood *(55–57)*. HBsAg does not cross the placenta, although HbeAg does, limiting its use in diagnosing congenital infection *(58)*. Likewise, serological detection of IgG against HBc, HbsAG, or HBe primarily measures transferred maternal immunity.

Hepatitis C

The hepatitis C virus (HCV) is a single-stranded RNA picornavirus belonging to the flaviviridae. Infection occurs through intravenous drug abuse, blood transfusions from infected donors, exposure to infected body fluids, and, more rarely, sexual contact. The prevalence of disease in the general population has been estimated at 1–4% *(59,60)*, and prevalences in pregnant women from western countries and Africa at 1.9% *(61)*, although higher prevalences of 3.5–5% have been found in patients attending sexually transmitted diseases (STD) clinics *(62)*.

The virus has an average window period of 6–8 wk prior to detectable sero-conversion, although this period may be extended to several months or a year in immunocompromised patients. Many individuals manifest no overt symptoms other than chronic fatigue. Approximately 80% of infected individuals become chronic carriers of HCV and are at risk of developing liver cirrhosis.

Vertical transmission has been associated with primary infection during pregnancy *(63)*. Transmission rates in HIV-negative, HCV-positive women have been estimated at 2.7–4.4% *(64)*, with rates increasing to 5.4–8.6% in HCV-positive women coinfected with HIV *(65)*.

Screening. Routine screening for HCV is indicated for HIV-positive women or women with risk factors such as intravenous drug abuse or multiple blood transfusions prior to 1990. However, clinical suspicion of underlying infection may be raised with elevated alanine aminotransferase or aspartate aminotransferase if these results are encountered during prenatal testing.

Third-generation ELISAs for detecting HCV IgG have improved specificity by detecting antibody against recombinant HCV antigens followed by recombinant immunoblot assay (RIBA) confirmation to determine reactivity with the nonstructural proteins NS3, NS4, and NS5 and viral core proteins (66). Analytic sensitivities of anti-HCV IgG ELISAs ranged from 98.8 to 100%, and specificities from 99.7 to 100% for commercially based assays including Roche's automated Cobas Core anti-HCV EIA and semi-automated Murex or Abbott anti-HCV EIAs (67). Other studies have demonstrated biological specificities among commercial kits to be 99% or more when assayed against healthy blood donors and known HCV-positive individuals (68).

Diagnosis. As described, positive serologies require confirmation by RIBA. Standard of care also indicates obtaining HCV viral load and performing viral genotyping to assess the susceptibility of the infecting strains to interferon (IFN)-α therapy. However, the efficacy of IFN-α therapy in HCV-positive pregnant women and its impact on the fetus have not been widely studied. Demand for rapid, sensitive tests to detect blood donors in the window period prior to sero-conversion has led to significant developments for nucleic acid-based testing for HCV and HCV core antigen tests that stand to allow earlier detection of viral infection than serological methods (69).

Neonatal Diagnosis. Detection of HCV RNA in the neonate provides the best means of diagnosing congenital infection (70,71). Rare HCV-infected infants may test negative within the first month, suggesting repeat testing of negative infants for HCV RNA from 2–10 mo of age in infants born to HCV-positive women (72).

Human Immunodeficiency Virus

Human immunodeficiency virus (HIV)-1 and -2 are single-stranded RNA retroviruses that have infected more than 30 million people worldwide. Since 1998, more than 3.7 million children have been infected with HIV, the majority by vertical transmission, and 2.7 million have died of acquired immunedeficiency syndrome (AIDS). In developing countries, congenital infection can account for up to 10% of all AIDS cases.

The ACTG 076 clinical trial first demonstrated the efficacy of antiretroviral therapy in preventing vertical transmission. Oral zidovudine (AZT) during weeks 14–34 of gestation followed by intravenous AZT during labor and delivery reduced the rate of *in utero* transmission by 67%, to 8.3% of infants born to HIV-positive women (73). Subsequent studies have endeavored to assess the impact of other antepartum regimens (e.g., AZT/3TC) and intrapartum therapies [e.g., single-dose maternal nevirapine followed by neonatal nevirapine within 72 h (74)] on vertical transmission to develop treatment protocols more suitable for implementation in developing countries (75).

Screening and Diagnosis. The Centers for Disease Control and Prevention, and American Medical Association, and other organizations have strongly encouraged routine screening for HIV in pregnant women because of the ability to reduce vertical transmission of the virus with appropriate intervention (76,77). Screening remains voluntary with informed patient right of refusal, because concerns have been raised of deterring women from seeking prenatal care if testing for HIV were mandatory. Selection of screening tests may vary with the situation, namely, in an ambulatory setting as opposed to more emergent situations involving women with no prenatal care.

Screening for anti-HIV IgG followed by confirmatory western blot or IFA remains the standard for diagnosis. Molecular tests should not be used to make an initial diagnosis, particularly in low-prevalence populations where the positive predictive values of such tests are poor *(78)*. Many commercial EIAs and ELISA kits are available for testing blood specimens for common subtypes of HIV-1 and HIV-2. A number of kits also exist for testing saliva specimens. Commercial EIAs for HIV-1 or HIV-1 and -2IgG commonly have sensitivities greater than 99% and specificities of 99.6%. Even with such high specificity, all positive tests should be confirmed because of the adverse impact of falsely positive results including social stigmata and unnecessary exposure of the fetus to antiretrovirals.

In selecting testing methodologies, the clinical setting must be considered. Ideally, all women should be tested at their initial prenatal care visit. Antiretroviral therapy initiated early in pregnancy has the greatest effect in preventing vertical transmission. Unfortunately, many HIV-infected women are among those receiving no or inadequate prenatal care. However, recent studies have shown that intrapartum antiretroviral therapies can reduce the transmission of HIV by up to 50%. In the setting of a woman presenting in labor and without prenatal care, rapid HIV testing should be considered. Many rapid-HIV kits have been introduced commercially over the past 10 years. In the United States, the OraQuick Rapid HIV-1 (Ora-Sure Technologies) test has recently been cleared by the Food and Frug Administration (FDA) as a Clinical Laboratory Improvement Act (CLIA)-waived test, which can be performed in many point-of-care locations *(10)*. The assay may be performed on whole blood from venipuncture or finger stick and takes about 20 min to obtain results. The test has a sensitivity of 99.6% and specificity of 100% when compared with standard EIAs. Subsequent to delivery, confirmation of results by Western blot or IFA must be obtained, as with other screening tests.

HIV-2 and some rare subtypes of HIV-1, such as Group O, may not be detected by many commercial EIA or ELISA kits *(79)*. In women with significant exposure to these subtypes [e.g., sexual contact with individuals from high-prevalence areas such as West-Central Africa *(80)*], tests with the ability to detect the rare subtypes should be selected *(81,82)*. Currently available western blots assay the host antibody response against polypeptides from the env and gag proteins. The CDC criteria for interpreting blots as positive calls for definitive banding patterns against the viral proteins p24, gp46, and gp120 or gp60. Reactive patterns that do not meet these criteria are reported as indeterminant *(83)*. As the majority of HIV-positive individuals with indeterminant results convert within 1 mo, testing should be repeated within this time frame *(84)*. However, this option is of limited utility in emergent situations. Pregnant women presenting emergently in whom indeterminant results occur with rapid serological or western blot assays should receive further testing with HIV p24 antigen or viral load assay, using a methodology other than B-DNA for detection, with the understanding that confirmatory testing will need to be performed to validate results obtained by these measures.

Fetal Diagnosis. Due to the risk of transmitting HIV and other potential infectious agents to the fetus, many groups advocate refraining from performing amniocentesis or other invasive procedures in pregnant HIV-positive women unless absolutely indicated *(85)*.

Neonatal Diagnosis. Detection of HIV viral load in the neonate provides the best means for diagnosing vertical transmission. Initial testing performed within 48 h of birth diagnoses 25–30% of congenitally infected neonates *(86)*. Subsequent viral load testing should be performed within 2 wk, and at 1, 2, and 6 mo of age. Single positive viral load results should be repeated and confirmed with a different assay and detection method on a new patient sample. This regimen has 100% sensitivity for diagnosing infected infants by 6 mo of age *(87)*. Additional confirmation of the HIV-negative status in these infants includes documenting the loss of maternally transferred anti-HIV IgG through 18 mo of age *(86)*.

Additional Testing Indicated in Pregnant, HIV-Positive Women. HIV infection has significant impact on maternal health and the risk of transmitting of other infectious agents to the fetus, including CMV, syphilis, and toxoplasmosis. Additional studies should be undertaken to assist with (1) the clinical assessment of maternal immune status, (2) response to antiretroviral therapy, (3) presence of underlying sexually transmitted diseases, and (4) immunity to additional pathogens. Table 3 lists recommended testing to follow these factors in pregnant HIV-positive women.

Measurement of plasma viral loads are recommended every 4 wk until virus has been suppressed to undetectable concentrations or the desired treatment goals have been attained, after which they may be performed every 3 mo, or as indicated, to monitor response to therapy. CD4+ T cell counts performed every 3–4 mo serve as an independent monitor of the patient's immune status and responses to antiretroviral therapy *(88)*. As with nonpregnant patients, chronically infected women with severely suppressed CD4+ T cell counts, may not elevate their counts greatly between readings in response to significant decreases in viral load.

HIV genotyping to identify resistance to AZT, nevirapine, or other drugs used in treatment regimens should be performed if infection with resistant strains or development of resistance is suspected. Viral genotyping assays have clearly matured to a state where they can reliably detect and predict resistance for more common characterized mutations such as the K103N mutation in viral reverse transcriptase that confers resistance to nevirapine *(89,90)*. Results are best obtained on patient samples with plasma HIV viral loads greater than 1000 copies/mL *(91)*. Commercially available assays that perform double-strand sequencing of patient virus and allow analysis against the most updated and validated HIV genotype databases provide the most reliable results. Testing should also be performed in laboratories with experience in performing DNA sequencing and that subscribe to proficiency testing in this area offered by the CAP. Interpretation of less-common mutations and their impact on viral resistance should be done in consultation with individuals having expertise in the performance and interpretation of genotyping assays.

Many laboratories use the Visible Genetics Trugene or Applied Biosystems ViroSeq HIV-1 genotyping kits that have been approved by the FDA. Although published studies indicated concordance of 92–99.7% among academic centers for detecting primary viral mutations in samples for proficiency testing *(92,93)*, recent CAP survey data indicated detection of primary mutations in a single proficiency sample among 73% of participating laboratories *(94)*. Significant variations in detection and identification of relevant mutations have also been demonstrated among commercially available kits and with the interpretation software used *(95)*.

Table 3
Screening Tests Recommended in Pregnant HIV-Positive Women

Reason	Test	Frequency of testing
Maternal immune status	Plasma viral load	Every 4 wk until goals for therapy attained, or to monitor disease status
	CD4+ T cell counts	Every 3–4 mo
	HIV genotyping	If suspected infection with resistant virus, or resistance developing to treatment
Maternal serostatus	CMV IgM and IgG	First prenatal visit, or after primary HIV diagnosis
	Group B streptococci	Third trimester
	HBsAg	Routine screening
	Hepatitis C serologies	First prenatal visit, or after primary HIV diagnosis
	Rubella	Routine screening
	RPR or VDRL	First trimester, 28 wk, and at delivery
	Toxoplasmosis IgG and IgM	First prenatal visit, or after primary HIV diagnosis
	VZV	First prenatal visit, or after primary HIV diagnosis
Presence of infection	Nucleic acid testing for *C. trachomatis*	First prenatal visit, or after primary HIV diagnosis
	Nucleic acid testing or culture for gonorrhea	First prenatal visit, or after primary HIV diagnosis

Adapted from refs. *88,96,97.*

Hepatitis serologies and serologies for CMV, varicella zoster virus (VZV), and *Toxoplasma gondii* should be obtained, in addition to screening for *Chlamydia trachomatis* and gonorrhea infection *(88,96,97)*. Other sections of this chapter describe appropriate screening and diagnostic testing to perform.

HERPES VIRUS I AND II

Transmission commonly occurs through sexual contact and exposure to infected bodily fluids. Herpes virus (HSV)-I, the etiology of herpes labialis, causes oral lesions and gingivalstomatitis. HSV-II is associated with genital infection. Primary maternal infection with HSV-II commonly presents with painful vesicular lesions at the site of inoculation. However, disease may remain subclinical in women, particularly in individuals with immunity to HSV-I. Both viruses establish a latent state and may be reactivated during pregnancy.

The sero-prevalence of HSV-I ranges from 61 to 75%, and HSV-II from 11 to 23% in industrialized countries *(98,99)*. Rates of positive sero-prevalence in other countries range from 75.7 to 95% for HSV-I and from 15 to 43% for HSV-II *(100)*.

Congenital infection with HSV-II is thought to occur in 1 in 2000–5000 deliveries. Intrapartum infection accounts for 75–80% of infection diagnosed in infants, with the remaining number comprising postpartum infections. *In utero* transmission early in pregnancy has been associated with fetal loss. Later infection may result in microcephaly or hydranencephaly, and ocular findings including microphthalmia, keratoconjunctivitis, and retinitis. Defects have been documented in women with both primary and reactivated infection *(101)*. Skin findings on the newborn are common and include the presence of vesicles and scarring. Without treatment, babies with disseminated HSV disease commonly succumb to HSV pneumonitis or disseminated intravascular coagulation.

Screening. Routine screening of pregnant women for HSV IgG is performed only in women with high risk factors for the disease to determine maternal exposure. Abbott, Roche, Diamedix, Zeus Scientific, and Wampole Laboratories produce available anti-HSV IgG assays in the EIA format. Source of the viral antigen used in assay systems determines specificity of the test and may permit detection only of exposure to HSV without distinguishing between HSV-I and -II. Most assays have sensitivities ranging from 85 to 100% and specificities of 79–97% *(102,103)*. Some assays use viral glycoproteins specific for each virus to determine immune status to HSV-I and -II. These assays have sensitivity of 95% for HSV-I and 98% for HSV-II. Specificity is 96% for HSV-I and 97% for HSV-II.

Diagnosis. Serological testing can identify maternal exposure but cannot determine presence of active disease, or asymptomatic viral shedding, or predict maternal transmission prepartum or intrapartum. Current recommendations indicate ceasarian delivery only for women with active lesions at the time of delivery *(104,105)*.

Direct culture of HSV from lesions is preferred for identifying active disease near the time of birth. Culture methods commonly use Vero cells or human foreskin fibroblasts. Standard shell viral culture techniques may permit detection of viral cytopathic effect within 24–48 h incubation, after which positive cultures are confirmed by direct fluorescence assay (DFA) or PCR specific for HSV-I or -II viral antigens *(106)*. Recently developed systems specific for HSV permit detection of virus or viral antigens within 24 h after inoculation.

Immunoperoxidase staining of inoculated mink lung cells for HSV-specific antigens after 16–24 h incubation allows more rapid detection and has reported analytical sensitivity of 99% *(107,108)*. The enzyme-linked viral inducible system (Diagnostic Hybrids, Inc.) uses genetically engineered cells containing an inducible β-galactosidase behind a herpesvirus-specific promoter *(109,110)*. HSV-I and -II transactivators VP16 and ICP10 induce specific expression of the β-galactosidase reporter gene, which is easily detected with available chromogenic substrates *(12)*. Follow-up fluorescent detection allows identification of HSV-I or HSV-II *(111)*. Reports have indicated a sensitivity of 88% and specificity greater than or equal to 99% for the enzyme-linked viral inducible system commercial assay *(112)*.

Neonatal Diagnosis. *In utero* infection is confirmed by culture of the virus within 48 h of birth, commonly with material swabbed from vesicular lesions.

HUMAN T-LYMPHOMA VIRUS I

Infection with the human T-lymphoma viruses (HTLV) I and II retroviruses is endemic in the Caribbean and southern Japan. Infections occur sporadically throughout South America, Asia, Africa, and the southeastern United States *(113)*. Transmission occurs primarily through sexual contact and intravenous drug abuse, although the virus may be transmitted vertically or in breast milk *(114)*. Studies have indicated 0.5–7% risk of vertical transmission of HTLV-I from infected mothers *(115)* and up to 25% transmission to infants via breast-feeding *(116).* Primary infection produces no overt symptoms although isolated reports have described childhood onset of T-cell leukemias and other cancers in individuals infected with HTLV-I as infants or *in utero (117).* Chronic infection with HTLV-I carries a 3–5% lifetime risk for developing adult T-cell leukemia or lymphoma or tropical spastic paralysis. The prevalence of HTLV-I and -II infection in the United States is approx 4.3 individuals per 10,000 and is as low as 0.01% throughout much of western Europe *(118).* However, higher rates exist in populations from endemic areas or in individuals engaging in high-risk behaviors.

Screening. Serological screening for HTLV-I immune status in pregnant women has become routine in endemic areas such as southern Japan and parts of South America *(119,120).* In other regions, screening is indicated only in individuals from endemic areas or with risk factors for exposure to the virus. Sero-positive women receive counseling to abstain from breast-feeding.

In the United States, screening and identification of individuals exposed to HTLV-I use ELISA-based assays for anti-HTLV IgG. Positive results are confirmed by Western blot analyses against HTLV-I and -II viral glycoproteins. Most newer generation commercial EIA assays use recombinant proteins as opposed to viral lysates. Commercially available assays include EIA tests manufactured by Abbott Laboratories, Murex Diagnostics, and Organon-Teknika. Most studies have indicated that ELISA followed by western blot confirmation has a sensitivity of 95–100% for HTLV-I and 80–94% for HTLV-II exposure *(121).* However, indeterminate results on western blot have been associated with coinfection with malaria *(122)* and primary VZV infection where VZV-specific IgM cross-reacted with HTLV antigens *(123).* Testing performed in Japan and other areas outside of the United States commonly use particle agglutination assays such as the Serodia HTLV-I assay that have reported sensitivities of 99–100% and specificities of 95–100% *(124).* The tests are inexpensive and easy to perform, but not currently licensed by the FDA for patient testing in the United States.

Parvovirus B19

Parvovirus B19 is a nonenveloped single-stranded DNA virus. The virus is highly infectious, spreading primarily via respiratory droplets. Infection in children causes erythema infectiosum, or Fifth's disease. Adult infection has been associated with postviral arthropathies but commonly produces subclinical disease. The virus is a common cause of life-threatening aplastic crises in patients with hemoglobinopathies and other red cell disorders. Exposure to the virus has been correlated with the number of siblings in a family and with known exposure to infected children. In the United States, approx 45% of all blood donors test positive for parvovirus IgG. In children under the age of 5, prevalences remain less than 50% but rise steadily with age to a prevalence of greater than 75% by age 50.

B19 binds the P red cell carbohydrate antigen on red blood cell precursors and subsequently lyses erythroblasts. *In utero* infection has been associated with nonimmune fetal hydrops, central nervous system defects, fetal loss, and stillbirths *(125).*

Studies in Denmark estimated the prevalence of sero-conversion for parvovirus B19 among pregnant women to be 1.5–13%. Many women sero-converting during pregnancy remained asymptomatic, without rash or other indications of clinical disease. Rates of *in utero* transmission remain ill defined, but 17–33% of studied cases demonstrated transmission of the virus to the fetus. Of infected babies, fetal hydrops occurred in 34%, and death occurred in 3% of cases. However, more than half of pregnancies complicated by primary parvovirus B19 infection resulted in healthy infants *(126)*.

Screening. Screening for B19 sero-negativity is not routinely indicated because no vaccination or therapeutic interventions exist.

Diagnosis. Parvovirus B19 is not readily cultured in vitro. Acute and convalescent serologies detecting IgG against viral capsid proteins remain the basis for identifying past exposure to the virus. Newer generation ELISAs using recombinant VP1 and VP2 caspid proteins have greatly increased the sensitivity and specificity of these tests to more than 90%. Older assays using crude cell or tissue lysates were plagued by low specificity and variable sensitivity among reagent lots.

In pregnant women exhibiting viral exanthems, diagnosis should focus on rapidly determining whether the etiology is parvovirus B19, rubella, measles, or possibly CMV. Infected patients may manifest reactive IgM against B19 just prior to the onset of rash and other symptoms. The reactivity persists for 2–3 wk, after which IgM concentrations fall in most individuals as IgG titers rise. The sensitivity of IgM alone is 60% or less for diagnosing acute disease *(127)*. Cross-reactivity with rubella and measles has been reported with B19 IgM assays *(128)*. Reactive IgG commonly appears within days of pathogen-specific IgM and remains detectable for years. However, a subset of patients maintain high IgM titers for months after the primary infection, although the presence of high IgG titers differentiates acute infection from convalescence. Commercial IgG avidity assays for parvovirus are not currently available and have not been standardized or validated extensively for diagnostic use.

PCR-based assays for parvovirus DNA have proven useful in diagnosing acute infection. High titer viremia, to the order of greater than 10^{12} copes/mL, can last for a window period of a week during symptomatic disease *(129)*. Lower concentrations of virus may persist in blood for months after infection, although reports vary in the ability of PCR methods to detect viral DNA after the acute phase of infection. If collected from symptomatic individuals, viral PCR has a sensitivity of 79%–93% and specificity of 100% *(127,130)*.

In symptomatic women for whom it is important to obtain a specific diagnosis, antiparvovirus B19 IgM and detection of DNA by PCR on blood samples provide the best combination of tests to identify acutely infected patients and rule out other infectious causes. Overall sensitivity of both tests has been estimated to be 90% or more in symptomatic individuals *(127)*. Many case reports have used parvovirus PCR on AF, cord blood, and, less frequently, on chorionic villi *(131)* to diagnose fetal infection *(132,133)*. However, studies have not been undertaken to define the sensitivity and specificity of these assays for rapidly diagnosing acute infection of the fetus.

RUBELLA

Rubella is a single-stranded RNA togavirus that causes German measles. Humans are the only known hosts. Infection occurs primarily during the winter and spring months. Children commonly present with rash while adults may have a prodromal illness of 1–5 d associated with lymphadenopathy and other constitutional symptoms before rash appears. However, infection frequently remains subclinical *(134)*. Implementation of childhood vaccination in 1969 in the United States and abroad has greatly impacted the number of congenital infections and birth defects attributed to maternal rubella infection. The prevalence of unimmunized women in vaccinated populations is around 1.8% *(135)* and 40% or higher in unvaccinated populations *(136)*.

During acute infection, the virus infects the placenta and is transmitted to the fetus. Viral replication may be sustained for months in placental tissue, providing chronic exposure of the fetus to the virus. High rates of fetal infection, from 80 to 100%, occur if primary maternal infection happens during the first 8 wk of pregnancy, during the critical period of fetal organogenesis. The most severe defects are associated with infection during this period and include significant eye, ear, and heart defects, leading to congenital blindness and deafness in the newborn. Fetal infection rates range from 24 to 47% in women infected primarily during the second trimester, and for the last three months, 35, 60, and up to 100%, respectively. Other studies have demonstrated the risk for development of defects to be 90% for infection acquired prior to 11 wk gestation, 33% for infection acquired from weeks 11 to 12, 11% during weeks 13–14, and 24% during weeks 15–16 *(137)*. Secondary exposure or infection in an immune mother is thought to carry less risk of birth defects because the disease is less severe and maternally transferred immune IgG likely plays a role in limiting the course of disease and effecting viral clearance from infected tissues in the fetus.

Screening. Serological testing for rubella-specific IgG provides the basis for determining maternal immune status. Commonly used commercial assays include kits from Abbott Laboratories, Becton-Dickinson, BioMérieux, Murex Diagnostics, and Wampole Laboratories *(138)*. Assays have reported sensitivities of 99–100% and specificities of 94–99%, although one study of 497 women, which included 9 seronegative individuals, demonstrated a specificity of only 78% for the Abbott AxSYM Rubella IgG Assay *(135,139)*.

Diagnosis. Diagnosis of acute primary maternal infection or secondary exposure relies on serological testing. A fourfold increase in IgG titers in paired acute and convalescent sera collected 14–21 d apart confirm recent maternal infection. Serum IgM may be assayed on a single acute sample to help identify primary infection, but clinical measures should not be instituted on the basis of results from a single IgM assay *(140)*. As with all IgM assays, results may be confounded by the time-course of the IgM response during infection and known cross-reaction of most rubella assays with IgM produced during infection with mumps, Epstein-Barr Virus, CMV, or parvovirus B19 *(141)*. Rubella-specific IgM has also been shown to persist for up to a year after primary infection or vaccination *(142,143)*. IgM assays have variable sensitivities from 63 to 92% and specificities ranging from 82 to 98% *(144)*. Many studies have recommended repeat testing of positive IgM samples with different assays followed by confirmatory IgM and IgG convalescent serologies drawn as described. Likewise, IgM serologies performed on cord blood have been of use in some cases but suffer from lower specificity.

IgG avidity assays using recombinant antigens, particularly the E1 epitope to which neutralizing antibody is produced, stand to provide a better measure for diagnosing recent or primary infection *(145,146)*. Commercially available IgG avidity assays for rubella are available from Labsystems (Helsinki, Finland) *(146)* and Tosoh (Rivoli, Italy) *(147)* but are used primarily in reference laboratories. Sensitivity of 92% and specificity of 100% have been reported for commercially available assays *(148)*. A new avidity assay performed on saliva had reported sensitivity of 94% and specificity of 88% but has not been widely tested *(149)*. However, ability to obtain accurate results is highly dependent on performance of the assays because incubation and washing steps for IgG avidity can greatly influence the results.

Culture is not recommended for maternal diagnosis given the low titers present. However, culture has value in diagnosing congenital infection in the neonate, given the chronic nature of the infection and high titer viremia present in multiple organs *(150)*. Swabs of posterior pharynx are preferred, but cerebrospinal fluid (CSF), buffy coat, conjunctival swabs, and urine have also been used to diagnose infection. The virus is heat labile and destroyed by freezing. Samples submitted for culture must thus be procured with care. The virus remains viable for up to a week if swabs are placed in appropriate transport media and stored at 4°C. Most laboratories performing culture use African green monkey cells to support growth. Confirmation of positive cultures uses antigen detection or neutralization of cultured virus with immune sera on inoculation of uninfected cell lines.

VARICELLA ZOSTER VIRUS

Varicella zoster virus (VZV) is a double-stranded DNA herpesvirus that causes varicella (chickenpox) and reactivated herpes zoster infection (shingles). In primary infection, the virus has an average of 14 d incubation prior to the onset of symptoms and rash, though this time may vary from 10 to 23 d. Low-grade viremia commonly occurs 4–6 d after exposure *(151)*. In industrialized countries, 91–95% of women have protective immunity to the virus from vaccination or primary disease acquired in childhood *(152)*. Maternal immunity can prevent or limit the development of infection *in utero*, even during episodes of viral reactivation. However, cases of congenital infection have been reported in women with known immunity to the virus. The prevalence of primary infections in pregnant women is approximately 0.04%, with zoster reactivations occurring in 0.2% of pregnancies.

Congenital infection with VZV has been associated with abortions, stillbirths, and prematurity. The virus is teratogenic, and primary infection acquired during the first 28 wk gestation has been associated with chromosomal abnormalities caused by DNA breakages in infected cells. *In utero* infection has been associated with resulting birth defects in 5–10% of cases *(153)*. Malformations and defects most commonly associated with congenital infection include cataracts, other eye and central nervous system defects, and skin scarring.

Screening. Screening for VZV immune status is recommended in women with risks for exposure, such as day-care or health-care workers, or for HIV-positive women. Immunity to VZV should ideally be determined prior to pregnancy so susceptible women may be offered vaccination. IgG serologies provide the basis for determining maternal immune status. Commonly used commercial assays include the VZV ELISA from Wampole Laboratories, BioMérieux, and other EIAs produced by Diamedix, Sigma Diagnostics, and Zeus Scientific *(154)*. Most methodologies use capture EIA and have sensitivities of 96–99% and specificities of 96–98% *(155,156)*.

Diagnosis. Detection of VZV viral antigens and PCR of vesicular fluid or skin scrapings have been recommended to diagnose primary infection or reactivation. Direct immunofluorescent antigen detection (DFA) kits manufactured by Chemicon, Viromed, and Meridian commonly recognize viral proteins GP1, early antigen, and membrane antigen. DFA has reported sensitivities of 82–92% and specificity of 76% *(157,158)*. These methods are considered superior to serological testing or Tzanck preparation of skin scrapings, which does not distinguish VZV from other herpesviruses. Culture of VZV from skin material has been reported to have sensitivity of 20%–56% and specificity of 100% *(159)*. PCR assays for VZV gag gene or gene 28 have reported sensitivities of 95–96%, although kits are not available commercially *(157,160)*.

PCR has proved superior to culture or antigen detection for fetal diagnosis *(161)*. PCR testing on AF, placenta, and chorionic villi from sero-negative women exposed to the virus has reported good specificity, although the numbers of cases in which these tests have been used is small. Caution should be used in interpreting positive PCR results because the presence of viral DNA in AF, placenta, or fetal material does not necessarily predict the development of congenital defects *(153,162)*.

Bacterial Infections

Chlamydia Trachomatis

C. trachomatis is an obligate intracellular pathogen transmitted via sexual contact. The organism is a primary cause of nongonococcal urethritis in men and causes a spectrum of diseases in women, including cervicitis and salpingitis, although 9–10% of healthy women *(163,164)* and up to 40% of individuals examined in STD clinics may have asymptomatic infection *(165)*. Vertical transmission is believed rare, but untreated genital infections have been associated with abortion, stillbirth, premature rupture of membranes, and maternal endometritis postpartum *(166)*. Exposure intrapartum can lead to the development of ophthalmia neonatorum, and chalmydial pneumonia, which may develop in up to 10% of infected neonates *(167)*.

Screening. The ACOG recommends screening only for women with risk factors for underlying chlamydial infection *(168)*. However, recommendations from the CDC have suggested that all women in the United States be screened at their first prenatal visit *(169)*. Studies have indicated positive predictive values of 80–90% with nucleic acid tests for *C. trachomatis* when the prevalence of disease drops below 5% *(170)*, suggesting confirmation of results or repeat testing to diagnose patients in low-prevalence populations *(169)*.

Nucleic acid amplification of clamydial sequences from endocervical swabs has the highest sensitivity of available methods for identifying the organism and more rapid turnaround time than culture-based assays, which may take up to a week and have considerable expense. However, in vitro culture of *C. trachomatis* remains the indicated test for cases involving medicolegal issues.

For nucleic acid testing, endocervical samples should be collected on plastic or metal shaft swabs with Dacron, rayon, or cotton tips; placed in appropriate transport media; and stored at 2–25°C for delivery to the testing laboratory *(171)*. The majority of clinical laboratories in the United States and Canada use molecular amplification assays produced by Abbott Laboratories (LCx ligase chain reaction), GenProbe [PACE™2, transcription-mediated amplification (TMA)], Roche (PCR), or a hybrid capture assay by Digene (Hybrid Capture II CT/GC) *(172)*. The GenProbe assay permits dual detection of *C. trachomatis* and *Neisseria gonorrhoeae* from a single specimen. Molecular methods have reported sensitivity of 97.4–99.8% and specificities of 99.6–100% on cervical swabs, which provide better results than urine *(173,174)*. Improved sensitivities of 99% or more have been reported with methods using PCR or LCR as the amplification schemes, as opposed to nonamplified assays *(175)*.

Diagnosis. Probe-based molecular methods are the standard for diagnosing sexually transmitted disease in women and conjunctivitis in neonates.

GONORRHEA

Neisseria gonorrhoeae is a sexually transmitted disease that produces purulent, painful urethritis in men. Women commonly present with endocervicitis and urethritis. Symptoms of pelvic inflammatory disease develop in 10–20% of women. However, in the general population, 0.4–2.3% of women have asymptomatic disease or do not develop symptoms for which they seek medical attention *(164,176)*. Rates of symptomatic and asymptomatic disease are higher in women with multiple sexual contacts *(177)*. Infection during pregnancy has been associated with stillbirths *(178)* and low birth weights *(179)*. Transmission at birth can cause ophthalmia neonatorum and gonococcal infection of the pharynx or anus. Gonococcal ophthalmia frequently leads to blindness if left untreated *(180)*.

Gonococcal infections have a general prevalence of 0.3% in the United States, but a prevalence of 2.5–3% in populations with risk factors including low socioeconomic status, intravenous drug abuse, multiple sexual partners, and sexual activity before age 16 *(181,182)*.

Screening and Diagnosis. The ACOG has recommended screening high-risk women early in pregnancy and at 28 wk gestation *(183)*. CDC recommendations suggest screening in all pregnant women *(169,184)*. Probe-based assays and culture are the most commonly performed tests. While Gram-stain of purulent material in men has diagnostic significance, staining purulent endocervical discharge from women has both low sensitivity and specificity. Nucleic acid detection kits from GenProbe, Abbott Laboratories, Roche, and Digene have sensitivities of 92–96.8% and specificities of 98–100% compared with typical sensitivity of 83% and specificity of 100% for culture *(185–187)*. The Roche COBAS Amplicor assay has reported cross-reactivity with some commensal lactobacilli and has specificity of 96.8% for endocervical swabs *(188)*.

Culture is indicated for cases not responding to therapy or in areas with high prevalence of resistant gonococcal strains. Approximately 10% of *N. gonorrhoeae* isolates reported in the United States are resistant to penicillin. Resistance to third-generation cephalosporins (Ceftriaxone, Cefotaxime) has remained very low *(189)*.

N. gonorrhoeae is a fastidious Gram-negative diplococcus. The organism may be cultured on selective media including Thayer-Martin or NYC media, although chocolate agar, routinely used in genital cultures, supports growth. Direct plating of samples onto media provides the best means of recovering organisms. However, for situations where direct plating is not possible, samples should be collected onto Dacron or rayon swabs with plastic or metal tips and placed in transport media or a swab transport system. Samples placed in swab transport systems should be delivered to the laboratory within 6 h of collection to facilitate maximal recovery of *N. gonorrhoeae (190)*. A single endocervical culture from symptomatic women typically has sensitivity of 80–95% and specificity of 100%. Positive samples typically grow within 1–2 d of collection, producing translucent, oxidase-positive colonies that demonstrate Gram-negative diplococci when stained. Identification may be further confirmed with DNA probes or biochemical characterization including sugar fermentation profiles.

GROUP B STREPTOCOCCI

Chapter 13 discusses screening of pregnant women for colonization with group B streptococci.

LISTERIA MONOCYTOGENES

L. monocytogenes infection commonly occurs through ingestion of unpasteurized milk and milk products, processed meats, or vegetables contaminated with animal wastes *(191,192)*. During pregnancy, women are 20 times more susceptible to infection and account for one-third of all cases of listeriosis reported in the United States. Infection occurs most commonly in the third trimester of pregnancy *(193)*. Maternal infection carries a 27% risk of morbidity to the fetus and can lead to miscarriages, chorioamnionitis, preterm labor, and septicemia and meningitis in the fetus *(194)*. Approximately 8.6 neonatal cases of listeriosis occur per 100,000 live births in the United States *(195)*.

L. monocytogenes invades the body through intestinal M cells overlying the localized lymphoid tissue in Peyer's patches of the intestine and disseminates hematogenously to remote sites, including the placenta. The infection produces gastrointestinal symptoms 9–48 h after ingestion and flulike symptoms 2–6 wk subsequently with invasive disease *(191)*. Placental infection commonly produces local abscesses and damage to the maternal–fetal barrier that may contribute to bacteria entering the fetal circulation. Infection of the fetus in asymptomatic women may also occur through colonization of the vagina.

Diagnosis. Blood cultures drawn in symptomatic women are the ideal means of diagnosing infection *(193)*. CSF cultures are also of diagnostic use in women presenting with headache, neck stiffness, or other neurological signs. Stool culture is not recommended because of the difficulty of isolating the organism from this specimen. If *L. monocytogenes* is clinically suspected and communicated to the laboratory, laboratory personnel may perform a cold enrichment to select for growth of the organism. Gram-stain and culture of AF obtained in febrile women with preterm labor has assisted with diagnosis in reported cases *(196,197)*.

L. monocytogenes stains Gram-positive as short rods or with a coccobacilliary morphology. Culture produces translucent colonies on sheep's blood agar with a thin zone of β-hemolysis surrounding the colony. The organism survives refrigeration at 4°C and produces a characteristic tumbling motility visible on wet mounts or an umbrella shape when cultured in motility medium at 25°C *(193)*. Cases have also been diagnosed with placental culture and with immunohistochemical staining using monoclonal antibody specific for serotypes 1 and 4 of *L. monocytogenes* on placental sections (198).

INVASIVE INTRACELLULAR BACTERIA

Congenital infection with *Brucella (199)*, *Salmonella (200,201)*, *Shigella (202)*, and *Campylobacter species (203)* have been rarely reported. Standard culture methods, particularly blood culture from symptomatic women and stool culture for enteric pathogens, are indicated.

SYPHILIS

The spirochete *Treponema pallidum* subspecies *pallidum* causes syphilis. The disease is transmitted primarily through sexual contact and intravenous drug abuse and from vertical transmission. Primary infection produces a painless ulcerating lesion, or chancre, at the site of infection. Progression to secondary disease occurs with systemic dissemination of the spirochete to other sites and frequently happens 2–8 wk after appearance of the chancre. Patients develop maculopapular rash, malaise, and a myriad of other symptoms. Latent syphilis is divided into early and late stages relative to the duration of asymptomatic disease in an individual with positive treponemal-specific tests. Unfortunately, many women are not diagnosed until the secondary or early latent stages of disease (204,205). Additional discussion of the disease and end sequelae have been reviewed in a variety of texts (206,207).

Prevalence of disease among pregnant women ranges from 0.2% to 2.4% in many parts of the world (208,209) and up to 7.5% among patients visiting STD clinics (210). Recent data indicate national rates of congenital syphilis at 13.4 cases per 100,000 live births (211). However, in some areas these rates are as high as 2 cases per 1000 live births (212).

Most congenital infections occur in utero although some may be contracted during birth. Vertical transmission of syphilis to the fetus may occur at any point in pregnancy, although it is more likely to occur during the primary and secondary stages of maternal syphilis. The likelihood of congenital infection in the fetus also increases as the pregnancy progresses. HIV-positive women are also more likely to transmit the disease in utero. Conversely, damage to the placental barrier, inflicted by infecting spirochetes, increases the chances for HIV transmission in utero (213).

Hollier et al. have hypothesized that the course and pathogenesis of congenital infection first produces dysfunction of the placenta and fetal liver, followed by detectable presence of spirochetes in AF and hematologic abnormalities including thrombocytopenia, anemia, and leukocytosis or leukocytopenia (214). Bone lesions and central nervous system defects may subsequently be detected by ultrasound. Screening, diagnosis, and treatment of infection can greatly reduce or prevent the development of congenital infection (215,216), particularly if the disease is detected and treated prior to 28 wk gestation (217).

Screening and Diagnosis. All women undergo routine screening for syphilis. Repeat screening is recommended in high-risk women at 28–30 wk gestation and again at delivery (218). Risk factors include intravenous drug abuse, multiple sexual partners, and previous diagnosis of STD. Screening assays use one of two nontreponemal tests, the reactive protein regain (RPR) or the Venereal Disease Research Labs test (VDRL). Positive results are confirmed with a treponemal-specific assay, commonly the fluorescent treponemal antibody absorption (FTA-abs) or microhemagglutination (MHA-TP) tests. Table 4 lists the specificity and sensitivities of these four assays with regard to the stage of disease (219–221). Studies in low-prevalence populations (1.04%) have demonstrated a positive predictive value of 88% for the RPR. Follow-up testing with the FTA-abs or MHA-TP was effective in diagnosing biological false positives and significantly raised the predictive value of testing (222).

The RPR and VDRL are considered nontreponemal because they test for reactivity to cardiolipin (diphosphatidylglycerol), an acidic lipid found in the membranes of mitochondria and many bacterial species, including Treponema. Despite the seemingly nonspecificity of this antigen, early studies of serum from syphilis patients consistently revealed reactivity with cardiolipin, which proved to be a sensitive marker of infection. Both the RPR and VDRL use agglutination of cardiolipin-lecithin-cholesterol particles by patient sera to indicate positive results (221). The RPR rapid slide agglutination assay has gained wider utilization in clinical laboratories because of its ease of use and lower cost. The assay can also be used to provide patient titers against cardiolipin, which have use in following response to therapy.

Less than 1% of otherwise healthy individuals undergoing screening will give a falsely positive RPR or VRDL result (222,223). False positives occur in patients with

Table 4
Average Sensitivities and Specificity of Treponemal and Nontreponemal Assays
for Different Stages of Syphilis

Test	Primary	Secondary	Early latent	Late latent	Treated	Specificity
RPR	86	100	98	73	58	98
VDRL	78	100	95	71		98
FTA-abs	86	100	100	96	97.5	97
MHA-TP	76	97	97	97		99

Adapted from refs. *219,220,221.*

anticardiolipin antibody present after postviral syndromes *(221)* and less frequently in patients with lupus and connective tissue diseases *(224)*. False positive rates are also increased in HIV-positive patients, possibly because of the production of anticardiolipin antibodies during primary infection *(225,226)*. High concentrations of immunoglobulin in patient sera can rarely produce nonspecific agglutination of particles (prozone effect). The loose appearance of the resulting aggregates should prompt retesting with diluted patient sera, and most samples demonstrate negative reactivity with titers of 1:16 or less *(223)*. Some studies have suggested that pregnancy increases the rate of false positivity with RPR and VDRL testing, although others have not demonstrated such an association *(227)*.

Confirmatory tests assay reactivity with treponemal antigens. The FTA-abs adsorbs patient sera against a nonpathogenic spirochete, *T. phagadenis*, prior to incubation with killed *T. pallidum* (Nichol's strain). Addition of fluorescently labeled antihuman globulin allows detection of the spirochetes by fluorescent microscopy. The MHA-TP measures the ability of adsorbed patient samples to agglutinate fixed sheep red blood cells coated with *T. pallidum* antigens. The assay is easier to perform and interpret than the FTA-abs but has lower sensitivity of detection during primary infection. Samples with inconclusive results obtained with the MHA-TP should be retested with the FTA-abs. The MHA-TP is also not indicated for testing on CSF samples, whereas the VDRL and FTA-abs may be used to screen and assist with the diagnosis of neurosyphilis *(221)*.

PCR on AF has been used to diagnose congenital infection in women at less than or equal to 20 wk gestation *(228,229)*. Assays have apparent sensitivities of 60–66% and specificity of 100% for diagnosing fetal infection, but limited numbers of samples were tested in published studies, each of which used different primer sets for amplification *(205,230,231)*. PCR for the 47kD membrane antigen of *T. pallidum* has assisted with diagnosing placental infection postpartum in some cases *(232)*. If available, direct detection of *T. pallidum* by darkfield microscopy on AF may yield positive results but has lower sensitivity than PCR. Microscopy should be performed immediately after collection to permit detection of motile spirochetes *(221)*. VDRL and anti-treponemal IgM all have limited utility in diagnosing *in utero* infection, particularly in a fetus with a gestational age less than 22 wk *(205)*. The tests also have higher rates of false positive and false negative results when performed on cord blood.

Protozoal Infections

With the exception of toxoplasmosis, congenitally acquired protozoal infections occur infrequently in industrialized countries, although they cause significant morbidity and mortality in developing countries.

Malaria

Four species of *Plasmodium* infect humans: *P. falciparum, P. malariae, P. ovalae,* and *P. vivax.* Transmission commonly occurs through bites from infected *Anopheles* mosquitoes, although transfusion-associated and congenital infections have been well described. Of these species, falciparum malaria is the most widespread and serious for the following reasons: the parasite can infect red cells of any age, vascular sequestration of parasites occurs as part of the life cycle, and damage may be inflicted in multiple organs including the uterus and placenta.

Prevalence of malaria is highest in sub-Saharan Africa. Up to 29% of pregnant women in endemic areas have detectable parasitemia during pregnancy *(233)*. Primigravidas in particular are susceptible to infection. Studies in Rwanda demonstrated parasitemia in 3.5% of healthy women and 8.0% of HIV-positive women *(234)*. Areas of Southeast Asia demonstrate prevalences of 3–35% in some populations with a predominance of falciparum malaria *(235)*.

In pregnant women, underlying malarial infection can contribute to maternal anemia and adversely impact uteroplacental blood flow *(236)* because parasite-infected red cells sequester in the intervillous spaces of the placenta *(237)*. Of note, 16–20% of women with placental malaria have negative blood smears when tested at delivery *(238)*. While vertical transmission to the fetus occurs infrequently, significant placental infection can contribute to low birth weight, intrauterine growth retardation, preterm birth, and stillbirth *(236,239)*. Large randomized trials have demonstrated the efficacy of pyrimethamine and mefloquine treatment on maternal anemia and placental infection *(240,241)*. Maternal diagnosis of malaria can thus have positive impact on the health of both the mother and the fetus.

Screening and Diagnosis. Screening of pregnant women is advocated in parts of sub-Saharan Africa. Programs recommend screening for anemia and malaria antenatally and at labor and delivery *(242)*. Most hospitals use Wright-Giemsa staining of peripheral blood smears to identify and speciate parasites. Thick and thin smears should be prepared, preferably from recently collected, EDTA-anticoagulated blood or immediately from a finger stick. Thick smears have an analytical sensitivity of 5–20 parasites/µL (0.0001–0.0004% parasitemia), whereas thin smears have an analytical sensitivity of 100 parasites/mL (0.002% parasitemia). Both values are associated with asymptomatic infections *(243)*. Multiple smears should be performed from pregnant women, given the possibility of falciparum sequestering in the placenta and other tissues and limiting detection of the parasite in peripheral blood. Fluorescent detection by staining with DNA-binding dyes such as acridine orange can improve the turnaround time of testing because the slides may be scanned more rapidly at lower magnification for intracellular parasites *(244,245)*. However, speciation is not as readily determined with fluorescent staining.

To diagnose women presenting with clinical signs of malaria, specimens should ideally be drawn during febrile episodes. *P. faciparum* characteristically has a 36–48-hour cycle between febrile episodes, *P. vivax* and *P. ovalae* have 48-hour cycles, and *P. malariae* a 72-hour cycle *(243)*.

Use of *Plasmodia* rapid antigen tests for screening pregnant women has promise in detecting asymptomatic infection or the presence of placental infection in the absence of findings in peripheral blood. A study of the immunochromatographic technology (ICT) rapid Pf malaria dipstick assay, which detects histidine-rich protein 2 produced by *P. falciparum*, demonstrated a sensitivity of 89% and specificity of 94.9% in detecting women with falciparum parasitemia and/or placental malaria. Similar results were found for Becton Dickinson's ParaSight-F and Makromed's Malaria Rapid Test dipstick assays, which also detect histidine-rich protein 2, although findings were correlated with smear or PCR results on peripheral blood and not presence of placental infection *(246,247)*. DiaMed's OptiMAL antigen assay, which recognizes plasmodial lactate dehydrogenase and speciates *Plasmodia* as falciparum or non-falciparum, demonstrated sensitivity of 76.2% and specificity of 99.7% in patients from areas endemic for malaria *(248)*. However, in our own experience in the United States, the assay requires careful interpretation because it can produce falsely positive results in patients with high underlying lactate dehyrogenase values and false speciation of *P. falciparum* in patients infected with *Babesia microti*. Other investigators have also noted poor sensitivity of the assay in detecting subclinical parasitemia *(249)*.

PCR-based methods are gaining acceptance and use as a means for rapidly diagnosing and speciating malaria. Assays amplify specific sequences in the rRNA of different species, merozoite surface proteins, or other targets and have the potential to identify drug resistance *(250)*. Single and multiplex PCR assays to identify and speciate parasites or distinguish *P. falciparum* from other species have reported sensitivities of 97–100% and specificities of 96–100% *(251–254)*. The limit of detection of many assays is less than 5 parasites/µL of blood.

TOXOPLASMOSIS

Toxoplasma gondii is the most common protozoal etiology of congenital infections. The organism is ubiquitous in nature, found commonly in the soil from warm, humid areas contaminated by animal feces. Feral cats remain the primary reservoir of disease, shedding oocysts into the environment during acute infection.

The sero-prevalence of toxoplasmosis varies widely among populations, correlating with exposure and ingestion of environmental oocysts or bradyzoite cysts in undercooked meat from infected animals. The prevalence of sero-positivity in North America and Australia remain 3% or less in most populations. In parts of Europe, South America, and Africa, rates of sero-prevalence frequently exceed 50% of the population.

In humans, acute disease commonly causes a self-limited mononucleosislike syndrome including lymphadenopathy and fatigue, although primary disease may remain asymptomatic. Parasitemia can occur prior to and during the symptomatic phase of the illness and before sero-conversion, although the duration and window period of parasitemia with regard to exposure are ill defined. Chronic parasitemia occurs more frequently in HIV-positive and other immunocompromised patients, particularly those with other T-cell defects or receiving steroids.

Fetal infection during the first trimester occurs rarely but carries higher risk of spontaneous fetal loss or development of birth defects. Infection later in pregnancy occurs more frequently but has lower risk of adverse sequelae in the neonate *(255)*. Risks for congenital infection can thus be summarized as, "sooner is worse, but later is more frequent." The highest risk of severe congenital disease occurs during 10–24 wk, but the highest rate of vertical transmission occurs over 26–40 wk. Primary maternal infection occurring just prior to conception through 10 wk has a fetal transmission rate of 2%, but 80% or more of infected fetuses will have severe infection with manifestations including microophthalmia, chorioretinitis, presence of intracranial calcifications, and hydrocephalus. From 24 to 30 wk, the presence of severe infection drops from 80 to 20%, and from 30 wk to term the number of neonates with severe congenital infection drops to 6%, although 80% or more of women primarily infected during this period will transmit the infection to the fetus *(256)*.

Screening. Screening of pregnant women for anti-*Toxoplasma* IgG and IgM is undertaken only in high-prevalence areas to identify sero-negative women and obtain baseline serologies. Testing should also be offered to HIV-positive patients who are at risk for fatal CNS involvement of the disease. Individuals with exposure risks may be offered testing, although prevalence rates were found to be no higher in veterinary or slaughterhouse personnel provided workers followed routine hygienic procedures *(257,258)*. Individuals with negative IgG and IgM results are defined as sero-negative, whereas those with positive IgG and negative IgM are considered sero-positive. Individuals with results positive for anti-*Toxoplasma* IgM require further evaluation, as described below, to evaluate the presence of active or recent infection and provide independent confirmation of results.

Commercial assays commonly used in clinical laboratories include EIAs and IFAs manufactured by Abbott Laboratories, BioMérieux, Diamedix, and Wampole Laboratories. ISAGA and IgG avidity assays have utility for confirmation of positive serologies but are used primarily in reference laboratories that have significant experience with their use and interpretation.

Currently available EIAs use partially purified *T. gondii* antigens from lysates or infected cell lines cultured in vitro *(259,260)*. Although these sensitivities and specificities compare with the gold-standard Sabin-Feldman dye and hemagglutination assays, identification and purification of immunodominant recombinant antigens stand to provide improved assays in the coming years *(261–263)*.

Commercial anti-*Toxoplasma* IgG assays have sensitivities ranging from 81.8 to 97.9% and specificities of 97–100%. Assays for IgM include EIAs by the same companies and an ISAGA produced by BioMérieux. Although newer IgM assays have specificities of 97–100%, sensitivities vary from 91 to 98% *(264,265)*. Furthermore, studies have demonstrated long-term persistence of anti-*Toxoplasma* IgM in up to 7% of pregnant women, thus limiting the predictive value of a single positive anti-*Toxoplasma* IgM as a measure for acute infection during pregnancy *(266)*.

In 1997, the FDA recommended that samples demonstrating equivocal or positive results for acute infection be confirmed at an outside reference laboratory with experience in toxoplasmosis testing *(267)*. Laboratories performing toxoplasmosis serologies are thus advised to contract with an appropriate reference laboratory for appropriate quality assurance and confirmation of positive results. Table 5 lists interpretation and appropriate follow-up testing for serologies.

Diagnosis. Diagnosis of acute maternal infection uses serological testing on paired acute and convalescent sera collected 2–3 wk apart and tested simultaneously. As with other conditions, a fourfold rise in IgG titers suggests primary infection or reactivation. IgM serologies can be used to assist in diagnosis of paired acute and convalescent serologies. However, interpretation of single IgM results are confounded by the long-term

Table 5
Intepretation and Follow-Up Actions for Toxoplasmosis Serological Testing

IgG results	IgM results	Interpretation	Follow-up
Negative	Negative	No evidence of infection.	
Positive	Negative	Indicative of prior infection with *T. gondii* ≥ 1 yr ago.	
Negative	Indeterminant	Possible acute infection but cannot rule out falsely positive IgM.	Obtain convalescent sample and repeat testing.
Negative	Positive	Possible acute infection but cannot rule out falsely positive IgM.	Obtain convalescent sample, and repeat testing.
Indeterminant	Negative	Indeterminate results concerning immune status to current or prior *T. gondii* infection.	Obtain new sample for testing. Consider using different method for assaying anti-*Toxoplasma* IgG.
Indeterminant	Indeterminant	Indeterminate results concerning immune status to current or prior *T. gondii* infection.	Obtain new sample for repeat testing of IgG and IgM.
Indeterminant	Positive	Possible acute infection.	Obtain convalescent sample and repeat testing. If results identical, or positive IgG obtained, send acute and convalescent sera to reference laboratory for confirmation.
Positive	Indeterminant	Prior *T. gondii* infection ≥ 1 yr or possible false-positive IgM	Obtain convalescent sample and repeat testing. If results repeated, send to reference laboratory for confirmation.
Positive	Positive	Possible infection within the past year.	Send sample to reference laboratory for confirmation of results.

Adapted from refs. *267,271,274.*

persistence of IgM in some sero-converted individuals *(266)* and by the presence of "natural" IgM antibodies against *Toxoplasma* antigens in individuals who have not been infected with the parasite *(268).*

Use of anti-*Toxoplasma* IgA in serum has reported sensitivity of 45% and specificity comparable to IgM, and is not routinely used *(269).* However, no studies have been undertaken to determine whether analysis of secretory IgA from saliva or other mucosal secretions permits better detection of toxoplasma-specific IgA.

Reference laboratories may undertake confirmation with different EIA and IFA assays and the Sabin-Feldman dye test, anti-*Toxoplasma* ISAGA, IgG avidity assays, and differential agglutination reactions that use panels of *Toxoplasma* antigens associated with early and convalescent antibody responses to assist in determining the development of the host's immune response to the pathogen.

The Sabin-Feldman dye test assesses the ability of patient sera to complement lyse the proliferative-phase tachyzoites of *T. gondii*. Patient sera, tachyzoites, and negative sera, serving as a source of complement, are incubated. Lysed tachyzoites take up methylene blue and stain darkly when observed by microscopy *(270)*. A newer variation of this test, adapted for use in 96-well plates, uses transgenic tachyzoites expressing β-galactosidase. Lysis of the parasites permits rapid biochemical detection of the released β-galactosidase *(271)*.

IgG avidity assays have been reported to indicate presence of infection within the past 3–5 mo, for individuals demonstrating a low avidity index of IgG reactivity with *T. gondii* antigens *(272–274)*. Commercially available IgG avidity assays include kits produced by LabSystems and Bio-Mérieux. Adaptation of the BioMérieux assay for the VIDAS platform allows automation of the procedure. However, results are best used in conjunction with other assays available within reference laboratories to make determinations concerning acute infection in pregnant women *(274)*.

PCR on AF provides the best test for determining fetal infection. Reported studies have used amplification of the B1 gene and other multicopy chromosomal targets to permit specific identification of *T. gondii* in AF. PCR on AF of women with serological results suggesting sero-conversion during pregnancy have sensitivity of 83–97.5% and specificity of 100% for detecting fetal infection *(275,276)*. Detection of anti-*Toxoplasma* IgM or IgA in cord blood has sensitivity of 80%, but low specificities of 91.2 and 87.7%, respectively *(277)*. For this reason, PCR on AF is preferred for fetal diagnosis of infection.

TRYPANOSOMA CRUZI

Trypanosoma cruzi is the cause of American trypanosomiasis, or Chagas's disease. The disease is endemic in many parts of Latin and South America, although an estimated 50,000–100,000 individuals in the United States have the disease *(278)*. The disease may be acquired from bites inflicted by infected reduvid beetles ("kissing bugs"), blood transfusions from infected individuals, and vertically from mother to child. In countries such as Argentina, congenital Chagas' disease has surpassed the number of acute vector-associated cases diagnosed each year *(279)*. Acute disease commonly produces nonspecific signs of malaise. Chronic sequelae of disease develop over years and include congestive heart failure, defects in the cardiac conduction system, and damage to the musculature of the gastrointestinal tract resulting in megacolon and megaesophagus.

The prevalence of sero-positivity in areas of rural Argentina has been reported to be as high as 38% *(280)*. A prevalence among pregnant Brazilian women of 0.9% was found, although the prevalence increases with age *(281)*. In Argentina, congenital infection rates of 0.12% have been described in live births. However, 0.5–11.7% of infants born to sero-positive women have congenitally acquired the infection, although this number is believed to grossly underrepresent the actual number of cases *(279)*.

Maternal parasitemia can lead to placentitis, premature labor, and spontaneous abortions. In vitro studies have indicated that the trypomastigotes can alter cellular actin filaments as a first step to invasion of syncytiotrophoblast cells *(282)*. Congenital infection results in severe defects in the neonate and has a high fatality rate if not treated promptly after birth *(283)*. Unfortunately, anti-parasite therapies are toxic or have unknown toxicity on the fetus, limiting treatment options prior to delivery. However, rapid diagnosis at or prior to birth, with subsequent treatment of the neonate, can greatly reduce the morbidity and mortality associated with congenital infection.

Screening. Routine screening programs for Chagas's disease have been implemented in high-prevalence areas using hemagglutination or ELISA-based methods to detect anti-trypanosomal IgG *(284)*. Assays using crude parasite lysates have lower sensitivities and specificities than newer generation tests using purified antigens and often demonstrate significant cross-reactivity with antigens from *Leishmania* and other parasites *(285,286)*. The need for highly sensitive and specific assays for ensuring safety of the blood supply has led to development of newer ELISAs using recombinant antigens from *T. cruzi*, or synthetic peptides. An assay against recombinant TcF protein has been reported to have a sensitivity of 100% and specificity of 98.94% in screening Brazilian blood donors *(287)* and is superior to assays using synthetic antigens *(288)*. A dipstick assay from InBios (*Trypanosoma* Detect™) uses the TcF protein to detect reactive serum antibody and stands to provide a needed rapid and easy-to-perform test for anti-trypanosomal IgG in an ambulatory setting *(289)*. However, extensive trials comparing the sensitivity and specificity of the dipstick assay with the ELISA in a patient setting, or in pregnant women, have not been published.

Diagnosis. Blood smears provide a cornerstone for diagnosing acute infection by identifying parasites. However, numerous reports have determined that PCR on venipuncture or cord blood has superior sensitivity and equivalent specificity to examination of blood smears for parasites to diagnose acute, chronic, or congenital infection *(290)*. Amplification of kinetoplast minicircle DNA sequences, present in excess of 100,000 copies per cell, have provided the most sensitive means of detection in chronically infected patients, in which the blood parasite burden is low *(291)*. However, availability of appropriate laboratory facilities for performing rigorous amplification reactions for clinical testing and the lack of commercially available kits limit widespread use of such assays where they are most needed.

REFERENCES

1. Primary health care approaches for prevention and control of congenital and genetic disorders (WHO/HGN/WG/00.1). Cairo, Egypt, December 6–8, 1999. http://www.who.int/ncd/hgn/hcprevention.htm#3.4%A0%20Avoiding%20maternal%20infections

2. Palmer AL, Rotbart HA, Tyson RW, Abzug MJ. Adverse effects of maternal enterovirus infection on the fetus and placenta. J Infect Dis 1997;176(6):1437–1444.

3. Strobino BA, Williams CL, Abid S, Chalson R, Spierling P. Lyme disease and pregnancy outcome: a prospective study of two thousand prenatal patients. Am J Obstet Gynecol 1993;169(2 Pt 1):367–374.

4. Abramowsky C, Beyer-Patterson P, Cortinas E. Nonsyphilitic spirochetosis in secondtrimester fetuses. Pediatr Pathol 1991;11(6):827–838.

5. [No authors listed]. Intrauterine West Nile virus infection, New York, 2002. Morb Mortal Wkly Rep 2002;51(50):1135–1136.

6. Edwards JF, Hendricks K. Lack of serologic evidence for an association between Cache Valley virus infection and anencephaly and other neural tube defects in Texas. 1997;3(2):195–197.

7. Mittendorf R, Pryde P, Herschel M, Williams M. Is routine antenatal toxoplasmosis screening justified in the United States? statistical considerations in the application of medical screening tests. Clin Obs Gyn 1999;42(1):163–173.

8. Flajnik MF. Comparative analyses of immunoglobulin genes: surprises and portents. Nat Rev Immunol 2002;2(9):688–698.

9. Notidis E, Heltemes L, Manser T. Dominant, hierarchical induction of peripheral tolerance during foreign antigen-driven B cell development. Immunity 2002;17(3):317–327.

10. OraQuick(tm) Rapid HIV-1 antibody test: summary of safety and effectiveness. Center for Biologics Evaluation and Research, Food and Drug Administration. 2002. Washington, D.C. Available online at: http://www.fda.gov/cber/pmasumm/P010047S.pdf

11. Commission on Laboratory Accreditation. Molecular pathology checklist. College of American Pathologists. 2002. Northfield, IL. Available online at: http://www.cap.org/html/checklist_html/MOL033103.html

12. Olivo P. Transgenic cell lines for detection of animal viruses. Clin Micro Rev 1996;9(3):321–334.

13. Alford CA, Stagno S, Pass RF, et al. Congenital and perinatal cytomegalovirus infections. Rev Infect Dis 1990;12:745–753.

14. Gaytant MA, Steegers EA, Semmekrot BA, Merkus HM, Galama JM. Congenital cytomegalovirus infection: review of the epidemiology and outcome. Obstet Gynecol Surv 2002;57(4):245–256.

15. Fowler KB, Stagno S, Pass RF. Maternal immunity and prevention of congenital cytomegalovirus infection. JAMA 2003;289(8):1008–1011.

16. Stagno, S. Cytomegalovirus. In Remington JS, Klein JO, eds. Infectious Diseases of the Fetus and Newborn, 5th ed. Philadelphia: W. B. Saunders, 2001.

17. Boppana SB, Pass RF, Britt WJ. Virus-specific antibody responses in mothers and their newborn infants with asymptomatic congenital cytomegalovirus infections. J Infect Dis 1993;167(1):72–77.

18. Dahle AJ, Fowler KB, Wright JD, Boppana SB, Britt WJ, Pass RF. Longitudinal investigation of hearing disorders in children with congenital cytomegalovirus. J Am Acad Audiol 2000;11(5):283–290.

19. Weber B, Fall EM, Berger A, Doerr HW. Screening of blood donors for human cytomegalovirus (HCMV) IgG antibody with an enzyme immunoassay using recombinant antigens. J Clin Virol 1999;14(3):173–181.

20. Donner C. Liesnard C, Brancart F, and Rodesch F.. Accuracy of amniotic fluid testing before 21 weeks' gestation in prenatal diagnosis of congenital cytomegalovirus infection. Prenatal Diagn 1994;14: 1055–1059.

21. Lipitz S, Yagel S, Shalev E, Achiron R, Mashiach S, and Schiff E. Prenatal diagnosis of fetal primary cytomegalovirus infection. Obstet Gynecol 1997;89:763–767.

22. Revello MG, Lilleri D, Zavattoni M, Furione M, Middeldorp J, Gerna G. Prenatal diagnosis of congenital human cytomegalovirus infection in amniotic fluid by nucleic acid sequence-based amplification assay. J Clin Microbiol 2003;41(4):1772–1774.

23. Lazzarotto T, Guerra B, Spezzacatena P, et al. Prenatal diagnosis of congenital cytomegalovirus infection. J Clin Microbiol 1998;36:3540–3544.

24. Bodeus M, Hubinont C, Bernard P, Bouckaert A, Thomas K, Goubau P. Prenatal diagnosis of human cytomegalovirus by culture and polymerase chain reaction: 98 pregnancies leading to congenital infection. Prenat Diagn 1999;19(4):314–317.

25. Lazzarotto T, Gabrielli L, Foschini MP, et al. Congenital cytomegalovirus infection in twin pregnancies: viral load in the amniotic fluid and pregnancy outcome. Pediatrics 2003;112(2):e153–e157.

26. Lazzarotto T, Varani S, Guerra B, Nicolosi A, Lanari M, Landini MP. Prenatal indicators of congenital cytomegalovirus infection. J Pediatr 2000;137(1):90–95.

27. Warren WP, Balcarek K, Smith RJ. Comparison of rapid methods of detection of cytomegalovirus in saliva with virus isolation in tissue culture. J Clin Microbiol 1992;30:786–789.

28. Yamamoto AY, Mussi-Pinhata MM, Pinto PC, Figueiredo LT, Jorge SM. Usefulness of blood and urine samples collected on filter paper in detecting cytomegalovirus by the polymerase chain reaction technique. J Virol Methods 2001;97(1–2):159–164.

29. Ordog K, Szendroi A, Szarka K, et al. Perinatal and intrafamily transmission of hepatitis B virus in three generations of a low-prevalence population. J Med Virol 2003;70(2):194–204.

30. Dawar M, Patrick DM, Bigham M, Cook D, Krajden M, Ng H. Impact of universal preadolescent vaccination against hepatitis B on antenatal seroprevalence of hepatitis B markers in British Columbia women. Can Med Assoc J. 200318;168(6):703–704.

31. Langer BC, Frosner GG, von Brunn A. Epidemiological study of viral hepatitis types A, B, C, D and E among Inuits in West Greenland. J Viral Hepat 1997;4(5):339–349.

32. Malcolm RL, Ludwick L, Brookes DL, Hanna JN. The investigation of a "cluster" of hepatitis B in teenagers from an indigenous community in North Queensland. Aust N Z J Public Health 2000; 24(4):353–355.

33. Euler GL, Wooten KG, Baughman AL, Williams WW. Hepatitis B surface antigen prevalence among pregnant women in urban areas: implications for testing, reporting, and preventing perinatal transmission. Pediatrics 2003;111(5 Part 2):1192–1197.
34. Levy M, Koren G. Hepatitis B vaccine in pregnancy: maternal and fetal safety. Am J Perinatol 1991;8(3):227–232.
35. Pavel A, Tirsia E, Maior E, Cristea A. Detrimental effects of hepatitis B virus infection on the development of the product of conception. Virologie 1983;34(1):35–40.
36. Wong S, Chan LY, Yu V, Ho L. Hepatitis B carrier and perinatal outcome in singleton pregnancy. Am J Perinatol 1999;16(9):485–488.
37. [No authors listed]. Program to prevent perinatal hepatitis B virus transmission in a health-maintenance organization:Northern California, 1990–1995. Morb Mortal Wkly Rep 19972;46(17):378–380.
38. Moore L, Bourne AJ, Moore DJ, Preston H, Byard RW. Hepatocellular carcinoma following neonatal hepatitis. Pediatr Pathol Lab Med 1997;17(4):601–610.
39. Robinson WS. Hepadnaviridae. In Mandell GL, Bennett JE, Dolin R, eds. Principles and Practice of Infectious Diseases, 5th ed. Philadelphia: Churchill Livingstone, 2000.
40. Weber B, Bayer A, Kirch P, Schluter V, Schlieper D, Melchior W. Improved detection of hepatitis B virus surface antigen by a new rapid automated assay. J Clin Microbiol 1999;37(8):2639–2647.
41. Weber B, Dengler T, Berger A, Doerr HW, Rabenau H. Evaluation of two new automated assays for hepatitis B virus surface antigen (HBsAg) detection: IMMULITE HBsAg and IMMULITE 2000 HBsAg. J Clin Microbiol. 2003;41(1):135–143.
42. Pfeifer K, Pelzer C, Coleman P, Pope M, Kapprell HP. Early detection of hepatitis B surface antigen: prototype of a new fully automated HBsAg microparticle enzyme immunoassay (MEIA). Clin Lab 2003;49(3–4):161–166.
43. Kfoury Baz EM, Zheng J, Mazuruk K, Van Le A, Peterson DL. Characterization of a novel hepatitis B virus mutant: demonstration of mutation-induced hepatitis B virus surface antigen group specific "a" determinant conformation change and its application in diagnostic assays. Transfus Med 2001;11(5):355–362.
44. Zaaijer HL, Vrielink H, Koot M. Early detection of hepatitis B surface antigen and detection of HBsAg mutants: a comparison of five assays. Vox Sang 2001;81(4):219–221.
45. Previsani N, Lavanchy D. "Hepatitis B vaccines." WHO Department of Communicable Disease Surveillance and Response, CSR (Document WHO/CDS/CSR/LYO/2002.2: Hepatitis B). 2002. Geneva, Switzerland. Available online at http://www.who.int/emc-documents/hepatitis/docs/whocdscsrlyo 20022/surveillance/vaccines.html
46. Zuckerman AJ. Effect of hepatitis B virus mutants on efficacy of vaccination. Lancet 2000;355 (9213):1382–1384.
47. Previsani N, Lavanchy D. "Hepatitis B virus mutants," WHO Department of Communicable Disease Surveillance and Response, CSR (Document WHO/CDS/CSR/LYO/2002.2: Hepatitis B). 2002. Geneva, Switzerland. Available online at http://www.who.int/emc-documents/hepatitis/docs/whocdscsrlyo 20022/surveillance/virus_mutants.html
48. Wilson JN, Nokes DJ, Carman WF. Predictions of the emergence of vaccine-resistant hepatitis B in The Gambia using a mathematical model. Epidemiol Infect 2000;124(2):295–307.
49. ID-B nucleic acid amplification survey final critique. Northfield, IL: College of American Pathologists, 2002.
50. Berger A, Doerr HW, Weber B. Human immunodeficiency virus and hepatitis B virus infection in pregnancy: diagnostic potential of viral genome detection. Intervirology 1998;41(4-5):201–207.
51. Ranger-Rogez S, Alain S, Denis F. Hepatitis viruses: mother to child transmission. Pathol Biol (Paris) 2002;50(9):568–575.
52. Xu DZ, Yan YP, Choi BC, et al. Risk factors and mechanism of transplacental transmission of hepatitis B virus: a case-control study. J Med Virol 2002;67(1):20–26.
53. Batayneh N, Bdour S. Risk of perinatal transmission of hepatitis B virus in Jordan. Infect Dis Obstet Gynecol 2002;10(3):127–132.
54. Crumpacker CS. Hepatitis. In Remington JS, Klein JO, eds. Infectious Diseases of the Fetus and Newborn Infant, 5th ed. Phildelphia: W.B. Saunders, 2001.
55. Qian XH. Monitoring of maternal–fetal hepatitis B virus transmission by molecular hybridization technique Zhonghua Fu Chan Ke Za Zhi. 1992;27(5):259–262, 315.
56. Sterneck M, Kalinina T, Otto S, et al. Neonatal fulminant hepatitis B: structural and functional analysis of complete hepatitis B virus genomes from mother and infant. J Infect Dis 1998;177(5):1378–1381.
57. Tamada K, Kohga M, Takeuchi Y, Masuda E, Hattori K, Kim NF. Serologically silent hepatitis B virus infection in infants. Pediatr Int 2000;42(4):375–379.

58. Wang JS, Zhu QR. Infection of the fetus with hepatitis B e antigen via the placenta. Lancet 2000;355(9208):989.

59. Mazzeo C, Azzaroli F, Giovanelli S, et al. Ten year incidence of HCV infection in northern Italy and frequency of spontaneous viral clearance. Gut 2003;52(7):1030–1034.

60. Yomtovian R, Praprotnim D. Adverse consequences of autologous transfusion practice. In Popovsky MA, ed. Transfusion Reactions, 2nd ed. AABB Press, Bethesda, MD, 2001.

61. Njouom R, Pasquier C, Ayouba A, et al. Hepatitis C virus infection among pregnant women in Yaounde, Cameroon: prevalence, viremia, and genotypes. J Med Virol 2003;69(3):384–390.

62. Romanowski B, Preiksaitis J, Campbell P, Fenton J. Hepatitis C seroprevalence and risk behaviors in patients attending sexually transmitted disease clinics. Sex Transm Dis 2003;30(1):33–38.

63. Agha S, Sherif LS, Allam MA, Fawzy M. Transplacental transmission of hepatitis C virus in HIV-negative mothers. Res Virol 1998;149(4):229–234.

64. Ferrero S, Lungaro P, Bruzzone BM, Gotta C, Bentivoglio G, Ragni N. Prospective study of mother-to-infant transmission of hepatitis C virus: a 10-year survey (1990–2000). Acta Obstet Gynecol Scand 2003;82(3):229–234.

65. Mazza C, Ravaggi A, Rodella A, et al. for the Study Group for Vertical Transmission. Prospective study of mother-to-infant transmission of hepatitis C virus (HCV) infection. J Med Virol 1998;54(1):12–19.

66. De Lamballerie X. Serological and molecular biology screening techniques for HVC infection. Nephrol Dial Transplant 1996;11(Suppl)4:9–11.

67. Lavanchy D, Steinmann J, Moritz A, Frei PC. Evaluation of a new automated third-generation anti-HCV enzyme immunoassay. J Clin Lab Anal 1996;10(5):269–276.

68. Vrielink H, Zaaijer HL, Reesink HW, van der Poel CL, Cuypers HT, Lelie PN. Sensitivity and specificity of three third-generation anti-hepatitis C virus ELISAs. Vox Sang 1995;69(1):14–17.

69. Widell A, Molnegren V, Pieksma F, Calmann M, Peterson J, Lee SR. Detection of hepatitis C core antigen in serum or plasma as a marker of hepatitis C viraemia in the serological window-phase. Transfus Med 2002;12(2):107–113.

70. Conte D, Fraquelli M, Prati D, Colucci A, Minola E. Prevalence and clinical course of chronic hepatitis C virus (HCV) infection and rate of HCV vertical transmission in a cohort of 15,250 pregnant women. Hepatology 2000;31(3):751–755.

71. Kassem AS, el-Nawawy AA, Massoud MN, el-Nazar SY, Sobhi EM. Prevalence of hepatitis C virus (HCV) infection and its vertical transmission in Egyptian pregnant women and their newborns. J Trop Pediatr 2000;46(4):231–233.

72. Healy CM, Cafferkey MT, Conroy A, et al. Outcome of infants born to hepatitis C infected women. Ir J Med Sci 2001;170(2):103–106; discussion 92–93.

73. Wiznia AA, Crane M, Lambert G, Sansary J, Harris A, Solomon L. Zidovudine use to reduce perinatal HIV type 1 transmission in an urban medical center. JAMA 1996;275(19):1504–1506.

74. Prevention of mother to child transmission of HIV: selection and use of nevirapine, technical notes. Document# WHO/HIV_AIDS/2001.03; WHO/RHR/01.21 2003 World Health Organization, Geneva Switzerland. Available online at http://www.who.int/reproductive-health/rtis/nevirapine.htm

75. Mother-to-child transmission of HIV. In Reproductive Tract Infections and Sexually Transmitted Infections Including HIV/AIDS. 2003, World Health Organization, Geneva Switzerland. Available online at http://www.who.int/reproductive-health/rtis/MTCT/index.htm

76. [No authors listed]. HIV testing among pregnant women: United States and Canada, 1998–2001. Morb Mortal Wkly Rep 2002;51(45):1013–1016.

77. Phillips KA, Bayer R, Chen JL. New Centers for Disease Control and Prevention's guidelines on HIV counseling and testing for the general population and pregnant women. J Acquir Immune Defic Syndr 2003;32(2):182–191.

78. Rich JD, Merriman NA, Mylonakis E, et al. Misdiagnosis of HIV infection by HIV-1 plasma viral load testing: a case series. Ann Intern Med 1999;130(1):37–39.

79. Koch WH, Sullivan PS, Roberts C, et al. Evaluation of United States-licensed human immunodeficiency virus immunoassays for detection of group M viral variants. J Clin Microbiol 2001;39(3):1017–1020.

80. Gurtler LG, Zekeng L, Tsague JM, et al. HIV-1 subtype O: epidemiology, pathogenesis, diagnosis, and perspectives of the evolution of HIV. Arch Virol Suppl 1996;11:195–202.

81. Hunt JC, Golden AM, Lund JK, et al. Envelope sequence variability and serologic characterization of HIV type 1 group O isolates from Equatorial Guinea. AIDS Res Hum Retroviruses 1997;13(12):995–1005.

82. de Mendoza C, Lu W, Machuca A, Sainz M, Castilla J, Soriano V. Monitoring the response to antiretroviral therapy in HIV-1 group O infected patients using two new RT-PCR assays. J Med Virol 2001;64(3):217–222.

83. Interpretation and use of the western blot assay for serodiagnosis of human immunodeficiency virus type 1 Infections. Morb Mort Wkly Rep 1989;38(S-7):1–7.

84. Revised guidelines for HIV counseling, testing and referral. Morb Mort Wkly Rep 2001;50:1–58.

85. Davies G, Wilson RD, Desilets V, et al. for the Society of Obstetricians and Gynaecologists of Canada. Amniocentesis and women with hepatitis B, hepatitis C, or human immunodeficiency virus. J Obstet Gynaecol Can 2003;25(2):145–148, 149–152.

86. Natural history, detection and treatment of HIV infection in pregnant women and newborns. In Stoto MA, Almario DA, McCormick MC, eds. Reducing the Odds: Preventing Perinatal Transmission of HIV in the United States. Washington: National Academy Press, 1999.

87. Bremer JW, Lew JF, Cooper E, et al. Diagnosis of infection with human immunodeficiency virus type 1 by a DNA polymerase chain reaction assay among infants enrolled in the Women and Infants Transmission Study. J Pediatr 1996;129(2):198–207.

88. Levine AM. Evaluation and management of HIV-infected women. Ann Intern Med 2002;136(3):228–242.

89. Durant J, Clevenbergh P, Halfon P, et al. Drug-resistance genotyping in HIV-1 therapy: the VIRADAPT randomised controlled trial. Lancet 1999;353(9171):2195–2199.

90. Eshleman SH, Mracna M, Guay LA, et al. Selection and fading of resistance mutations in women and infants receiving nevirapine to prevent HIV-1 vertical transmission (HIVNET 012). AIDS 2001;15(15):1951–1957.

91. Kuritzkes DR, Grant RM, Feorino P, et al. Performance characteristics of the TRUGENE HIV-1 genotyping kit and the opengene DNA sequencing system. J Clin Microbiol 2003;41(4):1594–1599.

92. Wilson JW, Bean P, Robins T, Graziano F, Persing DH. Comparative evaluation of three human immunodeficiency virus genotyping systems: the HIV-GenotypR method, the HIV PRT GeneChip assay, and the HIV-1 RT line probe assay. J Clin Microbiol 2000;38(8):3022–3028.

93. Grant RM, Kuritzkes DR, Johnson VA, et al. Accuracy of the TRUGENE HIV-1 genotyping kit. J Clin Microbiol 2003;41(4):1586–1593.

94. HIV-C: HIV viral load. final critique. CAP Survey 2002. Northfield, IL: College of American Pathologists, 2002.

95. Sturmer M, Doerr HW, Staszewski S, Preiser W. Comparison of nine resistance interpretation systems for HIV-1 genotyping. Antivir Ther 2003;8(3):239–244.

96. Beckerman KP. Pregnancy and prenatal care of women with HIV. In HIV InSite Knowledge Base, 1998. University of California San Francisco, San Francisco CA. Available online at: http://hivinsite.ucsf.edu/InSite.jsp?page=kb-03-01-13

97. Frenkel L. State of the art management of the HIV-infected pregnant woman. In Medscape coverage of the 7th Conference on Retroviruses and Opportunistic Infections. 2003. WebMD Medscape Health Network, New York, NY. Available online at: http://www.medscape.com/viewarticle/420614

98. Gaytant MA, Steegers EA, van Laere M, et al. Seroprevalences of herpes simplex virus type 1 and type 2 among pregnant women in the Netherlands. Sex Transm Dis 2002;29(11):710–714.

99. Crosby RA, DiClemente RJ, Wingood GM, Rose E. Testing for HSV-2 infection among pregnant teens: implications for clinical practice. J Pediatr Adolesc Gynecol 2003;16(1):39–41.

100. Cowan FM, French RS, Mayaud P, et al. Seroepidemiological study of herpes simplex virus types 1 and 2 in Brazil, Estonia, India, Morocco, and Sri Lanka. Sex Transm Infect 2003;79(4):286–290.

101. Hutto C, Arvin A, Jacobs R, et al. Intrauterine herpes simplex virus infections. J Pediatr 1987;110(1):97–101.

102. Prince HE, Ernst CE, Hogrefe WR. Evaluation of an enzyme immunoassay system for measuring herpes simplex virus (HSV) type 1-specific and HSV type 2-specific antibodies. J Clin Lab Anal 2000;14:13–16.

103. Arvaja M, Lehtinen M, Koskela P, Lappalainen M, Paavonen J, Vesikari T. Serological evaluation of herpes simplex virus type 1 and type 2 infections in pregnancy. Sex Transm Infect 1999;75(3):168–171.

104. Roberts SW, Cox SM, Dax J, Wendel GD Jr, Leveno KJ. Genital herpes during pregnancy: no lesions, no cesarean. Obstet Gynecol 1995;85(2):261–264.

105. Rudnick CM, Hoekzema GS. Neonatal herpes simplex virus infections. Am Fam Physician 2002;65(6):1138–1142.

106. Marshall DS, Linfert DR, Draghi A, McCarter YS, Tsongalis GJ. Identification of herpes simplex virus genital infection: comparison of a multiplex PCR assay and traditional viral isolation techniques. Mod Pathol 2001;14(3):152–156.

107. Johnson FB, Visick EM. A rapid culture alternative to the shell-vial method for the detection of herpes simplex virus. Diagn Microbiol Infect Dis 1992;15(8):673–678.

108. Herpes simplex virus (HSV). ARUP's Guide to Clinical Laboratory Testing, ARUP Laboratories, 2002, Salt Lake City, UT.

109. Stabell EC, Olivo PD. Isolation of a cell line for rapid and sensitive histochemical assay for the detection of herpes sinplex virus. J. Virol Methods 1992;38:195–204.

110. Patel N, Kauffmann L, Baniewicz G, Forman M, Evans M, Scholl D. Confirmation of low-titer, herpes simplex virus-positive specimen results by the enzyme-linked virus-inducible system (ELVIS) using PCR and repeat testing. J Clin Microbiol 1999;37(12):3986–3989.

111. Turchek BM, Huang YT. Evaluation of ELVIS HSV ID/typing system for the detection and typing of herpes simplex virus from clinical specimens. J Clin Virol 1999;12(1):65–69.

112. LaRocco MT. Evaluation of an enzyme-linked viral inducible system for the rapid detection of herpes simplex virus. Eur J Clin Microbiol Infect Dis 2000;19(3):233–235.

113. Siegel RS, Gartenhaus RB, Kuzel TM. Human T-cell lymphotropic-I-associated leukemia/lymphoma. Curr Treat Options Oncol 2001;2(4):291–300.

114. Bittencourt AL. Vertical transmission of HTLV-I/II: a review. Rev Inst Med Trop Sao Paulo 1998;40(4):245–251.

115. Denis F, Verdier M, Bonis J. Vertical transmission of HTLV-I. Pathol Biol (Paris) 1992;40(7):714–719.

116. Otigbah C, Kelly A, Aitken C, Norman J, Jeffries D, Erskine KJ. Is HTLV-1 status another antenatal screening test that we need? Br J Obstet Gynaecol 1997;104(2):258–260.

117. Lin BT, Musset M, Szekely AM, et al. Human T-cell lymphotropic virus-1-positive T-cell leukemia/lymphoma in a child report of a case and review of the literature. Arch Pathol Lab Med 1997;121(12):1282–1286.

118. Poljak M, Bednarik J, Rednak K, Seme K, Kristancic L, Celan-Lucu B. Seroprevalence of human T cell leukaemia/lymphoma virus type I (HTLV-I) in pregnant women, patients attending venereological outpatient services and intravenous drug users from Slovenia. Folia Biol (Praha) 1998;44(1):23–25.

119. Hino S, Katamine S, Miyata H, Tsuji Y, Yamabe T, Miyamoto T. Primary prevention of HTLV-I in Japan. J Acquir Immune Defic Syndr Hum Retrovirol 1996;13 Suppl 1:S199–S203.

120. dos Santos JI, Lopes MA, Deliege-Vasconcelos E, et al. Seroprevalence of HIV, HTLV-I/II and other perinatally-transmitted pathogens in Salvador, Bahia. Rev Inst Med Trop Sao Paulo 1995;37(4):343–348.

121. Thorstensson R, Albert J, Andersson S. Strategies for diagnosis of HTLV-I and -II. Transfusion 2002;42(6):780–791.

122. Mahieux R, Horal P, Mauclère P, et al. Human T-cell lymphotropic virus type 1 gag indeterminate western blot patterns in Central Africa: relationship to plasmodium falciparum infection. J Clin Microbiol 2000;38(11):4049–4057.

123. Sato A, Isaka Y, Morita F, et al. Human sera from varicella-zoster virus (VZV) infections cross-react with human T cell leukaemia virus type 1 (HTLV-1): common epitopes in VZV gene 22 protein and HTLV-1 p19 gag protein. J Gen Virol 1992;73:2969–2973.

124. Karopoulos A, Silvester C, Dax EM. A comparison of the performance of nine commercially available anti-HTLV-I screening assays. J Virol Methods 1993;45(1):83–91.

125. Gilbert GL. 1: Infections in pregnant women. Med J Aust 2002;176(5):229–236.

126. Török TJ. Human parvovirus B19. In Remington JS, and Klein JO, eds. Infections of the Fetus and Newborn Infant, 5th ed. Philadelphia: W.B. Saunders, 2001.

127. Gallinella G, Zuffi E, Gentilomi G, et al. Relevance of B19 markers in serum samples for a diagnosis of parvovirus B19-correlated diseases. J Med Virol 2003;71(1):135–139.

128. Thomas HI, Barrett E, Hesketh LM, Wynne A, Morgan-Capner P. Simultaneous IgM reactivity by EIA against more than one virus in measles, parvovirus B19 and rubella infection. J Clin Virol 1999;14(2):107–118.

129. Zerbini M, Gallinella G, Cricca M, Bonvicini F, Musiani M. Diagnostic procedures in B19 infection. Pathol Biol (Paris) 2002;50(5):332–328.

130. Manaresi E, Gallinella G, Zuffi E, Bonvicini F, Zerbini M, Musiani M. Diagnosis and quantitative evaluation of parvovirus B19 infections by real-time PCR in the clinical laboratory. J Med Virol 2002;67(2):275–281.

131 Dong ZW, Zhou SY, Li Y, Liu RM. Detection of a human parvovirus intrauterine infection with the polymerase chain reaction. J Reprod Med 2000;45(5):410–412.

132. Rodis JF, Borgida AF, Wilson M, et al. Management of parvovirus infection in pregnancy and outcomes of hydrops: a survey of members of the Society of Perinatal Obstetricians. Am J Obstet Gynecol 1998;179(4):985–988.

133. von Kaisenberg CS, Jonat W. Fetal parvovirus B19 infection. Ultrasound Obstet Gynecol 2001;18(3): 280–288.

134. Kimberlin, DW. Rubella virus. In Richman DD, Whitley RJ, Hayden FG, eds., Clinical Virology, 2nd ed. Washington DC: ASM Press, 2002.

135. Diepersloot RJA, Dunnewold-Hoekstra H, Kruit-den Hollander J, and Vlaspolder F. Antenatal screening for hepatitis B and antibodies to toxoplasma gondii and rubella virus: evaluation of two commercial immunoassay systems. Clin Diag Lab Immun 2001;8(4):785–787.

136. Mellinger AK, Cragan JD, Atkinson WL, et al. High incidence of congenital rubella syndrome after a rubella outbreak. Pediatr Infect Dis J 1995;14(7):573–578.

137. Cooper LZ, Preblud SR, Alford CA. Rubella. In, Infections Diseases of the Fetus and Newbord Infant, 5th ed. Philadelphia: W.B. Saunders, 2001;pp.347–375.

138. S-C diagnostic immunology; CAP survey 2002. Deerfield IL: College of American Pathologists, 2002.

139. Wampole Laboratories Rubella IgG ELISA. [Product insert] Cranbury, NJ: Wampole Laboratories, 1996.

140. Best JM, O'Shea S, Tipples G, et al. Interpretation of rubella serology in pregnancy: pitfalls and problems. Br Med J 2002;325(7356):147–148.

141. Thomas HIJ, Barrett E, Hesketh LM, Wynne A, Morgan-Capner P. Simultaneous IgM reactivity by EIA against more than one virus in measles, parvovirus B19 and rubella infection. J Clin Virol 1999;14:107–118.

142. Banatvala JE, Best JM, O'Shea S, Dudgeon JA. Persistence of rubella antibodies following vaccination: detection of viremia following experimental challenge. Rev Infect Dis 1985;7(suppl 1):S86–S90.

143. Thomas HIJ, Morgan-Capner P, Roberts A, Hesketh L. Persistent rubella-specific IgM reactivity in the absence of recent primary rubella and rubella reinfection. J Med Virol 1992;36:188–192.

144. Hudson P, Morgan-Capner P. Evaluation of fifteen commercial enzyme immunoassays for the detection of rubella-specific IgM. Clin Diagn Virol 1996;5:21–26.

145. Nedeljkovic J, Jovanovic T, Oker-Blom C. Maturation of IgG avidity to individual rubella virus structural proteins. J Clin Virol 2001;22(1):47–54.

146. Pustowoit B, Liebert UG. Predictive value of serological tests in rubella virus infection during pregnancy. Intervirol 1998;41(4–5):170–177.

147. Rubella IgG avidity assay. [product insert]. Rivoli, Italy: Tosoh Corporation, 2003. Available online at http://www.tosohbioscience.it/data/91095.htm

148. Gutierrez J, Rodriguez MJ, De Ory F, Piedrola G, Maroto MC. Reliability of low-avidity IgG and of IgA in the diagnosis of primary infection by rubella virus with adaptation of a commercial test. J Clin Lab Anal 1999;13(1):1–4.

149. Akingbade D, Cohen BJ, Brown DW. Detection of low-avidity immunoglobulin G in oral fluid samples: new approach for rubella diagnosis and surveillance. Clin Diagn Lab Immunol 2003;10(1):189–190.

150. Lie SO, Skrede S, Steen-Johnsen J, Flugsrud L. Congenital rubella: clinical, immunological and virological studies on three cases. Scand J Infect Dis 1970;2(2):145–149.

151. Gershon AA, Silverstein SJ. Vericella-zoster virus in ASM Press, clinical Virology, 2nd ed. Richman DD, Whitley RJ, Hayden FG, eds. Washington D.C.: ASM Press, 2002.

152. Sauerbrei A, Wutzler P. The congenital varicella syndrome. J Perinatol 2000;20(8 Pt 1):548–554.

153. Isada NB, Paar DP, Johnson MP, et al. In utero diagnosis of congenital varicella zoster virus infection by chorionic villus sampling and polymerase chain reaction. Am J Obstet Gynecol 1991;165(6 Pt 1): 1727–1730.

154. VR3-A: virology antibody detection. CAP Survey Results 2002. College of American Pathologists, 2002.

155. DIAMEDIX™ Immunosimplicity™ VZV-IgG test kit, [product insert]. Diamedix Corporation, Miami, FL, 2000.

156. Doern GV, Robbie L, St Amand R. Comparison of the Vidas and Bio-Whittaker enzyme immunoassays for detecting IgG reactive with varicella-zoster virus and mumps virus. Diagn Microbiol Infect Dis 1997;28(1):31–34.

157. Sauerbrei A, Eichhorn U, Schacke M, Wutzler P. Laboratory diagnosis of herpes zoster. J Clin Virol 1999;14(1):31–36.

158. Dahl H, Marcoccia J, Linde A. Antigen detection: the method of choice in comparison with virus isolation and serology for laboratory diagnosis of herpes zoster in human immunodeficiency virus-infected patients. J Clin Microbiol 1997;35(2):347–349.

159. Perez JL, Garcia A, Niubo J, Salva J, Podzamczer D, Martin R. Comparison of techniques and evaluation of three commercial monoclonal antibodies for laboratory diagnosis of varicella-zoster virus in mucocutaneous specimens. J Clin Microbiol 1994;32(6):1610–1613.

160. Weidmann M, Meyer-Konig U, Hufert FT. Rapid detection of herpes simplex virus and varicella-zoster virus infections by real-time PCR. J Clin Microbiol 2003;41(4):1565–1568.

161. Mouly F, Mirlesse V, Meritet JF, et al. Prenatal diagnosis of fetal varicella-zoster virus infection with polymerase chain reaction of amniotic fluid in 107 cases. Am J Obstet Gynecol 1997;177(4):894–898.

162. Kustermann A, Zoppini C, Tassis B, Della Morte M, Colucci G, Nicolini U. Prenatal diagnosis of congenital varicella infection. Prenat Diagn 1996;16(1):71–74.

163. Gaydos CA, Howell MR, Quinn TC, McKee KT Jr, Gaydos JC. Sustained high prevalence of Chlamydia trachomatis infections in female army recruits. Sex Transm Dis 2003;30(7):539–544.

164. Farley TA, Cohen DA, Elkins W. Asymptomatic sexually transmitted diseases: the case for screening. Prev Med 2003;36(4):502–509.

165. Jensen IP, Fogh H, Prag J. Diagnosis of Chlamydia trachomatis infections in a sexually transmitted disease clinic: evaluation of a urine sample tested by enzyme immunoassay and polymerase chain reaction in comparison with a cervical and/or a urethral swab tested by culture and polymerase chain reaction. Clin Microbiol Infect 2003;9(3):194–201.

166. Mardh PA. Influence of infection with Chlamydia trachomatis on pregnancy outcome, infant health and life-long sequelae in infected offspring. Best Pract Res Clin Obstet Gynaecol 2002;16(6):847–864.

167. Numazaki K, Asanuma H, Niida Y. Chlamydia trachomatis infection in early neonatal period. BMC Infect Dis 2003;3(1):2. Epub 2003 Apr 04.

168. Gonorrhea and chlamydial infections. ACOG Technical Bulletin, No. 190. Washington DC: American College of Obstetricians and Gynecologists, 1994.

169. Screening tests to detect *Chlamydia trachomatis* and *Neisseria gonorrhoeae* infections; 2002. Morb Mort Wkly Rep 2002;15(RR-15):1–39.

170. Zenilman JM, Miller WC, Gaydos C, Rogers SM, Turner CF. LCR testing for gonorrhoea and chlamydia in population surveys and other screenings of low prevalence populations: coping with decreased positive predictive value. Sex Transm Infect 2003;79(2):94–97.

171. Pace™2 Specimen Collection Guide for Chlamydia trachomatis and Neisseria gonorrhea. San Diego: Gen-Probe Corporation 1998.

172. Pfaller, M. Molecular approaches to diagnosing and managing infectious diseases: practicality and costs. Emerg Infect Dis. 2001;7(2):312–318.

173. Wylie JL, Moses S, Babcock R, Jolly A, Giercke S, Hammond G. Comparative evaluation of chlamydiazyme, PACE 2, and AMP-CT assays for detection of Chlamydia trachomatis in endocervical specimens. J Clin Microbiol 1998;36(12):3488–3491.

174. Modarress KJ, Cullen AP, Jaffurs WJ Sr, et al. Detection of Chlamydia trachomatis and Neisseria gonorrhoeae in swab specimens by the Hybrid Capture II and PACE 2 nucleic acid probe tests. Sex Transm Dis 1999;26(5):303–308.

175. Black CM, Marrazzo J, Johnson RE, et al. Head-to-head multicenter comparison of DNA probe and nucleic acid amplification tests for Chlamydia trachomatis infection in women performed with an improved reference standard. J Clin Microbiol 2002;40(10):3757–3763.

176. Nabarro JM, Grant AM, Simon RD, Beral V, Catterall RD. Screening for gonorrhoea in a central London family planning clinic. Fertil Contracept 1978;2(1):1–4.

177. Akerele J, Abhulimen P, Okonofua F. Prevalence of asymptomatic genital infection among pregnant women in Benin City, Nigeria. Afr J Reprod Health 2002;6(3):93–97.

178. Oppenheimer EH, Winn KJ. Fetal gonorrhea with deep tissue infection occurring in utero. Pediatrics 1982;69(1):74–76.

179. Elliot B, Brunham RC, Laga M, et al. Maternal gonococcal infection as a preventable risk factor for low birth weight. J Infect Dis 1990;161:531–536.

180. [No authors listed] Ophthalmia neonatorum. Afr Health. 1995;17(5):30.

181. Allard R, Robert J, Turgeon P, Lepage Y. Predictors of asymptomatic gonorrhea among patients seen by private practitioners. Can Med Assoc J 1985;133:1135–1139, 1146.

182. Rosenthal GE, Mettler G, Pare S, et al. A new diagnostic index for predicting cervical infection with either Chlamydia trachomatis or Neisseria gonorrhoeae. J Gen Intern Med 1990;5:319–326.

183. ACOG technical bulletin: Gonorrhea and chlamydial infections No. 190. Washington, DC: American College of Obstetricians and Gynecologists, 1994.

184. 1998 guidelines for treatment of sexually transmitted diseases. Morb Mort Wkly Rep 1998;47(RR-1): 1–118.

185. Carroll KC, Aldeen WE, Morrison M, Anderson R, Lee D, Mottice S. Evaluation of the Abbott LCx ligase chain reaction assay for detection of Chlamydia trachomatis and Neisseria gonorrhoeae in urine and genital swab specimens from a sexually transmitted disease clinic population. J Clin Microbiol 1998;36(6):1630–1633.

186. Darwin LH, Cullen AP, Arthur PM, et al. Comparison of Digene hybrid capture 2 and conventional culture for detection of Chlamydia trachomatis and Neisseria gonorrhoeae in cervical specimens. J Clin Microbiol 2002;40(2):641–644.

187. Van Der Pol B, Williams JA, Smith NJ, et al. Evaluation of the Digene Hybrid Capture II Assay with the Rapid Capture System for detection of Chlamydia trachomatis and Neisseria gonorrhoeae. J Clin Microbiol 2002;40(10):3558–3564.

188. van Doornum GJ, Schouls LM, Pijl A, Cairo I, Buimer M, Bruisten S. Comparison between the LCx Probe system and the COBAS AMPLICOR system for detection of Chlamydia trachomatis and Neisseria gonorrhoeae infections in patients attending a clinic for treatment of sexually transmitted diseases in Amsterdam, The Netherlands. J Clin Microbiol 2001;39(3):829–835.

189. Gonococcal isolate surveillance report, sexually transmitted disease surveillance 2001 Supplement. Atlanta, GA: Department of Health and Human Services, Centers for Disease Control 2001. Available online at: http://www.cdc.gov/std/GISP2001/

190. Neisseria species and Moraxella catarrhalis. In Diagnostic Microbiology, 5th ed, Koneman EW, Allen SD, Janda WM, Schreckenberger PC, Winn CW, eds., Philadelphia: Lippincott, 1997.

191. Leung TN, Cheung KL, Wong F. Congenital listeriosis: case reports and review of literature. Asia Oceania J Obstet Gynaecol 1994;20(2):173–177.

192. Voelker R. Listeriosis outbreak prompts action—finally. JAMA 2002;288(21):2675–2676.

193. The aerobic Gram positive bacilli. In Diagnostic Microbiology, 5th ed. Koneman EW, Allen SD, Janda WM, Schreckenberger PC, Winn CW, eds., Philadelphia: Lippincott 1997.

194. Svare J, Andersen LF, Langhoff-Roos J, Madsen H, Bruun B. Maternal-fetal listeriosis: 2 case reports. Gynecol Obstet Invest 1991;31(3):179–181.

195. Tappero JW, Schuchat A, Deaver KA, Mascola L, Wenger JD, for the Listeriosis Study Group. Reduction in the incidence of human listeriosis in the United States: effectiveness of prevention efforts? JAMA 1995;273(14):1118–1122.

196. Mazor M, Froimovich M, Lazer S, Maymon E, Glezerman M. Listeria monocytogenes: the role of transabdominal amniocentesis in febrile patients with preterm labor. Arch Gynecol Obstet 1992;252(2):109–112.

197. Benhaim Y, Aucouturier JS, Hillion Y, Moulies ME, Ville Y. The role of amniocentesis in the management of chorioamnionitis with Listeria monocytogenes. J Gynecol Obstet Biol Reprod (Paris) 2003;32(1):39–42.

198. Case records of the Massachusetts General Hospital. Weekly clinicopathological exercises, Case 15-1997: Respiratory distress and seizure in a neonate. N Engl J Med 1997;336(20):1439–1446

199. Lubani MM, Dudin KI, Sharda DC, et al. Neonatal brucellosis. Eur J Pediatr 1988;147(5):520–522.

200. Roll C, Schmid EN, Menken U, Hanssler L. Fatal Salmonella enteritidis sepsis acquired prenatally in a premature infant. Obstet Gynecol 1996;88(4 Pt 2):692–693.

201. Chin KC, Simmonds EJ, Tarlow MJ. Neonatal typhoid fever. Arch Dis Child 1986;61(12):1228–1230.

202. Rebarber A, Star Hampton B, Lewis V, Bender S. Shigellosis complicating preterm premature rupture of membranes resulting in congenital infection and preterm delivery. Obstet Gynecol 2002;100(5 Pt 2):1063–1065.

203. Wong SN, Tam AY, Yuen KY. Campylobacter infection in the neonate: case report and review of the literature. Pediatr Infect Dis J 1990;9(9):665–669.

204. Lee CB, Brunham, RC, Sherman E, Hardin CK. Epidemiology of an outbreak of infectious syphilis in Manitoba. Am J Epidemiol 1987;125:277–283.

205. Hollier LM, Harstad TW, Sanchez PJ, Twickler DM, Wendel GD Jr. Fetal syphilis: clinical and laboratory characteristics. Obstet Gynecol 2001;97(6):947–953.

206. Tramont EC. *Treponema pallidum*. In Mandell GL, Bennett JE, Dolin R, eds., Principles and Practice of Infectious Diseases, 5th ed., vol. 2. Philadelphia: Churchill Livingston, 2000.

207. Ingall D, Sánchez PJ. Syphilis. In Remington JS, Klein JO, eds., Infectious Diseases of the Fetus and Newborn 5th ed. Philadelphia: W.B. Saunders, 2001.

208. Sullivan EA, Abel M, Tabrizi S, et al. Prevalence of sexually transmitted infections among antenatal women in Vanuatu, 1999–2000. Sex Transm Dis 2003;30(4):362–366.

209. Cho YH, Kim HO, Lee JB, Lee MG. Syphilis prevalence has rapidly decreased in South Korea. Sex Transm Infect 2003;79(4):323–324.

210. Sellami A, Kharfi M, Youssef S, et al. Epidemiologic profile of sexually transmitted diseases (STD) through a specialized consultation of STD. Tunis Med 2003;81(3):162–166.

211. Congenital syphilis: United States, 2000. Morb Mort Wkly Rep 2001;50(27):573–577.

212. Risser JM, Hwang LY, Risser WL, Hollins L, Paffel J. The epidemiology of syphilis in the waning years of an epidemic: Houston, Texas, 1991–1997. Sex Transm Dis 1999;26(3):121–126.

213. Lee MJ, Hallmark RJ, Frenkel LM, Del Priore G. Maternal syphilis and vertical perinatal transmission of human immunodeficiency virus type-1 infection. Int J Gynaecol Obstet 1998;63(3):247–252.

214. Hollier LM, Harstad TW, Sanchez PJ, Twickler DM, Wendel GD Jr. Fetal syphilis: clinical and laboratory characteristics. Obstet Gynecol 2001;97(6):947–953.

215. Fitzgerald DW, Behets F, Preval J, Schulwolf L, Bommi V, Chaillet P. Decreased congenital syphilis incidence in Haiti's rural Artibonite region following decentralized prenatal screening. Am J Public Health 2003;93(3):444–446.

216. Wendel GD Jr, Sheffield JS, Hollier LM, Hill JB, Ramsey PS, Sanchez PJ. Treatment of syphilis in pregnancy and prevention of congenital syphilis. Clin Infect Dis 2002;35(suppl 2):S200–S209.

217. Tikhonova L, Salakhov E, Southwick K, Shakarishvili A, Ryan C, Hillis S. Congenital syphilis in the Russian Federation: magnitude, determinants, and consequences. Sex Transm Infect 2003;79(2):106–110.

218. Larkin JA, Lit L, Toney J, Haley JA. Recognizing and treating syphilis in pregnancy. Medscape Womens Health 1998;3(1):5.

219. Laboratory diagnosis of syphilis. In Canadian STD Guidelines, 1998 ed. Ottawa: Centre for Infectious Disease Prevention and Control, 1998, pp. 65–68.

220. Castro R, Prieto ES, Santo I, Azevedo J, Exposto Fda L. Evaluation of an enzyme immunoassay technique for detection of antibodies against Treponema pallidum. J Clin Microbiol 2003;41(1):250–253.

221. Spirochetal Infections. In Diagnostic Microbiology, 5th ed. Koneman EW, Allen SD, Janda WM, Schreckenberger PC, Winn WC, eds. Philadelphia: Lippincott, 1997.

222. Cade JE, Boozer CH, Leigh JE. Seropositivity of the rapid plasma reagin (RPR) test in a dental school patient population: a retrospective study. J Public Health Dent 2003;63(1):61–63.

223. el-Zaatari MM, Martens MG, Anderson GD. Incidence of the prozone phenomenon in syphilis serology. Obstet Gynecol 1994;84(4):609–612.

224. Koskela P, Vaarala O, Makitalo R, Palosuo T, Aho K. Significance of false positive syphilis reactions and anticardiolipin antibodies in a nationwide series of pregnant women. J Rheumatol 1988;15(1):70–73.

225. Gwanzura L, Latif A, Bassett M, Machekano R, Katzenstein DA, Mason PR. Syphilis serology and HIV infection in Harare, Zimbabwe. Sex Transm Infect 1999;75(6):426–430.

226. Leder AN, Flansbaum B, Zandman-Goddard G, Asherson R, Shoenfeld Y. Antiphospholipid syndrome induced by HIV. Lupus 2001;10(5):370–374.

227. Koskela P, Vaarala O, Makitalo R, Palosuo T, Aho K. Significance of false positive syphilis reactions and anticardiolipin antibodies in a nationwide series of pregnant women. J Rheumatol 1988;15(1):70–73.

228. Nathan L, Bohman VR, Sanchez PJ, Leos NK, Twickler DM, Wendel GD Jr. In utero infection with Treponema pallidum in early pregnancy. Prenat Diagn 1997;17(2):119–123.

229. Grimprel E, Sanchez PJ, Wendel GD, et al. Use of polymerase chain reaction and rabbit infectivity testing to detect Treponema pallidum in amniotic fluid, fetal and neonatal sera, and cerebrospinal fluid. J Clin Microbiol 1991;29(8):1711–1718.

230. Burstain JM, Grimpel E, Lukehart SA, Norgard MV, Radolf JD. Sensitive detection of Treponema pallidum by using the polymerase chain reaction. J Clin Microbiol 1991;29(1):62–69.

231. Nathan L, Bohman VR, Sanchez PJ, Leos NK, Twickler DM, Wendel GD Jr. In utero infection with Treponema pallidum in early pregnancy. Prenat Diagn 1997;17(2):119–123.

232. Genest DR, Choi-Hong SR, Tate JE, Qureshi F, Jacques SM, Crum C. Diagnosis of congenital syphilis from placental examination: comparison of histopathology, Steiner stain, and polymerase chain reaction for Treponema pallidum DNA. Hum Pathol. 1996;27(4):366–372.

233. Olowu JA, Sowunmi A, Abohweyere AE. Congenital malaria in a hyperendemic area: a revisit. Afr J Med Med Sci 2000;29(3-4):211–213.

234. Ladner J, Leroy V, Simonon A, et al. for the Pregnancy and HIV Study Group (EGE). HIV infection, malaria, and pregnancy: a prospective cohort study in Kigali, Rwanda. Am J Trop Med Hyg 2002;66(1):56–60.

235. Hung le Q, Vries PJ, Giao PT,. Control of malaria: a successful experience from Viet Nam. Bull World Health Organ 2002;80(8):660–666.

236. Dorman EK, Shulman CE, Kingdom J, et al. Impaired uteroplacental blood flow in pregnancies complicated by falciparum malaria. Ultrasound Obstet Gynecol 2002;19(2):165–170.

237. Achur RN, Valiyaveettil M, Alkhalil A, Ockenhouse CF, Gowda DC. Characterization of proteoglycans of human placenta and identification of unique chondroitin sulfate proteoglycans of the intervillous spaces that mediate the adherence of Plasmodium falciparum-infected erythrocytes to the placenta. J Biol Chem 2000;275(51):40344–40356.

238. Leke RF, Djokam RR, Mbu R, et al. Detection of the Plasmodium falciparum antigen histidine-rich protein 2 in blood of pregnant women: implications for diagnosing placental malaria. J Clin Microbiol 1999;37(9):2992–2996.

239. Menendez C, Ordi J, Ismail MR, et al. The impact of placental malaria on gestational age and birth weight. J Infect Dis 2000;181(5):1740–1745.

240. Shulman CE, Dorman EK, Cutts F, et al. Intermittent sulphadoxine-pyrimethamine to prevent severe anaemia secondary to malaria in pregnancy: a randomised placebo-controlled trial. Lancet 1999;353(9153):632–636.

241. Parise ME, Ayisi JG, Nahlen BL, et al. Efficacy of sulfadoxine-pyrimethamine for prevention of placental malaria in an area of Kenya with a high prevalence of malaria and human immunodeficiency virus infection. Am J Trop Med Hyg 1998;59(5):813–822.

242. Malaria: case management update. Harare, Zimbabwe: WHO-SMAC, June 2003.

243. Garcia, L. Malaria and babesiosis. In Diagnostic Medical Parasitology, 4th ed. Washington, DC: ASM Press, 2001.

244. Keiser J, Utzinger J, Premji Z, Yamagata Y, Singer BH. Acridine orange for malaria diagnosis: its diagnostic performance, its promotion and implementation in Tanzania, and the implications for malaria control. Ann Trop Med Parasitol 2002;96(7):643–654.

245. Htut Y, Aye KH, Han KT, Kyaw MP, Shimono K, Okada S. Feasibility and limitations of acridine orange fluorescence technique using a malaria diagnosis microscope in Myanmar. Acta Med Okayama 2002;56(5):219–222.

246. Kilian AH, Kabagambe G, Byamukama W, Langi P, Weis P, von Sonnenburg F. Application of the ParaSight-F dipstick test for malaria diagnosis in a district control program. Acta Trop 1999;72(3): 281–293.

247. Richardson DC, Ciach M, Zhong KJ, Crandall I, Kain KC. Evaluation of the Makromed dipstick assay versus PCR for diagnosis of Plasmodium falciparum malaria in returned travelers. J Clin Microbiol 2002;40(12):4528–4530.

248. Grobusch MP, Hanscheid T, Gobels K, Comparison of three antigen detection tests for diagnosis and follow-up of falciparum malaria in travellers returning to Berlin, Germany. Parasitol Res 2003;89(5): 354–357.

249. Coleman RE, Maneechai N, Ponlawat A, et al. Short report: failure of the OptiMAL rapid malaria test as a tool for the detection of asymptomatic malaria in an area of Thailand endemic for Plasmodium falciparum and P. vivax. Am J Trop Med Hyg 2002;67(6):563–565.

250. Cattamanchi A, Kyabayinze D, Hubbard A, Rosenthal PJ, Dorsey G. Distinguishing recrudescence from reinfection in a longitudinal antimalarial drug efficacy study: comparison of results based on genotyping of msp-1, msp-2, and glurp. Am J Trop Med Hyg 2003;68(2):133–139.

251. Mockenhaupt FP, Ulmen U, von Gaertner C, Bedu-Addo G, Bienzle U. Diagnosis of placental malaria. J Clin Microbiol 2002;40(1):306–308.

252. Patsoula E, Spanakos G, Sofianatou D, Parara M, Vakalis NC. A single-step, PCR-based method for the detection and differentiation of Plasmodium vivax and P. falciparum. Ann Trop Med Parasitol 2003;97(1):15–21.

253. Padley D, Moody AH, Chiodini PL, Saldanha J. Use of a rapid, single-round, multiplex PCR to detect malarial parasites and identify the species present. Ann Trop Med Parasitol 2003;97(2):131–137.

254. Kamwendo DD, Dzinjalamala FK, Snounou G, et al. Plasmodium falciparum: PCR detection and genotyping of isolates from peripheral, placental, and cord blood of pregnant Malawian women and their infants.Trans R Soc Trop Med Hyg 2002;96(2):145–149.

255. Gagne SS. Prim. toxoplasmosis. Care Update Ob Gyns 2001;8(3):122–126.
256 Remington JS, LcLeaod R, Thulliez P, Desmonts G. Toxoplasmosis. In Remington JS and Klein JO, eds., Infectious Diseases of the Infant and Newborn, 5th ed. Philadelphia: W.B. Sauders, 2001.
257. Sengbusch HG, Sengbusch LA. Toxoplasma antibody prevalence in veterinary personnel and a selected population not exposed to cats. Am J Epidemiol 1976;103(6):595–597.
258. Lings S, Lander F, Lebech M. Antimicrobial antibodies in Danish slaughterhouse workers and greenhouse workers. Int Arch Occup Environ Health 1994;65(6):405–409.
259. Toxoplasma IgG enzyme immunoassay test kit [product insert]. Miami: Diamedix Corporation 1998.
260. Pellouxa H, Bruna E, Vernetb G, et al. Determination of anti-Toxoplasma gondii immunoglobulin G avidity: adaptation to the vidas system (bioMérieux). Diagn Microbiol Infect Dis. 1998;32(2):69–73.
261. Beghetto E, Pucci A, Minenkova O, et al. Identification of a human immunodominant B-cell epitope within the GRA1 antigen of Toxoplasma gondii by phage display of cDNA libraries. Int J Parasitol 2001;31(14):1659–1668.
262. Li S, Galvan G, Araujo FG, Suzuki Y, Remington JS, Parmley S. Serodiagnosis of recently acquired Toxoplasma gondii infection using an enzyme-linked immunosorbent assay with a combination of recombinant antigens. Clin Diagn Lab Immunol 2000;7(5):781–787.
263. Lecordier L, Fourmaux MP, Mercier C, Dehecq E, Masy E, Cesbron-Delauw MF. Enzyme-linked immunosorbent assays using the recombinant dense granule antigens GRA6 and GRA1 of Toxoplasma gondii for detection of immunoglobulin G antibodies. Clin Diagn Lab Immunol 2000;7(4):607–611.
264. Dao A, Fortier B. Evaluation of the Immulite 2000 Toxoplasma quantitative IgG and Toxoplasma IgM for the diagnosis of human toxoplasmosis. Ann Biol Clin (Paris) 2001;59(2):157–164.
265. Decoster A, Lecolier B. Bicentric evaluation of Access Toxo immunoglobulin M (IgM) and IgG assays and IMx toxo IgM and IgG assays and comparison with Platelia Toxo IgM and IgG assays. J Clin Microbiol 1996;34(7):1606–1609.
266. Jenum PA, Stray-Pedersen B, Melby KK, et al. Eng J. Incidence of Toxoplasma gondii infection in 35,940 pregnant women in Norway and pregnancy outcome for infected women. J Clin Microbiol 1998;36(10):2900–2906.
267. Burlington DB. FDA public health advisory: limitations of toxoplasma IgM commercial test kits. Washington DC: Food and Drug Administration, 1997. Available online at: http://www.fda.gov/cdrh/toxopha.html
268. Konishi E. Naturally occurring immunoglobulin M antibodies to Toxoplasma gondii in Japanese populations. Parasitology. 1991;102 Pt 2:157–162.
269. Jenum PA, Stray-Pedersen B. Development of specific immunoglobulins G, M, and A following primary Toxoplasma gondii infection in pregnant women. J Clin Microbiol 1998;36(10):2907–2913.
270. Sabin AB, Feldman HA. Dyes as microchemical indicators of a new immunity phenomenon affecting a protozoan parasite (toxoplasma). Science 1948;108:660–663.
271. Dando C, Gabriel KE, Remington JS, Parmley SF. Simple and efficient method for measuring antitoxoplasma immunoglobulin antibodies in human sera using complement-mediated lysis of transgenic tachyzoites expressing beta-galactosidase. J Clin Microbiol 2001;39(6):2122–2125.
272. Alvarado-Esquivel C, Sethi S, Janitschke K, Hahn H, Liesenfeld O. Comparison of two commercially available avidity tests for toxoplasma-specific IgG antibodies. Arch Med Res 2002;33(6):520–523.
273. Sensini A, Pascoli S, Marchetti D, et al. IgG avidity in the serodiagnosis of acute Toxoplasma gondii infection: a multicenter study. Clin Microbiol Infect 1996;2(1):25–29.
274. Montoya JG, Liesenfeld O, Kinney S, Press C, Remington JS. VIDAS test for avidity of Toxoplasma-specific immunoglobulin G for confirmatory testing of pregnant women. J Clin Microbiol 2002;40(7):2504–2508.
275. Hohlfeld P, Daffos F, Costa JM, Thulliez P, Forestier F, Vidaud M. Prenatal diagnosis of congenital toxoplasmosis with a polymerase-chain-reaction test on amniotic fluid. N Engl J Med 1994;331(11):695–699.
276. Reischl U, Bretagne S, Kruger D, Ernault P, Costa JM. Comparison of two DNA targets for the diagnosis of toxoplasmosis by real-time PCR using fluorescence resonance energy transfer hybridization probes. BMC Infect Dis 2003;3(1):7.
277. Robert-Gangneux F, Gavinet MF, Ancelle T, Raymond J, Tourte-Schaefer C, Dupouy-Camet J. Value of prenatal diagnosis and early postnatal diagnosis of congenital toxoplasmosis: retrospective study of 110 cases. J Clin Microbiol 1999;37(9):2893–2898.
278. Leiby DA, Read EJ, Hall HJ, et al. Detection of antibodies to Trypanosoma cruzi among blood donors in the southwestern and western United States. II. Evaluation of a supplements enzyme immunoassay

and radioimmunoprecipitation assay for confirmation of seroreactivity. Transfusion 1995;35: 219–225.

279. Gurtler RE, Segura EL, Cohen JE. Congenital transmission of Trypanosoma cruzi infection in Argentina. Emerg Infect Dis 2003;9(1):29–32.

280. Gürtler RE, Chuit R, Cecere MC, Castañera MB, Cohen JE, Segura EL. Household prevalence of seropositivity for Trypanosoma cruzi in three rural villages in northwest Argentina: environmental, demographic, and entomologic associations. Am J Trop Med Hyg 1998;59:741–749.

281. Reiche EM, Morimoto HK, Farias GN, et al. Prevalence of American trypanosomiasis, syphilis, toxoplasmosis, rubella, hepatitis B, hepatitis C, human immunodeficiency virus infection, assayed through serological tests among pregnant patients, from 1996 to 1998, at the Regional University Hospital Norte do Parana. Rev Soc Bras Med Trop 2000;33(6):519–527.

282. Sartori MJ, Pons P, Mezzano L, Lin S, de Fabro SP. Trypanosoma cruzi infection induces microfilament depletion in human placenta syncytiotrophoblast. Placenta 2003;24(7):767–771.

283. Bittencourt AL, Vieira GO, Tavares HC, Mota E, Maguire J. Esophageal involvement in congenital Chagas' disease: report of a case with megaesophagus. Am J Trop Med Hyg 1984;33(1):30–33.

284. Blanco SB, Segura EL, Cura EN, et al. Congenital transmission of Trypanosoma cruzi: an operational outline for detecting and treating infected infants in north-western Argentina. Trop Med Int Health 2000;5(4):293–301.

285. Malchiodi EL, Chiaramonte MG, Taranto NJ, Zwirner NW, Margni RA. Cross-reactivity studies and differential serodiagnosis of human infections caused by Trypanosoma cruzi and Leishmania spp: use of immunoblotting and ELISA with a purified antigen (Ag163B6). Clin Exp Immunol 1994;97(3): 417–423.

286. Vexenat Ade C, Santana JM, Teixeira AR. Cross-reactivity of antibodies in human infections by the kinetoplastid protozoa Trypanosoma cruzi, Leishmania chagasi and Leishmania (viannia) braziliensis. Rev Inst Med Trop Sao Paulo 1996;38(3):177–185.

287. Ferreira AW, Belem ZR, Lemos EA, Reed SG, Campos-Neto A. Enzyme-linked immunosorbent assay for serological diagnosis of Chagas' disease employing a Trypanosoma cruzi recombinant antigen that consists of four different peptides. J Clin Microbiol 2001;39(12):4390–4395.

288. Peralta JM, Teixeira MG, Shreffler WG, et al. Serodiagnosis of Chagas' disease by enzyme-linked immunosorbent assay using two synthetic peptides as antigens. J Clin Microbiol 1994;32(4):971–974.

289. Trypanosoma Detect(tm) product sheet, Seattle: InBios Corporation 2003. Available online at http://www.inbios.com/tcruzi.html

290. Virreira M, Torrico F, Truyens C, et al. Comparison of polymerase chain reaction methods for reliable and easy detection of congenital Trypanosoma cruzi infection. Am J Trop Med Hyg 2003;68(5): 574–582.

291. Avila HA, Pereira JB, Thiemann O, et al. Detection of Trypanosoma cruzi in blood specimens of chronic chagasic patients by polymerase chain reaction amplification of kinetoplast minicircle DNA: comparison with serology and xenodiagnosis. J Clin Microbiol 1993;31(9):2421–2426.

13 Laboratory Testing for Group B Streptococcus in the Pregnant Patient

Sebastian Faro, MD, PhD

CONTENTS

INTRODUCTION

Streptococcus agalactiae (group B streptococcus [GBS]), colonizes the vagina and rectum in 25–30% of pregnant women *(1–5)*. GBS infection can cause septic abortion, premature rupture of amniotic membranes, chorioamnionitis, postpartum endometritis, neonatal pneumonia, meningitis, and sepsis. The gastrointestinal tract, in particular the rectum, serves as the natural reservoir for GBS and is the likely source of vaginal colonization via transperitoneal contamination. Once in the vagina, the bacterium can be transferred between a woman and man during sexual intercourse, but it should not be classified as a venereal disease because the bacterium appears to wax and wane among the endogenous vaginal microflora. A unique characteristic of vaginal colonization is its resistance to oral, intramuscular, and intravenous antibiotics. However, the administration of intravenous antibiotics during labor does have the ability to prevent neonatal colonization and infection. The benefit of intrapartum antibiotic prophylaxis is to suppress the growth of GBS and colonization of the upper genital tract (i.e., uterine contents) during labor.

SCREENING FOR GBS

Instituting guidelines for the prevention of GBS disease in pregnant patients has resulted in a steady decline of early-onset neonatal disease. Prior to the use of such prevention strategies, the incidence of early-onset neonatal disease was 2–3 per 1000 live births *(6)*. When GBS prevention guidelines were initially adopted in the early 1990s, the

From: *Current Clinical Pathology: Handbook of Clinical Laboratory Testing During Pregnancy*
Edited by: A. M. Gronowski © Humana Press, Totowa, NJ

Table 1
Risk Factors for Possible Transmission
of Perinatal Group B Streptococcus (GBS)

1.	Previously delivered an infant who had invasive GBS disease
2.	GBS bacteriuria during the current pregnancy
3.	Delivery at less than 37 wk gestation
4.	Duration of ruptured membranes $\geq$18 h.
5.	Intrapartum temperature $\geq$100.4°F ($\geq$38.0°C)

From ref. 9.

incidence of transmission declined to 1.8 per 1000 live births in the United States and the case fatality rate was 5% (6). By 1999, when the guidelines had been readily accepted, the incidence had decreased by 70% to 0.5 cases per 1000 live births (7,8).

The initial GBS strategy recommended by the Centers for Disease Control and Prevention (CDC) in the early 1990s, was based on a consensus between the American Academy of Pediatrics and the American College of Obstetricians and Gynecologists (9). The strategy initiated treatment on the basis of either the presence of risk factors or a positive culture. The risk assessment system was designed for patients who were not cultured for GBS or whose testing was not yet completed prior to the onset of labor. The patient with one or more risk factors (Table 1) was considered as a candidate for intrapartum antibiotic prophylaxis.

Using the risk-based system to determine who should receive intrapartum antibiotic prophylaxis did reduce the incidence of early-onset neonatal GBS disease. However, in 2002, the CDC reported a population-based surveillance for early-onset GBS disease among 600,000 live births and found that using a culture-based screening system was greater than 50% more effective than the risk-based system for preventing perinatal GBS disease (10).

Therefore, the most recent (2002) recommendation from the CDC is to screen all pregnant patients between 35 and 37 wk gestation for vaginal and rectal colonization (11). This gestation time is important because GBS colonization is transient and the predictive value of culture is too low to be clinically useful when cultures are obtained prior to 5 wk before delivery (12). In a study of 26 women with positive cultures between 35 and 37 wk gestation, all were found to be positive at the time of labor (5). All patients found to be positive should receive intravenous antibiotics during labor (Table 2). One benefit of the culture-based screening system is that it treats only women who are GBS-colonized. The culture screening system also treats infected women who do not have risk factors. This is important because in the CDC surveillance, 18% of all laboring mothers without risk factors were found to be GBS positive by culture (10).

ANTIBIOTIC PROPHYLAXIS

Intravenous penicillin G is the antibiotic of choice for GBS. Intravenous ampicillin is an acceptable alternative to penicillin G, but penicillin G is preferred because it has a narrow spectrum and is less likely to select for antibiotic-resistant organisms. Clindamycin or erythromycin may be used for women allergic to penicillin, although the efficacy of these drugs for GBS disease prevention has not been measured in controlled trials.

Table 2
Recommended Regimens for Intrapartum Antimicrobial Prophylaxis for Perinatal Group B
Streptococcus (GBS) Disease Prevention

1. Recommended:	Penicillin G, 5 million units IV initial dose, then 2.5 million units IV every 4 h until delivery
2. Alternative:	Ampicillin, 2 g IV initial dose, then 1 g IV every 4 h until delivery
3. If penicillin allergic Patients not at high risk for anaphylaxis:	Cefazolin, 2 g IV initial dose, then 1 g every 8 h until delivery
Patients at high risk for anaphylaxis:	Isolate not resistant to clindamycin and/or erythromycin: clindamycin, 900 mg IV every 8 h, or erythromycin, 500 mg IV every 6 h until delivery
GBS is resistant to clindamycin or erythromycin or susceptibility unknown:	Vancomycin 1 g IV every 12 h until delivery

From ref.*11*.

Table 3
Recommendations for Obtaining Specimens for the Prevention of Group B Streptococcus
(GBS) Perinatal Transmission in the Pregnant Patient in Preterm Labor[1]

1. Obtain a vaginal–rectal specimen for the detection of GBS
2. Initiate penicillin or suitable alternative IV antibiotic therapy for at least 48 h
3. GBS culture is negative: discontinue antibiotic
4. GBS culture is positive: continue IV penicillin for at least 48 h (during tocolysis) until labor is arrested
5. GBS-positive patient: resume antibiotic therapy during intrapartum period until delivery

From ref. *11*.

PREMATURE LABOR

Approximately 25% of neonatal GBS disease occurs in premature infants *(6)*. Because preterm (<37 wk) delivery is a significant risk factor for early-onset GBS disease, and because timing of treatment prior to delivery is crucial, intrapartum prophylaxis in patients with threatened preterm delivery is important. However, because GBS screening is recommended at 35–37 wk, culture results are not always available when labor or rupture of membranes occurs prematurely. This makes management of these patients difficult. A suggested approach to GBS chemoprophylaxis in the patient with threatened preterm delivery is outlined in Table 3. Essentially, prophylaxis is initiated until screen results are known. If the patient is GBS positive, antibiotics are continued for no less than 48 h until labor is arrested and then is resumed at the time of delivery.

SAMPLE COLLECTION

The current gold standard is to obtain a specimen from the vagina and the rectum using a cotton- or Dacron-tipped swab. One swab can be used to obtain both specimens; first it is used to swipe the lateral vaginal walls of the lower one-third of the vagina (Table 4). The swab is then inserted into the rectum just past the anal sphincter and then placed in appropriate transport medium because the specimen should not be transported in a dry state. If two separate vaginal and rectal swabs are obtained, they can both be placed into the same container of medium. Stuart's and Amies transport media are nonnutritive and will support viability of GBS for up to 4 d at room temperature or under refrigeration *(11)*.

The use of a vaginal–rectal swab does result in some discomfort to the patient. However, it has long been held that both a vaginal and a rectal specimen are needed to obtain the highest yield of those patients colonized by GBS. Orafu et al. screened 136 patients for GBS colonization *(13)*. Three samples were obtained: one from the perianal area without breeching the sphincter so the rectum was not entered, the second specimen obtained from the vaginal/perianal area, and the third specimen was an anorectal specimen. The swabs were placed in Stuart's transport medium and taken to the laboratory. The swabs were placed in LIM broth medium for selective growth of GBS. When comparing all three sampling sites, the vaginal/anal specimens were positive for GBS in 26.5% of the samples, the anorectal specimens were positive in 27.2% of samples, and the perianal specimens were positive in 28.7% of the samples *(13)*. There was no difference in the recovery rates from sampling any of the three sites. Therefore, it appears that obtaining a specimen from the vaginal/perianal area for the detection of GBS colonization is as good as obtaining a vaginal/rectal specimen. The former site is associated with less discomfort than inserting a swab into the rectum. However, vaginal–rectal specimens are currently the recommended specimen.

LABORATORY TESTS

The standard culture technique used to detect GBS in vaginal and rectal specimens is to place the specimen in an enrichment system, such as Todd-Hewitt broth supplemented with nalidixic acid (15 µg/mL) and either colistin (10 µg/mL) or gentamicin (8 µg/mL) selective broth medium. Commercially available options include TransVay broth supplemented with 5% defibrinated sheep blood or LIM broth. The CDC recommends incubation for 18–24 h at 37°C and subculture onto blood agar medium and incubation for an additional 18–24 h. Colonies thought to be GBS are confirmed either by the latex agglutination test or the CAMP method.

The CAMP test depends on the synergistic reaction of a diffusible, heat-stable protein (CAMP factor) produced by a majority of group B streptococci and a β lysin (sphingomyelinase C) produced by staphylococci *(14)*. The test is performed by placing a single streak of streptococcus isolate perpendicular to a streak of staphylococci (β-lysin-producing strain) leaving a space of 2 mm between the two streaks on a trypticase soy agar plate containing 5% sheep blood and incubated overnight at 35°C *(15)*. The β lysin binds to the erythrocyte membranes and, when exposed to the CAMP factor, the cells undergo hemolysis. A positive test is indicated by the presence of an arrowhead-shaped zone of complete β hemolysis developing in the area where the GBS CAMP factor and staphylococcal β-lysin have diffused and mixed (Fig. 1).

Table 4
Procedure for Collecting and Processing Clinical Specimens
for the Culture of Group B Streptococcus (GBS)

1. Obtain a specimen by swabbing the vaginal introitus and anorectum.
2. Place the swab in appropriate transport medium, such as Amies transport medium. The swab will maintain GBS viability for 4 d at room temperature or under refrigeration.
3. Remove the swab from the transport medium and inoculate into selective broth medium, such as Todd-Hewitt, Lim, or SBM broth.
4. Incubate selective broth 18–24 h. Subculture the broth to sheep blood agar plate.
5. Inspect and identify organisms suggestive of GBS (β-hemolytic or non-hemolytic, Gram-positive, and catalase negative). If GBS is not identified after incubation for 19–24 h on sheep blood agar plate, reincubate and inspect at 48 h to identify suspected organisms.
6. Various slide agglutination tests or other tests for GBS antigen detection (e.g., genetic probe or fluorescent antibody) may be used for specific identification, or the CAMP test may be employed for presumptive identification.
7. Direct specimen testing can now be performed with real-time PCR and the results can be available within 60 min of processing the specimen (not in the CDC recommendation because this technique received FDA approval after the CDC guidelines were published).

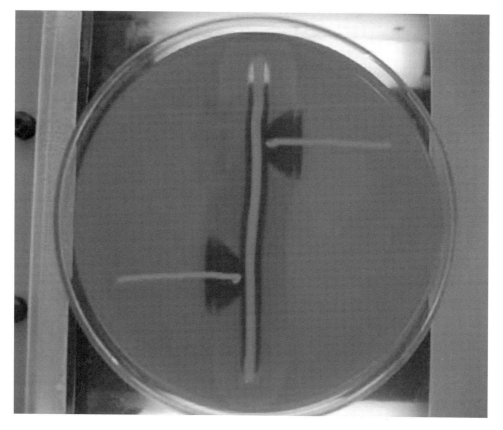

Fig. 1. Photograph of a CAMP test positive for Group B Streptococcus (GBS). Note presence of an arrowhead-shaped zone of complete β hemolysis in the area where the GBS CAMP factor and staphylococcal β-lysin have diffused and mixed.

An alternative culture technique that reduces the time from inoculation to identification has been described. Specimens obtained from the vagina and rectum are directly plated onto Granada agar, which that has been shown to be an effective method for identifying GBS (16). Grenada agar is a differential agar medium that allows presumptive identification of GBS based on production of a red-orange pigment by colonies of GBS.

In a study by Gil et al. (17), Granada broth medium was compared to Granada agar, Granada agar plate, selective blood agar, and LIM broth. No statistical differences in recovery of GBS between the Granada agar plate and selective Columbia blood agar were found. However, the advantage of the Granada agar plate is that the red-orange GBS colonies can readily be identified by the naked eye and no further identification is required, such as using the CAMP test or latex agglutination test. The Granada method can provide identification of GBS in a specimen obtained from the vagina and rectum within 18–24 h. Overman et al. (16) compared the Granada method to LIM broth enrichment, followed by culture on sheep blood agar, as well as to AccuProbe detection. The AccuProbe S. agalactiae system (Gen-Probe, San Diego, CA) detects bacterial rRNA by means of probe hybridization. In this study, specimens were directly plated onto Granada agar plates and then placed in LIM broth. The Granada agar plates were incubated anaerobically at 35°C for 24–48 h. GBS colonies were identified by the presence of red-orange pigmented colonies. The bacteria from these colonies were further tested using the Streptex latex agglutination reagent (Murex Biotech Ltd., Darford, England) to confirm GBS. The LIM broth was incubated at 35°C for 18–24 h. Specimens obtained from the broth were subcultured on sheep blood agar and incubated for 24 h. Colonies causing β-hemolysis were confirmed as GBS by testing with Streptex latex agglutination reagent. The remaining LIM broth was subjected to vortex mixing and a 50 µL aliquot was tested using the AccuProbe rRNA assay system. The broth-enhanced methods had similar sensitivities: LIM broth/sheep blood agar was 97.5% and the LIM broth/AccuProbe rRNA was 93.5%, compared to the Granada agar method, which had a sensitivity of 40%. Although the Granada method saves time, it does not appear to be as sensitive as the LIM broth enrichment.

Park et al. (18) reported on the feasibility of using a direct latex agglutination test for detection of the GBS antigen. This procedure involved obtaining vaginal–rectal specimens and placing them into LIM broth containing Todd-Hewitt broth with 10 µg of colistin per mL and 15 µg of nalidixic acid. The inoculated enrichment broth was incubated for 18–24 h, subcultured on blood agar plates, and incubated at 5% CO_2 for 18–24 h. All β-hemolytic and nonhemolytic colonies that morphologically suggest GBS were tested with the Phadebact® Streptococcus Test (Boule Diagnostics, Sweden) (18). These investigators also use the Phadebact assay to test LIM broth cultures directly after an 18–24 h incubation. They found that 20.6%, or 247, of the 1200 vaginal–rectal swab specimens were positive for GBS. The Phadebact (direct latex) system identified 244 GBS specimens, for a sensitivity of 98.8% and a specificity of 100%. The traditional method identified 130 as GBS, for a sensitivity of 93.1% (18). Although the Phadebact has both a high sensitivity and specificity, the vaginal–rectal specimen that is suspected of containing GBS must be cultured for at least 18 h to increase the number of GBS organisms present, and it cannot be performed on patient specimens directly. This delay is crucial because the inoculum size of GBS will increase from 10^2 bacteria/mL of amniotic fluid (AF) to at least 10^6 bacteria/mL of AF during 18 h of labor. The latter inoculum size is more than adequate to cause a de novo infection in the fetus and the mother.

Rapid Testing

One problem with the culture screening method is that it is not effective for patients who go into labor prior to screening, patients who do not have routine prenatal care, and/or women whose prenatal records are not available at the time of delivery. Because culture requires 18–24 hours to obtain results, the recommendations outlined in Table 3 have been set forth. However, many have advocated the use of a rapid method for GBS detection. Currently, two methods are available: immunoassay for GBS antigen and polymerase chain reaction (PCR).

IMMUNOASSAYS

Currently, there is one immunoassay test available to identify GBS colonization in the vagina and rectum of pregnant women. The Strep B OIA test (ThermoBioStar, Louisville, KY) is performed by extracting the GBS antigen from the swab used to obtain the vaginal–rectal specimen. The extraction reagent is added to a vial and the swab is immersed in the reagent and incubated for 5 min. A second extraction reagent is added and the mixture is incubated for another 5 min. The mixture is neutralized and the swab is pressed against the wall of the vial to release as much fluid as possible. Antigroup B streptococcal antibody is added to the mixture and incubated for 3–5 min. A few drops of the mixture is placed on the Strep B OIA cartridge and after 10 min, the surface is washed and blotted. If GBS is present, a blue to purple circle develops on the gold surface, indicating the presence of the GBS antigen *(19)*. The test takes approx 35 min.

Baker evaluated the Strep B OIA test and compared it to culture methods *(19)*. The prevalence of GBS vaginal colonization using the culture enrichment technique was 25%, and 17.3% using direct plating on blood agar. When compared to selective broth medium, the sensitivity of the Strep B OIA was 37%. This sensitivity rose to 53% when compared with nonselective blood agar medium results. Song et al. also found that the sensitivity of the Strep B OIA was not sufficient for this test to be used in the routine screening of pregnant women *(20)*. These investigators found that the negative predictive value was high, 88.9%, but the positive predictive value of the Strep B OIA was low, 51.5% *(20)*. Therefore, this test is clearly not suited for routine screening of pregnant women.

MOLECULAR METHODS

Progress toward the development of a DNA probe has been made. In 1999, Ryan et al. compared the diagnostic accuracy of a DNA probe to the traditional LIM broth enhancement, and blood agar to LIM broth and DNA probe *(21)*. For the comparison, two vaginal/perianal specimens were obtained from women in preterm labor. One sample was used to inoculate LIM broth and incubated for 8–24 hours and was then inoculated on blood agar. The second specimen was used to inoculate LIM broth, incubated for 8–24 h, and subsequently used for DNA probe testing. The traditional method revealed a prevalence of 32%. After 8 h incubation in LIM broth, the DNA probe had a poor sensitivity of 79%; however, the DNA probe had a sensitivity of 96% after 24 h incubation in LIM broth *(21)*. The DNA probe results were similar to the traditional LIM broth enhancement followed by plating on blood agar. However, the DNA probe provided results in a shorter period of time.

Recently, a real-time PCR test was developed that rapidly determines whether the lower genital tract or vaginal–rectal area is colonized in a pregnant patient admitted to labor and delivery. Bergeron et al. have reported that GBS colonization of the vagina/rectum can be ascertained within 30 to 60 min *(22)*. These investigators screened 172 women in labor and compared two PCR tests to the standard culture system. Specimens for GBS detection were collected from the vagina and rectum and 33, or 29.5%, were found to be positive. The sensitivity of the rapid PCR test compared to the standard culture technique was 97% and the negative predictive value was 98% *(22)*. Once the specimen is processed, this rapid PCR test requires approx 30–45 min to complete. Conventional PCR tests require approx 100 min to complete. Traditional enrichment culture in LIM broth followed by subculture on sheep blood agar and identification by either the CAMP tests or latex agglutination requires approx 24–36 h. The presence of blood, AF, or feces does not interfere with the rapid PCR test.

This new, real-time PCR assay, specific for GBS, was developed with a new rapid DNA amplification system (LC 32 LightCycler, Idaho Technology, Idaho Falls, ID). The system combines air thermal cycling with a fluorescence-based system of detection *(23)*. The procedure employs two pairs of adjacent hybridization probes labeled with a fluorescent reporter molecule that hybridizes to the GBS-specific amplicon or to the internal control *(24)*.

Rapid PCR GBS detection using SmartCycler® Real-Time PCR technology, known as the IDI-Strep B Assay (Infectio Diagnostic, Sainte Foy, Quebec, Canada), is also available for detection of GBS. The vaginal–rectal specimen is placed in 0.5 mL of Stuart's transport medium, which provides just enough medium to soak the cotton-tipped applicator. Ten μL of the transport medium is subjected to DNA extraction using a DNA extraction kit, and purified GBS genomic DNA is used as a positive control. The IDI-Strep B Assay can be completed within 1.5–2 h of obtaining the specimen in the laboratory.

In November 2002, the US Food and Drug Administration approved a real-time PCR test for GBS. Until that time, no truly reliable test for GBS detection existed that would be considered rapid. This real-time rapid PCR provides the practitioner with the opportunity to detect GBS in the genital tract of laboring women prior to their delivery. Mothers and newborns, in this scenario, who test negative can be spared the potential risk of receiving antibiotics. Thus, this technology not only provides rapid testing for GBS prior to the onset of labor or during labor, but also immediately after delivery. However, there are drawbacks to this rapid method. First, for this test to be effective, it must be offered 24 h per day, 7 d per week, which will require qualified personnel to be on hand at all times. The second is the cost of this method. Because samples are performed on receipt into the laboratory and not batched, several control samples must be performed with every test. This effectively raises the cost of each reportable test result. Certainly with time these problems will be overcome, but until then, the use of this test has been limited.

SUMMARY

GBS is a major cause of neonatal early-onset sepsis and maternal postpartum endometritis. Significant strides have been made in reducing the incidence of GBS early-onset neonatal sepsis by instituting a policy of universal antepartum screening of all pregnant women between 35 and 37 wk gestation. Identification of women colonized by GBS is best accomplished by obtaining a vaginal–rectal swab and placing the swab in appropriate transport media for either culture or PCR detection of GBS. The risk-assessment protocol is no longer recommended and should be discontinued. All women who are known to be colonized by GBS and in labor should receive penicillin prophylaxis. For patients stating that they are allergic to penicillin, when obtaining a specimen for GBS detection, it is important to write on the laboratory request form that the patient is allergic to penicillin and to have susceptibility testing of GBS isolates performed. This will allow the physician to choose an appropriate alternative to penicillin.

The culture-based method for detecting GBS requires approx 24–48 h to complete from the time the specimen is received in the laboratory and reported to the physician. The PCR method requires approx 2 h to complete from the time the specimen is received in the laboratory. The PCR-based system can detect the presence of one colony and therefore has greater sensitivity and specificity than any other detection system, including culture. The PCR-based detection system will reduce the number of false negatives, allowing rapid detection for women admitted to labor and delivery whose GBS status is unknown, such as women not having prenatal care and women admitted in preterm labor, that is, 36 wk or less.

REFERENCES

1. Anthony BF, Okada DM, Hobel CJ. Epidemiology of group B streptococcus: longitudinal observations during pregnancy. J Infect Dis 1978;137:524–30.
2. Regan JA, Klebanoff MA, Nugent RP, for the Vaginal Infections and Prematurity Study Group. epidemiology of group B streptococcal colonization in pregnancy. Obstet Gynecol 1991;77:604–610.
3. Yow MD, Leeds LJ, Thompson PK, Mason EO, Clark DJ, Beachler CW. The natural history of group B streptococcal colonization in the pregnant woman and her offspring. I. Colonization studies. Am J Obstet Gynecol 1980;137:34–38.
4. Dillon HC, Gray E, Pass MA, Gray BM. Anorectal and vaginal carriage of group B streptococci during pregnancy. J Infect Dis 1982;145:794–799.
5. Boyer KM, Gadzala CA, Kelly PD, Burd LI, Gotoff SP. Selective intrapartum chemoprophylaxis of neonatal group B streptococcal early-onset disease. II. Predictive value of prenatal cultures. J Infect Dis 1983;148:802–809.
6. Zangwill KM, Schuchat A, Wenger JD. Group B streptococcal disease in the United States, 1990: report from a multistate active surveillance system. Morb Mort Wkly Rep CDC Surveillance Summaries 1992;41:25–32.
7. Centers for Disease Control and Prevention. Early-onset group B streptococcus disease, United States, 1998–1999. Morb Mort Wkly Rep 2002;49:793–796.
8. Schrag SJ, Zywicki S, Farley MM, et al. Group B streptococcal disease in the era of intrapartum antibiotic prophylaxis. N Engl J Med 2000;342:15–20.
9. Centers for Disease Control and Prevention. Prevention of perinatal group B streptococcal disease: a public health perspective. Morb Mort Wkly Rep 1996;45:1–24.
10. Schrag SJ, Zell ER, Lynfield R, et al. A population-based comparison of strategies to prevent early-onset group B streptococcal disease in neonates. N Engl J Med 2002;347:233–239.
11. Schrag S, Gorwitz R, Fultz-Butts K, Schuchat A. Prevention of perinatal group B streptococcal disease; revised guidelines from CDC. Morb Mort Wkly Rep 2002;51(RR11):1–22.
12. Yancy MK, Schuchat A, Brown LK, Ventura VL, Markenson GR. The accuracy of late antenatal screening cultures in predicting genital group B streptococcal colonization at delivery. Obstet Gynecol 1996;88:811–815.
13. Orafu C, Gill P, Nelson K, Hecht B, Hopkins M. Perianal versus anorectal specimens: is there a difference in group B streptococcal detection? Obstet Gynecol 2002;99:1036–1039.
14. Facklan RR, Padula JF, Wortham EC, Cooksey RC, Rountree HA. Presumptive identification of group A, B, and D streptococci on agar plate media. J Clin Microbiol 1979;9:665–672.
15. Ruoff KL, Garner CV. Streptococcal infections. In Wentworth BB, Baselski VS, McArthur CP, et al. eds. Diagnostic Procedures for Bacterial Infections. Washington, DC: American Public Health Association, Inc., 1987, pp. 491–517.
16. Overman SB, Eley DD, Jacobs BE, Ribes JA. Evaluation of methods to increase the sensitivity and timeliness of detection of Streptococcus agalactiae in pregnant women. J Clin Microbiol 2002;40: 4329–4331.

17. Gil EG, Rodriguez MC, Bartolome R, Berjano B, Cabero L, Andreu A. Evaluation of the Granada agar plate for the detection of vaginal and rectal group B streptococci in pregnant women. J Clin Microbiol 1999;37:2648–2651.

18. Park CJ, Vandel NM, Ruprai DK, Martin EA, Gates KM, Coker D. Detection of group B streptococcal colonization in pregnant women using direct latex agglutination testing of selective broth. J Clin Microbiol 2001;39:408–409.

19. Baker CJ. Inadequacy of rapid immunoassays for intrapartum detection of group B streptococcal carriers. Obstet Gynecol 1996;88:51–55.

20. Song JY, Lin LL, Shott S, et al. Evaluation of the Strep B OIA test compared to standard culture methods for detection of group B streptococci. Infect Dis Obstet Gynecol 1999;7:202–205.

21. Ryan KM, Lencki SG, Elder BL, Northern WI, Khamis HJ, Bofill JA. DNA probe for beta-hemolytic group B streptococcus: diagnostic accuracy in threatened preterm labor. J Reprod Med 1999;44: 587–591.

22. Bergeron MG, Ke D, Menard C, et al. Rapid detection of group B streptococci in pregnant women at delivery. N Engl J Med 2000;343:175–179.

23. Wittwer CT, Ririe KM, Andrew RV, David DA, Gundry RA, Balis UJ. The LightCycler: a microvolume multisample fluorimeter with rapid temperature control. Biotechniques 1997;22:176–181.

24. Ke D, Menard C, Picard FJ, et al. Development of conventional and real-time PCR assays for the rapid detection of group B streptococci. Clin Chem 2000;46:324–231.

14 Immunologic Diseases of Pregnancy

William A. Bennett, PhD

Contents

INTRODUCTION

Obstetricians and reproductive immunologists have long recognized that the mother's immune response is significantly affected by pregnancy. Immunologic diseases of pregnancy are known to impact maternal, fetal, and neonatal well-being. Effective management of human pregnancy requires an understanding of both the normal maternal adaptations to pregnancy and immune-related disorders associated with gestation.

IMMUNOLOGIC CHALLENGE OF PREGNANCY

Pregnancy provides the following unique challenges to the mother's immune system *(1)*: (1) maternal tissues and blood are in intimate and prolonged contact with the semiallogeneic fetus; (2) pregnancy is established in the uterus, a specialized organ with its own mucosal barrier (the decidua); (3) impact of the fetal–placental unit on maternal immunity increases with advancing gestation; (4) hormones and cytokines released by the fetus and/or placenta impact maternal immune function; (5) deported placental and fetal cells are released into the maternal bloodstream. These challenges require appropriate adaptations of the maternal immune response for the establishment and maintenance of successful pregnancy.

NORMAL IMMUNOLOGIC ADAPTATIONS TO PREGNANCY

Humoral and Cellular Immune Responses in Pregnancy

Humoral immunity and B cell function remain relatively intact during normal human pregnancy *(1)*. In fact, the placenta facilitates maternal–fetal immunoglobulin G (IgG) transport while blocking transport of other immunoglobulin (Ig) classes. At birth, IgG

From: *Current Clinical Pathology: Handbook of Clinical Laboratory Testing During Pregnancy*
Edited by: A. M. Gronowski © Humana Press, Totowa, NJ

antibodies are present in the neonate but disappear at 3–6 mo of life. Maternal immune disorders involving IgG antibodies can impact the fetus because of transplacental passage of this Ig isotype.

In contrast, numerous changes in cellular immunity have been reported during pregnancy. These include a suppression of neutrophil chemotaxis, decreased natural killer cell activity, lowered CD4 to CD8 cell ratios, and reduced CD8 cytotoxic activity (1–5). Interferon (IFN)-γ-dependent T-cell cytotoxic activity and IFN-γ production by natural killer (NK) cells are also suppressed during pregnancy (6).

Pregnancy-Related Immune Adaptations and Maternal Health

A number of reviews have addressed the adaptations that occur in maternal systemic immunity during pregnancy (7–9). Severals studies have reported that pregnant women are more prone to various types of viral infections (10–22), consistent with the concept of suppressed cell-mediated immunity during human pregnancy. In addition, a trend has been noted toward a worsening of autoimmune diseases that are primarily antibody mediated and amelioration of those that are cell mediated.

Researchers have also analyzed the maternal response to vaccines and the ability to mount delayed-type hypersensitivity (DTH) responses. Both of these responses appear to be intact during human pregnancy (23,24). For example, maternal immunization with Neisseria meningitis in pregnancy is safe for both the mother and infant (25). In fact, maternal immunization provided infants with increased concentrations of specific IgG for 2–3 mo and oral IgA for 6 mo. An additional study found that immunization against tetanus toxoid during pregnancy was an effective and affordable way to protect against neonatal tetanus (26). It has been suggested that common infections and more serious conditions such as neonatal herpes simplex, cytomegalovirus, and the human immuno-deficiency virus may be prevented with maternal immunization (27).

Thus, although it is apparent that pregnancy may partially suppress cell-mediated immunity, the mother is normally able to mount an immunologic response to infection and foreign antigens.

Mechanisms of Fetal Immunoprotection

A question that has intrigued immunologists for decades is how the fetus escapes immune rejection by the maternal immune system (the "enigma of the fetal allograft" [28]). A key element in the answer to this question is the relative paucity of classical major histocompatibility (MHC) class I (human leukocyte antigen [HLA]-A or HLA-B) or class II antigens by the fetal trophoblast (trophoblast invisibility hypothesis). Although human extravillous trophoblast cells do not normally express classical MHC antigens, the nonclassical MHC antigen HLA-G is expressed. HLA-G is unique in that it does not stimulate cytotoxic T-cell activity (7) while actively inhibiting NK cells (29).

Increasing experimental evidence also indicates that maternal immune function during pregnancy can be altered by the local cytokine microenvironment. In 1986, two distinct and mutually inhibitory subsets of murine T-helper cells were described, each with characteristic cytokine profiles (30). The first group of cells, termed T_H1 cells, secrete interleukin (IL)-2, IFN-γ, and tumor necrosis factor-α. The second classification of cells (T_H2 cells) produce IL-4, IL-5, and IL-10 (31). T_H1-type cytokines have been associated with cell-mediated immunity and delayed hypersensitivity reactions, whereas T_H2 cytokines promote humoral immune responses and allergic reactions. Because T_H1

cytokines are viewed as harmful to human pregnancy, and T_H2 cytokines such as IL-4 and IL-10 can suppress their production, it has been proposed that successful pregnancy is a T_H2-dominated phenomenon *(32)*. Several different lines of clinical evidence support this hypothesis. For example, cell-mediated autoimmune conditions such as rheumatoid arthritis are often improved during pregnancy, whereas disorders associated with an autoimmune antibody response often worsen *(33)*. Various placental products including progesterone *(34)*, prostaglandin E_2 *(35)*, and cytokines such as IL-4 and IL-10 *(32)* suppress T_H1 responses. Given the dramatic changes in hormone and cytokine production during pregnancy, it is likely that immune function is affected by the microenvironment present at the maternal–fetal interface. However, despite the intriguing nature of the T_H2 dominance hypothesis of pregnancy immunotolerance, it should be noted that IL-10 "knockout" mice are able to reproduce successfully *(36)*.

In theory, pregnancy-related immunusuppression would be thought to increase the risk of bacterial infections, as has been reported in transplant patients receiving corticosteroids or other immunosuppressive therapies. Furthermore, the fetus is particularly susceptible to infection, with colonization of the membranes surrounding the fetus (chorioamnionitis) or decidua (deciduitis) being associated with miscarriage, premature labor, growth defects, and intrauterine death. Thus, we are faced with the following question: "How does the fetus suppress maternal rejection responses while maintaining the mother's resistance to bacterial infection?"

Role of the Maternal Innate Immune System During Pregnancy

Part of the answer to this question may lie in the adaptive changes that occur to the mother's innate immune system during human pregnancy. Increased numbers of monocytes and granulocytes have been reported from the first trimester of pregnancy onward. During pregnancy, circulating monocytes and granulocytes possess activated phenotypes similar to that observed in systemic sepsis *(37)*. Monocytes also display increased phagocytosis and respiratory burst activity in pregnancy *(38,39)*. In addition, monocyte surface expression of the endotoxin receptor CD14 is increased *(37)* and granulocyte activation occurs in normal progressing pregnancies *(40)*. Finally, cells of the innate immune system large granular lymphocytes, macrophages, and γ δ T cells rather than classical T or B cells are the principal components of the decidual leukocyte cell infiltrate.

A better understanding of the normal adaptive changes of the maternal immune response to pregnancy will provide important insights into the underlying etiologies of immune-related diseases of pregnancy.

IMMUNOLOGIC DISORDERS IN PREGNANCY

Immunologic disorders of pregnancy can be grouped into autoimmune and alloimmune conditions. In autoimmune diseases of pregnancy, there are humoral and cellular responses to self-tissues, reflecting a failure of self-tolerance. In contrast, alloimmune diseases of pregnancy are directed against cells or tissues antigenically distinct from the woman carrying the pregnancy. Autoimmune diseases influence pregnancy and are influenced by pregnancy. For example, sex steroids produced during pregnancy can affect the onset and severity of lupus during pregnancy. In addition, pregnancy can cause a remission of rheumatoid arthritis (RA) in a majority of patients.

Maternal and Fetal Hyperthyroidism

Clinical Symptoms, Etiology, and Treatment

Maternal hyperthyroidism occurs in approx 0.2% of pregnancies and is associated with an increased risk of severe preeclampsia, low birth weight, prematurity, intrauterine growth restriction, and perinatal mortality (41–44) (for more details, see Chapter 8). The most common cause of hyperthyroidism in pregnancy is Grave's disease, a condition associated with preeclampsia, heart failure, and maternal thyroid storm *(43,44)*. A severe fetal complication of Graves' disease is thyrotoxicosis, which is associated with a high rate of fetal and neonatal mortality (up to 30%) usually related to cardiac failure *(45)*. In Grave's disease, IgG antibodies are produced against the thyroid-stimulating hormone (TSH), or thyrotropin, receptor, which trigger excess production of thyroid hormone *(45)*. Maternal–fetal transport of these antibodies into the fetus can also activate the fetal and neonatal thyroid gland *(46,47)*. Fetal hyperthyroidism generally occurs during the second half of pregnancy, with symptoms sometimes persisting for weeks to months after birth until antibodies are cleared. Grave's disease can lead to fetal tachycardia, growth restriction, goiter formation, and nonimmune hydrops *(45,48)*. Complications including tachycardia, arrhythmia, cardiac insufficiency, irritability, and diarrhea also persist in the neonate *(45)*. Antithyroid drugs such as propylthiouracil and methimazole are first-line treatments for Grave's disease during pregnancy, readily crossing the placenta and blocking the synthesis of thyroid hormones *(49,50)*.

Laboratory Evaluation and Diagnosis

Detecting fetal hyperthyroidism is difficult because of the lack of correlation between maternal and fetal thyroid hormone concentrations. Generally, a third-trimester elevation in fetal T_4 concentrations from 2.5 to 5 times that of normal pregnancy is a significant risk factor for fetal complications *(51)*. Funipuncture and subsequent measurement of fetal thyroxine and TSH concentrations *(52)* can confirm suspicion of fetal hyperthyroidism because of maternal history. However, obtaining serial fetal hormone concentrations by this technique is not practical because of its relatively high mortality rate (approx 1%) *(52)*. Fetal ultrasound can also be applied to monitor thyroid size and detect goiter formation. However, at present the most effective management involves close monitoring of the fetus for signs of tachycardia and intrauterine growth restriction and observation of the mother for related symptoms. Neonates should also be monitored because of the relatively long half-life of IgG. Effective management may include the use of antithyroid therapy until TSH antibody concentrations decrease *(43)*; (see Chapter 9).

Systemic Lupus Erythematosis

Clinical Symptoms, Etiology, and Treatment

Systemic lupus erythematosis (SLE) is a chronic autoimmune disorder diagnosed clinically by systemic inflammatory symptoms first appearing in women during their childbearing years *(53,54)*. SLE tends to flare during pregnancy and during the postpartum period, with most of these episodes being mild. During pregnancy, women with SLE-associated antiphospholipid antibodies (APLA) are at increased risk for spontaneous abortions and stillbirths *(55)*. A serious fetal complication of SLE is congenital heart block (CHB), which forms a portion of the neonatal lupus syndrome (NLS). About half of infants with NLS develop CHB even with an absence of cutaneous lupus *(56)*. Doppler ultrasound or fetal echocardiography between 16 and 30 wk gestation usually detects CHB. Fetal findings associated with CHB include persistent fetal bradycardia leading to congestive heart failure or hydrops fetalis *(57)*. Neonates with CHB display approx a 20% mortality rate, with most surviving infants requiring implantation of a pacemaker during the first year of life *(58,59)*.

Maternal circulating APLAs are hypothesized to play a key role in the underlying etiology of CHB. Both peak transport of maternal IgG to the fetus and maturity of the conductive system of the fetal heart occur at 14–16 wk gestation *(56)*. Immunohistochemical studies have confirmed expression of the Ro/SSA and LA/SSB antigens in heart tissues of fetuses with CHB, because with specific antibodies to the LA antigen *(60)*. However, maternal antibodies alone may not fully explain the etiology of CHB, because both the Ro and LA antigens are not normally expressed on the cell surface in such a fashion that antibody recognition would occur. Some groups have theorized that physiological stresses, viral infections, hormones, and fetal apoptosis may increase cell-surface expression of the antigens *(61)*. Maternal APLAs apparently exert their effects on the heart by direct interference with calcium transport in the myocardial tissue *(62)*.

Treatments designed to prevent or reduce fetal CHB attempt to decrease passage of antibodies into the fetus and reduce the inflammation responsible for defective heart conduction. These types of treatments include corticosteroids, intravenous gammaglobulin, and plasmapheresis *(63)*. Although some studies have reported promising results in terms of preventing inflammatory processes (i.e., myocarditis or pericardial effusions), no solid evidence supports the concept that complete heart block is reversible *(61)*. Some researchers have recommended prophylactic treatment for high-risk mothers in order to prevent transport of immunoglobulins and to minimize the inflammatory process. However, these studies have been inconclusive, and risk–benefit ratios have not been clearly defined. Because the overall incidence of CHB is low even in high-risk pregnancies, prophylactic therapy is not advised *(63)*.

LABORATORY TESTING AND DIAGNOSIS

Pregnancy is not absolutely contraindicated in SLE patients with controlled, inactive disease *(51)*. However, antibody screening by enzyme-linked immunosorbent assay (ELISA) tests should be performed. In this respect, a positive test for anticardiolipin antibody has been shown to be a strong predictor for the presence of intraglomerular thrombi in SLE patients with renal involvement *(64)*. Other studies have shown that high concentrations of IgG antibodies to cardiolipin along with the presence of antibodies to lupus anticoagulating and/or β glycoprotein can be used to define a subset of patients with active SLE *(65)*. A positive ELISA test for these antibodies should be followed up with immunoblotting, which gives a higher predictive value. Although specific risk values have not been established, a direct correlation between maternal antibody concentrations and fetal risk has been proposed *(66)*. After antibody testing, serial fetal echocardiograms should be performed from 16 to 24 wk gestation for the early detection of myocarditis or heart block. CHB is diagnosed by the detection of persistent fetal bradycardia in the absence of anatomic abnormalities or infection.

Antiphospholipid Syndrome

CLINICAL SYMPTOMS, ETIOLOGY, AND TREATMENT

Antiphospholipid syndrome (APS) is an autoimmune disease characterized by recurrent venous or arterial thrombosis, fetal loss, thrombocytopenia, and other complications related to APLA (reviewed in ref. *67*). Although APS was first described in patients with SLE, it also may occur in the absence of any other disorder (primary APS). Several mechanisms have been proposed by which APLA may result in these complications of pregnancy including the following *(67)*: (1) activation of endothelial cells with up-regulation of adhesion molecules and subsequent increased endothelial adherence by platelets and monocytes; (2) shifts in the prostacyclin–thromboxane balance; (3) impaired antithrombin III activity caused by cross-reactivity with glycosaminoglycans; (4) inhibition of thrombomodulin protein C-protein S activation; (5) suppression of the functions of other coagulation inhibitors (β2-glycoprotein I and annexin V).

Patients with APS may experience a recurrence of a single complication or episodes of different clinical symptoms. For example, a woman with recurrent fetal losses may also develop deep vein thrombosis or thrombocytopenia. Widespread thrombosis in multiple organs can also occur in patients with APS, lasting over a period of days to weeks. This can occur as a result of discontinuing anticoagulant therapy or as a complication of surgery or infection. Patients with this type of catastrophic APS exhibit multiple organ failure, diminished mental status, and a 50% mortality rate *(68)*.

Recurrent spontaneous abortion has been cited as a frequent complication of APS *(67)*. The development of radioimmunoassays *(69)* and ELISAs *(70)* for APLAs has confirmed the association between the presence of APLAs and recurrent pregnancy loss *(71–76)*. Branch et al. *(77)* provided direct evidence of this association when they reported that passive transfer of IgG fractions from women with APS to pregnant Balb/c mice caused intrauterine fetal death. Subsequent immunohistochemical studies revealed decidual necrosis, prominent intravascular IgG APLA antibody, and fibrin deposition.

A number of retrospective studies have established a strong relationship between the presence of circulating lupus anticoagulant (LA) and anticardiolipin antibodies (aCL) and pregnancy loss *(68,71,78,79)*. The rate of fetal loss in untreated women with LA and previous pregnancy failure may be as high as 80% *(80–82)*. This relationship has been confirmed by cohort studies in unselected populations *(83–86)* and in women with APS *(81,84–86)*. Remarkably, APLA-related pregnancy losses often occur in the second or third trimester. This differs from fetal losses in general, in which only a small percent occur during mid to late gestation. In a cohort study of 76 women (333 pregnancies) with APS, 50% of losses were a results of second- or third-trimester fetal death *(87)*. In this cohort of women, 80% had suffered at least one previous fetal death. APLAs have also been associated with recurrent early pregnancy loss. Numerous cohort-control studies have documented positive tests for APLAs in a higher proportion of women with recurrent spontaneous abortion than in controls *(74,86,88–94)*. These studies have reported positive tests for APLA in 5–20% of women with recurrent pregnancy loss. In contrast to recurrent spontaneous abortions, APLAs are not associated with sporadic preembryonic or embryonic pregnancy loss *(95)* (also see Chapter 15).

Neurological complications associated with APS include stroke and transient ischemic attacks *(96,97)*. Less common complications include transverse myelopathy, chorea, seizures, and migraines *(98)*. Coronary complications in APS may present as ischemia or infarction of the ventricle secondary to coronary artery thrombosis. Most clinical symptoms of APS are associated with thrombosis or thromboembolic vascular occlusions *(96–98)*. Although some cell infiltration may occur, the vessel walls tend to remain intact. Veins and arteries of any size at any location in the body may be involved. The majority (60–65%) of thrombotic events are venous, but arterial thrombosis and stroke are common occurrences *(99,100)*. The most frequent site of venous thrombosis is in the lower extremities. However, up to a third of patients suffer at least one pulmonary embolus. APLAs are also associated with arterial thrombosis, which can occur in nontypical locations including retinal, subclavian, digital, or brachial arteries. The most common arterial event in APS is stroke and the most frequently involved vessel is the middle cerebral artery. Approximately 4–6% of otherwise healthy individuals who experience a stroke at less than 50 yr of age are positive for the presence of APLAs *(101,102)*.

Interestingly, a potential neuroendocrine–cytokine interrelationship has been proposed for the clinical manifestation of APS in pregnancy (reviewed in ref.*103*). According to this model, APLA suppresses the production of the cytokine IL-3, a cytokine important in the regulation of pregnancy-associated events including trophoblast invasion, placentation, and embryonic growth. In these studies, pregnant women with APS have been shown to have low concentrations of IL-3. Another important observation is that mice expressing antisense IL-3 RNA display serve neurologic dysfunction, suggesting that suppression of IL-3 could mediate both the pregnancy loss and central nervous system dysfunction observed in APS.

Pregnancy and estrogen-containing oral contraceptives (OCs) appear to increase the risk for thrombosis in women with APS. This is supported by studies in which the majority of APS women experiencing thromboses were pregnant or using OCs *(103)*. Furthermore, a large cohort study has shown that one-fourth of thrombotic events in women with APS occurred during pregnancy or during the postpartum period *(103)*. Finally, two prospective studies have shown a 5–12% risk of thrombosis during pregnancy or peripartum in women with APS *(81,104)*. Thus, the presence of well-characterized APS may be a contraindication for the use of estrogen-containing OCs.

Autoimmune thrombocytopenia is strongly associated with APLA, occurring in up to 40% of individuals with primary APS *(105,106)*. Thrombocytopenia in the setting of APLA is difficult to distinguish from idiopathic thrombocytopenia purpura (ITP). Pregnancy complications associated with APS include preeclampsia, fetal growth impairment, abnormal fetal heart rate tracings, and preterm birth. Utero–placental insufficiency is widely viewed as the common link in all these disorders. Preeclampsia is very common in women diagnosed with APS *(81,104)*. In a study conducted at the University of Utah, 50% of women with APS had preeclampsia and 25% exhibited severe preeclampsia *(81)*. APLA also has been cited by some research groups as a prospective risk factor for the development of preeclampsia *(83)*. An 11–17% rate of positive tests for APLA has been reported in women with preeclampsia *(107–110)*, and the association is strongest in women with severe, early onset (<34 wk gestation) disease *(107)*.

The presence of APLAs without clinical symptoms does not require treatment, but rather careful monitoring. Patients with thrombocytopenia associated with the APS are generally treated with prednisone. Thrombosis in APS requires heparin followed by oral anticoagulant (warfarin). Anticoagulation is continued indefinitely, with adequate doses of anticoagulant to achieve an international normalized ratio of 3.0 to 3.5, shown diminish the risk of recurrence *(111)*. Catastrophic APS requires treatment with intravenous heparin, corticosteroids, and cyclophosphamide. Treatment of patients at risk for pregnancy loss in the setting of APS remains controversial, particularly regarding the use of steroids for the prevention of fetal loss. There is some clinical evidence to support the use of aspirin and heparin throughout gestation to prevent abortion *(112)*.

Laboratory Testing and Diagnosis

On the basis of the 1998 workshop on the classification of APS, diagnosis of this condition requires that at least one of the following clinical criteria and laboratory criteria are met.

Clinical Criteria	*Laboratory Criteria*
1. Vascular thrombosis	1. Positive aCL and LA antibodies: 2 or more tests at least 6 wk apart
2. Pregnancy morbidity	2. Familial deficiencies of protein C, protein S, or antithrombin III
	3. Factor V resistance to protein C (Factor V Leiden)

A number of problems have been associated with laboratory testing for APLAs. These include the following *(113,114)*: (1) controversy and uncertainty about the exact nature and specificity of relevant antiphospholipid antibodies, (2) nonstandardized assays, (3) unacceptable interlaboratory variability, and (4) inadequate quality control. The two best-characterized and clinically useful APLAs are LA and aCL. Both of these APLAs have been independently associated with clinical manifestations of APS. Because some individuals with APS have either LA or aCL, but not both, testing for both antibodies is recommended.

LA is an APLA present both in patients with SLE and some individuals without this order. LA is actually a misnomer in that this antibody is associated with thrombosis, not anticoagulation. It is detected in plasma by a variety of phospholipid-dependent clotting assays including the activated partial thromboplastin time, kaolin clotting time, dilute Russel viper venom time, and plasma clotting time tests *(79)*. These tests are based on the observation that phospholipids serve as a template on which the enzymes and cofactors of the clotting cascade interact. LA present in patient samples binds to phospholipids, proteins, or epitopes created by phospholipid–protein interactions and interfere with the interaction of clotting factors and prolong clotting times. However, other nonrelated factors such as improper processing of samples, anticoagulant medications, and clotting factor deficiencies can prolong clotting times. The addition of normal plasma to patient samples can prevent false positive tests caused by clotting factor deficiencies. Regardless of the test used, LA is difficult to reliably quantify and results are generally reported as either present or absent.

Anticardiolipin antibodies are detected by ELISA using microtiter plates coated with cardiolipin in ethanol. For these assays, test serum is diluted in 10% bovine serum in phosphate-buffered saline. This assay has been successfully standardized and international calibrators for the assay and standard units for the antibody have been developed *(115)*. These standard sera have been assigned numeric values in terms of IgG anticardiolipin, IgM anticardiolipin, and IgA anticardiolipin (APL). Results are then reported as negative, low, medium, or high for the presence of each of these types of aCL. A high degree of cross-reactivity has been reported between antibodies to the different anionic phospholipids, suggesting that these antibodies may be generated to common shared epitoptes. For this reason, the term anticardiolipin has been replaced by the term antiphospholipid and the syndrome is therefore referred to as the antiphospholipid syndrome.

Low concentrations of IgG anticardiolipin and IgM anticardiolipin are sometimes found in healthy individuals (115) and can result from infection (116) or nonspecific binding. In contrast, moderate to high concentrations of aCLs have been correlated with a variety of APLA-related disorders (96,117,118). Thus, most laboratories regard only significantly elevated aCL or LA or both as sufficient laboratory criteria for the diagnosis of APS (96,119). Positive tests for APS can be transient and should be confirmed on two occasions at least several weeks apart (86,96).

Antibodies to other phospholipid antigens, especially antiphosphatidyl serine antibodies, are sometimes present in patients with clinical disorders such as APLA (94). However, most individuals positive for other APLAs also have aCL and/or LA. Because assays for other APLAs have not undergone quality control and standardization, they are not currently recommended for routine clinical use.

Thrombocytopenic Purpura

CLINICAL SYMPTOMS, ETIOLOGY, AND TREATMENT

Thrombocytopenic purpura is a platelet disorder often associated with purpuric and other hemorrhagic conditions (120). In ITP, IgG antibodies are produced against platelet glycoproteins including IIb-IIIa, GPIb-IX, and occasionally against GPIa-Iia or GPV. This disorder occurs more often in women than men, and more than 70% of these women are in their childbearing years (120). ITP is a relatively common complication of human pregnancy, occurring in approx 1 in 1000 live births (121).

Thrombocytopenia during pregnancy most often occurs because of increased platelet destruction rather than through decreased platelet production. Thrombocytopenia may occur as part of HELLP (hemolysis, elevated liver enzymes, and low platelets) syndrome, ITP, alloimmune thrombocytopenia, SLE, or in response to certain drugs (122) (see Chapter 10).

Although pregnancy does not heighten the symptoms of ITP in the mother, it can lead to postpartum neonatal complications. This is because antibodies from the ITP mother cross into the fetus, resulting in approx 30% of these newborns developing thrombocytopenia (123). Fetal risk of severe thrombocytopenia is prevalent in mothers with a platelet count of less than 75×10^9 platelets/L (124). The major maternal complication associated with ITP is hemorrhage during and following childbirth, particularly in association with cesarean sections. Perinatal thrombocytopenia is usually not life threatening and normally resolves within the first month of life (125).

Treatment of ITP with oral corticosteroids (1.0–1.5 mg/kg/d of prednisone) exerts its effects through increasing platelet production rather than reducing the activity of the antiplatelet antibodies (126). In patients who fail to respond to prednisone treatment, intravenous infusion of high doses of polyvalent, monomeric Ig has been reported to produce a rapid reversal of ITP (127). This therapy appears to act by interfering with phagocyte Fc-receptor-mediated immune clearance of IgG-coated platelets. The recommended treatment for ITP is 0.4 mg/kg/d administered over a period of 5 d (123). In cases where the fetus is determined to be suffering from severe thrombocytopenia, platelet infusions *in utero* may be required (125).

In contrast to ITP, alloimmune thrombocytopenia exerts its most dramatic effects on the fetus and neonate rather than the mother. This condition occurs in approx 1 in 1000 neonates. In alloimmune thrombocytopenia, maternal platelet antibodies develop that cross the placenta, causing fetal platelet destruction in fetuses expressing targeted platelet antigen. Hemorrhagic complications are more severe in fetuses or neonates of mothers with alloimmune thrombocytopenia compared to those with ITP, and, unfortunately, diagnosis usually does not occur until after delivery of an affected neonate. The risk of recurrence of alloimmune thrombocytopenia has been cited to be as high as 90% *(128)*.

LABORATORY TESTING AND DIAGNOSIS

Various ELISA systems have been used to measure serum platelet bindable IgG *(128–130)*. Although at one time accepted as a diagnostic characteristic of ITP, over the last decade it has been realized that platelet-associated IgG is not specific for this disorder and that increased concentrations are seen in several other disorders *(131)*. Although true platelet antibodies will increase the concentrations of platelet immunoproteins, other proteins can display adherence to platelets as well. There is now convincing evidence that several glycoproteins such as GP Iib/IIIa, GP Ib, and GP V found on platelet membranes act as target antigen sites for the attachment of antibodies to platelets *(131)*. This understanding has led to the development of direct, monoclonal antibody-specific immobilization of platelet antigens using monoclonal antibodies directed against the specific platelet antigens *(132,133)*. However, testing is still rather complex, requiring an experienced laboratory equipped to test for the different platelet antigens with appropriate positive and negative controls to confirm the specificity of the tests *(134)*.

Clinically, diagnosis of ITP is obtained by exclusion of other potential causes of thrombocytopenia. In this regard, a platelet count of less than $150 \times 10^9/L$ in the absence of HIV, splenomegaly, elevated liver enzymes, hypertension, or disseminated intravascular coagulopathy is suggestive of ITP *(128)*.

Myasthenia Gravis

CLINICAL SYMPTOMS, ETIOLOGY, AND TREATMENT

Myasthenia gravis (MG) is a condition that is manifested clinically by weakness of the striated voluntary muscles. MG particularly affects the muscles of the face and extremities and is obvious after repetitive activity. The weakness that occurs in MG patients is mediated by autoantibodies against adult muscle acetylcholine receptors (AChR) of the neuromuscular junction *(135)*. These antibodies destroy elements of the postsynaptic membrane of the myoneural junction in affected muscle groups *(136)*. This results in decreased nerve-impulse transmission and patients with MG exhibit diminished skeletal muscle strength and rapid fatigue with exercise.

The immune manifestations of MG include the following: (1) lymphocyte infiltration of skeletal muscles, (2) proliferative response to purified acethylcholine receptor, (3) decrease in acetylcholine receptors, and (4) antibody-dependent, complement-mediated lysis of the postsynaptic membrane *(137,138)*. Antibodies to the acetylcholine receptor are present in 85–90% of women with MG. These are IgG antibodies and thus can cross the placental barrier and affect the fetus.

Manifestations of MG in pregnancy are highly variable. It has been reported that approximately one-third of women experience greater symptoms of MG when pregnant, whereas the remaining two-thirds either remain the same or improve *(137,138)*. Worsening of the disease can occur at any stage of pregnancy, and the disease course in one pregnancy is not predictive of its course in subsequent pregnancies. During pregnancy, plasmapheresis has been used to treat women in MG crisis *(139)*, along with anticholinesterase drugs and corticosteroids.

Neonatal MG occurs in approx 20% of neonates whose mothers suffer from adult MG, and is condition lasts for 2–3 wk following birth. Symptoms in neonatal MG range from hypotonea to respiratory distress, which can be so acute so as to require mechanical ventilation *(140)*.

LABORATORY TESTING AND DIAGNOSIS

A variety of methods have been utilized to detect the presence of circulating antibodies to the AChR in pregnant women and neonates thought to be suffering from MG. Examples of these include radioimmunoassays *(141,142)*, immunoprecipitation tests *(143,144)*, and ELISA assays *(142,145)*. On the basis of the results of these assays, it is estimated that up to 90% of patients with MG are positive for the presence of AChR antibodies. More recently, an interesting relationship has been described between the ratio of antifetal muscle AChR: antiadult muscle AChR antibodies *(141–145)*. These studies have revealed that an increase in this ratio is predictive of the occurrence of neonatal MG in a first child. Thus, autoantibodies against the embryonic form of AChR could play a key role in the pathogenesis of neonatal MG.

Rheumatoid Arthritis

CLINICAL SYMPTOMS, ETIOLOGY, AND TREATMENT

RA is a chronic, systemic, autoimmune inflammatory disease that affects the joints of women of all age groups. Almost 75 yr ago, Hench et al. *(146)* reported improvement in a large percentage of women with RA during the course of their pregnancies. Subsequent studies have confirmed the decrease in symptoms of RA in a majority of pregnant women *(147–154)*. The conclusion drawn from these studies is that 75% of patients improve, whereas the rest stay the same or experience heightened symptoms. This improvement is reflected by the following: (1) 50% of patients report improvement during the first trimester *(147,150)*, (2) regression of subcutaneous nodules occurs in some patients *(152)*, (3) many patients are able to stop taking nonsteroidal antiinflammatory analgesics *(152)*. Pregnancy is not a cure for RA because reoccurrence of symptoms invariably occurs after delivery *(147–149)*. Symptoms of RA usually return at levels comparable to that observed before pregnancy *(147,152)* and require renewal of treatment *(149)*. Although the majority of RA patients report an improvement during pregnancy, a small portion report increased symptoms *(149)*. The physiology of the pregnancy-induced improvement in RA has not been clearly established. Early studies pointed to the potential role that increased adrenal hormone might play in this response *(146)*. Although free cortisol does rise during pregnancy, this elevation is not sufficient to have a clinical effect on joint inflammation. A number of other theories have been proposed to explain this ameliorating response in RA patients during pregnancy, which can be summarized as follows: (1) the effect of hormonal changes during pregnancy, such as increases in cortisol, estrogen, and progesterone *(155,156)*, (2) the suppression of cell-mediated immunity thought to occur during pregnancy, with a predominance of T_H2 over T_H1 cytokine responses *(157)*, and (3) altered neutrophil function during pregnancy (i.e., decreased neutrophil respiratory burst activity).

There is a paucity of studies on the effects of RA on pregnancy. Generally, women with RA have an uneventful pregnancy without significant complications. In addition, RA does not appear to adversely affect fetal outcome.

Laboratory Testing and Diagnosis

Laboratory studies for pregnant patients with RA are the same as for any pregnancy (i.e., hemotocrit, blood group studies). Because normocytic-normochromic anemia occurs in pregnant women with RA, closer monitoring of hemoglobin concentrations may be merited. If patients are on antirheumatic drugs, blood work may be required to monitor the adverse affects of the drugs. For example, in patients receiving sulfasalazine and nonsteroidal antiinflammatory drugs, a white blood cell count along with aspartate aminotransferase and alanine aminotransferase results should be obtained.

IMMUNODEFICIENCY DISORDERS AND HUMAN PREGNANCY

Common Variable Immunodeficiency

Clinical Symptoms, Etiology, and Treatment

Common variable immunodeficiencies (CVID) are a heterogeneous group of undifferentiated syndromes whose unifying characteristic is defective antibody production. These disorders are usually diagnosed from 20 to 30 yr of age and are characterized by the following: (1) recurrent bacterial infections, (2) decreased serum immunoglobulins, and (3) impaired antibody responses. The etiology of CVID is cited to include a failure of T-cell support required for B-cell survival and IgG production (158). Its genetic basis appears to be polygenic (159) with one susceptibility gene postulated to be either that encoding the HLA-DQ chain itself or located within the class III region (159).

Women with CVID have given birth to live children (160–162). The nature and severity of the related infections determine pregnancy outcome in women with CVID. During normal pregnancy, the fetus is usually well protected against most bacterial infections. However, if a CVID mother suffers from severe septicemia or worsening pulmonary disease, this can compromise the pregnancy. For this reason, it is recommended that infections in CVID patients should be treated early and aggressively with targeted antimicrobial therapy.

Early IgG therapy can arrest the cycle of recurrent infections and progressive lung disease that occurs in CVID pregnancies (163). However, IgG therapy has been associated with complications that include dyspnea, flank pain, hypotension, collapse, and death. Maternal IgG normally crosses the placenta into the fetus during the third trimester of pregnancy, which results in a marked reduction in the half-life of IgG, and concentrations in patients with CVID may fall below protective concentrations. Therefore, IgG therapy should be given more frequently to maintain maternal IgG concentrations above 200 mg/dL. Fetal losses caused by intrauterine or fetal infections have been reported in CVID mothers with inadequate circulating IgG concentrations (163,164). Maternal intravenous IgG infusion significantly increases the fetal IgG subclasses IgG1, IgG2, and IgG3 (165). Newborn infants born to CVID mothers do not display clinical manifestations of this disease (166). However, newborns born to CVID mothers are slow to achieve normal serum IgG concentrations for age, and antibody responses to various antigens are delayed.

Laboratory Testing and Diagnosis

One of the key laboratory criteria for diagnosing CVID is the detection of low concentrations of serum IgG (<500 mg/dL). Furthermore, IgM and IgA concentrations are undetectable in most patients, although a small subset of patients will display normal concentrations. Most CVID patients will display increased antibody responses to initial foreign antigen stimulation. However, these patients cannot switch the antibody production from IgM to IgG after repeated antigen challenges. Patients with CVID generally have normal peripheral blood B-cell numbers, with a small number of patients displaying a lack of circulating B cells. Some patients with normal B-cell numbers will have reduced numbers of T cells or T cells lacking the capacity to promote B-cell differentiation *(167)*.

Selective IgA Deficiency

Clinical Symptoms, Etiology, and Treatment

Selective IgA deficiency is the most common immunodeficiency in women of child-bearing age (incidence of from 1:400 to 1:800). The etiology of this disorder is thought to include defects in either the B-cell synthesis or release of IgA. Clinical manifestations of this disorder are related to a deficiency of secretory IgA, a major player in the secretory immune system that protects the body cavities (i.e., respiratory tract, gastrointestinal lumen, mammary gland, urinary tract, middle ear, and lacrimal tract). Chronic respiratory infections and diarrhea can occur, along with autoimmune conditions such as RA and SLE *(168,169)*. It is hypothesized that abnormal cytokine-induced switching occurs at the gene level, with an underlying T-cell defect providing a significant contribution to the etiology of this disease.

Genetically, an association has been reported between selective IgA deficiency and chromosomal abnormalities, including partial deletion of the short or long arm of chromosome 19 or a ring chromosome 18 *(170,171)*. Selective IgA deficiency exhibits familial expression and occurs frequently in the immediate relatives of individuals with CVID *(172)*.

There is significant variability in the onset and severity of the clinical symptoms of selective IgA deficiency. The basic defect in this disorder is thought to involve the terminal differentiation of IgA-secreting plasma cells, a process under the direction of the thymus. Most patients with IgA deficiency have allergic problems (e.g., asthma) that tend to be chronic and resistant to treatment. Patients with IgA deficiency also may present with celiac disease, intestinal nodular lymphoid hyperplasia, ulcerative colitis, regional ileitis, and pernicious anemia *(173)*.

Maternal selective IgA deficiency in pregnancy probably does not directly effect the fetal immune system, because IgA does not cross the placenta and neonates are normally deficient in IgA. IgA is the last Ig isotype to develop, which delays the diagnosis of this condition until adult concentrations are reached at between 10 and 12 yr of age. IgA-deficient women who become pregnant do not manifest particular complications over and above that which normally accompany this disease state.

Laboratory Testing and Diagnosis

Low serum concentrations of IgA (below 5 mg/dL) are the characteristic laboratory finding for women with selective IgA deficiency. In addition, patients with selective IgA deficiency display IgG subclass imbalances, and this combined IgG deficiency may increase susceptibility to infection in these patients.

Chronic Mucocutaneous Candidiasis

CLINICAL SYMPTOMS, ETIOLOGY, AND TREATMENT

Chronic mucocutaneous candidiasis (CMC) is a rare cellular immune deficiency manifested clinically by chronic fungal infections of the mucous membranes, nails, scalp, and skin. CMC is often associated with hypoadrenalism, hypothyrodism, diabetes mellitus, or hypoparathyroidism *(174)*. Women with CMC may carry a normal pregnancy to term in cases when associated endocrine disorders are not severe. The most critical of these complications are hypothyroidism and Addison's disease *(175)*.

Although CMC is widely considered a genetic disorder, its inheritance patterns are complex. An autosomal recessive form of inheritance has been proposed *(176)*, possibly linked to chromosome 22 *(177)*. The etiology of CMC is thought to include a failure of T-cell cytokine production, because treatment with proinflammatory mediator IL-2 has been shown to be beneficial *(178)*. Although the etiology of CMC is likely a T-cell defect, the molecular basis remains unknown *(179)*.

Laboratory Testing and Diagnosis

One of the problems associated with the laboratory diagnosis of patients with CMC is the extensive laboratory parameters observed with this disorder. However, a number of recent studies have examined the association between defective cell-mediated immune responses by lymphocytes from patients with CMC in response to candida antigen stimulation. In a recent study, de-Moraes-Vasconcelos and et al. *(180)* performed a panel of tests examining the cell-mediated immune response of lymphocytes from CMC patients and reported the following: (1) low to normal proliferative responses of lymphocytes to hytohemogglutinin, (2) suppressed lymphocyte proliferation in response to pokeweed mitogen, (3) lowered production of IL-2 and IFN-γ in response to stimulation with candida antigens, and (4) increased antigen-induced apoptosis in lymphocytes. In addition, recent flow cytometry studies have shown a decrease in the percentage of CD4+/CD9 T-helper inducer cells following candida antigen stimulation *(181)*. This group also reported an increase in IL-4 production and reduced IL-2 receptor production by stimulated lymphocytes. On the basis of these studies, it is possible that measurement of inflammatory cytokine production by ELISA techniques in cultures of lymphocytes stimulated with candida antigens may prove useful in the diagnosis of patients with CMC. Further studies are needed to determine whether the suppression of T_H1-mediated cellular immune responses is greater than that normally associated with pregnancy.

Hereditary Angiodema

CLINICAL SYMPTOMS, ETIOLOGY, AND TREATMENT

Hereditary angiodema (HAE) is a rare genetic disease inherited as an autosomal dominant trait. The etiology of HAE involves a lack of C1 inhibitor, a key regulatory protein for both the kallikrein–kinen system and early portions of the complement cascade *(182)*. Clinical manifestations of HAE include recurrent swelling of the extremities, face, larynx, bowel mucosa, and airways *(183)*. HAE patients are also at increased risk for developing immune-related conditions such as SLE, Sjogren's syndrome, autoimmune thyroid disease, mesangiocapillary glomerulonephritis, coronary arteritis, Chrohn's disease, and scleroderma.

Clinical symptoms of HAE occur in association with the patient's hormonal status, with increased severity during the menstrual period *(184)*. Interestingly, pregnancy has been found to be associated with a decrease in clinical symptoms of HAE. This response usually lessens the need for prophylactic therapy during pregnancy.

LABORATORY TESTING AND DIAGNOSIS

At present, there is no definitive, readily available laboratory test for the diagnosis of HAE. However, work by Verpy et al. *(185)* revealed the potential of new molecular-based techniques for identifying patients with this rare disorder. In this study, a complete mutational scan of the gene-coding region for the serpin C1 inhibitor was performed in 36 unrelated angioedema patients using fluorescence-assisted mismatch analysis. Remarkably, mutations accounting for the C1 inhibitor deficiency were identified in every 1 of 34 patients. This group suggested that fluorescence-assisted mismatch analysis may prove to be a rapid and robust mutation scanning procedure, with application to HAE and other genetic disorders.

Chronic Granulomatous Disease

CLINICAL SYMPTOMS, ETIOLOGY, AND TREATMENT

Chronic granulomatous disease (CGD) is a rare immunodeficiency disease occurring in from 1 in a 100,000 to 1 in 250,000 individuals. Clinically, patients with CGD develop serious infections early in life that affect the skin, lungs, liver, and bones. CGD patients also are at high risk for abscesses and septicemia. *Staphylococcus aureus* is the most common pathogen associated with CGD, but infections with Gram-negative organisms and fungi (*Candida* and *Aspergillis*) also occur.

The underlying etiology of CGD results from defects in any of the four genes encoding essential subunits of respiratory burst oxidase, the superoxide-generating enzyme complex in phagocytic leukocytes *(186)*. This prevents phagocytes from mounting a normal respiratory burst or generating hydrogen peroxide and oxygen radicals on stimulation *(187)*. Although current methods of management, including prophylactic use of antibiotics and IFN-γ, have improved the prognosis for these patients, CGD is still associated with significant morbidity and mortality from life-threatening infections and complications. Recent gene-expression studies of patients with the X-linked (X91) form of this disorder have revealed that different mechanisms of molecular quality control lead to the common phenotype of absence of mature membrane-bound nicotinamide adenine dinucleotide phosphate (NADP) oxidase complex in leukocytes *(188)*. These include the following: (1) aberrant intron splicing, creating a premature stop codon, (2) a frame-shift mutation, resulting in generation of a peptide with an aberrant and elongated C-terminus, and (3) a point mutation, creating a single amino acid change in the predicted FAD binding site of PG 91-phox. Similarly, a heterogeneous group of mutations in the gene encoding the P67-phox protein has been reported that results in the complete loss of NADPH oxidase activity *(189)*.

LABORATORY TESTING AND DIAGNOSIS

Laboratory diagnosis of CGD is made by demonstrating the inability of neutrophils to kill bacteria, especially staphylococci. Absent or reduced superoxide production as measured by the ferricytochrome c assay also is used to confirm CGD. Immunoblotting can also be useful in determining concentrations of the cytochrome b subunit in membrane fractions from disrupted neutrophils *(190)*. A convenient assay that is used to test for the defective respiratory burst in CGD is the nitroblue tetrazolium test, which turns blue when neutrophils are capable of killing bacteria.

CGD is not easily diagnosed from findings obtained at a physical exam. Mothers with CGD frequently also suffer from ulcers and gingivitis. Many patients have mild or moderate lymphadenopathy, splenomegaly, and hepatomegaly. Elevated erythrocyte sediment-ation rates, polyclonal gammopathy, and anemia are seen in most patients *(191)*. Successful, uneventful pregnancies have been reported in women with mild CGD *(191)*.

Hyperimmunoglobulin E Syndrome

CLINICAL SYMPTOMS, ETIOLOGY, AND TREATMENT

Hyperimmunoglobulin E syndrome (HIES) is an immune-based disorder characterized by the following: (1) remarkably high serum IgE, (2) recurrent staphylococcal infections, (3) cold subcutaneous abscesses, (4) chronic eczematous rashes, and (5) defects in neutrophil chemotaxis *(192,193)*. Major clinical features of this disease include recurrent bronchitis and severe pneumonias with pneumatoceles. The tendency for recurrent infections is usually well established at the age of 6 wk. *Staphylococcus aureus* is the major infection associated with HIES, followed by haemophilus influenza, group A streptococcus, *Escherichia coli*, and pseudomonas. In addition, chronic candidal infections can affect the mouth, nails, and skin.

Patients with HIES treated with IFNγ (0.05 mg, three times a week) exhibit a reduced severity of symptoms *(194)*. In addition, IgE production by peripheral blood mononuclear cells from these patients was reduced by approx 50%. Other therapeutic approaches involve prolonged therapy with intravenous antibiotic therapy *(195)*.

The type of genetic inheritance underlying HIES is unclear. Some groups have reported a familial occurrence, which may be related to an autosomal dominant form with incomplete penetrance. The underlying immunologic defect is also unknown, although lack of T-cell suppressor function may mediate increased IgE production.

LABORATORY TESTING AND DIAGNOSIS

Laboratory features of HIES include mild to moderate eosinophilia and an elevated erythrocyte sedimentation rate. By definition, patients with HIES have serum IgE concentrations in excess of 2000 IU/mL *(192,193)* and exhibit an impaired leukocyte chemotactic response *(196)*.

Acrodermatitis Enteropatheca

CLINICAL SYMPTOMS, ETIOLOGY, AND TREATMENT

Acrodermatitis enteropatheca is a rare autosomal disease that manifests itself clinically by the following: (1) failure to thrive, (2) skin lesions, (3) alopecia, (4) stomatitis, (5) glossitis, (6) paroncychia, and (7) secondary bacterial and fungal infections. Severe dermatitis and diarrhea may occur beginning in early infancy *(197)*. Acrodermatitis enteropatheca occurs because of a deficiency in zinc absorption linked to abnormal enterocytes in the intestinal lining. In these patients, the enterocytes lack expression of an oligopeptidase that normally destroys an oligopeptide involved in the chelation of zinc. With the presence of this peptide, zinc is chelated and cannot be absorbed, resulting in the patient becoming zinc deficient *(198)*.

Jamison *(199)* reported that lower maternal zinc concentrations were associated with several different diseases of pregnancy including abnormal labor, atonic bleeding, and premature birth. AF zinc concentrations also increase during the third trimester of pregnancy and it has been suggested that they play an important role in its antibacterial and antiviral activities *(200)*.

LABORATORY TESTING AND DIAGNOSIS

The most sensitive indicator of mild deficiencies of zinc is the measurement of plasma or zinc concentrations in a carefully collected sample *(201)*. During the course of normal pregnancy, there is a clear decrease in maternal serum zinc concentrations to about 50% of normal values, whereas concentrations in fetal cord blood and AF increase in normally progressing pregnancies. Treatment of acrodermatitis enteropatheca during pregnancy requires the daily supplementation of zinc (300 mg/d) in order to maintain concentrations within the range of 72–137 mg/dL *(202)*.

Pure Red Cell Aplasia

CLINICAL SYMPTOMS, ETIOLOGY, AND TREATMENT

Pure red cell aplasia (PRCA) is a rare disorder in which production of red cell precursors in the bone marrow is suppressed. PRCA is characterized clinically by severe anemia, reticulocytopenia, and a selective reduction of bone marrow erythroid precursors *(203)*. PRCA is not restricted to age, race, or gender and may occur as a congenital disorder or in an acquired fashion. The acquired form of PRCA has been associated with other disease states such as chronic lymphocytic leukemia, chronic granulocytic leukemia, Hodgkin's lymphomas, non-Hodgkin's lymphomas, multiple myeloma, acute lymphoblastic leukemia, or idiopathic myelofibrosis. Viral and bacterial infections have been associated with PRCA including human parvovirus B19 and HIV.

The mechanisms involved in autoimmune PRCA are not well understood. The suppression of erythroid colony formation may occur secondary to cellular rather than humoral inhibitory factors *(204)*. Successful pregnancies have been reported in women with PRCA *(203,205)*. Some groups have reported that PRCA can occur as a distinct disorder of pregnancy *(203)*. In these patients, anemia begins early in pregnancy and prompt recovery is seen soon after delivery. This can occur in any pregnancy and may relapse in subsequent pregnancies.

LABORATORY TESTING AND DIAGNOSIS

Diagnosis of PRCA is based on the determination of reticulocyte counts of less than 1% with normocellular marrow possessing 0.45% mature erythroblasts *(205)*. In vitro diagnosis studies also have been performed in which serum and purified IgG from patients suffering from PRCA specifically inhibited erythroid colony formation *(203)*. This effect reportedly disappears with remission of the disease.

SUMMARY

As outlined in this chapter, pregnancy imposes a number of unique challenges to the mother's immune system. First, in order for the developing fetus to survive, the maternal immune system must not mount lethal immunologic responses to placental antigens expressed at the maternal–fetal interface. This response is likely mediated through the lack of expression of classical transplantation antigens by the fetal trophoblast along with the effects of cytokines and hormones in the local microenvironment that suppress cell-mediated immunity. The second challenge that pregnancy presents is that of preservation of sufficient maternal immune function to provide protection against infection. Our current understanding is that preservation of the humoral immune response, combined with activation of the innate immune system, provides the needed immunologic protection in normal pregnancies.

Failure of the pregnant mother to properly adapt to pregnancy can result in the development or worsening of a variety of immune-based disorders, and in some cases (e.g., RA) actually can lead to an amelioration of symptoms. As reproductive immunologists and obstetricians more fully understand the ways in which alloimmune and autoimmune disorders complicate human pregnancy, new methods of diagnosis and treatment will be available to improve the course of pregnancy in these women and lessen the detrimental effects on the fetus and neonates.

REFERENCES

1. Sacks G, Sargent I, Redman C. An innate view of human pregnancy. Immunol Today 1999;20:114–118.
2. Krause PJ, Ingardia CJ, Pontius LT, Malech HL, LoBello TM, Maderazo EG. Host defense during pregnancy: Neutrophil chemotaxis and adherence. Am J Obstet Gynecol 1987;157:274–280.
3. Şalmeron O, Vaquer S, Salmeron I, et al. Pregnancy is associated with a reduction in the pattern of the cytotoxic activity displayed by lymphokine-activated killer cells. Am J Reprod Immunol 1991;26:150–155.
4. Hidaka Y, Amino N, Iwatani Y, et al. Changes in natural killer cell activity in normal pregnant and postpartum women: increases in the first trimester and postpartum period and decreases in late pregnancy. J Reprod Immunol 1991;20:73–83.
5. Castilla J, Rueda R, Vargas, M, Gonzalez-Gomez F, Garcia-Olivares E. Decreased levels of circulating CD4+ T lymphocytes during normal human pregnancy. J Reprod Immunol 1989;7:103–111.
6. Nakamura N, Miyazaki K, Kitano Y, Fujisaki S, Okamura H. Suppression of cytotoxic lymphocyte activity during pregnancy. J Reprod Immunol 1993;23:119–130.
7. Sargent IL. Maternal and fetal immune responses during preganancy. Exp Clin Immunogenet 1993; 10:85–102.
8. Feinberg BB, Gonik B. General precepts of the immunology of pregnancy. Clin Obstet Gynecol 1991;34:3–16.
9. Weinberg ED. Pregnancy: associated depression of cell-mediated immunity. Rev Infect Dis 1984;6:814–831.
10. Brabin BJ. Epidemiology of infection in pregnancy. Rev Infect Dis 1985;7:579–603.
11. Drutz DJ, Cantanzara A. Coccidiodomycosis. Am Rev Resp Dis 1978:117:727–771.
12. Stagno S, Reynolds DW, Huang ES, Thames SD, Smith RJ, Alford CA. Congenital cytomegalovirus infection: occurrence in an immune population. N Engl J Med. 1977;296:1254–1258.
13. Siegel M, Greenberg M. Incidence of poliolyelitis in pregnancy. N Engl J Med. 1955;253:841–847.
14. Weinstein I, Aycock WL, Feemster RF. The relation of sex, pregnancy and menstruation to susceptibility to poliomyelitis. N Engl J Med 1951; 245:54–58.
15. Priddle HD, Lenz WR, Young DL, Stevenson CS. Poliomyelitis in pregnancy and the puerperium. Am J Obstet Gynecol 1952:63:408–413.
16. D'Cruz IA, Balani SG, Iyer LS. Infectious hepatitis and pregnancy. Obstet Gynecol 1968;31:449–455.
17. Borhanmanesh F, Haghighi P, Hekman K, et al. Viral hepatitis during pregnancy. Gasteroenterology, 1973;64:304–312.
18. Morrow RH, Smetana HF, Sai FT, Edgecomb JK. Unusual features of viral hepatitis in Accra, Ghana. Ann Intern Med 1968;68:1250–1264.
19. Greenberg M, Jocobziner H, Parker J, et al. Maternal mortality in the epidemic of Asian influenza, New York City, 1957. Am J Obstet Gynecol 1958;76:897–902.
20. Freeman DW, Barno A. Deaths from Asian influenza associated with pregnancy. Am J Obstet Gynecol 1959;78:1172–1175.
21. Diro M, Beydoun SN. Malaria in pregnancy. South Med J 1982;75:959–962.

22. Hedvall E. Pregnancy and tuberculosis. Acta Med Scand 1953;147(suppl 286):3–101.

23. Murray DL, Imagawa DT, Okada DM, St. Geme JW. Antibody response to monovalent A/New Jersey/8/76 influenza vaccine in pregnant women. J Clin Microbiol 1979;10:184–187.

24. Lichtenstein MR. Tuberculin reaction in tuberculosis during pregnancy. Am Rev Tuber 1942:46:89–92.

25. Shahid NS, Steinhoff MC, Roy E, Begum T, Thompson CM, Siber GR. Placental and breast transfer of antibodies after maternal immunization with polysaccharide meningococcal vaccine: a randomized, controlled evaluation. Vaccine 2002;20:2404–2409.

26. Maral I, Cerak M, Aksakal FN, Baykan Z, Kayikcioglu F, Bumin MA. Tetanus immunization in pregnant women: serum levels of antitetanus antibodies at the time of delivery. Eur J Epidemiol 2001;17:661–665.

27. Munoz FM, Englund JA. Vaccines in pregnancy. Infect Dis Clin North Am 2001;150:253–271.

28. Medawar PB. Some immunological and endocrinological problems raised by evolution of viviparity in vertebrates. Symp Soc Exp Biol 1953;320–323.

29. Munz C, Holmes N, King A, et al. Human histocompatibility leukocyte antigen (HLA)-G molecules inhibit NKAT3 expressing natural killer cells. J Exp Med 1997;185:385–391.

30. Mosmann TR, Cherwinshi H, Bond MW, Giedlin MA, Coffman RL. Two types of murine helper T-cell clones. I. Definition according to profiles of lymphokine activities and secreted proteins. J Immunol 1986;136:2348–2357.

31. Mosmann TR, Coffman RL. Th1 and Th2 cells: different patterns of lymphokine secretion according to profiles of lymphokine activities and secreted proteins. J Immunol 1989;136:2348–2357.

32. Wegmann TG, Lin H, Guilbert L, Mossman TH. Bidirectional cytokine interactions in the materno-fetal relationship: successful allopregnancy is a Th2 phenomenon. Immunol Today 1993;14:353–355.

33. Varner MW. Autoimmune disorders and pregnancy. Semin Perinatol 1991;15:238–250.

34. Piccini MP, Giudizi MG, Biagiotti R, et al. Progesterone favors the development of human T-helper cells producing Th2-type cytokines and promotes both IL-4 production and membrane CD30 expression in established Th1 cell clones. J Immunol 1995;155:128–133.

35. Kelly RW, Critchley HO. A T-helper-2 bias in decidua: the prostaglandin contribution of the macrophage and trophoblast. J Reprod Immunol 1997;33:181–187.

36. Kuhn R, Lohler J, Rennick D, et al. Interleukin-10-deficient mice develop chronic enterocolitis. Cell 1993;75:263–274.

37. Sacks GP, Studena K, Sargent IL, Redman CWG. Normal pregnancy and preeclampsia both produce inflammatory changes in peripheral blood leukocytes akin to those of sepsis. Am J Obstet Gynecol 1998;179:80–86.

38. Koumandakis E, Koumandaki L, Kaklamani E, Sparos L, Aravantinos D, Trichopoulos D. Br J Obstet Gynecol 1986;93:1150–1154.

39. Shibuya T, Izuchi K, Kuroiwa A, Okabe N, Shirakawa K. Study on nonspecific immunity in pregnant women: increased chemi-luminescence response of peripheral blood phagocytes. Am J Reprod Immunol Microbiol 1987;15:19–23.

40. Shillingford AJ, Weinger S. Maternal issues affecting the fetus. Clin Perinatol. 2001;28:31–70.

41. Davis LE, Lucas MJ, Hankins GD, Roark ML, Cunningham FG. Thyrotoxicosis complicating pregnancy. Am J Obstet Gynecol 1989;160:63–70.

42. Burrow GN. The management of thyrotoxicosis in pregnancy. N Eng J Med 1985;313:562–565.

43. Mestman JH. Hyperthyroidism in pregnancy. Endocrinol Metab Clin North Am 1998;27:127–149.

44. Mulder JE. Thyroid disease in women. Med Clin North Am 1998;82:103–125.

45. Polak M. Hyperthyroidism in early infancy: pathophysiology, clinical features, and diagnosis with a focus on neonatal hyperthyroidism. Thyroid 1998;8:1171–1177.

46. Krude H, Bierbermann H, Krohn HP, Dralle H, Gruthers A. Congenital hyperthyroidism. Exp Clin Endocrinol Diabetes 1997;105:6–11.

47. Mestman JH. Hyperthyroidism in pregnancy. Endocrinol Metab Clin North Am 1998;27:127–149.

48. Zimmerman D. Fetal and neonatal hyperthyroidism. Thyroid 1999;9:727–733.

49. Messer PM, Hauffa BP, Olbright T, et al. Antithyroid drug treatment of Grave's disease in pregnancy: long-term effects on somatic growth, intellectual development and thyroid function in offspring. Acta Endocrinol (Copenh) 1990;123:311–316.

50. McKenzie JM, Zakarija M. Clinical review 3: the clinical use of thyrotropin receptor antibody measurements. J Clin Endocrinol Metab 1989;69:1093–1096.

51. Mestman JH, Goodwin M, Montoro MM. Thyroid disorders of pregnancy. Endocrinol Metab Clin North Am 1995;24:41–71.

52. Wenstrom KD, Weiner CP, Williamson RA, Grant SS. Perinatal diagnosis of fetal hyperthyroidism using funipuncture. Obstet Gynecol 1990;76:513–517.

53. Ruiz-Irastorza G, Khamashta MA, Castellino G, Hughes GRV. Systemic lupus erythematosus. Lancet 2001;357:1027–1032.

54. Sontheimer RD, Gilliam JN. Systemic lupus erythematosus and the skin. In Lahita RG ed. Systemic Lupus Erythematosus and the Skin, 2nd ed. New York: Churchill Livingstone, 1992, p. 657.

55. Carmona F, Font J, Cervera R, Munoz F, Cararach V, Balasch J. Obstetrical outcomes of pregnancy in patients with systemic lupus erythematosus: a study of 60 cases. Eur J Obstet Gynecol Reprod Biol 1999;83:137–142.

56. Brustein D, Rodriguez JM, Minkin W, Rabhan NB. Familial lupus erythematosus. 1977;238:2294–2296.

57. Bunyon JP, Hebert R, Copel J, et al. Autoimmune-associated congenital heart block: demographics, mortality, morbidity, and recurrence rates obtained from a national lupus registry. J Am Coll Cardiol 1998;31:1658–1666.

58. Bunyon JP, Waltuck J, Klein C, Kleinman C, Capel J. In utero identification and therapy of CHB. Lupus 1995;4:116–121.

59. Julkunen H, Kaaja R, Wallgren E, Teramo K. Isolated congenital heart block: fetal and infant outcome and familial incidence of heart block. Obstet Gynecol 1993;82:11–16.

60. Horsfall AC, Venables PJW, Taylor PV, Maini RN. Ro and La antigens and maternal anti-La idiotype on the surface of myocardial mibres in congenital heart block. J Autoimmun 1991;4:165–176.

61. Scott JS, Maddison PJ, Taylor PV, Esscher E, Scott O, Skinner RP. Connective tissue disease, autoantibodies to ribonucleoprotein and cogenital heart block. N Engl J Med 1983;309:209–212.

62. Boutjdir M, Zhang Z, Chen L, et al. Electrophysiologic characterization of purified IgG from a mother whose child has congenital heart block (CHB) on L-type calcium currents (Ica). Arthritis Rheum 1995;38:S230.

63. Copel JA, Bunyon JP, Kleinman CS. Successful in utero therapy of fetal heart block. Am J Obstet Gynecol 1995;173:1384–1390.

64. Bhandari S, Harnden P, Brownjohn AM, Turney JH. Association of anticardiolipin antibodies with intraglomerular thrombi and renal dysfunction in lupus nephitis. QJM 1998;91:401–409.

65. Swadzba J, DeClerck LS, Stevens WJ, et al. Anticardiolipin, anti-beta (2) glycoprotein I antiprothrombin antibodies and lupus anticoagulant in patients with systemic lupus erythematosus with a history of thrombosis. J Rheum 1997;24:1710–1715.

66. Provost TT, Watson R. Anti-Ro (SSA) HLA-DR3-positive women: the interrelationship between serum ANA negative, SS, SCLE, and NLE mothers and S/LE overlap female patients. J Invest Dermatol 1993;100:14S–20S.

67. Levine JS, Branch DW, Rauch J. The antiphospholipid syndrome. N Engl J Med:2002;346:752–763.

68. Asherson RA. The catastrophic antiphospholipid syndrome. J Rheum 1992;19:508–512.

69. Harris EN, Gharavi AE, Patel SP, Hughes GRV. Evaluation of the anticardiolipin antibody test: report of an international workshop, 4 April 1986. Clin Exp Immunol 1987;68:215–222.

70. Gharavi AE, Harris EN, Asherson RA, Hughes GRV. Antiphospholipid antibodies: isotype distribution and phospholipid specificity. Ann Rheum Dis 1987;46:1–6.

71. Branch DW, Scott JR, Kochenour NK, Hershgold E. Obstetric complications associated with the lupus anticoagulant. N Engl J Med 1985;313:1322–1326.

72. Cowchock S, Smith JB, Gocial B. Antibodies to phospholipids and nuclear antigens in patients with repeated abortions. Am J Obstet Gynecol 1986;155:1002–1010.

73. Unander AM, Norberg R, Hahn L, Arfors L. Anticardiolipin antibodies and complement in 99 women with habitual abortions. Am J Obstet Gynecol 1987;156:114–119.

74. Barbui T, Cortelazzo S, Galli M, et al. Antiphospholipid antibodies in early repeated abortions: a case-controlled study. Fertil Steril 1988;50:589–592.

75. Deleze M, Alarcon-Segovia D, Valdes-Macho E, Oria CV, Ponce de Leon S. Relationship between antiphospholipid antibodies and recurrent fetal loss in patients with systemic lupus erythematosus and apparently healthy women. J Rheumatol 1989;16:768–772.

76. Parke A, Maier D. Habitual fetal loss may indicate autoimmune disease. Fertil Steril 1989;51:280–285.

77. Branch DW, Dudley DJ, Mitchell MD, et al. Immunoglobulin G fractions from patients with antiphospholipid antibodies cause fetal death in Balb/c mice: a model for autoimmune fetal loss. Am J Obstet Gynecol 1990;163:210–216.

78. Beaumont JL. Syndrome hemorrhagique acquuis du a un anticoagulant circulant. Sangre 1964;25:1–15.

79. Vinter D, Dufour P, Cosson M, Houpcau JL. Antiphospholipid syndrome and recurrent miscarriages. Eur J Obstet Gynecol Reprod Biol 2001;96:37–50.

80. Branch DW, Scott JR. Clinical implications of antiphospholipid antibodies: the Utah experience. In Harris EN, Exner T, Hughes GRV, Asherson RA, eds, Phospholipid Binding Antibodies. Boca Raton, FL: CRC Press, 1991, pp. 335–346.

81. Branch DW, Silver RM, Blackwell JL, Reading JC, Scott JR. Outcome of treated pregnancies in women with antiphospholipid syndrome: an update of the Utah experience. Obstet Gynecol 1992;80:614–620.

82. Rai RS, Clifford K, Cohen H, Regan L. High prospective fetal loss rate in untreated pregnancies of women with recurrent miscarriage and antiphospholipid antibodies. Hum Reprod 1995;10: 3301–3304.

83. Lockwood CJ, Romero R, Feinberg RF, Clyne LP, Coster B, Hobbins JC. The prevalence and biologic significance of lupus anticoagulant and anticardiolipin antibodies in a general obstetric population. Am J Obstet Gynecol 1989;161:369–373.

84. Pattison NS, Chamley LW, McKay EJ, Liggins GC, Butler WS. Antiphospholipid antibodies in pregnancy: prevalence and clinical associations. Br J Obstet Gynaecol 1993;100:909–913.

85. Lynch A, Marlar R, Murphy J, et al. Antiphospholipid antibodies in predicting adverse pregnancy outcome. Ann Intern Med 1994;120:470–475.

86. Yasuda M, Takakuwa K, Tokunga A, Tanaka K. Prospective studies of the association between anticardiolipin antibody and outcome of pregnancy. Obstet Gynecol 1995;86:555–559.

87. Out HJ, Bruinse HW, Christianens GC, et al. A prospective, controlled multicenter study on the obstetric risks of pregnant women with antiphospholipid antibodies. Am J Obstet Gynecol 1992;167:26–32.

88. Rai RS, Regan L, Clifford K, et al. Antiphospholipid antibodies and beta2-glycoprotein-I in 500 women with recurrent miscarriage: results of a comprehensive screening approach. Hum Reprod 1995;10:2001–2005.

89. Oshiro BT, Silver RM, Scott JR, Yu H, Branch DW. Antiphospholipid antibodies and fetal death. Obstet Gynecol 1996;87:489–493.

90. Petri M, Hopkins. Lupus pregnancy center: 1987 to 1996. Rheum Dis Clin North Am 1997;23:1–13.

91. Out HJ, Bruinse HW, Derksen RH. Antiphospholipid antibodies and pregnancy loss. Hum Reprod 1991;6:889–897.

92. Parazzini F, Acaia B, Faden D, Lovotti M, Marelli G, Cortelazzo S. Antiphospholipid antibodies and recurrent abortion. Obstet Gynecol 1991;77:854–858.

93. Parke AL, Wilson D, Maier D. The prevalence of antiphospholipid antibodies in women with recurrent spontaneous abortion, women with successful pregnancies, and women who have never been pregnant. Arthritis Rheum 1991;34:1231–1235.

94. MacLean MA, Cumming GP, McCall F, Walker ID, Walker JJ. The prevalence of lupus anticoagulant and anticardiolipin antibodies in women with a history of first trimester miscarriages. Br J Obstet Gynecol 1994;101:103–106.

95. Balasch J, Creus M, Fabregues F, et al. Antiphospholipid antibodies and human reproductive failure. Hum Reprod 1996;11:2310–2315.

96. Harris EN, Chan JK, Asherson RA, Aber VR, Gharavi AE, Hughes GR. Thrombosis, recurrent fetal loss and thrombocytopenia: predictive value of the anticardiolipin antibody test. Arch Intern Med 1986;146:2153–2156.

97. Hughes GRV, Harris EN, Gharavi AE. The anticardiolipin syndrome. J Rheumatol 1986;13:486–489.

98. Brey RL, Gharavi AE, Lockshin MD. Neurological complications of antiphospholipid antibodies. Rheum Dis Clin North Am 1993;19:833–850.

99. Rosove MH, Brewer PMC. Antiphospholipid thrombosis: clinical course after the first thrombotic event in 70 patients. Ann Intern Med 1992;117:303–308.

100. Khamashta MA, Cuadrado MJ, Mujic F, Taub NA, Hunt BJ, Hughes GR. The management of thrombosis in the antiphospholipid-antibody syndrome. N Engl J Med 1995;332:993–997.

101. Brey RL, Hart RG, Sherman DG, Tegeler CH. Antiphospholipid antibodies and cerebral ischemia in young people. Neurology 1990;40:1190–1196.

102. Ferro D, Quintarelli C, Rasura M, Antionini G, Violi F. Lupus anticoagulant and the fibrinolytic system in young patients with stroke. Stroke 1993;24:368–370.

103. Chapman J, Shoenfeld Y. Neurological and neuroendocrine-cytokine inter-relationship in the antiphospholipid syndrome. Ann NY Acad Sci 2002;966:415–424.

104. Lima F, Khamashta MA, Buchanan NMM, Kerslake S, Hunt BJ, Hughes GR. A study of sixty pregnancies in patients with the antiphospholipid syndrome. Clin Exp Rheumatol 1996;14:131–136.

105. Harris EN, Asherson RA, Gharavi AE, Morgan SH, Derue G, Hughes GRV. Thrombocytopenia in SLE and related autoimmune disorders: association with anticardiolipin antibody. Br J Hematol 1985;59:227–250.

106. Asherson RA, Khamashta MA, Ordi-Ros J, et al. The "primary" antiphospholipid syndrome: major clincial and serological features. Medicine 1989;68:366–374.

107. Branch DW, Andres R, Digre KB, Rote NS, Scott JR. The association of antiphospholipid antibodies with severe preeclampsia. Obstet Gynecol 1989;73:541–545.

108. Milliez J, Delong F, Bayani N, et al. The prevalence of autoantibodies during third trimester pregnancy complicated by hypertension or idiopathic fetal growth retardation. Am J Obstet Gynecol 1991;165:51–56.

109. Sletnes KE, Wislof F, Moe N, Dale PO. Antiphospholipid antibodies in preeclamptic women: relation to growth retardation and neonatal outcome. Acta Obstet Gynecol Scand 1992;71:112–117.

110. Moodley J, Bhoola V, Cuursma J, Pudfin D, Byrne S, Kenoyer DG. The association of antiphospholipid antibodies with severe early onset preeclampsia. S Afr Med J 1995;85:105–107.

111. Rivier G, Herranz MT, Khamashta MA, Hughes GR. Thrombosis and antiphospholipid syndrome: a preliminary assessment of three antithrombotic treatments. Lupus 1994;3:85–90.

112. Rai R, Cohen H, Dave M, Regan I. Randomized controlled trial of aspirin and asprin plus heparin in pregnant women with recurrent miscarriage associated with phospholipid antibodies (or antiphospholipid antibodies). Br Med J 1997;314:253–257.

113. Coulam CB, McIntyre JA, Wagenknecht D, Rote N. Interlaboratory inconsistencies in detection of anticardiolipin antibodies. Lancet 1990;335:865.

114. Peaceman AM, Silver RK, MacGregor SN, Socol ML. Interlaboratory variation in antiphospholipid antibody testing. Am J Obstet Gynecol 1992;166:1784–1787.

115. Harris EN, Spinnato JA. Should anticardiolipin tests be performed in otherwise healthy pregnant women? Am J Obstet Gynecol 1991;165:1272–1277.

116. Vaarala O, Palusuo T, Kleemola M, Aho K. Anticardiolipin response in acute infections. Clin Immunol Immunopathol 1986;41:8–15.

117. Silver RM, Porter TF, van Leeuwen I, Jeng G, Scott JR, Branch DW. Anticardiolipin antibodies: clincial consequences of "low titers." Obstet Gynecol 1996;87:494–500.

118. Alarcon-Segovia D, Perez-Vasquez ME, Villa AR, Drenkard C, Cabiedes J. Preliminary classification criteria for the antiphospholipid syndrome with systemic lupus erythematosus. Semin Arthritis Rheum 1992;21:275–286.

119. Branch DW, Silver RM, Pierangeli SS, van Leeuwen I, Harris EN. Antiphospholipid antibodies in women with recurrent pregnancy loss, fertile controls, and antiphospholipid syndrome. Obstet Gynecol 1997;89:549–555.

120. Silver R, Branch W, Scott J. Maternal thrombocytopenia in pregnancy: time for reassessment. Am J Obstet Gynecol 1995;173;479–482.

121. Burrow R, Kelton J, Thrombocytopenia in delivery: a prospective study of 6715 deliveries. Am J Obstet Gynecol 1990;162:731–734.

122. Biswas A, Arulkumaran S, Ratnam S. Disorders of platelets in pregnancy. Obstet Gynecol Surv 1994;49:585–594.

123. Al-Mofada S, Osman M, Kides E, al Momen AK, al Herbish AS, al Mobaireck K. Risk of thrombocytopenia in the infants of mothers with idiopathic thrombocytopenia. Am J Perinatol 1994;6:423–426.

124. Paides M, Haut M, Lockwood C. Platelet disorders in pregnancy: implications for mother and fetus. Mt Sinai J Med 1994;61:389–403.

125. Mennell J, Bussel J. Antenatal management of the thrombocytopenias. Clin Perinatol 1994;21:591–614.

126. Jaff M. Medical aspects of pregnancy. Cleveland Clin J Med 1994;61:263–271.

127. Rose V, Gordon I. Idiopathic thrombocytopenia purpura in pregnancy: successful management with immunoglobulin infusion. JAMA 1985;254:2626–2628.

128. Howe SE, Lynch DM, Lynch JM. An enzyme-linked immunosorbent assay for the quantification of serum platelet-bindable IgG. Transfusion 1984;24:348–352.

129. Hedge UM, Ball S, Zuiable A, Roter BL. Platelet-associated immunoglobulins (PAIgG and PaigM) in autoimmune thrombocytopenia. Br J Haematol 1985;59:221–226.

130. Lynch DM, Lynch JM, Howe SE. A quantitative ELISA procedure for the measurement of membrane-bound platelet-associated IgG (PAIgG). Am J Clin Pathol 1985;83:331–336.

131. Hegde UM. Platelet antibodies in immune thrombocytopenia. Blood Rev 1992;6:34–42.
132. Joutsi-Korhonen L, Javela K, Hormila P, Kekomaki R. Glycoprotein V-specific platelet-associated antibodies in thrombocytopenic patients. Clin Lab Hematol 2001;23:307–312.
133. Garner SF, Campbell K, Metcalfe P, et al. Glycoprotein V: the predominant target antigen in gold-induced autoimmune thrombocytopenia. Blood 2002;100:344–346.
134. Bussel JB. Immune thrombocytopenia in pregnancy: autoimmune and alloimmune. J Reprod Immunol 1997;37:35–61.
135. Plauche W. Myasthenia gravis in mothers and their newborns. Clin Obstet Gynecol 1991;34:82–99.
136. Rowland L. Controversies about the treatment of myasthenia gravis. J Neurol Neurosurg Psych 1980;43:644–659.
137. Vernet-der Garbedian B, Lacokova M, Eymard B, et al. Association of neonatal myasthenia gravis with antibodies against the fetal acetylcholine receptor. J Clin Invest 1994;94:555–559.
138. Matthews I, Sims G, Ledwidge S, et al. Antibodies to acetylcholine receptor in parous women with myasthemia: evidence for immunization by fetal antigen. Lab Invest 2002;82:1407–1417.
139. Plauche WC. Myasthenia gravis in mothers and their newborns. Clin Obstet Gynecol 1991;34:82–99.
140. Vincent A, Newsom-Davis J. Acetylcholine receptor antibody as a diagnostic test for myasthenia gravis: results in 153 validated cases and 2967 diagnostic assays. J Neurol Neurosurg Psych 1985;48:1246–1252.
141. Hinman CL, Ernstoff RM, Montgomery IN, Hudson RA, Rauch HC. Clinical correlates of enzyme-immunoassay versus radioimmunoassay measurements of antibody acetylcholine receptor in patients with myasthenia gravis. J Neurol Sci 1986;75:305–316.
142. Howard FM Jr. Lennon VA, Finley J, Matsumato J, Elveback LR. Clinical correlations of antibodies that bind, block or modulate human acetylcholine receptors in myasthenia gravis. Ann. NY Acad Sci 1987;505:526–538.
143. Jailkhani BL, Asthana D, Jafferey NF, Khajuria A, Subbalaxmi B, Ahuja GK. ELISA for detection of IgG and IgM antibodies to human nicotinic acetylcholine receptor in myasthenia gravis. Ind J Med Res 1986;83:187–195.
144. Vernet-der Garabedian B, Lacokova M, Eymard B, et al. Association of neonatal myasthenia gravis with antibodies against the fetal acetylcholine receptor. J Clin Invest 1994;94:555–559.
145. Gardnerova M, Eymard B, Morel E, et al. The fetal/adult acetylcholine receptor antibody ratio in mothers with myasthenia gravis as a marker for transfer of the disease to the newborn. Neurology 1997;48:50–54.
146. Hench PS. The ameliorating effect of pregnancy on chronic atrophic (infectious rheumatoid) arthritis, fibrositis and intermittent hydraarthrosis. Proc Staff Meet Mayo Clin 1938;3:161–167.
147. Oka M, Vainio U. Effect of pregnancy on the prognosis and serology of rheumatoid arthritis. Acta Rheum Scand 1966;12:47–52.
148. Neely NT, Persellin RH. Activity of rheumatoid arthritis during pregnancy. Texas Med 1977;73:59–63.
149. Persellin RH. The effect of pregnancy on rheumatoid arthritis. Bull Rheum Dis 1977;27:992–997.
150. Ostensen M, Husby G. A prospective clinical study of the effect of pregnancy on rheumatoid arthritis and ankylosing spondylitis. Arch Rheum 1983;26:1155–1159.
151. Ostensen M, Husby G. Pregnancy and rheumatic disease: a review of recent studies in rheumatoid arthritis and ankylosing spondylitis. Klin Wochenschr 1984;62:891–895.
152. Bulmash JM. Rheumatoid arthritis and pregnancy. Obstet Gynecol 1985;8:223–276.
153. Ostensen M, Aune LB, Husby G. Effect of pregnancy and hormonal changes on the activity of rheumatoid arthritis. Scand J Rheumatol 1983;12:69–72.
154. Takeuchi A, Persellin RH. The inhibitory effect of pregnancy serum on polymorphonuclear leukocyte chemotaxis. J Clin Lab Immunol 1980;3:121–124.
155. Lahita RG. Sex steroids and the rheumatic diseases. Arthritis Rheum 1985;28:121–126.
156. Talal N, Ahmed SA. Immunomodulation by hormones: an area of growing importance. J Rheumatol 1987;14:191–193.
157. Muller B, Gimsa U, Mitchison NA, Radbruch A, Sieper J, Yin S. Modulating the Th1/Th2 balance in inflammatory arthritis. Sem Immunopathol 1998;20:181–196.
158. Lane P. Common variable immunodeficiency: does life begin at 40? Clin Exp Immunol 1994;95:201–203.
159. Hammarstrom L, Gilner M, Smith C. Molecular basis for human immunodeficiencies. Curr Opin Immunol 1993;5:579–584.

160. Holland N, Holland P. Immunological maturation in an infant of an agammaglobulinemic mother. Lancet 1966;2:1152–1155.

161. Laursen H, Christensen M. Immunoglobulins in normal infant born of severe hypogammaglobulinemic mother. Arch Dis Child 1973;48:646–648.

162. Kobayashi R, Hyman C, Stiehm E. Immunologic maturation in an infant born to a mother with agammaglobulinemia. Am J Dis Child 1980;1334:942–944.

163. Dams E, Van der Meer J. Subcutaneous immunoglobulin replacement in patients with primary antibody deficiencies. Lancet 1995;345:864.

164. Hauser C, Buriot D. Gamma globulin therapy during pregnancy in mothers with hypogammaglobulinemia. Am J Obstet Gynecol 1982;144:112.

165. Madsen D, Catanzarite V, Varela Gittling F. Common variable hypogammaglobulinemia in pregnancy: treatment with high dose immunoglobulin infusions. Am J Hematol 1986;21:327–329.

166. Slade H. Human immunoglobulins for intravenous use and hepatitis C viral transmission. Clin Diag Lab Immunol 1994;6:613–619.

167. Report of a WHO Scientific Group. Primary immunodeficiency disease. Immunodef Rev 1992;3:195.

168. Ammann A, Hong R. Selective IgA deficiency: presentation of 30 cases and a review of the literature. Medicine 1971;50:223–236.

169. Bluestone R, Goldberg L, Katz R, Marchesano JM, Calabro JJ. Juvenile rheumatoid arthritis: a serologic survey of 200 consecutive patients. J Pediatr 1970;77:98–102.

170. Finley S, Finley W, Noto R, et al. IgA absence associated with a ring-18 chromosome. Lancet 1968;1:1095–1096.

171. Stewart JM, Go S, Ellis E, Robinson A. Absent IgA and deletions of chromosome 18. J Med Genet 1970;7:11–19.

172. Volankis JE, Zhu ZB, Schaffer FM, et al. Major histocompatibility complex III genes and susceptibility to immunoglobulin A deficiency and common variable immunodeficiency. J Clin Invest 1992;89: 1914–1922.

173. Douglas SD, Goldberg LS, Gudenberg HH, et al. Agammaglobulinemia and co-existent pernicious anemia. Clin Exp Immunol 1970;6:181–187.

174. Kirkpatrick C. Chronic mucocutaneous candidiasis. J Am Acad Dermatol 1994;31:S14–S17.

175. Oyefara B, Kim H, Danziger RN, Carroll M, Greene JM, Douglas SD. Autoimmune hemolytic anemia in chronic mucocutaneous candidiasis. Clin Diagn Lab Immunol 1994;1:38–43.

176. Bentur L, Nisbet-Brown E, Levison H, Roifman CM. Lung disease associated with IgG subclass deficiency in chronic mucocutaneous candidiasis. J Pediatr 1991;118:82–86.

177. Aaltonen J, Komulainen J, Vikman E, et al. Autoimmune polyglandular disease type I: exclusion map using amplifiable multiallelic markers in a microtiter well format. Eur J Human Genet 1993;1: 164–171.

178. Sander E, Prolla A, Marques R, Zelmanowitz T, Zampese M, Schwartsmann G. Reversal by interleukin-2 of alopecia universalis, mucocutaneous candidiasis, and sexual impotence in a patient with malignant thymoma. J Natl Cancer Inst 1993;85:673.

179. Noh L, Hussein S, Sukumaran K, Rose I, Abdullah N. Chronic mucocutaneous candidiasis with deficient CD2 (E receptor) but normal CD3 mononuclear cells. J Clin Lab Immunol 1991;35:89–93.

180. De Padova-Elder S, Detre C, Kantor G, et al. Candidiasis endocrinopathy syndrome. Arch Dermatol 1994;130:19.

181. De Morales-Vasconcelos D, Orii NM, Romano CC, Iqueoka RY, Duarte AJ. Characterization of the cellular immune function of patients with chronic mucocutaneous candidiasis. Pathology 2001;54: 81–83.

182. Nielsen E, Johansen H, Holt J, et al. C1 inhibitor and diagnosis of hereditary angiodema in newborns. Pediatr Res 1994;35:184–187.

183. Srinivasan J, Beck P. IgA nephropathy in heriditary angioedema. Postgrad Med J 1993;69:95.

184. Frank M, Gelfand J, Atkinson J. Heriditary angiodema: the clinical syndrome and its management. Ann Int Med 1984;84:580.

185. Verpy E, Biasotto M, Brai M, Misiano G, Meo T, Tose M. Exhaustive mutation scanning by fluorescence-assisted mismatch analysis discloses new genotype–phenotype correlations in angiodema. Am J Hum Genetics 1996;59:308–319.

186. Kume A, Denauer MC. Gene therapy for chronic granulomatous disease. J Lab Clin Med 2000;135: 122–128.

187. Smith R, Curnutte J. Molecular basis of chronic granulomatous disease. Blood 1991;77:673–686.

188. Lin SJ, Huang YE, Chen JY, et al. Molecular quality control machinery contributes to the leukocyte NADPH oxidase deficiency in chronic granulomatous disease. Biophysica Acta 2002;1586:276–286.

189. Patino PJ, Rae J, Noack D, et al. Molecular characterization of autosomal recessive chronic granulomatous disease caused by a defect of the nicotinamide adenine dinucleotide phosphate (reduced form) oxidase component p67-phox. Blood 1999;94:2505–2614.

190. Hopkins P, Bemiller L, Curnutte J. Chronic granulomatous disease: diagnosis and classification at the molecular level. Clin Lab Med 1992;2:277–304.

191. Veille J, Bigley R. Chronic granulomatous disease in pregnancy. Obstet Gynecol 1985;66:8S–9S.

192. Yamada H, Magoaka I, Takamori K, Ogawa H. Double filtration plasmapheresis enhances neutrophil chemotactic responses in hyperimmunoglobulin E syndrome. Artif Organs 1995;19:98–102.

193. Bulengo-Ransby S, Headington J, Cantu-Gonzalez G, Rasmussen JE. Staphylococcal botryomycosis and hyperimmunoglobulin E (Job's) syndrome in an infant. J Am Acad Dermatol 1993;54:109–111.

194. Pung YH, Vetro SW, Bellanti JA. Use of interferons in atopic (IgE-mediated) diseases. Ann. Allergy 1993;71:234–238.

195. Donabedian H, Gallin JI. The hyperimmunoglobulin E recurrent-infection (Job's) syndrome: a review of the NIH experience and the literature. Medicine 1983;62:195–208.

196. Leung DY, Geha RS. Critical and immunologic aspects of the hyperimmunoglobulin E syndrome. Hematol Oncol Clin North Am 1988;2:81–100.

197. Sandstrom B, Cederblad A, Lindblad B, Lonnerdal B. Acrodermatitis enteropathica, zinc metabolism, copper status, and immune function. Arch Pediatr Adolesc Med 1994;148:980–985.

198. Fitzpatrick J. Self assessment 1993: acrodermatitis enteropathica. J Cutan Pathol 1994;21:566–567.

199. Jamison S. Effects of zinc deficiency in human reproduction. Acta Med Scand 1976;593:5–89.

200. Kynast G, Saling E. The relevance of zinc in pregnancy. J Perinat Med 1980;8:171–182.

201. Ruz M, Cavan KR, Bettger WJ, Thompson L, Berry M, Gilson RS. Development of a dietary model for the study of mild zinc deficiency in humans and evolution of some biochemical and functional indices of zinc status. Am J Clin Nutr 1991;53:1295–1303.

202. Taylor A. Detection and monitoring of disorders of essential trace elements. Ann Clin Biochem 1996;33:486–510.

203. Baker R, Manoharan A, DeLuca E, Begley CG. Pure red cell aplasia of pregnancy: a distinct clinical entity. Br J Haematol 1993;85:619–622.

204. Maung Z, Norden J, Middleton P, Jack FR, Chandler JE. Pure red cell aplasia: further evidence of T cell clonal disorder. Br J Haematol 1994;87:189–192.

205. Itoh Y, Aizawa S, Nehashi Y, et al. Pure red cell aplasia combined with pregnancy. Am J Hematol 1993;43:79.

15 Recurrent Pregnancy Loss

Carolyn B. Coulam, MD

CONTENTS

INTRODUCTION
CAUSES OF RECURRENT PREGNANCY LOSS
DIAGNOSIS OF RECURRENT PREGNANCY LOSS
TREATMENT OF RECURRENT PREGNANCY LOSS
CONCLUSION
REFERENCES

INTRODUCTION

Normal human reproduction is an inefficient process with only 22.8% of conceptive matings resulting in live birth (Fig. 1) *(1,2)*. Miscarriages are the most common complication of pregnancy, affecting 15% of women *(3)*. Loss of pregnancy is a physically and emotionally challenging ordeal. When pregnancy loss is repetitive, these feelings are magnified and the result is a distressing and frustrating problem for both the patients and the physicians. Recurrent pregnancy losses can occur early or late in the pregnancy. Early pregnancy losses are losses of embryos during the first trimester of pregnancy and have been termed abortions or miscarriages. Although most miscarriages are sporadic and not repetitive, there is a subset of couples that suffer recurrent miscarriage. Although the risk of miscarriage increases with maternal age, overall 15% of pregnancies miscarry. Approximately 13% of all recognized first pregnancies are lost. The risk of a second consecutive miscarriage is only slightly increased to 17%. However, the risk of miscarriage after two consecutive pregnancy losses rises to between 35 and 40% and continues to rise with each subsequent miscarriage *(4)*. As many as 5% of all couples conceiving experience two consecutive miscarriages and 2% have three or more consecutive losses. Late pregnancy losses are losses of fetuses after the first trimester of pregnancy. Late pregnancy losses occur far less frequently than early pregnancy losses and comprise only 1% of pregnancies. Late pregnancy losses are usually associated with incompetent cervix, premature rupture of membranes, preterm labor, intrauterine growth retardation, or placental abruption.

Whereas in the past a cause for recurrent pregnancy loss could be determined in only a minority of couples, more recent studies have shed a great deal of light on the reasons for recurrent pregnancy loss. With advancing technology to aid in the diagnosis of various proven and suspected causes of recurrent pregnancy loss, the proportion of unexplained recurrent losses is diminishing, allowing for more rational methods of treatment.

From: *Current Clinical Pathology: Handbook of Clinical Laboratory Testing During Pregnancy*
Edited by: A. M. Gronowski © Humana Press, Totowa, NJ

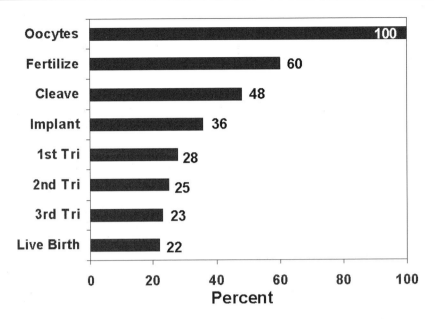

Fig. 1. Life table analysis of reproductive inefficiency in the human (drawn from data taken from refs. *1* and *2*).

CAUSES OF RECURRENT PREGNANCY LOSS

There are two major reasons for recurrent pregnancy loss. One is that there is something wrong with the pregnancy itself, such as a chromosomal abnormality that prohibits the pregnancy from implanting or growing properly. The other reason is a problem within the environment in which the pregnancy grows that does not allow an otherwise normal embryo to implant or grow properly. Problems within the environment or lining of the uterus have been classified as anatomic, hormonal, and immunologic.

Problems With the Pregnancy

Problems with the pregnancy are most often characterized by the presence of an abnormal chromosome analysis of the conceptus. Chromosomal abnormalities occur in about 60% of eggs retrieved for in vitro fertilization (IVF) that have been studied with preimplantation genetic diagnosis *(5)*, 50% of all products of conception from first trimester miscarriages *(6)*, 5% of late pregnancy losses, and 0.5% of live births *(7)*. When products of conception from more than 200 miscarriages of women with recurrent pregnancy loss were tested with chromosomal analysis, 55% were abnormal *(6)*. Of interest, only 35% of products of conception from women experiencing recurrent pregnancy loss after a live birth were chromosomally abnormal *(6)*. Some pregnancy losses associated with abnormal chromosomes such as trisomy have been reported to have a high risk of repeating *(8)*. However, if such chromosomal "accidents" explained all recurrent miscarriages, the probability of three or more miscarriages in a row resulting from "accidents" would account for 5% or less of the observed incidence of losses *(2)*. Therefore, although chromosomal abnormalities play a major role in earlier pregnancy losses, other causes account for most late pregnancy losses as well as approximately half of all miscarriages.

A number of studies have suggested the existence of a paternal (sperm-derived) effect on human embryo quality and pregnancy outcomes that are not reflected as a chromosomal abnormality *(9)*. Damaged sperm DNA can have a negative impact on fetal development and present clinically as occult or early clinical miscarriage. The sperm DNA integrity assay (discussed in detail later) serves as a tool for identifying those at risk for such damage (Coulam, Roussev, unpublished data, 2002).

Problems With the Environment

Problems within the environment in which the embryo implants and fetus grows have been classified as anatomic, hormonal, and immunologic.

ANATOMIC ABNORMALITIES

Anatomic abnormalities are lesions inside the uterus that, if present, would mechanically inhibit normal implantation and hence normal embryo and/or fetal growth. Anatomic abnormalities include endometrial polyps, submucosal fibroids, uterine synechiae, and Mullerian duct defects.

HORMONAL RESPONSE

Hormonal response of the endometrium in the past was measured by taking a biopsy of the lining of the uterus and correlating endometrial status with serum concentrations of progesterone. If the biopsy was "out of phase" by 2 or more days, a diagnosis of luteal phase defect was made. However, endometrial biopsy has failed to correlate with pregnancy outcome *(10)*. Although hormonal imbalances such as luteal phase defect have been associated with occult pregnancy loss, they do not play a role in clinically recognized pregnancy loss *(10)*.

Blood flow to the endometrial lining, measured as uterine artery resistance (pulsatility index) and subendometrial flow, is under hormonal control and has been shown to correlate with pregnancy outcome *(11,12)*. If resistance of flow through the uterine artery is elevated, or if flow of blood through the spiral arteries leading to the endometrium is low, successful pregnancy outcome is not expected *(11,12)*.

IMMUNOLOGIC MECHANISMS

Immunologic mechanisms have recently been recognized as a major cause of recurrent pregnancy loss associated with the loss of chromosomally normal pregnancies. Forty-five percent of miscarriages and 95% of late pregnancy losses from women experiencing recurrent pregnancy loss are chromosomally normal. Literature is developing that suggests a role of the immune system in the majority of these losses *(13,14)*. The result of the immunologic processes that lead to loss of the pregnancy frequently involves interference of the blood supply to the pregnancy. Interference of blood supply among early and late pregnancy losses is manifested by clotting of the placental–fetal vessels. Clotting of these vessels can be caused by (1) cytokines that are produced by immunologic cells within the lining of the uterus, (2) antiphospholipid antibodies produced by circulating B cells, (3) a genetic predisposition contributed by thrombophilia genes.

Cytokines. Miscarriages can be caused by cytokines secreted by cells within the uterus. The activities of these cytokines have been characterized as proinflammatory and anti-inflammatory. Although initial exposure to proinflammatory cytokines is necessary to stimulate invasion of the blastocyst and formation of new blood vessels at the time of implantation, prolonged exposure of proinflammatory cytokines to the pregnancy is detrimental. Thus, for pregnancy to be successful, a change in balance of secretion of cytokines from proinflammatory to anti-inflammatory cytokines must occur. Three major types of immune cells within the endometrium contribute to the proinflammatory and anti-inflammatory responses: T cells, natural killer (NK) cells, and macrophages. Macrophages and NK cells infiltrate implantation sites destined to miscarry *(15)*. Both of these cells are sources of proinflammatory cytokines that can activate production of the prothrombinase fgl2 *(15)*. Fgl2 leads to deposition of fibrin and activation of polymorphonuclear leukocytes (PMN) that can destroy the vascular supply to the placenta. Blood supply to the embryo is compromised and the pregnancy essentially "withers on the vine." Increased expression of fgl2 has been s hown association with miscarriage of chromosomally normal embryos as contrasted with chromosomally abnormal embryos *(15)*. Assays for clinical testing of fgl2 are not as yet available.

Not all losses associated with increased clotting may be caused by proinflammatory cytokine stimulation of fgl2. There is a growing emphasis on the role of antiphospholipid antibodies and genetic causes of blood clotting such as hyperhomocysteinemia, prothrombin mutations, and factor V Leiden among women experiencing recurrent pregnancy loss. Assays for these risk factors are clinically available.

Antiphospholipid Antibodies. Antiphospholipid antibodies (APLA) have been shown to be associated with both early and late pregnancy loss. The action of APLA on the blood vessel cells results in blood clotting within the vessels *(16,17)* and thus blood supply to the pregnancy is impaired. Of the APLAs tested, ethanolamine and serine have been shown to target blood vessel cells *(16,17)*. Testing for APLA is discussed in detail later.

Thrombophilia Genes. Recently, interest has focused on genetic causes of blood clotting. A number of genes involved in blood clotting have been shown to be associated with abnormal clotting and a history of thrombosis. Deficiencies of antithrombin III, protein S or C, are usually associated with a previous history of thromboses. Other gene mutations are not associated with such a high risk of blood clots, but are associated with recurrent pregnancy loss. These genetic risk factors include factor V Leiden, prothrombin, and methylenetetrahydrofolate reductase (MTHFR) gene mutations *(18)*. All of these mutations have been associated more with second- and third-trimester loss than first-trimester loss. However, it appears that the more mutations there are, the higher the risk for early pregnancy loss. In one study *(19)*, about 8% of women with a history of recurrent miscarriage had combined thrombophilic defects compared with 1% of controls. Testing for thrombophilic genes is presented in the next section.

Summary

In summary, immunologically mediated losses of pregnancies result from impairment of blood supply to the pregnancy. Stimuli that lead to impairment of blood supply to the pregnancy include cytokines, APLAs, and thrombophilia genes. With multiple mechanisms contributing to immunologic causes of recurrent pregnancy loss, advanced diagnostic tools are necessary for diagnosis and treatment of unexplained losses of chromosomally normal embryos.

Table 1
Diagnosis and Management of Recurrent Pregnancy Loss

Etiology	Diagnostic evaluation	Therapy
Problems with the pregnancy		
Genetic	Karyotype partners	Genetic counseling
	Karyotype product of conception	Donor gametes
	Preimplantation genetic diagnosis	Preimplantation selection
Endocrine	Endometrial biopsy/serum progesterone	Progesterone
	FSH/estradiol/inhibin B	Donor oocytes
	Sperm DNA integrity	Donor sperm
	hCG/progesterone/inhibin A	None
	Blood flow to endometrium-color Doppler	Asprin/Viagra
Problems with the environment		
Anatomic	Hysterosalpingogram	Septum transection
	Hysteroscopy	Myomectomy
	Hysterosonography	
Immunologic	Antiphospholipid antibodies	Aspirin and heparin
	Antithyroid antibodies	IVIg
	Antinuclear antibodies	Glucocorticoids
	Natural killer cell activation	IVIg
	Reproductive immunophenotype	IVIg
Hematologic	Coagulation assays	
	Genetic testing for:	Aspirin/heparin
	• hyperhomocysteinemia	plus folic acid and vitamin B
	• factor V Leiden	
	• factor II prothrombin mutation	
Microbiologic	Cervical cultures	Antibiotics
Psychological	Patient history	Counseling
	Interview/questionnaire	
Iatrogenic	Patient history	Eliminate exposure
	Toxicological screen	

DIAGNOSIS OF RECURRENT PREGNANCY LOSS

Establishing the correct diagnosis is an important component in treating couples with recurrent pregnancy loss. Diagnostic tests useful in identifying causes of recurrent spontaneous abortion and potential treatments are shown in Table 1.

Problems With the Pregnancy

CHROMOSOMAL ANALYSIS

Chromosomal analysis of the fetal tissue from previous pregnancy losses and both parents is useful in determining those pregnancies that are lost as a result of problems within the pregnancy itself. Whereas the frequency of abnormal chromosomal analyses among couples experiencing recurrent pregnancy loss is 5 to 6% *(3)*, chromosomal aberrations are found in 55% of abortuses from women with a history of recurrent pregnancy loss *(5)*. There is a subset of couples having recurrent loss of pregnancy that have an increased risk of repeated aneuploidy. Currently, no ways other than karyotyping products of conception are available to identify women with losses caused by chromosomal abnormalities. We have, therefore, advocated that all losses after a first miscarriage should be karyotyped.

ASSESSING OVARIAN RESERVE

The development of diminished ovarian reserve generally reflects the processes of follicular depletion and decline in oocyte quality. Low ovarian reserve has been associated with a significant increase in pregnancy loss (Fig. 2) *(20)*. Older women have an increased risk of having a pregnancy with chromosomal abnormalities. A spontaneous abortion rate (after documentation of fetal cardiac activity) of 2% has been observed for maternal ages 35 yr or less, but increases to 16% for women 36 yr or older *(21)*.

Follicle-Stimulating Hormone and Estradiol. Basal serum follicle-stimulating hormone (FSH) and estradiol measurements have been the screening test of choice for assessing ovarian reserve. The rise in basal FSH is an excellent indicator of ovarian aging.

- *Indications for testing*: Women aged 35 yr or older, women of any age experiencing unexplained infertility who have a poor response to ovulation induction, women presenting for other tests of ovarian reserve including clomiphene challenge test, and women experiencing recurrent pregnancy losses should be tested.
- *Detection method*: Standard enzyme-linked immunosorbent assay (ELISA).
- *Interpretation of results*: In general, day 3 FSH concentrations 20–25 IU/L or more are considered to be elevated and associated with poor reproductive outcome *(22)*. Concomitant measurement of serum estradiol adds to the predictive power of an isolated FSH determination. Basal estradiol concentrations greater than 75–80 pg/mL are associated with poor outcome *(22)*.

Inhibin B. Inhibins are a family of protein hormones that control the secretion of FSH via a negative feedback mechanism. Inhibins are heterodimeric glycoproteins consisting of an α subunit covalently linked to either a β_A subunit (inhibin A) or to a β_B subunit (inhibin B). In the female, inhibin B is produced by the developing follicles, and concentrations peak in the follicular phase. Inhibin A is produced by the dominant follicle and the corpus luteum, and concentrations peak in the luteal phase. It is also produced by the fetoplacental unit during pregnancy. Inhibin B can be used in conjunction with serum FSH and estradiol to assess ovarian function. Because inhibin is produced by gonadal tissue, it is thought to be a more direct marker of gonadal activity and ovarian reserve than pituitary hormones. In addition, cycle day 3 inhibin B concentrations may demonstrate a decrease before day 3 FSH concentrations *(23)*.

- *Indications for testing*: Same as that for FSH and estradiol.
- *Detection method*: The first immunoassay for inhibin was known as the Monash assay. This was a radioimmunoassay using a polyclonal antiserum raised against purified inhibin. However, the antibodies were directed toward epitopes on the α subunit and therefore could not distinguish between inhibin A, inhibin B, or free α subunits. Currently, there are ELISA-based assays specific for inhibin A or inhibin B.
- *Interpretation of results*: Seifer et al. reported that women undergoing IVF with day 3 inhibin B concentration less than 45 pg/mL had a pregnancy rate of 7% and spontaneous

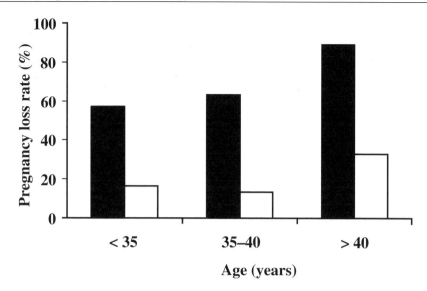

Fig. 2. Women with abnormal ovarian reserve (FSH > 14.2 IU/L) had a significantly higher rate of reproductive loss compared to patients with normal ovarian reserve. $p < 0.01$ for all groups. Solid bars, abnormal ovarian reserve; open bars, normal ovarian reserve. (Reprinted from ref. *20,* with permission from American Society for Reproductive Medicine.)

abortion rate of 33% compared to a pregnancy rate of 26% and abortion rate of 3% in women with day 3 inhibin B concentrations more than 45 pg/mL *(24)*. Women who are diagnosed with diminished ovarian reserve should be counseled regarding options such as oocyte donation or adoption.

PREDICTING EMBRYONIC FAILURE

Many biomarkers in serum have been studied for their ability to detect viable vs nonviable pregnancies including human chorionic gonadotropin (hCG), progesterone, estradiol, and inhibin A.

hCG and Progesterone. hCG and progesterone are inexpensive screening tests that can identify patients who need to undergo further testing.

- *Indications for testing*: Women over the age of 40 yr and women with a history of recurrent pregnancy loss should be tested during the first trimester (7–12 wk gestation).
- *Detection method*: hCG and progesterone are detected by standard ELISA assays.
- *Interpretation of results*: Serum hCG concentrations during the first 8 wk of pregnancy double in concentration every 2 d. Abnormal pregnancies have impaired hCG production and hence a prolonged doubling time. Serial hCG measurements can be used to assess the viability of pregnancy. If hCG is more than 1500 IU/L and the pregnancy is intrauterine, a gestational sac should be visible by transvaginal ultrasound. By transabdominal ultrasound, the gestational sac may not be visible until serum hCG concentrations are more than 6000 IU/L *(25)*. Viable pregnancy can be predicted with 97.5% sensitivity if serum progesterone concentrations are greater than 25 ng/mL. Nonviable pregnancies are detected with 100% sensitivity if serum progesterone concentrations are less than 5ng/mL. Pregnancies with progesterone concentrations between 5 and 25 ng/mL should have ultrasound performed *(25)*.

Inhibin A. Inhibin A is made by the fetoplacental unit during pregnancy *(26)*. A number of studies have reported that measurement of inhibin A may be an early predictor of embryonic failure. Serum concentrations of inhibin A have been shown to be lower as early as 4 wk gestation in pregnancies destined to fail compared with those that continue to deliver normal infants *(26–28)*.

- *Indications for testing*: Same as for hCG and progesterone.
- *Detection method*: Inhibin A is detected by standard ELISA assay.
- *Interpretation of results*: Lockwood et al. was among the first to demonstrate that inhibin A concentrations were correlated with embryonic demise *(26)*. These authors reported that clinical IVF pregnancies (with *in utero* sac present at 6 wk) that were subsequently diagnosed as missed abortions had significantly lower inhibin A concentrations at the time of the first pregnancy test (at 4 wk gestation). Inhibin A concentrations were 63.1 ± 17 pg/mL (mean ± SEM) for missed abortions and 129.6 ± 20 pg/mL for viable singletons and less than 5 pg/mL for "biochemical pregnancies" (no evidence of implantation, but positive hCG at 4 wk) (Table 2). Muttukrishna et al. reported similar findings of lower inhibin A concentrations in missed abortions (71.1 ± 12.1 pg/mL; mean ± SD) than in controls (193 ± 48 pg/mL) *(28)*. In a study by Vanderpuye et al. that examined the association of inhibin A concentrations with aneuploidy, from 7 to 12 wk gestation, all trisomies were associated with inhibin A concentrations below 175 pg/mL, and 60% of trisomy pregnancies were undetectable *(27)*. Phipps et al. *(29)* reported that the addition of inhibin A measurement to progesterone or progesterone and hCG increased specificity but not sensitivity (Tables 3 and 4). A cutoff has not yet been established to diagnose nonviable pregnancies, but clearly, lower inhibin A concentrations are associated with poor outcome. Further studies are needed to establish cutoffs.

SPERM DNA INTEGRITY

Sperm DNA Integrity (SDI) assay measures the percentage of DNA fragmentation of sperm. Damaged DNA in the single sperm cell that fertilizes a female oocyte can have a dramatic negative impact on fetal development and health of the offspring. Data on human sperm have established a threshold measurement that is predictive of low fertility potential. If 30% or more of the sperm have fragmented DNA detected, then approx 40% of miscarriages can be attributed to the male partner's genetic contribution *(30)*.

- *Indication for testing*: Male partners of couples with a history of unexplained infertility, poor embryo quality after IVF, implantation failure after IVF, recurrent chemical or occult pregnancy losses, or recurrent early spontaneous abortions should be tested with the SDI assay.
- *Detection method*: The SDI assay utilizes acridine orange (AO), a DNA probe, and the principles of flow cytometry. The assay measures the susceptibility of DNA to denaturation *in situ* following low pH treatment. This procedure denatures protamine-associated DNA in sperm cells but does not denature histone-associated DNA. Spermatozoa with normal chromatin structure do not demonstrate DNA denaturation. AO that intercalates into normal dsDNA fluoresces green, whereas AO that associates with denatured ssDNA fluoresces red when excited by a 488 nm light source.
- *Interpretation of test results*: The control group studies indicate the thresholds of the sperm DNA fragmentation index of 0–15%, 16–29%, and 30% or more relate to high, good to fair, and low to poor fertility potential, respectively *(30)*.

Table 2
Inhibin A (pg/mL) and hCG (IU/L) Concentrations in Different Types
of IVF Pregnancy With Fresh ET[a]

| | Gestation | Biochemical | Type of pregnancy | | |
			Missed abortion	Singleton	Multiple
Inhibin A	4 wk	<5	63.1 (17)*	129.6 (20)*	282.3 (47)
hCG	4 wk	175.2 (37)	372.5 (30)**	651.00 (67)**	1707.0 (112)
Inhibin A	6 wk	<5	71.9 (5.6)***	154.2 (21)***	231.7 (31)
hCG	6 wk	<5	5600.0 (128)**	7350.0 (140)**	9589.0 (452)

[a]Data presented are means, with SEM in parentheses.
*$p < 0.01$.
**not significant.
***$p < 0.05$.
Data from ref. 26.

Table 3
Estimated Specificity at Given Sensitivity
for Biomarker Combinations

Sensitivity	P	P + I	P + H	P + I + H
0.95	0.29	0.57	0.66	0.69
0.90	0.70	0.83	0.87	0.87
0.85	0.88	0.87	0.94	0.93
0.80	0.90	0.95	0.97	0.97
0.75	0.97	0.99	> 0.99	> 0.99

P, progesterone alone; P + H, progesterone plus serum hCG; P + I, progesterone plus inhibin A; P + I + H, progesterone plus inhibin A plus serum hCG.
Reprinted from ref. 29, with permission from the American College of Obstetricians and Gynecologists.

Table 4
Estimated Sensitivity at Given Specificity
for Biomarker Combinations

Sensitivity	P	P + I	P + H	P + I + H
0.95	0.83	0.82	0.83	0.83
0.90	0.89	0.85	0.87	0.89
0.85	0.92	0.90	0.92	0.92
0.80	0.93	0.91	0.93	0.93
0.75	0.93	0.92	0.93	0.93

P, progesterone alone; P + H, progesterone plus serum hCG; P + I, progesterone plus inhibin A; P + I + H, progesterone plus inhibin A plus serum hCG.
Reprinted from ref. 29, with permission from American College of Obstetricians and Gynecologists.

Table 5
The Frequency of Problems Within the Environment Contributing
to Recurrent Pregnancy Loss

Anatomic	10%
Blood flow	6%
Immunologic	75%
Unexplained	9%

Problems With the Environment

The cause of recurrent pregnancy losses caused by problems with the environment are summarized in Table 5.

EVALUATION OF THE UTERINE CAVITY

This procedure can reveal any anatomic cause of pregnancy loss or failure. Anatomic abnormalities within the uterus include the following:

- *Endometrial polyps*: benign lesions within the uterine cavity that are attached to the cavity wall by a stalk. Endometrial polyps usually form as a result of irregular shedding of the lining during menses.
- *Submucosal fibroids*: benign muscular tumors that protrude from the muscular layer of the uterus into the uterine cavity.
- *Endometrial adhesions*: scar tissue that forms inside the uterine cavity as a result of previous infection, operation, or pregnancy.
- *Congenital anomalies*: Congenital anomalies of the uterus are the result of lack of unification of the Mullerian ducts during embryologic development. Included in Mullerian duct abnormalities are septate uterus, bicornuate uterus, and double uterus. Although all of these anomalies have been associated with late pregnancy loss, their role in early and occult loss has been questioned and remains controversial *(31)*.
- Abnormalities within the uterine cavity are found in 10% of women experiencing pregnancy loss. The frequencies of each of the abnormal findings are shown in Table 6.

UTERINE BLOOD FLOW

Evaluation of uterine blood flow measures resistance of blood flow into the uterus through the uterine arteries (uterine artery pulsatility index) and blood flow to the lining of the uterus (subendometrial peak systolic velocity). Elevated uterine artery pulsatility index *(32)* or low subendometrial peak systolic velocity *(33)* implies that blood supply to the endometrium is insufficient to support pregnancy. Abnormal uterine blood flow is found in 6% of women experiencing recurrent pregnancy loss.

IMMUNOLOGIC TESTING

Immunologic testing identifies immunologic factors contributing to recurrent pregnancy loss or failure. Among women experiencing unexplained recurrent miscarriages, 75% demonstrate an immunologic factor *(34)*. The frequency of abnormalities of the immunologic tests among women experiencing recurrent pregnancy loss are shown in Fig. 3. Immunologic tests shown to be useful in diagnosing the cause of reproductive failure are discussed below.

Table 6
The Frequencies of Each of the Anatomic Abnormalities Found
Within the Uterus Among Women Experiencing Recurrent Pregnancy Loss

Endometrial polyps	36%
Endometrial adhesions	6%
Submucous fibroids	75%
Congenital anomalies	9%

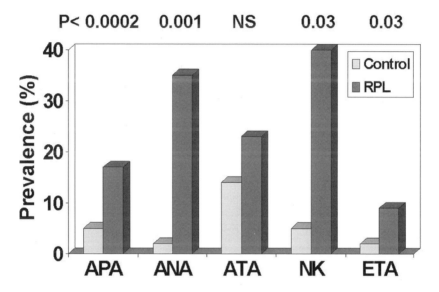

Fig. 3. Prevalence of abnormal immunologic test results among patients experiencing recurrent pregnancy failures. ANA, antinuclear antibodies; APA, antiphospholipid antibodies; ATA, antithyroid antibodies; ETA, embryotoxicity assay; NK, natural killer cells; RPL, recurrent pregnancy loss. (Drawn from data from ref. *24*.)

APLAs. APLAs are a family of autoantibodies that bind to both anionic and zwitterionic phospholipids. Their presence has been associated with both early and late pregnancy losses as well as with thrombosis. APLA causes clotting in placental blood vessels, which can result in placental insufficiency and subsequent pregnancy wastage. APLA can inhibit invasion of placental cells into the lining of the uterus at the time of implantation *(35)*. Eighty percent of women experiencing peri-implantation pregnancy loss have elevated circulating concentrations of APLA *(36)*.

- *Indication for testing*: All patients experiencing two or more consecutive pregnancy losses, endometriosis, IVF failure suspected to represent implantation failure, premature ovarian failure, or unexplained infertility and patients who have systemic lupus erythematosus (SLE), or another collagen vascular disease should be tested for the presence of APLA. In addition, previous borderline or positive APLA results should be repeated.

- *Detection method*: In the past, tests for APLA included coagulation assays for lupus anticoagulant (LA) and an ELISA for anticardiolipin antibodies (aCL). Although some studies described a correlation between LA and specific aCL measured by ELISA *(37)*, others have demonstrated discordance between the prevalence of LA and APLA *(38)*. The term LA is a misnomer because most patients with LA do not have SLE, and in vivo, these antibodies are a procoagulant rather than an anticoagulant. In vitro, LA inhibits phospholipid-dependent coagulation, so there is a prolongation of the dilute Russell viper venom time and activated partial thromboplastin time. Two additional tests must be performed to confirm the presence of LA. First, a mixing study must be done to demonstrate that there is inhibitor present instead of a factor deficiency. This is done by mixing the patient's plasma with normal plasma. The activated partial thromboplastin time should not be correct in the presence of LA. Second, a phospholipid-neutralizing procedure should be performed to demonstrate phospholipid dependence. The prevalence of circulating LA among women experiencing reproductive failure is low (<3%) *(34)*. Even though other autoimmune diseases have been shown to involve polyclonal rather than monoclonal B-cell activation *(39)*, most studies of antiphospholipid syndrome (APS) have examined only antibodies to cardiolipin. Several investigators have advocated a panel of APLAs to screen for APS *(40–43)*. This panel of tests includes not only antcardioilipin but also antiphosphatidylethanolamine, antiphosphatidylcholine, antiphosphatidylinositol, antiphosphatidic acid, antiphosphatidylglycerol, and antiphosphatidylserine. It has been reported that the aCL is less specific for risk of thromboembolism than LA because aCL antibodies can also be found in nonthrombotic conditions such as syphilis, Lyme disease, hepatitis C, human immunodeficiency virus, Q fever, tuberculosis, and parvovirus B19. However, among women experiencing recurrent pregnancy loss, several studies have indicated that 40 to 80% of women evaluated for APS would have the diagnosis missed if only aCL is measured *(41–44)*. Moreover, these aCL-negative but APA-positive patients present with clinical signs and symptoms indistinguishable from their aCL-positive counterparts *(45,46)*. APLAs have been shown to have a direct effect on the preembryo *(47)*, trophoblasts *(17,35)*, and endothelial cells *(16,17)*. Of the APLA's tested, antiphosphatidyl serine, -choline, -glyerol, -inositol, and -ethanolamine, but not anticardiolipin, have been shown to target the preembryo *(47)*, antiphosphatidylserine, and antiphosphatidylethanolamine, but not anticardiolipin, to target trophoblastic cells *(17,35)*, and antiphosphatidylserine and antiphosphatidylethanolamine as well as anticardiolipin to target endothelial cells *(16,17,48)*. Difficulty in interpretation and comparison of results from one laboratory to another arises from the lack of standardization of the assays, and calibrators are not available *(49,50)*. Substances such as anti-β_2GP1 have also been shown to be present in patients with pregnancy loss *(37,49)*. However, tests for the substances identify only the negatively charged APLAs and not the zwitterionic APLAs.
- *Interpretation of results*: For a diagnosis of APS to be made, a patient must test positive for LA and aCL on two separate occasions at least 6 to 8 wk apart. Results are reported as negative, borderline, or positive. A normal result is negative (see also Chapter 14).

Antinuclear Antibodies. Antinuclear antibodies (ANA) are autoantibodies to nuclear antigens. A number of autoimunne diseases are associated with elevated circulating concentrations of ANA including SLE and other collagen and vascular diseases, and reproductive autoimmune failure syndrome (RAFS). RAFS is the association of recurrent pregnancy loss, unexplained infertility, or endometriosis with the presence of circulating autoantibodies including ANA. ANA and APLA, but not antithyroid antibodies

(ATA) have been shown to have a direct toxic effect on preimplantation embryos *(47)*. The frequent association of the presence of elevated APLA and ANA in the same individual can be explained by the recently proposed hypothesis that they result from antibodies being formed to cell products after cell death *(50)*.

- *Indications for testing*: Individuals with a history of symptoms of SLE and/or collagen vascular disease as well as all women experiencing two or more unexplained consecutive pregnancy losses, unexplained infertility, or symptoms associated with endometriosis should be tested for the presence of ANA.
- *Detection method*: ANA to eight nuclear antigens can be screened for the immunoglobulin G isotype to single-stranded DNA, double-stranded DNA, Smith antigen, ribonucleoprotein, Sjogrens antigen A, Sjogren's antigen B, scleroderma 70, and histones.
- *Interpretation of results*: Results are reported as negative or positive. A normal value is negative.

ATA. ATA include antithyroglobulin (ATG) and microsomal antibodies also known as antithyroperoxidase (TPO) antibodies. Thyroid autoantibodies have been shown to be independent markers for pregnancies at risk for loss *(51–53)*. Women who have ATA miscarry at approximately twice the rate of women who have no ATA (Fig. 4). ATA are associated with an increase in proinflammatory cytokines secreted by T cells within the uterine lining *(54)*. Thus, the presence of ATA may represent a marker of an underlying T-cell dysfunction that directly affects implantation and subsequent miscarriage.

- *Indication for testing*: All patients who have a history of thyroid abnormalities and/or a history of two or more pregnancy losses or unexplained infertility should be tested for the presence of ATA. Because women having ATA during the first trimester of pregnancy have a 50% chance of either miscarrying or developing thyroid dysfunction in the postpartum period, testing all women during the first trimester has been recommended *(52)*.
- *Detection method*: The ATG and TPO tests are based on agglutination assays with gelatin particles that have been sensitized with either thyroglobulin or the thyroid microsomal antigen or use standard ELISA assays.
- *Interpretation of results*: Negative antibody titers are considered normal. Stagnaro-Green et al. reported that thyroid antibodies are an independent marker of at-risk pregnancy. However, the presence of a positive ATG or TPO test was able to predict these at-risk pregnancies with only 34% sensitivity and 81% specificity *(52)*. Similarly, LeJeune at al. *(53)* reported 23% sensitivity and 95% specificity for detecting first-trimester miscarriage and 29% sensitivity and 84% specificity for detecting early and late miscarriage.

Reproductive Immunophenotype. Reproductive Immunophenotype (RIP) measures the circulating percentages of NK cells. Elevated percentages of circulating NK cells predict loss of a chromosomally normal pregnancy *(55)*.

- *Indication for testing*: All women who have unexplained infertility or who fail to conceive after IVF and embryo transfer of apparently normal embryos or who experience two or more consecutive pregnancy losses should be tested for the presence of elevated percentage of circulating CD56+ cells. Elevated percentage of circulating CD56+ cells should be monitored during pregnancy to aid in management of treatment.
- *Detection method*: The percentage of mononuclear cells expressing CD3, CD4, CD8, CD19, CD16, and CD56 is detected by flow cytometry using an immunofluoroescence technique.

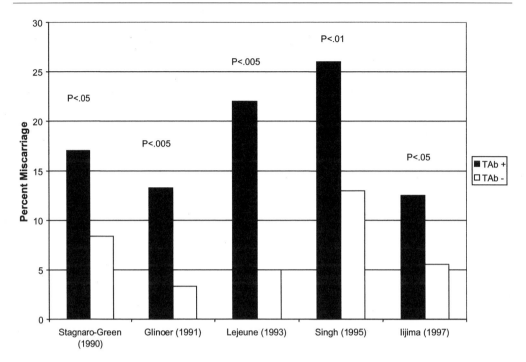

Fig. 4. The percentage of miscarriages in unselected pregnancies in women who were thyroid antibody positive (TAb+) and thyroid antibody negative (TAb–). (Reprinted with permission from ref. *51*.)

- *Interpretation of test results*: Normal values in blood of percentage of lymphocytes are CD3, 51–79%; CD4, 30–52%; CD8, 16–40%; CD19, 5–17%; CD56+/16, 3–16%; CD56+/16+, 0–11% *(34)*.

Natural Killer Activation. The Natural Killer activation (NKa) assay tests the killing function of circulating NK cells and the ability of intravenous immunoglobulin (IVIg) to suppress that activity. Increased NK killing activity has been demonstrated among women experiencing reproductive failure including recurrent pregnancy loss. Preconceptually measured abnormal NKa predicts postconceptual miscarriage *(56)*.

- *Indications for testing*: All women who have unexplained infertility, endometriosis, or other pelvic pathology such as pelvic adhesions, a history of recurrent IVF failures, or elevated APLA or ATA and are undergoing an IVF procedure, or a history of two or more consecutive pregnancy losses, should be tested with the NK Cell Activation Assay.
- *Detection method*: The percentage of lysed K562 cells is detected by flow cytometry using an immunofluorescence technique.
- *Interpretation of results*: Normal NK activity is less than 10% activated NK cells *(57)*. In the presence of IVIg, a decreased activity of at least 50% should be observed if the NK activity is elevated *(58)*.

Embryotoxicity Assay. Embryotoxicity assay detects factors that kill embryos. Circulating embryotoxic factors have been associated with recurrent pregnancy loss *(59)*. Most embryotoxic factors appear to be proinflammatory cytokines.

- *Indication for testing*: All women experiencing unexplained infertility, implantation failure after IVF, infertility associated with endometriosis, or two or more consecutive pregnancy losses should be tested for circulating embryotoxins.
- *Detection method*: Embryotoxins are identified by screening the patient's serum using a mouse blastocyst bioassay controlling for variability among mice *(59)*. Two cell embryos are collected from superovulated mated CB6F1/J mice and cultured in media supplemented with fetal bovine serum or 10% serum at 37°C with 5% CO_2 and high humidity. Each sample is assayed in triplicate using three mice, with at least five embryos from the same mouse per well. Embryonic development is evaluated at 72 h and the frequency of atretic embryos is recorded. Intrasample (interassay) variation yields a coefficient of variation of 10%. When repeated samples from a given individual are evaluated, the coefficient of variation is 9.7%. Interoperator variability is 4% interassay and 2% intra-assay.
- *Interpretation of results*: A normal value is negative for or shows an absence of circulating embryotoxins.

Ig Panel. The Ig Panel detects low concentrations of IgA. Low concentrations of IgA can be a contraindication to the use of IVIg. Thus, an Ig panel should be performed on all individuals prior to receiving IVIg therapy. Anyone who displays a low IgA concentration should be tested for anti-IgA antibodies.

- *Indications for testing*: An Ig panel should be performed on all individuals prior to receiving IVIg therapy to rule out hypogammaglobulinemic serum concentrations of IgA.
- *Detection method*: Total IgG, IgM, and IgA concentrations are determined by standard nephelometric technique.
- *Interpretation of results*: Normal serum concentrations for IgA, IgG, and IgM are as follows: IgA, 68–378 mg/dL; IgG, 694–1618 mg/dL; and IgM, 60–263 mg/dL. Any IgA concentration less than 68 mg/dL should be followed up with an anti-IgA.

Anti-IgA Antibody. Anti-IgA Antibody measures antibodies directed toward IgA. Low concentrations of IgA can be the result of lack of production of IgA or increased destruction of IgA by antibodies. It is important to distinguish between these two causes because the presence of anti-IgA puts an individual at risk for an adverse reaction to IVIg.

- *Detection method*: Anti-IgA antibodies are detected by standard immunoradiometric assay for the IgG isotype to IgA.
- *Indication for testing*: All individuals who are hypogammaglobulinemic for IgA should be tested for anti-IgA.
- *Interpretation of results*: Negative, less than 150% of negative control; limited specificity or low titer class-specific antibodies, 151–200% of negative control; class-specific or high titer limited specificity antibodies greater than 200% of negative control.

Thrombophilia Panel. The thrombophilia panel detects genetic risk factors for thrombosis or abnormal blood clotting. The specific genes tested are hyperhomocysteinemia, factor V Leiden, and prothrombin mutations. All three of these gene mutations have more frequently been associated with late rather than early pregnancy loss *(18)*.

- *Indications for testing*: Women with a history of blood clots and reproductive loss, especially late pregnancy losses, should be tested with the thrombophilia panel to rule out any genetic cause.
- *Detection method*: Thrombophilic gene mutations are detected by standard polymerase chain reaction.
- *Interpretation of results*: Results are reported as normal, heterozygote, or homozygote.

Summary

There are numerous diagnostic tests to help determine the cause of recurrent miscarriages. In addition, there are tests available to help monitor the progress of pregnancy in a woman who has had frequent pregnancy loss.

TREATMENT OF RECURRENT PREGNANCY LOSS

Treatment for recurrent pregnancy loss depends on the underlying causes. The two major reasons for loss of pregnancy are problems with the pregnancy itself or problems within the environment in which the pregnancy grows.

Problems With the Pregnancy

Problems with the pregnancy are usually characterized by the presence of an abnormal chromosome analysis of the conceptus. When pregnancies are lost with repeated abnormal karyotypes, the options for further treatment include preimplantation genetic diagnosis (PGD) and egg donation.

PGD

PGD is a procedure whereby the preimplantation embryo can be tested for genetic or chromosomal abnormalities before transfer into the uterus. In other words, it serves as a prepregnancy test of genetic normality. Because chromosomal abnormalities may result in miscarriage, a prepregancy test may also avoid pregnancy failures caused by chromosomal abnormalities. The technique is based on assisted reproductive technology procedures and allows selection and transfer of normal embryos into the uterus *(60,61)*.

Egg Donation

For women experiencing recurrent pregnancy loss as a result of repeated chromosomal abnormalities who are still childless after PGD, egg donation is another option. Egg donation involves preparing the uterus of the embryo recipient with hormonal replacement while stimulating the egg donor's ovaries with fertility drugs and harvesting and then fertilizing her eggs in the embryology laboratory with designated sperm (usually derived from the partner of the prospective embryo recipient). The embryos are then transferred to the uterus of the embryo recipient, who carries and delivers the pregnancy.

Sperm Donation

When recurrent pregnancy losses are associated with a sperm contribution measured as sperm DNA fragmentation greater than 30%, artificial insemination with donor sperm is an option for treatment.

Problems With the Environment

Problems within the environment in which the embryo implants and fetus grows have been classified as anatomic, hormonal, and immunologic.

Anatomic Abnormalities

Anatomic abnormalities are lesions inside the uterus that, if present, would mechanically inhibit normal implantation and hence normal embryo and/or fetal growth. Anatomic abnormalities include endometrial polyps, submucosal fibroids, uterine synechia, and Mullerian duct defects. Treatment for anatomic abnormalities of the uterus involve removal of the abnormality. Successful pregnancy rates after removal of endometrial polyps have be reported to be increased by three- to fourfold compared to before removal, and submucosal fibroids and endometrial adhesions by two- to threefold *(62)*. The advantage of correcting Müllerian duct defects to enhance live birth rates remains controversial *(31)*.

BLOOD FLOW

Blood flow has been shown to correlate with pregnancy outcome. If resistance of flow through the uterine artery is elevated or if flow of blood though the spiral arteries leading to the endometrium is low, successful pregnancy outcome is not expected. Aspirin *(63)* and sildenafil (Viagra) *(64)* have been shown to increase blood flow to the uterus and increase pregnancy rates in these patients.

Aspirin Therapy. Among women with increased resistance of blood flow through their uterine arteries who were treated with aspirin for a minimum of 2 wk, the miscarriage rate decreased from 60 to 15% *(63)*. An increase in subendometrial flow has also been noted with aspirin therapy. The usual dose of aspirin is 80 mg/d (one baby aspirin). However, occasionally, as much as 360 mg (one adult aspirin) has been required to see a beneficial effect on uterine blood flow.

Sildenafil (Viagra) Therapy. When aspirin is unsuccessful in improving uterine blood flow or if the miscarriages are associated with a thin (<9 mm) uterine lining, sildenafil (Viagra) has been used successfully to increase uterine blood flow. Viagra in the form of vaginal suppositories (25 mg four times a day) has been shown to increase uterine blood flow and the thickness of the uterine lining. To date, we have seen significant improvement in the thickness of the uterine lining in about 70% of women treated. Successful pregnancy resulted in 42% of women who responded to the Viagra *(64)*.

IMMUNOLOGIC CAUSES

Immunologic causes of recurrent pregnancy loss or failure can be treated with immunotherapy. Various forms of immunotherapy have been introduced to treat couples experiencing recurrent pregnancy loss. At least 70% of pathologies leading to recurrent pregnancy failures are manifest as a pre-existing excess of inflammation *(34)*. Treatments for recurrent pregnancy loss have included aspirin, heparin, glucocorticoids, IVIg all four, or a combination of two or three of these, and pentoxifylline.

Aspirin. Low-dose aspirin alone has been advocated in the treatment of recurrent miscarriage associated with APLA. However, results of clinical trials have shown aspirin alone to be half as effective as other treatments including heparin and glucocorticoids. Two studies have shown that in women receiving treatment for recurrent pregnancy loss associated with APLA, heparin plus aspirin provided a significantly better outcome than aspirin alone (live birth rate of 80 vs 44%) *(43,65)*.

A rationale for the use of low-dose aspirin therapy during pregnancy for women with APLA is to decrease blood clots from forming in the placental vessels. The mechanisms by which aspirin prevents blood clots are through its antiprostaglandin and antiprostacyclin effects and inhibition of platelet adhesiveness and aggregation.

Heparin and Aspirin. Heparin has also been used in conjunction with aspirin to prevent placental clotting. The rational for using heparin is that it is a blood thinner and inhibits clot formation by a different pathway than the aspirin. The combination of both heparin and aspirin given to women experiencing recurrent pregnancy loss who had

APLA is associated with a live birth rate of 80% compared with a live birth rate of 44% in women receiving aspirin alone *(43,65)*. Live birth rates with heparin, aspirin, and prednisone are 74% *(66)*. Thus, no enhancement of live birth rates is noticed when prednisone is added to heparin and aspirin therapy for treatment of recurrent pregnancy loss.

Glucocorticoids. Steroid therapy in the forms of prednisone, prednisolone, and dexamethasone has been used to treat recurrent pregnancy losses. Historically, recurrent postimplantation pregnancy loss associated with APLA was treated with combinations of prednisone and aspirin. The rationale for prednisone therapy is suppression of autoantibodies such as APLA and ANA. A randomized controlled trial confirmed the efficacy of prednisone and aspirin for treatment of recurrent spontaneous abortion associated with APLA *(67)*. In this study, women treated with prednisone and aspirin had a live birth rate of 77% compared with nontreated control women, who had a live birth rate of 8%. However, risks associated with the dosages of prednisone used to treat recurrent spontaneous abortion associated with APLA include signs of Cushing's syndrome, severe acne, increased risk of gestational diabetes, osteopenia, posterior capsule cataract, listeriosis, pneumonia, and even maternal death from military tuberculosis *(68–75)*. Early preeclampsia is more common in pregnancy in women receiving prednisone therapy, and premature rupture of membranes and associated preterm birth were almost always observed after prednisone treatment *(76,77)*. A study comparing live birth rates in women treated with heparin and aspirin and those treated with prednisone and aspirin showed 75% live births in both groups *(76)*. However, both maternal complications and preterm delivery with premature rupture of membranes and toxemia of pregnancy were significantly higher in pregnant women treated with prednisone and aspirin compared to those treated with heparin and aspirin *(76)*. Therefore, the current recommendation for "first attempt" treatment for recurrent pregnancy loss associated with APLA is heparin and aspirin.

IVIg. IVIg therapy has been used as treatment for recurrent pregnancy loss associated with APLA, elevated circulating NK cells, abnormal NK cell activity, and presence of circulating embryotoxins, as well as unexplained recurrent pregnancy losses.

The mechanisms by which IVIg is believed to enhance implantation rates include the following: IVIg decreases killing activity of NK cells, increases the activity of suppressor T cells, suppresses B-cell production of autoantibodies, and contains antibodies to antibodies or anti-idiotypic antibodies. Originally, IVIg therapy was used to treat women with postimplantation pregnancy losses who had not been successful in pregnancies previously treated with aspirin and prednisone or heparin *(68–70,77)*. The rationale for the use of IVIG in the original studies was the suppression of LA in a woman being treated for severe thrombocytopenia. IVIg was often given with prednisone or heparin plus aspirin. The estimated success rate of 71% for women at very high risk for failure with a history of previous treatment failures suggested that IVIg treatment was effective *(68–70,77)*. More recently, IVIg therapy alone has been used to successfully treat women with APLA as well as women who become refractory to conventional autoimmune treatment with heparin or prednisone and aspirin *(70–74)*.

Proinflammatory cytokines at the maternal–fetal surface can cause clotting of the placental vessels and subsequent pregnancy loss. One source of these cytokines is the NK cell. Biopsies of the lining of the uterus from women experiencing recurrent pregnancy loss reveal an increase in activated NK cells *(78)*. Peripheral blood NK cells are also elevated in women with recurrent pregnancy loss compared with women without a history of pregnancy loss *(55,79)*. IVIg has been used to successfully treat women with recurrent pregnancy loss and elevated circulating concentrations of NK cells, NK cell killing activity, and embryotoxins with live birth rates between 70 and 80% *(79)*. IVIg has also been used to treat women with unexplained recurrent pregnancy loss. Four randomized, controlled trials of IVIg for treatment of recurrent pregnancy loss have been published with conflicting results *(80–83)*. None of the studies took into account the pregnancies lost as a result of chromosomal abnormalities except the US-based trial, which showed a significant improvement in live birth rates in women treated with IVIg *(81)*. Approximately 60% of the pregnancies lost in the clinical trial would be expected to have chromosomal abnormalities that would not be corrected by IVIg *(6)*.

Leukocyte Immunization Therapy. Clinical trials evaluating leukocyte immunization therapy (LIT) have both supported and challenged the efficacy of this treatment for recurrent miscarriages. To address the uncertainties caused by these conflicting results, a worldwide collaborative study was undertaken *(84)*. The results of that very large study showed the difference between live birth rates in the treatment and control groups was 8 to 10% in favor of the treated group. This study also showed a negative effect of treatment in women with positive autoantibodies and no benefit of treatment among women who had a prior live birth. Because of the low rate of effectiveness in enhancing live birth, the FDA has at the time of this writing imposed a ban on LIT. A proposal for an investigational new drug application has been submitted to the FDA to further investigate the safety and efficacy of LIT. It is hoped that the application will be approved soon and LIT will again be clinically available.

Pentoxifylline. Pentoxifylline (Trental) is a methyl xanthine derivative that has nonspecific phosphodiesterase inhibitory activity. The phosphodiesterases are responsible for enzymatic degradation of the biologically active cyclic adenosine monophosphate (cAMP) and cyclic guanosine monophosphate (cGMP) to the biologically inactive molecules adenosine monophosphate and guanosine monophosphate. Thus, pentoxifylline would increase intracellular cAMP. Pentoxifylline has been shown to have anti-inflammatory effects mediated by two major actions: (1) reduction of production of cytokines by phagocytes and (2) inhibition of adhesion of neutrophils, monocytes, and lymphocytes to endothelial cells. Animal studies have demonstrated that pentoxifylline prevents miscarriages in abortion-prone mice *(85)*. Efficacy of pentoxifylline for treatment of recurrent pregnancy loss in human beings remains to be established.

Summary

Success rates for immunotherapy depend on the age of the woman and her diagnosis. Overall live birth rates in women with a history of recurrent pregnancy loss treated with various forms of immunotherapy is between 70 and 80%.

CONCLUSION

Recurrent pregnancy loss is a health-care concern that needs effective treatment. Before effective treatment can be instituted, a diagnosis must be made. The most common causes of recurrent pregnancy losses are chromosomal abnormalities within the pregnancy itself and immunologic risk factors within the uterus or the environment in which the pregnancy grows. The majority of patients experiencing immunologic recurrent pregnancy loss demonstrate a pre-existing "abnormal" inflammatory condition, and the physiology of recurrent pregnancy losses involves the vascular system as well as the immune system. Once an accurate diagnosis is made and appropriate immunotherapy administered, a live birth rate of 70 to 80% can be expected.

REFERENCES

1. Roberts CJ, Lowe CR. Where have all the conceptions gone? Lancet 1975;I:498–499.
2. Clark DA. Is there any evidence for immunologically mediated or immunologic modifiable early pregnancy failure? J Assist Reprod Genet 2000;20:63–72.
3. Daya S. Habitual abortion. In Copeland LJ, Jarrel J, eds. Textbook of Gynecology, 2nd ed. Philadelphia: WB Saunders, 2000, pp. 227–271.
4. Coulam CB. Epidemiology of recurrent spontaneous abortion. Am J Reprod Immunol 1991;26:23–27.
5. Munne S, Alikani M, Tomkin G, Grifo J, Cohen J. Embryo morphology, developmental rates, and maternal age are correlated with chromosomal abnormalities. Fertil Steril 1995;64:382–391.
6. Coulam CB, Stephenson M, Stern JJ, Clark DA. Immunotherapy for recurrent pregnancy loss: analysis of results from clinical trials. Am J Reprod Immunol 1996;35:330–337.
7. Warburton D, Fraser FC. Spontaneous abortion risks in man: data from reproductive histories collected in a medical genetics unit. Am J Hum Genet 1964;16:1–25.
8. Hassold T, Chen N, Funkhouser J, Joss T, Manuel B, Matsuura J. A cytogenetic study of 1000 spontaneous abortions. Ann Hum Genet Lond 1980;44:151–178.
9. Evenson DP, Jost LK, Zinaman MJ, et al. Utility of the sperm chromatin structure assay (SCSA) as a diagnostic and prognostic tool in the human fertility clinic. Hum Reprod 2000;14:1039–1049.
10. Peters AJ, Lloyd RP, Coulam CB. Prevalence of out-of-phase endometrial biopsy specimens. Am J Obstet Gynecol 1992;166:1738–1745.
11. Coulam CB, Bustillo M, Soenksen DM, Britten S. Ultrasonographic predictors of implantation after assisted reproduction. Fertil Steril 1994;62:1004–1010.
12. Battaglia C, Artini PG, Giulini S, et al. Colour Doppler changes and thromboxane production after ovarian stimulation with gonadotropin-releasing hormone agonist. Hum Reprod 1997;12:2477–2482.
13. Clark DA, Lea RG, Podor T, Daya S, Banwatt D, Harley C. Cytokines determining the success or failure of pregnancy. Ann N Y Acad Sci 1009;626:504–534.
14. Raghupathy R. Th1 type immunity is incompatible with successful pregnancy. Immunol Today 1997;18:478–482.
15. Clark DA, Chaouat G, Ding JW, August C, Coulam CB, Levy GA. Fgl2 in pregnancy: a novel prothrombinase at the fetomaternal interface may prevent bleeding and cause abortions. Am J Reprod Immunol 1999;41:374–379.
16. Roubey RAS, Hoffman M. From antiphospholipid syndrome to antibody mediated thrombosis. Lancet 1997;350:1491–1492.
17. Rand JH, Wu XX, Andree HAM, et al. Pregnancy loss in the antiphospholipid syndrome: a possible thrombogenic mechanism. N Enl J Med 1997;337:154–160.
18. Buchholz T, Thaler CJ. Inherited thrombophilia: impact on human reproduction. Am J Reprod Immunol 2003;50:20–32.
19. Mandel H, Brenner B, Berant M, Rosenberg N, Lanir N, Jakobs C. Coexistence of hereditary homocystinuria and factor V von Leiden: effect on thrombosis. N Engl J Med 1996;334:763–776.
20. Levi AJ, Raynault MF, Bergh PA, Drews MR, Miller BT, Scott RT. Reproductive outcome in patients with diminished ovarian reserve. Fertil Steril 2001;76:666–669.
21. Smith KE, Buyalos RP. The profound impact of patient age on pregnancy outcome after detection of fetal cardiac activity. Fertil Steril 1996;5:35–40.
22. Klein J, Sauer MV. Assessing fertility in women of advanced reproductive age. Am J Obstet Gyn 2001;185:758–770.
23. Seifer DB, Scott RT, Bergh PA, et al. Women with declining ovarian reserve may demonstrate a decrease in day 3 follicle-stimulating hormone. Fertil Steril 1999;72:63–65.
24. Seifer DB, Lambert-Messerlian G, Hogan JW, Gardiner AC, Blazar AS, Beck CA. Day 3 serum Inhibin B is predictive of assisted reproductive technologies outcome. Fertil Steril 1997;67:110–114.
25. Simpson JL. Fetal wastage. In: Gabbe SG, Niebyl JR, Simpson JL, eds. Obstetrics: Normal and Problem Pregnancies, 3rd ed. New York: Churhill Livingston, 1996, pp. 717–742.

26. Lockwood GM, Ledger WL, Barlow DH, Groome NP, Muttukrishna S. Measurement of inhibin and activin in early human pregnancy: demonstration of fetoplacental origin and role in prediction of early-pregnancy outcome. Biol Reprod 1997;57:1490–1494.

27. Vanderpuye OA, Goodman C, Randall HT, Rooussev RG, Tsao D, Coulam CB. Aneuploidy diagnosis in the first trimester: serum PAPP-A, free beta hCG and Inhibin A. Am J Reprod Immunol 2000;43:341

28. Muttukrishna S, Jauniaux E, Greenwold N, et al. Circulating levels of inhibin A, activin A and follistatin in missed and recurrent miscarriages. Hum Reprod 2002;17:3072–3078.

29. Phipps MG, Hogan JW, Peipert JE, Lambert-Messerlain GM, Canick JA, Seifer DB. Progesterone, inhibin, and hCG multiple marker strategy to differentiate viable from non-viable pregnancies. Obstet Gynecol 2000;95:227–231.

30. Evenson DP, Larson KL, Jost LK. Sperm chromatin structure assay: its clinical use for detecting sperm DNA fragmentation in male infertility and comparisons with other techniques. J Androl 2002;23:25–42.

31. Kirk EP, Chuong CJ, Coulam CB, Williams TJ. Pregnancy after metroplasty for uterine anomalies. Fertil Steril 1993;59:11641168.

32. Steer CV, Campbell S, Tan SL, et al. The use of transvaginal color flow imaging after in vitro fertilization to identify optimum uterine conditions before embryo transfer. Fertil Steril 1992;57:372–376.

33. Serafini P, Bartzolin J, Nelson J. Uterine power Doppler sonography: a prognosticator of pregnancy in IVF. J Assis Reprod Genet 1997;14:525.

34. Kaider AS, Kaider BD, Janowicz PB, Roussev RG. Immunodiagnostic evaluation in women with reproductive failure. Am J Reprod Immunol 1999;42:335–346.

35. Rote NS, Vogt E, De Vere G, Obringer AR, Ng AK. The role of placental trophoblast in pathophysiology of the antiphospholipid antibody syndrome. Am J Reprod Immunol 1998;39:125–36.

36. Coulam CB, Roussev RG. Chemical pregnancies: immunologic and ultrasonographic studies. Am J Reprod Immunol 2002;48:323–328.

37. Keswani S, Chauhan N. Antiphospholipis syndrome. R Soc Med 2002;95:336–342.

38. Triplett DA. Antiphospholipid antibodies and recurrent pregnancy loss. Am J Reprod Immunol 1989;20:53–67.

39. Shoenfeld Y, Schwartz RS. Genetic and immunologic factors in autoimmune diseases. N Engl J Med 1984;311:101–108.

40. Gleicher N, El-Roeiy A. The reproductive autoimmune failure syndrome. Am J Obstet Gynecol 1998;159:213–217.

41. Yetman DL, Kutteh WH. Antiphospholipid antibody panels and recurrent pregnancy loss: prevalence of anticardiolipin antibodies compared with other antiphosphlipid antibodies. Fertil Steril 1996;66: 540–546.

42. Coulam CB, Kaider BD, Kaider AS, Janowicz P, Roussev RG. Antiphospholipid antibodies associated with implantation failure after IVF/ET. J Assist Reprod Genet 1997;14:603–608.

43. Kutteh WH. Antiphospholipid antibodies associated with recurrent pregnancy loss: treatment with heparin and low-dose aspirin is superior to low-dose aspirin alone. Am J Obstet Gynec 1996;174: 1584–1589.

44. McIntyre JA. Antiphospholipid antibodies in implantation failures. Am J Reprod Immunol 2003;49: 221–229.

45. McCarty GA, Baddour VT, Giesler L, Wagenknecht DR, McIntyre JA. Antiphospholipid antibody syndrome (APS) patients with antiphosphatidylethanolamine antibodies have APS clinical symptoms. J Autoimmun 2000;15:A58

46. McCarty GA, Wagenknecht DR, McIntyre JA. Antiphospholipid antibody syndrome (APS) patients with antiphosphatidylcholine antibodies have APS clinical criteria. J Autoimmun 2000;15:A59.

47. Kaider BD, Coulam CB, Roussev RG. Murine embryos as a direct target for some human autoantibodies in vitro. Hum Reprod 1999;2556–2561.

48. Sugi T, McIntyre JA. Autoantibodies to kininogen-phosphatidylethanolamine complexes augment thrombin-induced platelet aggregation. Thromb Res 1996;84:97–109.

49. Pierangeli SS, Gharavi AE, Harris EN. Testing for antiphospholipid antibodies: problems and solutions. Clin Obstet Gyn 2001;44:48–57.

50. Bach JF, Koutouzou S. New clues to systemic lupus. Lancet 1997;350:11.

51. Abramson J, Stagnaro-Green A. In our view...thyroid antibodies and fetal loss: an evolving story. Thyroid 2001;11:57–63.

52. Stagnaro-Green A, Roman SH, Cabin RH, Harvey E, Alvarez-Marfany M, Davies TF. Detection of at risk pregnancy by means of highly sensitive assays for thyroid autoantibodies. JAMA 1990;264: 1422–1425.

53. Lejeune B, Grun JP, DeNayer PH, Servais G, Glinoer D. Antithyroid antibodies underlying thyroid abnormalities and miscarriage or pregnancy induced hypertension. Br J Obstet Gynaecol 1993;100:669–672.

54. Stewart-Akers AM, Krasnow JS, Brekosky J, Deloia JA. Endometrial leukocytes are altered numerically and functionally in women with implantation defects. Am J Reprod Med 1998;39:1–11.

55. Coulam CB, Goodman C, Roussev RG, Thomason EJ, Beaman KD. Systemic CD56+ cells can predict pregnancy outcome. Am J Reprod Immunol 1995;33:40–46.

56. Aoki K, Kajijura S, Matsumoto Y, Okada S, Yaghami Y, Gleicher N. Preconceptual natural killer cell activation as a predictor of miscarriage. Lancet 1995 135:1340–1342.

57. Kane KL, Ashton FA, Schmitz JL, Folds JD. Determination of natural killer cell function by flow cytometry. Clin Diagn Lab Immunol 1996;3:295–300.

58. Kwak JY, Kwak JM, Ainbinder SW, Ruiz AM, Beer AE. Elevated peripheral blood natural killer cells are effectively downregulated by immunoglobulin G infusion in women with recurrent spontaneous abortions. Am J Reprod Immunol 1996;35:363–369.

59. Roussev RG, Stern JJ, Thorsell L, Thomason EJ, Coulam CB. Validation of an embryotoxicity assay. Am J Reprod Immunol 1994;32:1–5.

60. Verlinsky Y, Cieslak J, Ivakhnenko V, et al. Prevention of age related aneuploidies by polar body testing of oocytes. J Assist Reprod Genet 1999;16:165–169.

61. Munne S, Magit C, Cohen J, et al. Positive outcome after preimplantation diagnosis of aneuploidy in human embryos. Hum Reprod 1999;14:2191–2199.

62. Varasteh NN, Neuwirth RS, Levin B, Keltz LB. Pregnancy rates after hysteroscopic polypectomy and myomectomy in infertile women. Obstet Gynecol 1999;94:168–171.

63. Wada I, Hsu CC, Williams G, Macnamee MC, Brinsden PR. The benefits of low-dose aspirin therapy in women with impaired uterine perfusion during assisted conception. Hum Reprod 1994;7:1954–1957.

64. Sher G, Fisch JD. Effect of vaginal sildenafil on the outcome of in vitro fertilization (IVF) after multiple IVF failures attributed to poor endometrial development. Fertil Steril 2002;78:1073–1076.

65. Rai R, Cohen H, Dave M, Regan L. Randomised controlled trial of aspirin and aspirin plus heparin in pregnant women with recurrent miscarriage associated with phospholipid antibodies (or antiphospholipid antibodies). Br Med J 1997;314:253–257.

66. Kwak JYH, Gilman-Sachs A, Beaman KD, Beer AE. Reproductive outcome in women with recurrent spontaneous abortions of alloimmune and autoimmune causes: preconception versus postconception treatment. Am J Obstet Gynecol 1992;166:1787–1795.

67. Hasegawa I, Takauwa K, Goto S, et al. Effectiveness of prednisone/aspirin for recurrent aborters with antiphospholipid antibody. Hum Reprod 1992;7:203–107.

68. Branch DW, Scoll JR, Kochenour NK, Hershgold E. Obstetric complications associated with the lupus anticoagulant. N Engl J Med 1985;313:1322–1326.

69. Alarcon-Segovia D, Deleze M, Oria CV, et al. Antiphospholipid antibodies and the antiphospholipid antibody syndrome in systemic lupus erythematosus. Medicine 1989;68:353–365.

70. Lubbe WF, Liggins CG. Lupus anticoagulant and pregnancy. Am J Obstet Gynecol 1985;153:322–327.

71. Carreras KO, Perez GN, Vega HR, Maclouf J. Lupus anticoagulant and recurrent fetal loss: successful treatment with gammaglobulin. Lancet 1988;2:393.

72. Francois A, Freund M, Reym P. Repeated fetal losses and the lupus anticoagulant. Ann Int Med 1988;109:933–934.

73. Scott JR, Branch DW, Knochenour NK, Ward K. Intravenous treatment of pregnant patients with recurrent pregnancy loss caused by antiphospholipid antibodies and Rh immunization. Am J Obstet Gynecol 1988;159:1055–1056.

74. Parke A, Maier D, Wilson D, Andreole J, Ballow M. Intravenous immunoglobulin, antiphospholipid antibodies, and pregnancy. Ann Int Med 1989;110:495–496.

75. MacLachlan NA, Letsky E, De Sweit M. The use of intravenous immunoglobulin therapy in the management of antiphospholipid antibody associated pregnancies. Clin Exp Rheumatol 1990;8:221–224.

76. Cowchock FS, Resse EA, Balaban D, Branch DW, Plouffe L. Repeated fetal losses associated with antiphospholipid antibodies: a collaborative trial comparing treatment with prednisone to low dose heparin. Am J Obstet Gynecol 1992;166:1318–1323.

77. Ramsdon CF, Faquharson RG. A woman with twelve first trimester losses in whom lupus anticoagulant was detected and treated with steroids, sandoglobulin and heparin. Clin Exp Rheumat 1990;8:221.

78. Lachapelle MH, Miron P, Hemmings R, Roy DA. Endometrial T, B and NK cells in patients with recurrent abortion: altered profile and pregnancy outcome. J Immunol 1996;156:4227–4234.

79. Coulam CB, Goodman C. Increased pregnancy rates after IVF/ET with intravenous immunoglobulin treatment in women with elevated circulating CD56+ cells. Early Pregnancy 2000;4:90–98.

80. Mueller-Eckhart G, Mallmann P, Neppert J, et al. for the German RSA/IVIG Trialist Group. Immunogenetic and serological investigations of nonpregnancy and pregnant women with a history of recurrent spontaneous abortion. J Reprod Immunol 1994;27:95–109.

81. Coulam CB, Krysa LW, Stern JJ, Bustillo M. Intravenous immunoglobulin for treatment of recurrent pregnancy loss. Am J Reprod Immunol 1995;34:333–337.

82. Christiansen OB, Pedersen B, Rosgaard A, Husth M. A randomized, double-blind, placebo controlled trial of intravenous immunoglobulin in the prevention of recurrent miscarriage: evidence for a therapeutic effect in women with secondary recurrent miscarriage. Hum Reprod 2002;17:809–816.

83. Stephenson MD, Dreher K, Houlihan E, Wu V. Prevention of unexplained recurrent spontaneous abortion using intravenous immunoglobulin: a prospective, randomized, double-blinded, placebo-controlled trial. Am J Reprod Immunol 1998;39:82–88.

84. Recurrent Miscarriage Immunotherapy Trialists Group (RMITG). Worldwide prospective observational study and meta-analysis on allogeneic leukocyte immunotherapy for recurrent spontaneous abortion. Am J Reprod Immunol 1994;32:55–72.

85. Chaouat G, Assai-Meliani A, Martal J, et al. IL-10 prevents naturally occurring fetal loss in the CBA X DBA/2 mating combination, and local defect in IL-10 production in this abortion-prone combination is corrected by in vivo injection of INF-tau. J Immunol 1995;154:4261–4268.

16 Multifetal Gestations

Isaac Blickstein, MD *and*
Louis G. Keith, MD, PhD

Contents

INTRODUCTION
MATERNAL ADAPTATION TO A MULTIFETAL PREGNANCY
SPECIAL CIRCUMSTANCES IN MULTIPLE PREGNANCIES
LABORATORY ASSESSMENT DURING MULTIPLE PREGNANCIES
REFERENCES

INTRODUCTION

Multifetal pregnancies are high-risk pregnancies—a sweeping statement underlying the day-to-day challenge of caring for the mother and her multiples. Remarkable changes have occurred in the clinical picture and outcomes of multiple gestations during the past 25 yr. First and foremost, the frequency of multifetal pregnancies, primarily attributed to infertility treatment, has reached epidemic dimensions in most developed countries *(1)*. Second, as a consequence of the ability of modern infertility technology to compensate for the reduced fecundity of older age, mothers of multiples are quite often past what was formerly thought to be "old" in terms of pregnancy and parturition. Third, the rapid improvements in neonatal care of the last two decades have pushed the limits of viability to gestational ages that were once considered as late miscarriages. Finally, the revolutionary technological achievements in imaging and genetic testing for singleton pregnancies have been adopted in the management of multifetal gestations to the point that some of the most advanced intrauterine interventions are currently performed exclusively in complicated multifetal pregnancies.

The following generalizations can be made regarding the current status of multifetal pregnancies:

- The overall rate of multiple births in most developed countries is currently as high as 2–4%, a figure two to four times higher than the natural rate during the late 1970s (prior to the implementation of assisted reproduction) or the rate in developing countries that do not have assisted reproduction *(1)*.
- Because the reduced fecundity of women over 35 yr of age significantly increases the need for infertility treatment, and thus the risk of a multiple pregnancy, the age of the mother of multiples is increasing in parallel with the increased use of infertility treatment. For example, the ratio between triplet births in the United States in two time periods

(1971–1977 and 1997–1998) demonstrates a stepwise, up to 10-fold increase, for women aged 35–44 yr *(2)*. At the same time, the frequency of women over 44 yr who delivered triplets during the period 1997–1998 was 50 times higher than the frequency during the period 1971–1977 *(2)*.

- According to a population-based survey, the ratio of induced to spontaneous twins increased from 1 to 46 in the 1970s to 1 to 2 in the late 1990s *(3)*. This trend is even more obvious in medical centers with busy infertility clinics, where induced conceptions presently comprise the majority of multiple pregnancies. It is currently estimated that the vast majority of triplets result from infertility treatment.

Although often underappreciated, maternal complications are quite common in multiple pregnancies (Table 1). Serious morbidity such as hypertensive disorders, eclampsia, complications of treatment for premature contractions, prolonged bedrest, prolonged hospitalization, and operative deliveries are significantly higher in twins and high-order multiples (HOMPs) than in singletons. Moreover, the epidemic of iatrogenic HOMPs confirmed that maternal morbidity increases with plurality. It is therefore expected that maternal morbidity would decrease following multifetal pregnancy reduction (MFPR). Indeed, Skupski et al. *(4)* found that severe preeclampsia was more common among in vitro fertilization (IVF) triplet pregnancies compared with IVF triplets reduced to twins and with nonreduced twins. In addition, Sivan et al. *(5)* found that gestational diabetes mellitus (GDM) was significantly higher in the triplets than in the triplets reduced to twins group.

Maternal morbidity should also be considered in the context of maternal age, because assisted reproduction initiates conceptions beyond the range of reproductive years when underlying diseases and pregnancy complications are more frequent and/or intensified. One study of 74 IVF patients, ages 45–59, reported 29 (39.2%) multiple gestations, including 20 twins, 7 triplets, and 2 quadruplets *(6)*. Antenatal complications occurred in 28 women (37.8%) including preterm labor, hypertension, diabetes, preeclampsia, HELLP (hemolysis, elevated liver enzymes, and low platelets count) syndrome, and fetal growth retardation. Cesarean section was performed in 64.8% *(6)*. Many of these complications represent serious pathology antecedents to maternal mortality, a fact that is often either overlooked or ignored.

Generally, there is not much specific difference between laboratory tests ordered for singletons and multiple gestations; however, in the case of multiples, the frequency and timing of these tests are often different. This chapter focuses on some distinctive features related to physiological changes characteristic of and peculiar to a mother of twins or a HOMP, followed by a discussion of various laboratory tests that have specific connotation for the multifetal pregnancy.

MATERNAL ADAPTATION TO A MULTIFETAL PREGNANCY

Multiple pregnancy represents a unique situation whereby the uterine milieu, composed of utero–placental, maternal, and fetal components, needs to provide for more fetal mass than is required in a singleton gestation. For example, the total masses of twins and triplets achieve the singletons 40 wk gestation 50th birth weight percentile (approx 3500 g) by 32 and 29 wk, respectively. Both the total twin birth weight at 36 wk (2 × 2500 g = 5000 g) and the total triplet birth weight at 33 wk (3 × 1700 g = 5100 g) exceed by far the 90th percentile of singletons at term *(7)*. The remarkable adaptation to the

Table 1
Complications That Are More Frequently Seen in Multifetal Pregnancies

Hypertensive diseases
    Preeclamptic toxemia
        HELLP syndrome
        Acute fatty liver
    Pregnancy-induced hypertension
        Chronic hypertension
        Eclampsia
Anemia
Gestational diabetes mellitus (?)
Premature contractions and labor
    Complications associated with tocolysis
Delivery-associated complications
    Cesarean section
    Operative delivery
    Premature rupture of membranes
    Postpartum endometritis
    Placental abruption

demands of these large fetal masses at early gestational age is seen in all maternal systems. Unfortunately, however, these demands frequently overwhelm the individual mother's physiologic capacity, leading to relative or absolute failure of adaptation (i.e., insufficiency) of certain components of the uterine environment.

The best example of the preceding cautionary statement is the change in cardiovascular system during pregnancy. Multiple gestation places increased demands on the maternal circulation, and, as expected, cardiac output in the second and third trimesters is greater during twin than during singleton pregnancy (8). Cardiac output is increased primarily by heart rate (9) and, during the third trimester, also by stroke volume and increased contractility (8). These changes suggest that the cardiovascular reserve is reduced during a multiple pregnancy. Expansion in plasma volume, necessary for the increased demand for nutrient supply, is exaggerated in women with twin pregnancies (10). The combination of multiple gestation, labor, and volume overload more than triples the cardiac output in twin gestation compared to the nonpregnant state (11) and may cause serious maternal complications, especially during β-mimetic tocolysis (12).

Another example of the maternal adaptation is the increased carbohydrate demand in a multifetal pregnancy (13). One of the theories proposed in the past to explain why multiple pregnancies were more prone to GDM was that the increased placental size (hyperplacentosis) was thought to increase certain hormone concentrations (primarily human placental lactogen) and, in turn, increased susceptibility to GDM. Casele et al. (14) conducted a 40-h metabolic study in nondiabetic gestations and compared the metabolic response to normal meal eating and the vulnerability to starvation ketosis in 10 twin versus 10 singleton gestations matched for age and prepregnancy weight. Their observations suggested that twin gestations are more vulnerable to the accelerated starvation of late normal pregnancy than is the case with singletons. Marconi et al. evaluated glucose disposal rate in 11 singleton, 5 twins, and 1 triplet pregnancy to show that the differences between multiples and singletons may be the result of a plurality-dependent increase in the metabolic demands of the multiple gestation, *(15)* All these observations point to the tremendous shift of nutrients from the maternal to the fetal compartment. The greater nutritional requirements caused by greater need and metabolism in multiple pregnancies is perhaps best demonstrated in the studies of Luke et al., who showed that early weight gain may prolong length of gestation and result in increased birth weights of twins *(16)* and triplets, *(17)*.

The laboratory assessment of maternal adaptation to a multifetal pregnancy differs little from the assessment of a singleton gestation. In general, interpretation of laboratory results should not be different from that in singletons. A vivid example is higher physiological demand for iron during a multiple pregnancy, frequently leading to maternal anemia *(18,19)*. Despite the fact that hemoglobin concentrations are significantly lower during twin gestations, frank maternal anemia should not be considered as a physiological adaptation and thus overlooked. Rather, anemia should be treated more aggressively because of the increased likelihood of peripartum hemorrhage.

SPECIAL CIRCUMSTANCES IN MULTIPLE PREGNANCIES

Diagnosis of Pregnancy

From the early days of pregnancy diagnosis using human chorionic gonadotropin (hCG) in urine or blood, it was clear that higher concentrations of these hormones are found in a multiple than in a singleton pregnancy. This laboratory finding often led to the consideration of a differential diagnosis between a multiple pregnancy and hydatidiform mole, because both were associated with an increased uterine size on pelvic examination, early onset hyperemesis gravidarum, and first-trimester bleeding. In the past, confusion led to many induced abortions of normal twin pregnancies; however, with the advent of sonography, the distinction between a mole and twins should be very simple. Moreover, because there is no accepted threshold that clearly distinguishes twins from singletons, the clinical utility of hCG as a diagnostic test is limited. Even the trend of β-hCG concentrations, usually obtained following assisted reproductive technologies, should not be used as evidence for or against a multiple pregnancy, because sonography is the diagnostic gold standard.

Biochemical Screening for Trisomy 21

Although each of the fetuses in a multiple gestation has the same chance for a chromosomal aberration, as does a singleton with similar risk variables, the risk for the mother that one of her multiples will be affected is approximately doubled if she carries twins. Thus, a 31-yr-old mother of dizygotic twins carries a similar risk of having one twin with Down syndrome as a 35-yr-old mother of a singleton *(20)*. Biochemical maternal serum screening for aneuploidy in older women is particularly attractive given the fact that multiples are commonly seen in older mothers and that invasive cytogenetic procedures (amniocentesis or chorionic villus sampling) carry a much higher risk of pregnancy loss when performed in multiples. Therefore, there is a genuine advantage to minimizing the use of invasive procedures in these premium, advanced maternal age pregnancies.

Screening for trisomy 21 (Down syndrome) is presently accomplished by the "triple" test composed of second-trimester maternal serum hCG or free β-hCG, α-fetoprotein (AFP), and unconjugated estriol (uE$_3$). The triple test yields a 67% detection rate for a 5% false-positive rate *(21)*. Inhibin A increases the detection rate by 7% for the same false-positive rate. In the first trimester, similar models predict that a combination of preg-nancy-associated plasma protein A (PAPP-A), free β-hCG, AFP, and uE_3 will yield a 70% detection rate, increasing to 88% if sonographic nuchal translucency (NT) thickness is added to the screening protocol *(21)*. In twin gestations, however, the contribution of each member of the set cannot be differentiated, and the total free β-hCG and PAPP-A values are 2.1 and 1.86 times greater than in singletons, yielding a 52% and 55% detection rate in twins discordant or concordant for trisomy 21 *(22)*. This detection rate, which is not significantly changed by chorionicity *(23)*, is less than the 75% attainable using NT thickness. However, the combination of NT thickness and maternal serum biochemistry provided detection rates approaching 80% *(22)*.

One should also consider that biochemical markers change following spontaneous or iatrogenic demise of one fetus, probably by release of tissue or serum from the dead fetus(es). For example, first-trimester MFPR causes elevated maternal serum AFP com-pared with normal twin values, and that maternal serum AFP concentration demonstrates a positive correlation with the number of dead fetuses and a negative correlation with the number of weeks elapsed since MFPR *(24)*. It follows that sonography should be per-formed to exclude fetal anomalies such as open neural tube and abdominal wall defects because abnormal maternal serum AFP concentrations cannot be used in these patients for screening.

Coagulopathy

As pointed out previously, fetal demise in a multiple pregnancy may be either spon-taneous or iatrogenic. Spontaneous death may occur early in pregnancy, giving rise to the so-called "vanishing twin" syndrome *(25)*, or later, during the subsequent trimesters. The iatrogenic counterpart of the "vanishing twin" syndrome is MFPR, a procedure primarily intended to reduce the number of multiples. At a later stage, selective fetocide is per-formed mainly for discordant anomalies detected by antenatal diagnostic testing.

In contrast to the dead fetus syndrome in singletons, which allegedly is associated with maternal disseminated intravascular coagulation (DIC), embryonic or fetal demise in multiples is seldom associated with clinical manifestations of coagulation defects. None-theless, many clinicians follow such pregnancies with biweekly coagulation profiles. Laboratory evidence of mild DIC after MFPR can be seen albeit uncommonly, but it will likely resolve spontaneously *(24)*.

In this respect, it should be remembered that normal pregnancy is a hypercoaguable state, with elevated plasma concentrations of coagulation factors VII, VIII, and X and fibrinogen and the increased concentrations of plasminogen activator inhibitors. It has been suggested that multifetal gestations represent an exaggerated imbalance in hemo-stasis, mimicking low-grade DIC *(26)*. For example, D-dimers, formed by plasmin-mediated proteolysis of cross-linked fibrin, were significantly higher in normal twin than in singleton gestations. These data suggest that for the majority of women with multifetal gestation, the coagulopathy observed in the laboratory may not be clinically apparent *(26)* and should be substantiated by additional laboratory testing for such conditions as decreased fibrinogen concentrations and thrombocytopenia.

Another example is coagulopathy associated with premature separation of the placenta (placental abruption), which occurs more frequently in multiple gestations *(12)*. The higher frequency of abruption may be simply a result of more placentas per pregnancy or because of a higher risk of acute decompression of the overdistended uterus (i.e., after rupture of the membranes of a gestational sac containing polyhydramnios, or following the delivery of the presenting fetus). In addition, abruption is associated with severe preeclamptic toxemia (PET), a well-known complication of multiple pregnancies. Placental abruption is a direct cause of pregnancy-related maternal death *(12)* mainly because of acute blood loss. DIC, however, may be much more profound than the associated blood loss would indicate.

Hypertensive Disorders

Hypertensive disorders, including PET, pregnancy-induced hypertension (PIH), and choronic hypertension are not only serious but often life-threatening maternal complications during multiple pregnancies *(12)*. PET occurs earlier and in a more severe form than in singleton pregnancy *(27)*, and eclampsia is a leading cause in maternal mortality among mothers of twins *(12)*. The range of relative risk of PIH, PET, and eclampsia for twin compared to singleton gestations is 1.2 to 2.7, 2.8 to 4.4, and 3.4 to 5.1, respectively *(28,29)*. Moreover, the risk of hypertensive disorders is plurality dependent and reduced following MFPR *(30)*.

Regrettably, there is no laboratory test that accurately predicts PET, which is generally diagnosed by elevated blood pressure, proteinuria, and edema. However, elevated serum uric acid concentrations, attributed to decreased renal urate excretion, are frequently found in pregnancies complicated with PET. Furthermore, uric acid concentrations of 6 mg/dL (0.35 mmol/L) or more measured at 30–31 wk of gestation in twin mothers predict the onset of preeclampsia with a sensitivity of 73% and a specificity of 74% *(28)*. Higher maternal serum uric acid concentrations observed in the third trimester of non-PET twin gestations result in part from increased uric acid production, as reflected in the increased daily uric acid excretion *(31)*, and presumably from higher adenosine concentrations *(32)*. A positive correlation is found, irrespective of maternal size, between the concentration of serum uric acid and the number of fetuses, suggesting that for clinical purposes, the uric acid cutoff concentration should be adjusted using 5.2, 7.2, and 7.6 mg/dL for singleton, twin, and triplet gestations *(33)*.

Finally, the involvement of the liver in variants of severe PET such as acute fatty liver and HELLP syndrome is more common in multiple than in singleton pregnancies because multiples may further stress the fatty acid oxidation capabilities of the susceptible woman *(34)*. Laboratory assessment in these cases would include frequent evaluations of liver enzymes, bilirubin, albumin, and ammonia concentrations, as well as serological tests to exclude hepatitis, similar to that of singleton pregnancies.

Gestational Diabetes Mellitus

Critical analysis of the data in the literature does not support a clear-cut association between GDM and multiple pregnancies. Moreover, several reservations concerning the available data are meritorious *(13)*. First, published studies are quite old and do not include multiples resulting from the current epidemic of iatrogenic conceptions, which exhibit a remarkable shift toward older maternal age *(13)*. Second, there is clear lack of population-based data. As a result, prospective studies are flawed because of a small sample size and insufficient statistical power. Third, there is a striking paucity of studies related to triplet pregnancies, which were once notoriously rare and of negligible importance. Finally, the balance between fetal growth-promoting effects of GDM and the inherent growth-restricting effects of the limited and overwhelmed uterine milieu is absolutely unknown.

In practice, clinicians tend to screen pregnant women irrespective of plurality. The laboratory assessment, including fasting plasma glucose concentrations or concentrations following one of the standardized glucose challenge tests, is not different from that in a singleton pregnancy.

LABORATORY ASSESSMENT DURING MULTIPLE PREGNANCIES

Multiple pregnancy merits close antenatal supervision. In practical terms, this means frequent antenatal visits to assess maternal and fetal well-being. Frequent repeated laboratory tests are expected during such gestations. After birth, neonatal assessments are usually double for twins, triple for triplets, etc. It is therefore safe to assume that a multiple gestation keeps the laboratory busy during the antenatal as well as during the postnatal period. In addition, pregnancy complications are either more frequent or of specific nature in a multifetal gestation (Table 1).

The prominent and well-established differences, especially in terms of fetal growth, between one member of a multiple set and a singleton, often led scholars to consider differently growth and growth aberrations in multiples. For example, it has been suggested that twins and triplets grow differently *in utero*, and therefore, twin- or triplet-specific growth curves should be employed in assessing multiples *(7)*. By the same token, it is possible that the overwhelmed maternal–fetal unit behaves differently in a multiple gestation. Hence, there is perhaps a need to adjust some laboratory reference intervals to the number of fetuses, but as yet this possibility has not been tested with large comparative studies *(33)*.

Laboratory tests undoubtedly complement other diagnostic modalities and clinical judgment in managing these challenging pregnancies. The laboratory assessment during a multiple pregnancy is not complete without a thorough understanding of the underlying condition.

REFERENCES

1. Blickstein I, Keith LG. The spectrum of iatrogenic multiple pregnancy. In: Blickstein I, Keith LG, eds. Iatrogenic Multiple Pregnancy: Clinical Implications. New York: Parthenon Publishing, 2001, pp. 1–7.
2. Kiely JL, Kiely M. Epidemiologic trends in multiple births in the United States, 1971–1998. Twin Res 2001;4:131–133.
3. Loos R, Derom C, Vlietinck R, Derom R. The East Flanders prospective twin survey (Belgium): a population-based register. Twin Res 1998;1:167–175.
4. Skupski DW, Nelson S, Kowalik A, et al. Multiple gestations from in vitro fertilization: successful implantation alone is not associated with subsequent preeclampsia. Am J Obstet Gynecol 1996;175:1029–1032.
5. Sivan E, Maman E, Homko CJ, et al. Impact of fetal reduction on the incidence of gestational diabetes. Obstet Gynecol 2002;99:91–94.
6. Sauer MV, Paulson RJ, Lobo RA. Oocyte donation to women of advanced reproductive age: pregnancy results and obstetrical outcomes in patients 45 years and older. Hum Reprod 1996;11:2540–2543.
7. Blickstein I. Normal and abnormal growth of multiples. Semin Neonatol 2002,7:177–185.
8. Veille JC, Morton MJ, Burry KJ. Maternal cardiovascular adaptations to twin pregnancy. Am J Obstet Gynecol 1985;153:261–263.
9. Robson SC, Hunter S, Boys RJ, Dunlop W. Hemodynamic changes during twin pregnancy. A Doppler and M-mode echocardiographic study. Am J Obstet Gynecol 1989;161:1273–1278.
10. Campbell DM, MacGillivray I. The importance of plasma volume expansion and nutrition in twin pregnancy. Acta Genet Med Gemellol 1984;33:19–24.
11. Skupski DW. Maternal complications of twin gestation. The Female Patient 1996;6:16–21.

12. Blickstein I. Maternal mortality in twin gestations. J Reprod Med 1997;42:680–684.
13. Hazan Y, Blickstein I. Diabetes and multiple pregnancies. In: Hod M, Jovanovic L, Di Renzo GC, De Leiva A, Langer A, eds. Textbook of Diabetes and Pregnancy. London: Martin Dunitz, 2003, pp. 502–507.
14. Casele HL, Dooley SL, Metzger BE. Metabolic response to meal eating and extended overnight fast in twin gestation. Am J Obstet Gynecol 1996;175:917–921.
15. Marconi AM, Davoli E, Cetin I, et al. Impact of conceptus mass on glucose disposal rate in pregnant women. Am J Physiol 1993;264:514–518.
16. Luke B, Min SJ, Gillespie B, et al. The importance of early weight gain in the intrauterine growth and birth weight of twins. Am J Obstet Gynecol 1998;179:1155–1161.
17. Luke B, Bryan E, Sweetland C, Leurgans S, Keith L. Prenatal weight gain and the birth weight of triplets. Acta Genet Med Germellol 1995;44:81–91.
18. Lurie S, Blickstein I. Age distribution of erythrocytes population in women with twin pregnancy. Gynecol Obstet Invest 1993;36:163–165.
19. Blickstein I, Goldschmit R, Lurie S. Hemoglobin levels during twin versus singleton pregnancies: parity makes the difference. J Reprod Med 1995;40:47–50.
20. Meyers C, Adam R, Dungan J, Prenger V. Aneuploidy in twin gestations: when is maternal age advanced? Obstet Gynecol 1997;89:248–251.
21. Cuckle H. Biochemical screening for Down syndrome. Eur J Obstet Gynecol Reprod Biol 2000;92: 97–101.
22. Spencer K. Screening for trisomy 21 in twin pregnancies in the first trimester using free beta-hCG and PAPP-A, combined with fetal nuchal translucency thickness. Prenat Diagn 2000;20:91–95.
23. Spencer K. Screening for trisomy 21 in twin pregnancies in the first trimester: does chorionicity impact on maternal serum free beta-hCG or PAPP-A levels? Prenat Diagn 2001;21:715–717.
24. Lynch L, Berkowitz RL. Maternal serum alpha-fetoprotein and coagulation profiles after multifetal pregnancy reduction. Am J Obstet Gynecol 1993;169:987–990.
25. Landy HJ, Keith LG. The vanishing twin: a review. Hum Reprod Update 1998;4:177–183.
26. Bar J, Blickstein D, Hod M, et al. Increased D-dimer levels in twin gestation. Thromb Res 2000;98: 485–489.
27. Blickstein I, Ben-Hur H, Borenstein R. Perinatal outcome of twin pregnancies complicated with preeclampsia. Am J Perinat 1992;9:258–260.
28. Krotz S, Fajardo J, Ghandi S, Patel A, Keith LG. Hypertensive disease in twin pregnancies: a review. Twin Res 2002;5:8–14.
29. Campbell DM, MacGillivray I. Preeclampsia in twin pregnancies: incidence and outcome. Hypertens Pregnancy 1999;18:197–207.
30. Skupski DW, Nelson S, Kowalik A, et al. Multiple gestations from in vitro fertilization: successful implantation alone is not associated with subsequent preeclampsia. Am J Obstet Gynecol 1996;175: 1029–1032.
31. Fischer RL, Weisberg LS, Hediger ML. Etiology of third-trimester maternal hyperuricemia in nonpreeclamptic twin gestations. Obstet Gynecol 2001;97:62–65.
32. Suzuki S, Yoneyama Y, Sawa R, Araki T. Relation between serum uric acid and plasma adenosine levels in twin pregnancies. Obstet Gynecol 2000;96:507–510.
33. Cohen SB, Kreiser D, Erez I, Kogan I, Seidman DS, Schiff E. Effect of fetal number on maternal serum uric acid concentration. Am J Perinatol 2002;19:291–296.
34. Davidson KM, Simpson LL, Knox TA, D'Alton ME. Acute fatty liver of pregnancy in triplet gestation. Obstet Gynecol 1998;91:806–808.

17 Diabetes in Pregnancy

Jonathan W. Dukes, BS, Albert C. Chen, BS, and Lois Jovanovic, MD

CONTENTS

INTRODUCTION

With the advent of injectable insulin in the 1920s, physicians were finally given the ability to treat the symptoms of diabetes mellitus (DM). Despite this success, the lack of rapid-acting insulin and self-blood glucose monitoring meant that the available insulin therapy could do little to maintain glucose at physiological concentrations. The effects of large glycemic excursions were readily seen as diabetic women had extensive obstetric complications as a result of their poorly controlled diabetes. Until the 1980s, physicians actively counseled diabetic women to avoid pregnancy *(1)*. Since that time, advancements in insulin therapies and diagnostic tests have allowed for near-normal glucose concentrations throughout pregnancy and produced dramatic improvements in the outcome of diabetic pregnancies. Despite these improvements, there is still a threefold increase in congenital anomalies in pregnancies complicated by diabetes in comparison to the background population *(2)*. Through better use of current therapies, this unnecessarily high number of complications can be lowered.

This chapter outlines the clinical laboratory tests available to physicians and patients for use in the management and treatment of diabetes during pregnancy. The miniaturization of some tests has brought them down to a scale where they can now be performed in the patient's own home. This breakthrough has been essential in the development of therapies for diabetes because proper management requires blood glucose testing several times each day. In addition, tests used to assess the maternal–fetal well-being need to be performed frequently in order to guide treatment decisions. Despite the magnitude of the task, it is possible to produce healthy babies through the judicious use of clinical tests. In light of new and more modern techniques, some older tests are of questionable efficacy so care should taken when choosing tests for patient management. This chapter assists in making those decisions and demonstrates target ranges for a variety of laboratory tests.

From: *Current Clinical Pathology: Handbook of Clinical Laboratory Testing During Pregnancy*
Edited by: A. M. Gronowski © Humana Press, Totowa, NJ

Diabetes Background

Three different forms of DM can complicate pregnancy: Type 1, type 2, and gestational diabetes mellitus (GDM). Type 1 and type 2 DM are conditions of hyperglycemia that exist before pregnancy. In type 1 diabetes, the immune system attacks the pancreatic β cells through an autoimmune disease; in most cases there appears to be an immunological cross-reaction with a virus possessing similar antigenic markers to β cells. Over time, the β cells are destroyed. Treatment for this type of DM requires daily insulin injections. In type 2 DM, the person continues to produce insulin, but his or her body develops insulin resistance. This type of DM is found in varying degrees of severity and can often be controlled through a combination of diet, exercise, and drug therapies that augment the body's insulin production and glucose uptake. GDM is defined as any degree of carbohydrate intolerance with onset or recognition during pregnancy *(3)*. GDM is an insulin-resistant state, similar to type 2 DM. It is manifested when the pancreatic production of insulin cannot keep up with the increasing anti-insulin hormones of pregnancy (cortisol, prolactin, human placental lactogen, and progesterone), the increased food intake and the increased adiposity, decreased physical activity, and increased insulin metabolism via placental insulinases during pregnancy *(1)*.

Complications of the fetus from pregnancies affected by diabetes can be divided into two main groups: congenital anomalies resulting from abnormal metabolic conditions in the first trimester, and macrosomia from these conditions in the second and third trimesters. During the first 11 wk of pregnancy, hyperglycemia has been shown to be a major teratogen *(4,5)*. Congenital anomalies may occur in up to 27% of pregnancies with severely uncontrolled hyperglycemia *(6)*. Macrosomia is clinically defined as birth weight greater than the 90th percentile (4000 to 4500 g in most populations) and occurs through the overnourishment of the fetus by maternal hyperglycemia. Most of the excess weight is body fat that accumulates in the shoulder, face, and waist regions. Macrosomia, although seemingly benign, can be very serious because it diverts developmental energy to the production of adipose tissue and increases the risk of birth trauma during delivery. Shoulder dystocia, or difficult delivery of the infant because the shoulders are too large to pass through the pelvic outlet of the mother, can lead to permanent neurological damage referred to as Erb's palsy, clavicular fracture, fetal distress, low Apgar scores, and birth asphyxia. To circumvent these problems, a macrosomic fetus needs to be delivered via cesarean section if it is deemed too large for the birth canal. Diagnosis of this condition is difficult because of the inability of ultrasonography to accurately image body fat *(7)*. Other methods of fetal weight determination, such as the state of maternal glycemic control, must be addressed in order to make a proper determination of delivery route, thus avoiding the excessive use of prophylactic cesarean section.

Excellent glycemic control during pregnancy is essential to the health of the unborn baby. Studies focusing on achieving normoglycemia during pregnancy have had great success in normalizing pregnancy outcome *(8,9)*. To achieve this goal, most programs use comprehensive patient training and treatment programs, such as physiologic insulin therapy, to significantly reduce the fetus's exposure to hyperglycemia *(8)*. Despite the intensity of the logistics, high success rates are possible through the proper use and interpretation of the available diagnostic tests and the highly motivated nature of the gravid patient population.

SCREENING FOR GDM

Background

Screening for GDM is essential to the proper health of the infant because GDM can be asymptomatic in the mother but cause serious problems to the fetus. Despite the relatively long period of time that the impact of GDM has been recognized, screening procedures have been a topic of frequent debate. Currently, there are more than 14 different published guidelines for use in screening for GDM. These guidelines vary in the criteria for the oral glucose tolerance test (OGTT) and their use of selective vs universal screening, fasting plasma glucose vs random plasma glucose, and other factors *(10)*. The most accepted of these guidelines are the World Health Organization (WHO), American Diabetes Association (ADA), and National Diabetes Data Group (NDDG) guidelines, with the latter two being the most used in the United States *(11)*. Each of these guidelines has varying degrees of sensitivity to detect potentially problematic pregnancies and there is much debate over which is most beneficial and cost effective. As a result of this lack of consensus, the decision of what test to use is at the discretion of the individual clinician. The choice should be made only after considering which test most benefits the patient and the fetus. Any rise in the postprandial glucose concentration should not be overlooked, and closer monitoring must be instituted to lower the risks of obstetric complications *(1)*.

Current Guidelines

WHO GUIDELINE

The WHO guideline stipulates the use of a 2-h, 75 g OGTT identical to that recommended for nonpregnant adults. Two plasma glucose readings are taken: fasting and 2 h postload. Elevated plasma glucose from either reading is considered diagnostic for GDM. The diagnostic values are identical to the lower criteria used for identifying impaired glucose tolerance in nonpregnant adults (Table 1) *(11a)*. Because of the severity of the obstetric complications that can occur, any degree of glucose intolerance is classified as GDM. This test should be administered at the first obstetric visit. If negative, it is reordered during the 24th to 28th wk of gestation.

The glucose load can be purchased premixed in solution or made in the office. The glucose load is made by mixing either 75 g of anhydrous glucose or 82.5g of glucose monohydrate in 250–300 mL water. If these compounds are not available, a partial hydrolysate of starch or the equivalent carbohydrate content may also be used.

The OGTT is performed with the patient in a fasting state (8–14 h). In the 3 d prior to the OGTT, the patient should follow an unrestricted carbohydrate diet with normal physical activity. A moderate carbohydrate meal (30–50 g) is consumed the evening before the OGTT and the patient should be advised that water may be consumed after the fast begins. Following the collection of the fasting blood sample, the patient should drink the prepared glucose load over the course of 5 mins. Two h after the patient has started to drink the glucose load, the second plasma glucose measurement is taken. Any two plasma glucose concentrations over that shown in Table 1 are diagnostic of GDM. During the course of the test, the patient must not be allowed to smoke and should remain seated. The person giving the test must note any factors that may influence the interpretation of the test results such as medications, inactivity, or infection *(3,12)*.

Table 1
Comparison of Diagnosis Guidelines for Gestational Diabetes Mellitus
With the Oral Glucose Tolerance Test

Glucose load	ADA[a] 100 g[b]	NDDG 100 g	WHO 75 g
Fasting	95 mg/dL	105 mg/dL	110 mg/dL
1 h	180 mg/dL	190 mg/dL	—
2 h	155 mg/dL	165 mg/dL	140 mg/dL
3 h	140 mg/dL	145 mg/dL	—

[a]Any two glucose concentrations over those shown are diagnostic of GDM.
[b]A 75 g load can be used in place of the 100 g. In that case, only the fasting, 1 h, and 2 h values are used. (Adapted from ref. *11a*.)

NDDG AND ADA GUIDELINES

The NDDG and ADA guidelines are the GDM diagnosis guidelines most commonly used in the United States. Both utilize the same test format and differ only in their diagnosis threshold values (Table 1). These tests are based on the O'Sullivan and Mahan statistical OGTT originally proposed in 1964 and modified in 1973 *(13)*. They both utilize a 1 h, 50 g glucose screening test (GCT) for at-risk patients followed by a fasting 3 h, 100 g OGTT for those who have a high plasma glucose reading on the 50 g GCT. Plasma glucose readings are taken every hour during the OGTT.

The NDDG guideline follows the O'Sullivan and Mahan cutoffs. These cutoffs were derived through a statistical calculation, with the high values being any concentration greater than two standard deviations above the calculated mean of the pregnant population (Table 1) *(14)*. After years of debate, this older guideline has been superseded in the United States by the newer ADA guideline. The ADA guideline uses the lower concentrations recommended in 1982 by Carpenter and Coustan *(3)*.

The current ADA protocol requires a risk assessment to determine the necessity of the OGTT (Table 2). Those of low-risk status are not required to undergo any form of glucose testing. Women considered at low-risk are those who are under 25 yr of age, have normal weight before pregnancy, are members of an ethnic group with a low prevalence of GDM, have no known diabetes in first-degree relatives, no history of abnormal glucose tolerance, and no history of poor obstetric outcome. All high-risk women should undergo an OGTT as soon as possible during the pregnancy, and then be retested between the 24th and 28th wk of gestation if the first test is negative. Those women considered to be of high-risk status have any one of the following characteristics: marked obesity, personal history of GDM, glycosuria, or a strong family history of diabetes. Women not falling into either of these groups are considered to be of average risk and should be tested sometime between the 24th and 28th wk of gestation.

The OGTT can be administered in two ways. First, it can be administered to all patients of high or average risk without a prior glucose screen. This type of universal testing can be more cost effective in a few homogeneous high-risk populations, but it will result in a large number of unnecessary tests in a low-risk population. In order to reduce this number in mixed-risk environments, the ADA suggests using a two-step approach *(3)*. This method utilizes a challenge test to identify those women who will most likely have

Table 2
ADA Risk Factors for GDM

Low risk: (all of the following)
                    < 25 yr of age
                    Ethnicity of low prevalence (those not listed below)
                    Normal weight before pregnancy
                    No known diabetes in first degree relatives
                    No history of abnormal glucose tolerance
                    No history of poor obstetric outcome

High risk: (any one of the following)
                    Marked obesity
                    Personal history of gestational diabetes
                    Glycosuria
                    Strong family history of diabetes
                    Ethnicity of high prevalence (Hispanic, African, Native
                    American, South or East Asian, Pacific Islands, and indigenous
                    Australian)

Average risk:
                    Individuals not falling in either group

Adapted from ref. *17*.

a high 100 g OGTT. All high- or average-risk patients are given a 50 g glucose challenge with plasma glucose concentrations measured 1 h postload consumption. This glucose challenge does not need to be done following an overnight fast, but the patient should remain seated and not smoke over the course of the hour. Those with a 1-h plasma glucose concentration above the chosen screen threshold value must return for a follow-up 100 g OGTT (Table 3).

The choice of a challenge threshold value is at the discretion of the individual clinician, although 140 mg/dL is the most commonly used. The pros and cons of each value must be weighed, because a lower threshold will increase the sensitivity of the challenge to GDM cases, but at the price of decreasing its specificity (specificity is the percentage of women who are referred to the OGTT that will test positive for GDM). For example, a threshold of 140 mg/dL will identify 79% of women who will be diagnosed with GDM by the follow-up OGTT and will have a specificity of 87%. A threshold of 130 mg/dL will increase the sensitivity of the test to 100%, but drop the specificity to 78% *(15)*. The choice of the challenge threshold depends on whether the goal of the clinician is to identify all women with GDM, or refer the fewest healthy patients to the time-intensive OGTT. These factors must be taken into account when choosing a threshold value for the 50 g challenge (Table 4).

The OGTT is performed in the same way, regardless of whether a glucose challenge test is used as a screen. The OGTT is given the morning after an overnight fast (8–14 h), following 3 d of an unrestricted diet with typical physical activity. The glucose load is bought prepackaged or made by mixing 100 g of anhydrous glucose in 250–300 mL water. Following the collection of the fasting blood sample, the patient should drink the prepared glucose load over the course of 5 min. Timing of the test begins as the patient starts to drink. Plasma blood samples are then taken every hour for 3 h. Two samples with

Table 3
Steps to Diagnosing Gestational Diabetes

1. Assess patient risk status on first prenatal visit.
2. Perform one- or two-step OGTT (see text) according to risk status.
     Low risk: No OGTT required.
     Average risk: Perform OGTT at 24–28 wk gestation.
     High risk: Perform OGTT as soon as possible. If negative, repeat at 24–28 wk or with signs of hyperglycemia.
3. If the two-step OGTT is used, screen patients to receive OGTT with a 50 g glucose load. All those with a 1-h value above the chosen threshold (see text) return for 100 g OGTT.
4. Compare 100 g OGTT results to values shown on Table 1. Any two samples above those shown are diagnostic of GDM.

Adapted from ref. *17*.

Table 4
**Sensitivity and Specificity of the 1-h 50 g Screen
for Gestational Diabetes**

Threshold	*130 mg/dL*	*135 mg/dL*	*140 mg/dL*
Sensitivity	100%	98%	79%
Specificity	78%	80%	87%

From ref. *15*.

glucose concentrations above those indicated in Table 1 are diagnostic of GDM. During the course of the test, the patient must not be allowed to smoke and should remain seated. The person giving the test must note any factors that may influence the interpretation of the test results such as medications, inactivity, or infection *(3,12)*. Some have suggested carbohydrate loading (>150 g carbohydrate daily) in the 3 d prior to the test. The authors do not advise this course of action because it produces artificial testing conditions.

The ADA suggests two alternatives to the above OGTT format. First, a woman can be diagnosed as having GDM without an OGTT if on two sequential days her fasting plasma glucose concentration is above 126 mg/dL or casual plasma glucose concentration is above 200 mg/dL (for more information, refer to the "Fasting Plasma Glucose," section). Second, the ADA also allows for a 2 h, 75 g OGTT to be used with the same cutoff values as those used for the 100 g GCT. This alternate test may be used in place of the 100 g OGTT, but ADA considers the body of evidence supporting the 100 g test to be much more substantial *(15)*.

CHOOSING A GUIDELINE

The current lack of consensus means that the choice of guideline is left up to the individual clinician. There are many factors that must be taken into account when choosing a guideline, and that choice should be made with careful attention to the needs of the clinician's patient population. The two most critical factors are cost and test sensitivity.

Much of the current debate is centered on which guideline is the most cost effective. Testing every pregnant woman for GDM with a 3-h OGTT can be a large undertaking that gives few returns in a low-risk population. The ADA and NDDG try to lower those costs by using risk-factor testing. Risk-factor testing divides the patient population into three risk groups: low, average, and high. Patients are put into one of these three groups by virtue of their age, body mass index, ethnicity, obstetric history, and family history of diabetes (Table 2). Risk-factor testing attempts to lower the number of tests given by assuming that those in a low-risk group are at negligent risk. Depending on the patient population, around 20% of pregnant women would fall into this group *(16)*. A 1 h, 50 g GCT is also used to limit the number of 3-h, 100 g GCTs that are given to healthy women. This screen is given to women of average risk and is intended to identify women who are most likely have a high OGTT. It has the benefit of allowing a large number of people to be screened at relatively low cost and effort. Only those who have a 1-h plasma glucose value above the chosen threshold will be referred to the 3-h, OGTT *(17)*.

Risk-based testing and the 1-h, 50 g GCT help make the ADA and NDDG guideline tests less costly to administer. Most studies have confirmed this, but there is debate as to the amount of money that is saved by the ADA criteria. Lavin et al. looked at the direct costs per test, and average time spent was lower with the NDDG compared to the WHO criteria. His group saw that each test would cost $7.88 for the NDDG compared to $10.88 for the WHO. The average time in testing would be 1.5 h for the NDDG because the majority of women would not have to take the 3-h OGTT. The average time with the WHO criteria is 2 h because every woman will take the 2-h OGTT *(18)*. Poncet et al. found in a 2002 French cost analysis study that the ADA risk-based 50 g challenge and 100 g OGTT is more cost effective than the universal WHO 75 g OGTT when looking at total treatment costs (not just the cost of testing as above, but also the cost of treating those women the tests identify as having GDM). They found that the risk-based ADA guideline cost €5588.32 per case of macrosomia prevented, whereas the universal WHO guideline cost €5708.00 *(19)*. These two studies show that the WHO criteria are more expensive to administer ($2 per test) and manage (€119.68 per case of macrosomia prevented) compared to the ADA/NDDG criteria. The higher cost per case of macrosomia prevented with the WHO guideline is most likely the result of the decreased specificity of the WHO criteria to at-risk births because of its lower diagnostic values. This means that more women who are not at risk for obstetric complication are treated for GDM with the WHO guideline, and that decreases the cost benefits. Although a risk-based test with a 50 g glucose challenge is the most cost effective, Poncet et al. readily admit that the universal WHO guideline is more efficient at identifying GDM cases *(19)*.

The sensitivity of each guideline relies on three factors: universal vs risk-factor testing, diagnostic cutoff values, and the number of high readings necessary to diagnose GDM. Risk-factor testing was instigated by the ADA and NDDG guidelines to decrease the number of tests administered. Opting not to test those women considered to be of low risk can reduce the number of tests by 10 to 20%. This is beneficial as long as those in the low-risk group have a negligible prevalence of GDM. Numerous studies have shown that this is not the case. Moses et al. showed that GDM in a low-risk Australian population has a prevalence of 2.8% and makes up 8.7% of the total GDM population *(20)*. Coustan et al. looked at the GDM population in Southern California and found that 22% of patients were under 25 and had no risk factors *(16)*. Giffin et al. saw that risk-factor testing missed 11.4% of patients that were identified using a universal test in an Irish population *(9)*. Each of these studies found a sizable number of cases in a segment of the pregnant population considered to be at low risk. In each case, the prevalence is lower, but it is not negligible. Kitzmiller notes that many of these studies are finding a prevalence of 3% in the low-risk populations. Of great significance is that the same prevalence was thought to exist in the entire North American population 30 yr ago, and that prompted the initial drive for a GDM test in the pregnant population *(21)*. Risk-based testing would be prudent only if those with GDM in the low-risk group had better obstetric outcomes than those with GDM in the higher risk groups *(19)*.

The diagnostic cutoffs and number of high results needed to diagnose GDM differ between the guidelines as well. The WHO has the lowest cutoff values compared to the ADA and NDDG, whereas the NDDG values are the oldest and highest. The newer ADA values stand between the WHO and NDDG (Table 1). The lower values of the WHO are problematic for some clinicians because they label more women as having GDM, and a number of these women may be misdiagnosed. Misdiagnosis means that these women would have had normal births without diabetic treatment, and this increases their health care costs because they receive unnecessary GDM treatment. Additionally, it labels them as being high-risk for type II DM later in life. Another safety measure the ADA criteria uses to prevent misdiagnosis is the necessity of two high glucose values out the four samples in order to diagnose GDM. The WHO criteria require only one high sample in order to diagnosis GDM. The requirement of two high samples is an artificial constraint because any high blood glucose concentration can affect the fetus and should not be treated as an isolated event.

These two factors both play a part in making the WHO guideline more sensitive in the identification of pregnancies with adverse outcomes. Pettitt et al. found that in the Pima Indian population, the NDDG criteria identified only 18% of the cases of GDM that were reported by the WHO criteria. The addition of these cases in the Pima Indian study was beneficial because the WHO guideline identified 38% of the women with macrosomic infants while the NDDG identified only 6%. The WHO guideline also identified 57% of those who needed delivery via cesarean section, whereas the NDDG identified none *(11)*. Deerochanawong et al. found similar results. They noted that the GDM prevalence using the WHO criteria is 15.7% in a Thai population, whereas the prevalence with the NDDG criteria is 1.7%. The WHO guideline also identified 6 out of 14 macrosomic infants in the study population compared to the 3 out of 14 that the NDDG identified *(22)*. Poncet et al., in their cost analysis study, noted that the WHO guideline is more efficient than the new ADA guideline at identifying problem pregnancies. The largest decrease was in perinatal mortality: from 0.940 cases per 100 births with ADA guideline to 0.695 with the WHO *(18)*. In these studies, the WHO guideline identified the same macrosomia cases as the NDDG and ADA guidelines, but it also identified a significant number of cases that were not identified by the other guidelines.

The WHO guideline has other advantages. The 75 g load is more palatable than the 100 g, is only a one-step test, and is the same test that the women will take 6 wk postpartum for reclassification. In the study of the Pima Indian population by Pettitt et al., 31% of women with an abnormal 1-h test failed to appear for the 3-h 100 g OGTT *(11)*. Compliance with follow-up OGTT is a necessity because the screen is not considered to be diagnostic by the ADA. Besides this difficulty, the 50 g GCT has other problems in that it is only moderately reproducible. Sacks et al. found that a challenge with a 135-mg/dL threshold is inconsistent with 33% of cases *(23)*. The 1-h, 50 g glucose challenge test causes more problems than it fixes.

Simplicity of use and greater sensitivity make the WHO guideline an ideal choice as a GDM screen. Adoption of this guideline in the United States has been slow for two reasons: cost and clinician's comfort. Some physicians are not convinced that the cost of increased testing is worth the small number of obstetric complications prevented, and the clinicians are comfortable with the NDDG protocol they have used for years. Despite the difficulty in acceptance, a transition to the WHO criteria would be better for the overall health of the infant population because more at-risk women will be identified. Also, it is possible that the WHO guideline, combined with the intensified insulin therapy, will be more cost effective in the long term. This combination will find more women who are at risk for obstetric complications and reduce the number of cesarean sections for macrosomic infants through proper insulin therapy. Unfortunately, no study to date has added the price of the cesarean sections and long-term treatment of macrosomic infants resulting from misdiagnosis to the cost-analysis of diabetes screening. Thus, there are significant human and monetary expenses that merit consideration in both a cost analysis study and in the decision-making process.

Alternate Testing Methods

With all of the risks of diabetes to both the developing infant and the pregnant mother, an accurate screening method is necessary. Ideally, the test should be quick, efficient, and easy to administer. Currently, the most widely used guidelines all utilize some form of the OGTT, which has proven to be highly specific and sensitive in all populations. However, this test has proven to be time consuming and costly to health care providers and induces discomfort in patients. Because of these shortfalls, there has been a strong desire to find an accurate replacement for the OGTT using alternative methods of screening that would be more convenient to both the patient and the medical staff.

Fasting Plasma Glucose

One alternate method currently being considered is the fasting plasma glucose (FPG). Some clinicians propose expanding the use of FPG to be the chosen screening test. Because the FPG tends not to vary significantly during normal pregnancy, many scientists believe this could be a more efficient test that could be administered as early as the first trimester *(24)*.

An FPG screen requires that the patient fast for at least 8 h prior to the test. In order to confirm diabetes, the test must be repeated to give two different days with high fasting blood glucose values. The current ADA guidelines state that any FPG above 126 mg/dL is considered diabetes, whereas the normal glucose concentration for pregnant women is less than 105 mg/dL *(25)*. This cutoff is supported by the study of Coustan and Imarah, who showed in a study of 445 patients that the mean FPG concentration in pregnancy is 94 ± 16 mg/dL *(26)*. The European Association of Perinatal Medicine has established guidelines with a lower normal concentration of 95 mg/dL *(27)*. Many clinicians feel that a high cutoff value would be highly specific but fear that it may not be sensitive enough to diagnose all of the cases of carbohydrate intolerance. Therefore, there have been many studies to find cutoff values that maximize both sensitivity and specificity, but no consensus has been reached.

Sacks et al. *(24)* first proposed the usefulness of FPG. They concluded that the test was sensitive enough to detect diabetes but could not reach the sensitivity of the 50 g GCT. However, FPG did provide substantial savings in time to the patient and the medical staff. The research of Atilano et al. *(28)* provides additional support for the FPG. In their analysis of OGTT results, the FPG had a positive predictive value of 96%, and surprisingly, the researchers noted that women with elevated FPG concentrations were more likely to have insulin therapy (which clearly was not well managed). However, Shushan et al. *(29)* concluded that the FPG in the first trimester has no correlation with the result of the glucose challenge test in the second trimester, so they do not recommend testing in the first trimester.

One approach that is shared by many studies is to perform the 50 g GCT with both an FPG and a 1-h glucose determination. This FPG–1-h 50 g GCT combination would allow doctors to counteract one of FPGs deficiencies (inability to detect high postprandial blood glucose values) with the oral glucose challenge test, without taking hours to administer. Then, the main goal of FPG focuses merely on the reduction in the total number of OGTTs required. Agarwal et al. *(30)* proposed using FPG in a rule-in, rule-out system. Because universal screening with the GCT and OGTT is costly for health care systems, their research focused on determining cutoffs that could minimize the amount of OGTT testing needed. Using this strategy eliminates the need for 50.9% of the OGTT. However, they concluded that the FPG unfortunately does not detect those with impaired glucose tolerance or postprandial hyperglycemia. Alternatively, a Swiss study by Perucchini et al. *(31)* revealed that the FPG eliminated 70% of the required OGTTs and had a 22% higher sensitivity than that of the GCT using a cutoff of 140 mg/dL. They state that the advantages of the FPG are its independence of gestational age, lower variation between tests, and reproducibility. They advocate using a universal screen utilizing FPG during 24–28 wk gestation with a 75 g OGTT as a follow-up.

Kraemer et al. *(32)* determined that the Brazilian health care system could save $1.50 per test if an FPG cutoff of 93 mg/dL was used for testing. This value correlated best with the first and second hour of the OGTT. They believe that the FPG is easier and cheaper to use than the GCT and saves a significant amount of money in health costs. Reichelt et al. *(33)* concluded for the Brazilian Study of Gestational Diabetes Working Group that the FPG leads to results similar to those from the GCT. They found FPG to be advantageous because of its presence worldwide, its ease of use, its affordability, and its ability to be reproduced. An OGTT was used to confirm diabetes if the FPG was between 85 mg/dL and 126 mg/dL (Table 5).

On the basis of current literature, we conclude that an FPG–1-h 50 g GCT is the optimal screening and diagnostic tool for gestational diabetes.

RANDOM PLASMA GLUCOSE

Also called the casual plasma glucose, this test has the benefit of being administered any time of the day. Because no fasting must be done prior to this test, the cutoff concentrations are much higher. In pregnant women, the ADA recommends diagnosing diabetes when the random plasma glucose reaches a concentration of greater than 200 mg/dL *(25)*. If it is confirmed on the subsequent day, the patient is considered diabetic. However, an additional advantage of random plasma glucose is its positive correlation to capillary whole blood glucose. In a study by Carr et al. *(34)*, some point-of-care glucose instruments have enough precision and accuracy to be able to correlate with laboratory-measured plasma glucose concentrations. With this method, results could be achieved almost instantaneously. Therefore, a physician could diagnosis the patient within minutes. However, the diagnosis of diabetes cannot be done on the basis of one positive result. Confirmation must still be obtained by testing on the subsequent day. However, since random plasma glucose is most likely to miss many diabetic patients with a milder form of carbohydrate intolerance, it is not recommended as a screening method of GDM.

Table 5
Published Studies on the Use of Fasting Plasma Glucose

Name	Study	Cutoff	Sensitivity	Specificity
Sacks et al. (24)	US	88 mg/dL	80.0%	40.0%
		84 mg/dL	90.0%	21.0%
		81 mg/dL	95.0%	11.0%
Agarwal et al. (30)	UAE	>79 mg/dL[a]	94.7%	94.0%
		<95 mg/dL[a]		
Perucchini et al. (31)	Switzerland	86 mg/dL[a]	81.0%	76.0%
Kraemer et al. (32)	Brazil	93 mg/dL	81.3%	74.4%
Reichelt et al. (33)	Brazil	85 mg/dL	94.0%	66.0%
		89 mg/dL	88.0%	78.0%

[a]Values converted from mmol/L to mg/dL (1 mg/dL = 0.05551 mmol/L).

GLYCATED PROTEINS

There is much hope that tests of glycated proteins, such as hemoglobin A1C and fructosamine, which are indirect indicators of blood glucose concentrations, could be used to screen for GDM. Because the landmark Diabetes Control and Complications Trial (DCCT) showed the significance of glycated proteins and their correlation to blood glucose concentrations, their place in monitoring has already been established (35). Many physicians hope that this utility could be applied to screening as well. Because this test would not rely on the patient to fast or take any special precautions before coming to the doctor's office, the pretest procedure is less rigorous than that of the OGTT. Likewise, the same sample of blood drawn for FPG could be also used for these glycated protein tests. However, the approach of utilizing these proteins is hindered by the high cost of testing and some inherent deficiencies in the tests' assays.

A1C. Glycosylated hemoglobin has been a mainstay of glucose monitoring for decades. Measuring the amount of glycosylated hemoglobin proteins, which have a life span of 120 d, has proven to be an accurate indicator of the degree of glucose control for the preceding 2–3 mo. The percent of glycosylation is directly proportional to the amount of glucose present in the blood stream. However, there has been much confusion in past literature because results were measured as either hemoglobin A_1 or hemoglobin A1C. Furthermore, because there was no standardization between assays, test results were very unreliable and confusing. With the medical community's consensus on measuring solely hemoglobin A1C culminating in the institution of the National Glycohemoglobin Standardization Program, physicians have hoped that a cutoff percentage of glycated A1C could be established as a convenient screen for gestational diabetes.

Some studies have shown deficiencies even with the new standard of hemoglobin A1C Artal et al. (36) tested 82 women in their third trimester of pregnancy with hemoglobin A1C vs OGTT. Their goal was to find a percent hemoglobin A1C that had similar or better sensitivity than the GCT. These researchers found that there was a significant correlation between A1C and the 3-h OGTT. However, even using the best-established cutoff of 7%, the test did not detect all of the cases of GDM. Therefore, these researchers do not recommend using A1C for screening. Joshi and Bharadwaj (37) agree with this conclusion. With a cutoff of 6%, they found a positive predictive value of 0%. They acknowledged that A1C has a high specificity (92.9%), but in order to increase sensitivity, specificity decreased. If a cutoff of 5% was used, the specificity decreased to 65.7% while the sensitivity increased to 42%. Without a high correlation between the two tests, the study recommended against using A1C for screening. Agarwal et al. *(38)* applied the rule-in, rule-out criteria (<5% and >6.5%) to hemoglobin A1C in their study in the United Arab Emirates. While the sensitivity of their test was high, their criteria ruled in only 21% of their diabetic patients. They surmise that the A1C test is more sensitive than specific, which curbs its usefulness as a diagnostic test. Cefalu et al. *(39)* examined the feasibility of A1C as a screening test, but the A1C values proved too insensitive to detect GDM (Table 6).

In his commentary, Goldstein *(40)* argues that hemoglobin A1C testing would be more widespread if the costs of A1C were close to those of the FPG. He agrees that A1C has the benefit that samples can be drawn at any time of day. However, because FPG is currently less expensive to measure than A1C, it is currently more cost effective to use FPG to screen. Of note, at a recent American Association of Clinical Endocrinologists Consensus Conference, it was agreed that when hemoglobin A1C is abbreviated, the abbreviation will not have subscripts. Thus, by convention, the abbreviation should be A1C.

Fructosamine. The fructosamine assay uses the ketoamine reduction of nitroblue tetrazolium method to indirectly measure glycated serum proteins that have a half-life of 8–14 d. Unfortunately, the concentration of serum proteins varies diurnally *(41)*. The additional debate over fructosamine's place in screening considers its benefits and deficiencies. In the past, this assay was less expensive to perform than the hemoglobin A1C assay and it also had the benefits of standardization. However, with the standardization of A1C testing and new advances in diagnostic technology, the fructosamine test has been replaced by the more reliable hemoglobin A1C assay because fructosamine lacks the strong correlation with blood glucose concentration that hemoglobin A1C has. Even with serum protein correction, fructosamine lacks good correlation to other indices of control. Therefore, it does not appear as though fructosamine should be used to screen for GDM.

In the most recent study, Agarwal et al. *(38)* examined fructosamine in their study of 430 pregnant women in the United Arab Emirates. Using the rule-in, rule-out system, their cutoff values were less than 210 µmol/L and greater than 240 µmol/L. Unfortunately, this system led to a significant number of false-negatives. The researchers concluded that fructosamine is not specific enough to rule in diabetic patients and therefore should not be used as a screen. This study supported the idea by Comtois et al. *(42)*, who first questioned the notion of fructosamine screening for GDM. In a study of 100 pregnant women in Canada, the researchers found no significant differences between diabetic patients and normal controls. However, they concluded that the difference in the normal and diabetic population's fructosamine–protein ratio was less significant than their fasting serum glucose concentrations. Cefalu et al. *(39)* also believed that fructosamine had low sensitivity. The researchers confirmed that fructosamine lacks the sensitivity to be a screening test but had the potential for use in monitoring glycemic status during pregnancy because it clearly distinguished those with good and poor glycemic control.

Hofmann et al. *(43)* also examined fructosamine concentrations in pregnant women. Their study of 678 pregnant control subjects in Austria had a 95th percentile of 2.59 mmol/L. They concluded that fructosamine is not sensitive enough to detect people with

Table 6
Published Studies on the Use of Hemoglobin A1C to Screen
for Gestational Diabetes

Name	Study location	Cutoff	Sensitivity	Specificity
Artal et al. (36)	US	7.0%	69.0%	—
Joshi and Bharadwaj (37)	US	6.0%	0.0%	92.9%
		5.0%	42.0%	65.7%
Agarwal et al. (38)	UAE	<5.0%	92.1%	98.1%
		>6.5%		
Cefalu et al. (39)	US	5.2%	23.0%	86.9%

All studies indicate that hemoglobin A1C is not sensitive enough to be used to screen for GDM.

Table 7
Published Studies on the Use of Fructosamine to Screen for Gestational Diabetes

Name	Study location	Cutoff	Sensitivity	Specificity
Agarwal et al. (38)	UAE, cFRA	<210 umol/L	92.2%	76.0%
		>240 umol/L		
Comtois et al. (42)	Canada	2.54 mmol/L	18.0%	99.0%
Cefalu et al. (39)	US	2.48 mmol/L	15.4%	97.6%
Hofmann et al. (43)	Austria	2.59 mmol/L	—	—
Roberts et al. (44)	England	2.48 mmol/L	27.0%	90.0%
		2.52 mmol/L	7.0%	95.0%

All studies indicate that fructosamine is not a feasible method of screening for gestational diabetes.

impaired glucose tolerance, but can differentiate the severity of diabetes (those requiring insulin therapy have elevated concentrations). With this data, they concluded that fructosamine should not be used for screening in pregnancy.

Roberts et al. (44), pioneers of the fructosamine screening method, conducted a final study in 1990 to determine the viability of their fructosamine screen. Looking at 507 women, they used a cutoff at the 95th percentile (2.55 mmol/L). However, the GCT proved to be a better screen than serum fructosamine at both the 28- and 36-wk intervals. They concluded by saying that fructosamine is better suited for management and should not be used for screening, thus ending the debate (Table 7).

Combined Screening. Because the FPG tends to have high sensitivity but moderate specificity and the glycated proteins have high specificity but low sensitivity, there have been some studies that combined elements of both tests. The goal is to have a screening type that would prove to be less of a burden on the patient while still retaining the high accuracy that the OGTT maintains. However, the only studies published excluded pregnant women specifically.

In a study by Herdzik et al. *(45)*, the authors concluded that the best correlations were found between (1) fructosamine and the 2-h postprandial concentration of the OGTT and (2) the fasting capillary glucose (FCG) concentration and the percent hemoglobin A1C. The fructosamine and the FCG were the best tests to identify impaired glucose tolerance, because the FCG alone was not adequate to do so. Fructosamine could be used as an indicator of the high postload glucose concentrations in conjunction with the FCG normally used to monitor the fasting glucose concentrations. Having a test using all three protocols (fructosamine, A1C, and FCG) led to no improvements. They believed that the A1C test had high specificity but very low sensitivity in detecting diabetes. Their final conclusion recommended that the FCG still be used in conjunction with the OGTT because that was the highest correlation combination of any test.

Ko et al. *(46)* studied the use of FPG combined with either hemoglobin A1C or fructosamine in a study in Hong Kong. They concluded that FPG could not be used alone to screen for diabetes (mainly because it would miss those with abnormal postprandial states) but advocated using one of the glycated protein tests in conjunction. In their study, they reported that the fructosamine test was less sensitive when compared with hemoglobin A1C. Anyone with an incredibly high risk would be confirmed with an OGTT. Their values of FPG greater than 5.6 mmol/L and A1C greater than 5.5% were found to be five times more likely in the diabetic patient than in the normal one. Fructosamine (>235 μmol/L) could also be used, mainly because compared to A1C, it is less labor intensive, quicker, and less expensive to perform (Table 8).

GLYCOSURIA

Once considered the mainstay of GDM testing, urine testing for glucose has largely been replaced by blood glucose testing. Glycosuria is based on the principle that some blood glucose will filter into the urine once concentrations exceed the renal threshold. For normal healthy individuals, this threshold is 180 mg/dL. However, in pregnancy, the renal threshold normally decreases, so that glycosuria increases in prevalence and may not always be indicative of any carbohydrate intolerance. Because of the lack of solid correlation between blood and urine glucose, urine glucose has limited value as a screen.

Some studies have indicated that glycosuria is present in many normal pregnancies, so using this as a screening test would lead to poor specificity. Fine *(47)* reported that urine glucose is found in almost all pregnancies, with the reference interval about 1–15 mg/100 mL (with a mean of 7 mg/100 mL). He speculates that such a decrease in the renal threshold could be traced to increased concentrations of adrenocorticotropic hormone, which could cause impaired reabsorption of glucose. In addition, glycosuria tends to peak after food intake. In his study of 1547 patients in England, he found such a low incidence of diabetes (0.28%) that he could not justify universal glycosuria screening. Furthermore, Sutherland et al. *(48)* concluded that only a small percentage of pregnant women with glycosuria have abnormal glucose tolerance. In a study of 1418 patients in England, they report that a fasting glycosuria is more sensitive (15%) than a random glycosuria, which found zero cases. They recommend that any pregnant woman who has glycosuria undergo an OGTT because the presence of fasting glycosuria does not always reflect a high fasting blood glucose concentration or correlate with abnormal glucose tolerance. A study by Gribble et al. *(49)* concluded that elimination of glycosuria screening would have no significant impact. Other studies have reached the same conclusion. Lind and Anderson *(50)* concluded that relying on the appearance of glycosuria to refer OGTT

Table 8
Published Studies Regarding Combined Screening Methods to Detect Diabetes Mellitus

Name	Study	Cutoff values	Sensitivity	Specificity
Herdzik et al. (46)	FCG (in mmol/L)	>5.2	80.7%	80.2%
	or 0.02 × value	>5.5	71.1%	95.2%
	of fructosamine	>5.4	74.3%	93.5%
	(in μmol/L)			
Ko et al. (46)	A1C and FPG	5.5% A1C and	83.8%	83.6%
		100.8 mg/dL	81.5%	83.2%
	Fructosamine and	235 μmol/L		
	FPG	fructosamine		
		and 97.2 mg/dL		

FCG, fasting capillary glucose; FPG, fasting plasma glucose.

Table 9
Studies About Glycosuria

Name	Study	Time	Sensitivity	Specificity
Sutherland et al. (48)	UK	3rd trimester,	0.0% (fasting)	
		using dipsticks	15.0% (random)	—
Gribble et al. (49)	US	1st trimester,		
		using dipsticks	7.1%	98.5%
Lind and Anderson (50)	UK	3rd trimester,		
		using dipsticks	25.0%	—

could miss diabetic patients. When random blood glucose (abnormal result defined as above the 99th percentile) to screen for diabetes, none of the diabetic patients were missed, with 25 false-positives. However, only 25% of the diabetic patients would have been referred to an OGTT on the basis of glycosuria. Therefore, glycosuria does not prove to be a cost-effective screen (Table 9).

In addition, certain drugs can significantly affect dipstick measurements of urine glucose. As reported by Rotblatt et al. (51), the test strips used in urine analysis use the glucose oxidase enzyme. This enzyme can be affected by reducing agents such as ascorbic acid and salicylates to lead to a large number of false positive results and, hence, lower its effectiveness.

In summary, with the advent of more advanced diagnostic techniques, glycosuria should be phased out of screening for GDM.

MANAGEMENT OF DIABETES DURING PREGNANCY

Background

The management of diabetes during pregnancy is possible through the extensive and frequent use of clinical testing. In all cases of diabetes, preexisting or gestational, management differs only in when it begins. Patients with preexisting type 1 and type 2 DM must bring their blood glucose concentration into tight control before conception and continue that level of control throughout pregnancy. Any diabetic woman planning a pregnancy should consult with her physician prior to conception to limit the risk of congenital anomalies. Management of patients with GDM begins at the point of diagnosis with the same clinical laboratory targets as those for patients with type 1 and type 2 DM. In all cases, the continual rise in hormonal growth factors as the pregnancy progresses will make the woman increasingly resistant to insulin. Constant monitoring of the glycemic state through self-monitored blood glucose (SMBG) is required to follow the increasing insulin requirements, and treatment regimens must be adapted accordingly. Other clinical tests specific to diabetes, such as A1C and glucosamine, should be used as quality-control markers because they are a reflection of overall glucose control.

Blood Glucose

Glucose Target Values

Blood glucose is the single most important factor to monitor during a diabetic pregnancy because it has a profound effect on the health and development of the fetus. Excessive blood glucose concentrations during the first trimester can result in debilitating congenital anomalies, whereas increased blood glucose concentration during the third trimester exponentially raises the risk for macrosomia *(1)*. In order to reduce the risk of obstetric complications, blood glucose must be kept at concentrations as close to normal as possible. Optimal obstetric outcome will be achieved with the fasting blood glucose concentration below 90 mg/dL and the 1-h postprandial concentration below 120 mg/dL. These values are lower than those suggested by the ADA in 1996 (fasting, 105 mg/dL; 2 h postprandial, 120 mg/dL); however, numerous studies have shown that lower values can negate the risks for obstetric complications *(52–57)*. The lower postprandial concentrations also bring the fasting blood glucose concentrations down to the normal range seen in nondiabetic pregnant women (60–90 mg/dL). This range is lower than the normal fasting glucose range for a nongravid woman and is caused by the caloric draw from the developing fetus. This is an important factor to take into account when setting a fasting glucose target value *(1)* (Table 10).

Optimal obstetric outcome is achieved when the 1-h postprandial glucose concentration is less than 120 mg/dL. Combs et al. showed that moving the 120 mg/dL from 2 h to 1 h postprandial negated the risk for macrosomia (zero observed out of nine cases) and was accompanied by only a minimal risk for small for gestational age infants (one case observed) *(52)*. Hod et al. also reported that lower blood glucose targets decrease the rate of macrosomia to that of the control population. In his study, a FPG concentration of 105 mg/dL and a 2-h postprandial glucose concentration of 140 mg/dL had a 17.9% macrosomia rate. Lowering the target glucose concentrations to 95 mg/dL and 120 mg/dL further reduced the rate of macrosomia to 8.8%. This is comparable to the 6.1% macrosomia rate in the nondiabetic controls *(53)*. Langer et al. also demonstrated that women who keep their fasting blood glucose in the 96–105 mg/dL range are at increased risk for macrosomia. By applying active insulin treatment for those women with an FPG concentration of 96–105 mg/dL, he lowered the rate of macrosomia from 28.6% (diet-treated) to 10.3% (insulin-treated) *(54)*.

Glucose Testing

Laboratory Testing. Traditional laboratory testing for blood glucose is not the principal management method for a diabetic pregnancy because of the time and expense involved. The necessity of daily fasting and postprandial measurements means that most

Table 10
Blood Glucose Targets

Test	Fasting	1-h postprandial
Capillary blood Glucose	90 mg/dL	120 mg/dL

measurements will be done at home on small portable blood glucose meters. Clinical laboratory blood glucose testing is used only during GDM diagnosis and as a quality-control measure during obstetric consultations to verify the accuracy of the patient's own measurements.

The type of blood used in laboratory glucose analysis affects the glucose reading. Three different types are used in glucose analysis: serum, plasma, and whole blood. Ideally, samples for use by clinical laboratories should be either serum or plasma. The laboratory will dictate its recommended sample method. Most clinical laboratories use the hexokinase/glucose-6-phosphate dehydrogenase reaction. This test has become the standard for laboratory glucose testing because of its broad linearity (verified up to 600 mg/dL), low standard deviation between samples (2 mg/dL), and high glucose recovery (> 99.3% of glucose in solution). It is also relatively unaffected by anticoagulants and hemoglobin so plasma samples can be used. Plasma is a preferable sample because there is no delay waiting for blood samples to clot and more plasma than serum can be obtained from a single sample. Whole blood, like the finger-prick sample used in SMBG, is seldom used today in clinical laboratory glucose tests because its accuracy can be affected by variations in the hematocrit and is subject to contamination. If whole blood is used, it is important to remember that it gives a measurement that is 15% lower than a serum or plasma sample *(58)*. Because most guidelines are based on the plasma/serum values, it is important to take into account the type of blood used in the glucose measurement in order to accurately interpret the laboratory results.

Another important consideration to take into account when taking blood samples for clinical analysis is the amount of time that will pass between sampling and testing. Over time, glycolytic enzymes found in blood cells will decrease the glucose concentration in the sample. At room temperature, glycolysis can decrease serum glucose concentrations by approx 5 to 7% (5–10 mg/dL) per hour in uncentrifuged blood. In order to maintain clinical accuracy, any sample that is not going to be immediately analyzed should be collected into a tube containing a substance that inhibits glycolysis, such as sodium fluoride, and steps to minimize hemolysis should be taken. Separated serum and plasma samples can be stored in a refrigerator for up to 3 d. If a longer delay is necessary, the samples should be frozen *(58)*.

SMBG. SMGB utilizes small, automated blood glucose meters that allow the diabetic patient to monitor and manage his or her own diabetes treatment. This management technique is essential in a diabetic pregnancy because fluctuations in blood glucose concentrations have profound effects on obstetric outcome. Proper management requires the patient to test herself frequently during the day so that her insulin regimen can be regulated in order to achieve normal glycemia.

Modern SMGB instruments are quite simple to operate. A small amount of blood is obtained by pricking the patient's finger with a lancet. The blood is then applied to a disposable test strip. The glucose in the blood sample is oxidized enzymatically by glucose oxidase and is measured in one of two ways. In one method, the oxidation reaction produces a small electric current that is measured by an electrode embedded in the test strip. Alternatively, the oxidation reaction is coupled to a second reaction that produces a colored product. A reflectance meter measures the intensity of the produced color. In both methods, the electric current or color intensity is proportional to the amount of glucose present (59).

The amount of blood necessary to obtain a measurement differs according to the instrument used. Instruments using older technology need as much as 15 μL of blood in order to take a proper reading. This requires that samples be taken from easily accessible and well-vascularized tissues, such as the fingertips. Newer technologies have reduced the blood needed to make a measurement to as little as 0.3 μL. This means that less sensitive sites such as the forearm or thigh can be utilized to obtain a blood sample (60).

Numerous studies have attempted to correlate readings taken at alternate body sites to readings taken at the fingertips. These studies vary slightly in their findings. One shows no difference, whereas another finds that nonfingertip sites give values up to 7.9% lower than the fingertips (60–62). Most studies consider these differences to be of negligible significance, but care should still be used in the interpretation of results from alternate testing sites because capillary blood glucose readings from alternate testing sites are temporally delayed because compared to fingertip measurements. Ellison et al. showed that nonfingertip postprandial capillary blood glucose peaks 30 min later and at a slightly lower concentration compared to the fingertip capillary blood glucose. If the patient feels hypoglycemic, or if her blood glucose concentrations are changing rapidly, a fingertip should be used in order to get the most accurate view of the current glycemic state (63).

There are several sources of error in SMBG. The nonuser-dependent errors arrive from the meters and test strips. Several studies have shown portable blood glucose meters to be of varying accuracy. A study done by the College of American Pathologists in 1993 found that only 58 and 78% of meters were within 10 and 15% of the clinical laboratory results, respectively (64). Another study by Ryan et al. in 2001 showed similar results, with only 53% of measurements within 10% of their corresponding laboratory-measured reference interval. Twenty-six percent of measurements exceeded 20% variance (65). These studies are separated by 8 yr, and there has been very little progress in reducing measurement variation, despite a call in 1994 by the ADA to reduce SMBG analytical error to 5% (59).

There are many sources of analytical error. These include hematocrit, altitude, humidity, temperature, inaccuracy with extreme hyper/hypoglycemia, and user error. The hematocrit problem is amplified in pregnancy because capillary percent hematocrit falls below that of nongravid patients (65). This is more of an issue for reflectance meters because they can produce results that are 10 to 20% higher than normal when confronted with low hematocrit situations (66). The accuracy of some electrode meters does not appear to be affected as significantly by low hematocrit (only 3.5% variance), making them a better choice for use in pregnancy (67).

It is also important to remember that the finger prick sample used in SMBG is capillary whole blood and its value is 15% lower than that of a serum or plasma sample. Some portable blood glucose meters are calibrated to give a reading that corresponds to the plasma or serum value, whereas others do not. It is important to know how the patient's blood glucose meter reports results in order to make proper treatment decisions. Because of the importance of accurate SMBG in the management of a diabetic pregnancy, glucose meter selection should be made after a careful consideration of its variance from the reference laboratory test *(58)*.

Discrepancies between plasma glucose concentrations and SMBG-measured concentrations can be attributed to both accidental and intentional causes. Intentional misreporting arises because patients are afraid to report poor management to their doctors. Mazze et al. reported that 26% of the written logbook entries were different than the values recorded in the memory of the patient's glucose meter. When the patients were made aware of the memory capacity of the glucose meter, there was a significant increase in patient's logbook accuracy *(68)*. These results indicate that patients must understand that the purpose of a logbook is not to "grade" their performance, but to enable physicians to make adjustments in their treatment regimen in order to normalize glucose concentrations.

Despite the significant sources for error, SMBG is the only method for the daily management of diabetes. The potential for congenital anomalies and obstetric complications in a diabetic pregnancy means that each patient must perform daily testing individually. The best way to limit measurement error is by a thorough patient education system. Because much of the diabetes management comes from personally administered tests and treatments, patients must understand and learn how to properly perform SMBG. Patients need to feel that they are not alone in their struggle and that all the tools and resources necessary for their success are available to them. With the proper training and motivation, they will be able to give birth to a normal healthy child.

A1C

BACKGROUND

Glycosylated hemoglobin, or more specifically, the variant known as A1C, has long been a mainstay of glucose monitoring. On the basis of results of the Diabetes Control and Complications Trial (DCCT) *(34)* and the United Kingdom Prospective Diabetes Study (UKPDS) *(69)*, there is evidence directly linking an individual's percent hemoglobin A1C to his or her risk of long-term complications of diabetes. Hemoglobin A1C is defined by the International Federation of Clinical Chemistry (IFCC) as hemoglobin irreversibly glycated at one or both N-terminal valines of the α chain *(70)*. When the Schiff base is formed, an irreversible Amadori rearrangement will result in a glycated protein. Because the primary factor of glycosylation is the blood glucose concentration, the percent hemoglobin A1C is believed to reflect mean blood glucose concentrations over the previous 2–3 mo. However, it has been shown that percent hemoglobin A1C is a "weighted average," with the most recent month's blood glucose concentrations attributing 50% of the percent hemoglobin A1C's value *(71)*. Hemoglobin A1C percentages can change quickly if there is a sudden normalization of blood glucose concentrations *(72)*. In addition, trend analysis can be applied to percent hemoglobin A1C measurement to indicate the effectiveness of a given treatment. A constant decrease could take just 3 wk to be statistically significant, instead of 2 to 3 mo *(73)*. Thus, measuring the percent hemoglobin A1C every 2 to 3 wk and comparing it to the patient's own previous result can be used to verify the glucose concentrations recorded by the self-blood glucose testing *(74)*.

Table 11
Reference Intervals for Percent Glycated Hemoglobin A1C

Normal, nonpregnant range	Normal, pregnant range	Abnormal range for pregnancy
4.0–6.0%[a]	4.0–5.0%[b]	>5.0%[b]

[a]Ref. *35.*
[b]Ref. *39.*

USE IN PREGNANCY

In pregnancy, there is an overall decrease in percent hemoglobin A1C. In a study by Gunton and McElduff, pregnant women have a mean glycated hemoglobin A1C of 4.5 ± 1.3% whereas nonpregnant women had a mean glycated hemoglobin A1C of 7.6 ± 2.4% (Table 11). There are many theories to explain this phenomenon. One study proposes that pregnancy is associated with lower blood glucose and higher lactate dehydrogenase concentrations, which results in less glycosylation *(75).* The consensus is that there is a decline in basal glucose concentrations in pregnancy *(76–78).* In addition, the rate of erythrocyte formation increases in pregnancy. Therefore, the overall volume of erythrocytes is increased, making the proportion of glycosylated hemoglobin smaller *(74).* In normal pregnancy, the percent of glycosylated hemoglobin is decreased from the 11–14 wk value until reaching its lowest point at 23–26 wk before returning to the baseline at 31–34 wk gestation *(79).*

RISKS

Maternal hyperglycemia is associated with congenital malformations and other risks of fetal distress. If the percent hemoglobin A1C is greater than 2 standard deviations (SD) above the mean, the relative risk of major malformations increases *(80).* This supports the ADA's recommendation for diabetic women planning to become pregnant to achieve an A1C value within 3 SD of the mean *(81).* A study of insulin-dependent diabetic pregnancies showed that those mothers with smaller sized fetuses all had higher percent glycated A1C *(82).* This suggested that poor glycemic control, especially in the early stages of pregnancy, would lead to early fetal growth delay and thereby increase the risk of malformation. A study by Rosenn et al. *(83)* showed that mothers with glycated hemoglobin A1 higher than 12–13% (equivalent first-trimester blood glucose concentration of 120–130 mg/dL) were at an increased risk of abortion and malformation (Table 11).

STANDARDIZATION

There are some problems with the A1C measurement that question its reliability. Multiple assays are used, which requires some form of standardization to relate their results to each other. The National Glycohemoglobin Standardization Program (NGSP) requires that assay results be aligned with the results of the DCCT and the UKPDS studies *(84).* Current calibration material often fails because of matrix effects *(84,85).* By using fresh (<1-wk-old) blood from the central laboratory of the NGSP, these effects can be minimized and the machines can be uniformly calibrated *(84).* Capillary blood samples can be mailed without a loss in accuracy or stability *(86).*

PHYSIOLOGICAL FACTORS

Many abnormalities in hemoglobin status have been shown to alter percent glycated hemoglobin to A1C. Therefore, it is necessary to obtain a clinical history of any hemoglobinopathies, alternations in red blood cell turnover, or conditions favoring the chemical modification of hemoglobin *(70)*. The effect of hemoglobin variants is method dependent *(87)*. It is known that hemolytic anemia, chronic blood loss, splenectomy, and renal dialysis will affect percent of glycated hemoglobin A1C by altering hemoglobin concentrations *(88)*. Therefore, correcting for serum hemoglobin concentration is recommended.

ASSAYS

Cation-Exchange High-Performance Liquid Chromatography. This assay separates hemoglobin based on charge differences. N-terminal glycation of α- or β-chains will change the pK_a of the amino group of the valine *(89)*. Hemoglobin species elute from the cation-exchange column at different times with the application of buffers that have increasing ionic strength *(70)*. It is susceptible to hemoglobinopathies, but its long-term stability (CV of 1.2% and 1.7% over 8 yr) lead to its selection as the standard assay for the NGSP *(84,85)*. In addition, although some hemoglobin variants can alter results, the chromatogram will indicate the presence of variants *(87)*. However, the system is not specific for A1C and will tend to include α/β dimers, mono- and multiple-glycated hemoglobin, carbamylated hemoglobin, and acetylated hemoglobin *(90)*. Likewise, urea reacts with hemoglobin at the same site as glucose. Therefore, the isoelectric point of carbamylated hemoglobin is similar to A1C and will coelute to lead to falsely high percentages *(91)*. The percent A1C for high-performance liquid chromatography (HPLC) methods is measured as A1C to total A_0, not total hemoglobin *(92)* (Table 12).

Boronate Affinity Chromatography. This assay depends on the binding of the sugar groups on the hemoglobin molecule *(92)*. *M*-aminophenylboronic acid reacts with the *cis*-diol groups of glucose bound to hemoglobin to form a reversible five-member ring complex. This complex can be eluted and measured quantitatively. This method is used by more than 50% of the laboratories surveyed by the College of American Pathologists in 1999 *(70)*. This assay is not affected by pH, temperature, or hemoglobin variants *(93)*. Therefore, the results have clinically reasonable ranges for all hemoglobin variants *(87)*. However, this method measures total glycated hemoglobin, not A1C specifically, so percent A1C is estimated *(70,93)*. In addition, the results are usually higher than the results from the HPLC *(70)* (Table 12).

Immunoassays. Immunoassays rely on an antibody against glycosylated hemoglobin A1C *(93)*. They depend on the presence of an epitope that includes glucose and N-terminal amino acids of the β chain of hemoglobin *(92)*. They are known to be unaffected by the most common hemoglobin variants, except those with alternations at the N-terminal amino acids *(70)*. Unlike HPLC, however, there is no recognition of hemoglobin variants in the event they are present *(87,92)*. However, immunoassays are run on testing machines portable enough that they can be in the doctor's office to receive results in minutes *(93)*. These assays report percent A1C as A1C to total hemoglobin *(92)* (Table 12). Because of its accuracy, portability, and ease of use, the immunoassay method of measuring A1C values is strongly recommended.

Electrophoresis. Electrophoresis also separates hemoglobin molecules by charge. It is used infrequently, mainly because of its susceptibility to hemoglobin variants *(70)*.

Table 12
Summary of Hemoglobin A1C Assays

Assay	Summary	Advantages	Disadvantages
Ion-exchange HPLC	Separates by charge	Method used in the DCCT trial; low CV in long-term studies	Affected by common and rare hemoglobin variants (sometimes listed)
Boronate Affinity	Separates by structure	Fully automated; not affected by any hemoglobin variants	Measures total glycosylated hemoglobin, not A1C, so it tends to underestimate
Immunoassay	Separates by affinity for antibody structure	Not affected by common hemoglobin variants; portable	Higher CV when compared to other methods; will not identify interferences
Electrophoresis	Separates by charge	Older method that is cheap to run	Affected by hemoglobin variants; not automated
Mass Spectrometry	Separates by mass/charge ratio	Fully automated; not affected by hemoglobin variants; low coefficient of variance	Needs large amount of expertise; high initial cost; lower reference ranges

When urea concentrations are approx 15–30 mmol/L, the presence of carbamylated hemoglobin (1–2%) is sufficient to elevate percent A1C in this assay (85). With other more sophisticated assays available, this assay is not recommended (Table 12).

Mass Spectrometry. Pursued by the International Federation of Clinical Chemistry, mass spectrometry relies on a separation of ions based on their mass-to-charge ratio (70). It is being developed to replace the HPLC method because of its low CV (1–2%) (94). Mass spectrometry would require only the measurement of four peaks (α and β chains, and glycated α and β chains) (95). This method would measure total glycoslyation of hemoglobin, not just the terminal valines of the α chain. This method is attractive because it is not affected by hemoglobin variants and in fact is currently used to identify such variants (70). The equipment cost is prohibitively high, but the reagent cost is comparable to current methodologies (95). However, the large amount of technical expertise to operate and the high cost of acquiring the equipment make it unappealing to most clinical laboratories (96). In addition, using results from mass spectrometry would require adjusting the target values and the reference intervals because this assay has results lower than those of the DCCT (85). Clearly, there needs to be an evaluation of long-term stability before it could be considered for replacing the HPLC standard in the NGSP (84) (Table 12).

Table 13
Reference Intervals for Glycosylated Proteins

Test	Normal, nonpregnant range	Normal, pregnant range	Abnormal range for pregnancy
Fructosamine (uncorrected)	2.0–2.7 mmol/L[a]	2.06–2.62 mmol/L[b,d]	> 2.62 mmol/L[b]
Glycosylated Plasma Proteins	17.0–23.6%[c]	19.64–25.56%[c]	>23%[c]

[a]Ref. *41.*
[b]Ref. *99.*
[c]Ref. *101.*
[d]range given as mean ± 2SD.

Fructosamine

BACKGROUND

The fructosamine assay has often been used as an alternative to percent A1C monitoring because of its shorter half-life (2–3 wk compared to A1C's 2–3 mo) and its insensitivity to hemoglobinopathies *(75,93)*. Fructosamine acts like a memory and reflects nonenzymatic protein glycosylation *(42)*. Therefore, it can be used to reflect the blood glucose concentrations in the last 2–3 wk. There is little day-to-day variation, and the test can be performed without any patient preparation *(97)*. The assay is based on the ketoamine's ability to reduce nitroblue tetrazolium at an alkaline pH *(98)*. It should be measured every 2–3 wk, because the serum protein's life span is equivalent to that time period. Fructosamine concentrations are averages that are weighted according to the past week. It has relative stability at different times of the day and from one day to the next. In a normal pregnant population, the concentration of fructosamine was found to be 2.34 ± 0.14 mmol/L *(99)*. Serum total protein and albumin concentrations fall after the first trimester of pregnancy and may contribute to the 6.1% reduction. This change leads to significant differences found among the first-, second-, and third-trimester concentrations *(100)* (Table 13). However, after the first-trimester, values do not change with increasing gestation *(17,79)*. Normally, the assay is measured at 2-wk intervals in pregnancy *(38)*.

USE IN PREGNANCY

Fructosamine's usefulness in pregnancy is debatable. Roberts et al. conclude that GDM patients with normal fructosamine by 35–37 wk gestation had babies that were smaller and less obese than those with abnormal values. These babies also had lower cord insulin and C-peptide concentrations *(99)*. Another study showed that there is a higher risk of miscarriage with higher concentrations of fructosamine *(97)*. Schrader et al. showed that using a combination of more than 23% glycosylated plasma proteins and a FPG greater than 90 mg/dL was 100% sensitive in detecting macrosomia *(101)*. However, a study by Ghosh et al. found no correlation between glycated serum proteins and the birth weight *(102)*. Without a clear consensus, fructosamine should not be the primary test used to monitor glycemic status in diabetic pregnancies.

INTERFERENCES

The fructosamine assay is a reduction reaction; thus, antioxidants have the potential to interfere with this method. Not surprisingly, high concentrations of vitamin C have been known to affect results. In addition, because the assay requires a specific pH of 10.35 (maintained with a carbonate buffer), it is very sensitive to pH and must be carefully maintained at that pH *(40)*. Low albumin concentrations are known to interfere with the assay, but only if the serum albumin concentration is less than 38 g/L *(103)*. There is also some interference from maternal hypertriglyceridemia when there is gross maternal obesity *(100)*. Lastly, there are some problems with standardization that has led to much debate on the merits of correcting for proteins.

Correcting for albumin has been shown to improve the predictive power of fructosamine, but correcting for total proteins has not *(104)*. Corrected fructosamine has higher correlation with other glycemic indices than uncorrected values *(98)*. Therefore, laboratories should indicate whether results have been corrected (the corrected value tends to be lower than the uncorrected). Correcting comes with increased cost, but the increase in accuracy is important to the patient.

24-H Urine Protein Testing

BACKGROUND

One consequence of prolonged diabetes is nephropathy, which can lead to end stage renal failure. In pregnancies complicated with diabetes, the consequences of nephropathy are greater because of the additional risk to the infant. Kidney trouble can also be a sign of preeclympsia, which endangers the life of the mother and the unborn child. An easily detectible symptom of both kidney disorders is proteinuria. The prevalence of proteinuria varies among ethnic groups. However, patients with high blood pressure and a family history of diabetes have a greater risk *(105)*.

DIAGNOSIS

Because nephropathy is a chronic symptom of diabetes, it is important that urine protein monitoring be initiated during prenatal planning, if possible, or at least at the first visit to the obstetrician, in order to establish baseline. For those patients with preexisting diabetes, testing should be performed every trimester unless an abnormal result warrants closer attention. Those with type 1 DM are at a higher risk, because the possibility of previously uncontrolled hyperglycemia cannot be ruled out.

There are three tests for proteinuria that measure three different analytes: albumin, total protein, and creatinine clearance. Microalbuminuria, a misnomer, does not describe small protein, but finding minute amounts of albumin in the urine. Normally, the kidney does not filter protein, but with kidney damage, these serum proteins can leak through. In order to make a diagnosis for microalbuminuria, urinary albumin excretion rates must be between 30 and 300 mg/24 h in a 24-h collection *(106)*. Because albumin follows a circadian rhythm, excretion rates during the day are variable, and it is imperative that 24-h urine samples be collected *(107,108)*. For normal healthy pregnancies, albumin concentrations in the urine should not exceed 30 mg/dL *(109)* (Table 14). Furthermore, total protein concentrations can also be determined from the same sample used to test for microalbuminuria. Another measurement is a test of the "cleaning power of the kidney," or the creatinine clearance. In pregnancies, the creatinine clearance in 24 h is approx 100–150 mg/min *(110)*. It remains constant during the last quarter of pregnancy *(111)*. Crea-

Table 14
Reference Intervals for Urine Microalbumin, Creatinine, and Total Protein

Test	Normal, nonpregnant range	Normal, pregnant range	Abnormal range for pregnancy
Microalbumin	Equal or <30 mg/24 h	Equal or <30 mg/24 h	> 30 mg/24 h
Creatinine	75–115 mL/min	100–150 mL/min[b]	< 90 mL/min[b]
Total protein	<138 mg/24 h	<138 mg/24 h	>260 mg/24 h[a]

[a]Ref. 107.
[b]Ref. 110.

$$\text{Creatinine clearance} = \frac{[\text{Creatinine}_{urine}]}{[\text{Creatinine}_{plasma}]} \times \text{Urine Volume (24 hours)}$$

Fig. 1. Creatinine clearance measures concentration of creatinine in the blood vs amount in the urine.

tinine clearance measures the concentration of creatinine in the blood vs the amount in the urine (Fig. 1). Therefore, a blood sample is needed to calculate clearance concentrations of creatinine in the blood, which usually does not vary in pregnancy.

TESTING

In-office testing using the dipstick method is not recommended because it uses a qualitative measuring system with low sensitivity (109,112). It is recommended that urine samples be collected and tested using more quantitative methods, either with point-of-care instruments or sent to the laboratory. Because collecting a 24-h sample of urine is a rather tedious task, it is suggested that all three tests be ordered at once, in order to avoid having the patient undergo multiple collections.

Importance of Thyroid Testing

The normal changes in thyroid function that occur during pregnancy are discussed in detail in Chapter 8. GDM, type 2 diabetic, and normal pregnant women have no significant differences in thyroid-stimulating hormone (TSH) and FT4 concentrations (113). However, up to 50% of type 1 diabetic pregnancies have abnormal thyroid function. This dysfunction is usually attributed to the autoimmune disorder that is present in patients with type I diabetes. The risk is increased if proteinuria is also present, because thyroid-binding globulin is lost to the urine (114). With lower concentrations of thyroid binding globulin, these women lose a significant amount of their reserve T_4 (115). When concentrations of T_4 fall, the pituitary will attempt to compensate by increasing the concentration of TSH in the blood. Therefore, monitoring TSH concentrations in the diabetic patient will indicate any thyroid imbalance. Refer to Chapter 8 for symptoms, risks, diagnosis, and treatment of the thyroid.

β-*Hydroxybutyrate*

Ketones are an alternate fuel source and increase in the body as a response to low insulin concentrations. They are intended delay the effects of starvation, but high concentrations of ketones put the body into states of ketoacidosis and ketosis that further complicate the body's metabolic state. There are two main ketone bodies: β-hydroxybutyrate (β-OHB) and acetoacetate. β-OHB is the ketone that should be followed during ketoacidosis because it is the most dynamic and abundant. During ketoacidosis, concentrations of β-OHB raise from parity to 10 times the concentration of acetoacetate *(116)*. Once therapy begins, β-OHB concentrations are the first fall as the β-OHB is converted in to acetoacetate *(117)*. Several quantitative tests specific to β-OHB are currently available and require only finger stick blood or urine samples. Urine and blood tests using the nitroprusside reaction should not be used because they are specific for acetoacetate *(116)* and are susceptible to positive interference by a number of endogenous substances *(118)*.

Testing for β-OHB is performed in order to monitor the progress of ketosis and distinguish it from simple hyperglycemia. It should be measured when glucose concentrations are greater than 270 mg/dL. Few studies have been made to determine the reference intervals for β-OHB. Wallace et al. published a guideline correlating β-OHB values to ketosis risk. Their study found that those with a β-OHB concentration below 1 mM/L have no risk for ketosis and need to be treated only for the hyperglycemia. Patients with β-OHB concentrations between 1 and 3 m*M*/L are at moderate risk and should be tested again after 1 h. Any concentration above 3 m*M*/L necessitates immediate medical treatment for ketosis (Table 15). Once effective treatment is initiated, β-OHB concentrations should fall at a rate of approximately 1 m*M*/L per hour *(117)*.

There is some question over the necessity of incorporating regular β-OHB testing into the management of a diabetic pregnancy. Experimental findings in rat models suggest that the ketones might be involved in congenital anomalies *(119–121)*. The direct effect of β-OHB on a diabetic pregnancy is difficult to determine because it is just one of the potentially teratogenic substances that are elevated in diabetes *(122,123)*. The most extensive study of the connection between β-OHB and obstetric outcome in humans is the Diabetes in Early Pregnancy Study (DIEP). This study showed no significant difference between the β-OHB concentrations in pregnancies that resulted in good obstetric outcomes and those that resulted in stillbirths or congenital anomalies. In fact, there was a slight decrease in the β-OHB concentrations of women with malformed infants. The DIEP study also demonstrated a positive correlation between β-OHB concentrations and glucose concentrations in diabetic mothers, and a negative correlation during week 6 in nondiabetic mothers. The reason for this is unclear and may be because of the degree of glycemic control in diabetic patients. Higher glucose concentrations reflect insufficient insulin in type I diabetic patients, and increased fat oxidation occurs as a result. The negative correlation in the nondiabetic mothers may be caused by sporadic eating patterns of pregnant women in the first trimester.

Most of the women in the DIEP study maintained near-normal glycemia throughout the pregnancy. As a result, the highest concentrations of β-OHB in the diabetic group were 20- to 40-fold lower than the β-OHB concentrations that induced congenital anomalies in rats *(124)*. Rat models produced moderate congenital anomalies at 10 m*M*/L *(121)*, whereas while the highest average β-OHB concentrations in the DIEP diabetic women was 0.32 m*M*/L *(124)*. The good diabetic control maintained in the DIEP study kept β-OHB and glucose concentrations down, thereby preventing any congenital anomalies.

Table 15
Correlation of β-OHB Concentrations With Risk for Ketosis

β-OHB Concentration	< 1 mM/L	> 1 mM/L and <3 mM/L	>3 mM/L
Ketosis risk	Low	Moderate	High
Treatment	Treat hyperglycemia	Treat hyperglycemia; repeat test in 1 h	Immediate ketosis treatment

[a]Measure ketones if glucose > 270 mg/dL. (Modified from ref. *117*.)

β-OHB concentrations should not be a concern during a well-managed diabetic pregnancy because β-OHB concentrations are directly related to and follow glucose concentrations. Direct β-OHB testing is unnecessary because it is merely a reflection of overall glucose control. Both SBGM and A1C serve equally well in that capacity and should already be used in the management a diabetic pregnancy. Through those tests and proper insulin treatment, the risk for malformation will be normalized *(123,124)*. Direct testing for β-OHB is necessary only in cases of severe hyperglycemia (blood glucose >270 mg/dL) in order to monitor the progress of ketoacidosis.

ACKNOWLEDGMENTS

The authors would like to thank Dr. Albert Svoboda for his advisory role in this project, Ms. Lucy Thomas and the library staff at Santa Barbara Cottage Hospital for their assistance, and the Coeta and Donald R. Barker Foundation Grant to The Sansum Medical Research Institute.

REFERENCES

1. Jovanovic L. Insulin therapy in pregnancy. In: Laehy JL, Cefalu WT, ed. Insulin Therapy. New York: Marcel Dekker, 2002:139–151.
2. Vääräsmäki M, Gissler M, Ritvanen A, Hartikainen A-L. Congenital anomalies and first life year surveillance in type 1 diabetic births. Diabet Med 2002;19:589–593.
3. Metzger BE, Coustan DR. Summary and recommendations of the fourth international workshop-conference on Gestational Diabetes Mellitus. Diabetes Care. 1998;21:B161–B167.
4. Ylinen K, Aula P, Stenman U-H, Kesäniemi-Koukkanen T, Teramo K. Risk of minor and major fetal malformations in diabetics with high haemoglobin A_{1C} values in early pregnancy. Br Med J 1984;289:345–346.
5. Miller E, Hare J, Cloherty J, Dunn P. Elevated maternal hemoglobin A_{1C} in early pregnancy and major congenital anomalies in infants of diabetic mothers. N Eng J Med 1981;304:1331–1334.
6. Reece EA, Homko C. Why do diabetic women deliver malformed infants? Clin Obstet Gynecol 2000;43:132–145.
7. Uvena-Celebrezze J, Catalano P. The infants of the women with gestational diabetes mellitus. Clin Obstet Gynecol 2000;43:127–139.
8. Howorka K, Pumprla J, Gabriel M, et al. Normalization of pregnancy outcome in pregestational diabetes through functional insulin treatment and modular out-patient education adapted for pregnancy. Diabet Med 2001;18:965–972.
9. Giffin ME, Coffey M, Johnson H. Universal vs. risk factor-based screening for gestational diabetes mellitus: detection rates, gestation at diagnosis and outcome. Diabet Med 2000;17:26–32.

10. Vogel N, Burnand B, Vial Y, Ruiz J, Paccaud F, Hohlfeld P. Screening for gestational diabetes: variation in guidelines. Eur J Ob Gyn Reprod Bio 2000;91:29–36.

11. Pettitt DJ, Bennett PH, Hanson RL, Narayan KMV, Knowler WC. Comparison of World Health Organization and National Diabetes Data Group procedures to detect abnormalities of glucose tolerance during pregnancy. Diabetes Care 1994;17:1264–1268.

11a. Jovanovic L, Pettitt D. Gestational diabetes mellitus. JAMA 2001;289:2516–2518.

12. WHO Consultation. Definition, diagnosis and classification of diabetes mellitus and its complications: report of a WHO consultation. Part 1: Diagnosis and classification of diabetes mellitus. WHO/NCD/NCS/99.2. Geneva: World Health Organization, 1999.

13. O'Sullivan JB, Mahan CM, Charles D. Screening criteria for high-risk gestational diabetic patients. Am J Obstet Gynecol 1973;116:895–900.

14. National Diabetes Data Group. Classification and diagnosis of diabetes mellitus and other categories of glucose intolerance. Diabetes 1979;28:1039–1057.

15. Carr SR. Screening for gestational diabetes mellitus: a perspective in 1998. Diabetes Care 1998;21 (suppl 2):B14–B18.

16. Coustan DR, Nelson C, Carpenter MW. Maternal age and screening for gestational diabetes: a population based study. Obstet Gynecol 1989;73:557–560.

17. ADA. Gestational diabetes mellitus. Diabetes Care 2000;23(suppl 1):S77–S79.

18. Lavin JP Jr, Lavin B, O'Donnell N. A comparison of costs and reimbursement associated with screening for gestational diabetes utilizing the National Diabetes Data Group (NDDG) or the World Health Organization (WHO) techniques. Obstet Gynecol 1999;93(suppl):72S.

19. Poncet B, Touzet S, Rocher L. Cost-effectiveness analysis of gestational diabetes mellitus screening in France. Eur J Obstet Gyn Reprod Bio 2002;103:122–129.

20. Moses RG, Moses J, Davis WS. Gestational diabetes: do lean young Caucasian women need to be tested? Diabetes Care 1998;21:1803–1806.

21. Kitzmiller JL. Cost analysis of diagnosis and treatment of gestational diabetes mellitus. Clin Ob Gyn 2000;43:140–153.

22. Deerochanawong, Putiyanun C, Wongsuryrat M. Comparison of National Diabetes Data Group and World Health Organization criteria for detecting gestational diabetes mellitus. Diabetologia 1996;39:1070–1073.

23. Sacks DA, Abu-Fadil S, Greenspoon JS. How reliable is the fifty-gram, one-hour glucose screening test? Am J Obstet Gynecol 1989;161:642–645.

24. Sacks DA, Greenspoon JS, Fotheringham N. Could the fasting plasma glucose assay be used to screen for gestational diabetes? J Reprod Med 1992;37:907–909.

25. The Expert Committee on the Diagnosis and Classification of Diabetes Mellitus. Report of the expert committee on the diagnosis and classification of diabetes mellitus. Diabetes Care 2002;25(suppl 1): S5–S20.

26. Coustan DR, Imarah J. Prophylactic insulin treatment of gestational diabetes reduces the incidence of macrosomia, operative delivery, and birth trauma. Am J Obstet Gynecol 1984;150:836–842.

27. European Association of Perinatal Medicine—Working Group on Diabetes and Pregnancy. Diabetes and Pregnancy, Update and Guidelines. European Association of Perinatal Medicine, 2002.

28. Atilano LC, Lee-Parritz A, Lieberman E, Cohen AP, Barbieri RL. Alternative methods of diagnosing gestational diabetes. Am J Obstet Gynecol 1999;181:1158–1161.

29. Shushan A, Samueloff A. Correlation between fasting glucose in the first trimester and glucose challenge test in the second. obstet gynecol. 1998;91:596–599.

30. Agarwal MM, Hughes PF, Punnose J, Ezimokhai M. Fasting plasma glucose as a screening test for gestational diabetes in a multi-ethnic, high-risk population. Diabet Med 200;17:720–726.

31. Perucchini D, Fischer U, Spinas GA. Using fasting plasma glucose concentrations to screen for gestational diabetes mellitus: prospective population based study. Br Med J 1999;319:812–815.

32. Kraemer de Aguiar LG, Jose de Matos H, de Brito Gomes M. Could fasting plasma glucose be used for screening high-risk outpatients for gestational diabetes mellitus? Diabetes Care 2001;24:954–955.

33. Reichelt AJ, Spichler ER, Branchtein L. Fasting plasma glucose is a useful test for the detection of gestational diabetes. Diabetes Care 1998;21:1246–1249.

34. Carr SR, Slocum J, Tefft L. Precision of office-based blood glucose meters in screening for gestational diabetes. Am J Obstet Gynecol 1995;173:1267–1272.

35. The Diabetes Control and Complications Trial Research Group. The effect of intensive treatment of diabetes on the development and progression of long term complications in the diabetes control in insulin dependent diabetes mellitus. N Engl J Med 1993;329:977–986.

36. Artal R, Mosley GM, Dorey FJ. Glycohemoglobin as a screening test for gestational diabetes. Am J Obstet Gynecol 1984;146:412–414.

37. Joshi R, Bharadwaj A. Gestational diabetes screening: can hemoglobin A1C measurement replace the glucose challenge test? Am J Obstet Gynecol 2002;99(suppl.):93S.

38. Agarwal MM, Hughes PF, Punnose J. Gestational diabetes screening of a multiethnic, high-risk population using glycated proteins. Diabetes Res Clin Pract 2001;51:67–73.

39. Cefalu WT, Prather KL, Chester DL. Total serum glycosylated proteins in detection and monitoring of gestational diabetes. Diabetes Care 1990;13:872–875.

40. Goldstein DE. Glycohemoglobin testing in patients with diabetes: it may be underutilized now, but that is certain to change. Diabetes Tech 1999;1:421–423.

41. Baker J, Johnson RN. Response to Baines. Br Med J 1985;291:1050.

42. Comtois R, Desjarlais F, Nguyen M. Clinical usefulness of estimation of serum fructosamine concentration as screening test for gestational diabetes. Am J Obstet Gynecol 1989;160:651–654.

43. Hofmann HM, Weiss PA, Pürstner P. Serum fructosamine and amniotic fluid insulin levels in patients with gestational diabetes and healthy control subjects. Am J Obstet Gynecol 1990;162:1174–1177.

44. Roberts AB, Baker JR, Metcalf P, Mullard C. Fructosamine compared with a glucose load as a screening test for gestational diabetes. Obstet Gynecol 1990;76:773–775.

45. Herdzik E, Safranow K, Ciechanowski K. Diagnostic value of fasting capillary glucose, fructosamine and glycosylated hemoglobin in detecting diabetes and other glucose tolerance abnormalities compared to oral glucose tolerance test. Acta Diabetol 2002;39:15–22.

46. Ko GT, Chan JC, Yeung VT. Combined use of a fasting plasma glucose concentration and Hb A1C or fructosamine predicts the likelihood of having diabetes in high risk subjects. Diabetes Care 1998;21:1221–1225.

47. Fine J. Glycosuria of pregnancy. Br Med J 1967;8:205–210.

48. Sutherland HW, Stowers JM, McKenzie C. Simplifying the clinical problem of glycosuria in pregnancy. Lancet 1970;1:1069–1071.

49. Gribble RK, Meier PR, Berg RL. The value of urine screening for glucose at each prenatal visit. Obstet Gynecol 1995;86:405–410.

50. Lind T, Anderson J. Does random blood glucose sampling outdate testing for glycosuria in the detection of diabetes during pregnancy? Br Med J 1984;289:1569–1571.

51. Rotblatt MD, Koda-Kimble MA. Review of drug interference with urine glucose tests. Diabetes Care 1987;10:103–110.

52. Combs CA, Gunderson I, Kitzmiller JL. Relationship of fetal macrosomia to maternal postprandial glucose control during pregnancy. Diabetes Care 1992;15:1251–1257.

53. Hod M, Bar J, Peled Y. Antepartum management protocol: time and mode of delivery in gestational diabetes. Diabetes Care 1998;21:B133–B117.

54. Langer O, Berkus M, Brustman L. Rationale for insulin management in gestational diabetes mellitus. Diabetes 1991;40(suppl 2):186–190.

55. Howorka K, Pumprla J, Gabriel M. Normalization of pregnancy outcome in pregestational diabetes through functional insulin treatment and modular out-patient education adapted for pregnancy. Diabet Med 2001;18:965–972.

56. de Veciana M, Major C, Morgan M. Postprandial versus preprandial blood glucose monitoring in women with gestational diabetes mellitus requiring insulin therapy. N Eng J Med 1996;333:1237–1241.

57. Jovanovic-Peterson L, Peterson C, Reed G. Maternal postprandial glucose levels and infant birth weight: the Diabetes in Early Pregnancy Study. Am J Obstet Gynecol 1991;164:103–111.

58. Cooper GR, Mullins RE, Myers GL. Methodology of measuring glucose, glycated serum proteins and hemoglobin, and lipids and lipoprotines. In: Davidson JK, ed. Clinical Diabetes Mellitus: A Problem-Oriented Approach, 3rd ed. New York: Thieme, 2000, pp. 189–212.

59. American Diabetes Association. Self-monitoring of blood glucose. Diabetes Care 1994;17:81–85.

60. Koschinsky T, Heidkamp P, Vogt H. FreeStyle: technical evaluation of a new blood glucose meter for self-monitoring of blood glucose (abstract). Diabetes 2000;49:A114.

61. Lock JP, Szuts EZ, Malomo, KJ. Whole-blood glucose testing at alternate sites. Diabetes Care 2002;25:337–341.

62. Bohannon N. Accuracy and replicability of blood glucose determinations using the FreeStyle glucose monitor (abstract). Diabetes 2000;49(suppl 1):A98.

63. Ellison JM, Stegmann JM, Colner SL. Rapid changes in postprandial blood glucose produce concentration differences at finger, forearm, and thigh sampling sites. Diabetes Care 2002;25:961–964.

64. Jones BA, Bachner P, Howanitz PJ. Bedside glucose monitoring. Arch Pathol Lab Med 1993;117: 1080–1087.
65. Ryan EA, Nguyen G. Accuracy of glucose meter use in gestational diabetes. Diabetes Technol Ther 2001;3:91–97.
66. Harmelin D, Molyneaux L, Fowler P. Reflectance meter type and management of gestational diabetes. Lancet 1990;335:735–736.
67. Stenger P, Allen ME, Lisius L. Accuracy of blood glucose meters in pregnant subjects with diabetes. Diabetes Care 1996;19:268–269.
68. Mazze RS, Shamson H, Pasmantier R. Reliability of blood glucose monitoring by patients with diabtes mellitus. Am J Med 1984;77:211–217.
69. United Kingdom Prospective Diabetes Study Group. Relative efficacy of randomly allocated diet, sulphonylurea, insulin, or metformin in patients with newly diagnosed non-insulin dependent diabetes followed for three years. Br Med J 1995;310:83–88.
70. Bry L, Chen PC, Sacks DB. Effects of hemoglobin variants and the chemically modified derivatives on assays for glycohemoglobin. Clin Chem 2001;47:153–163.
71. Tahara Y, Shima K. The response of GHb to stepwise plasma glucose changes over time in diabetic patients. Diabetes Care 1993;16:1313–1314.
72. Rohlfing CL, Wiedmeyer HM, Little RR. Defining the relationship between plasma glucose and Hb A1C: analysis of glucose profiles and Hb A1C in the Diabetes Control and Complications Trial. Diabetes Care 2002;25:275–278.
73. Cefalu WT, Parker TB, Johnson CR. Validity of serum fructosamine as index of short-term glycemic control in diabetic outpatients. Diabetes Care 1988;11:662–664.
74. Madsen H, Ditzel J, Hansen P. Hemoglobin A1C determinations in diabetic pregnancy. Diabetes Care 1981;4:541–546.
75. Gunton JE, McElduff A. Hemoglobinopathies and Hb A1C measurement. Diabetes Care 2000;23: 1197–1198.
76. Widness JA, Schwartz HC, Kahn CB. Glycohemoglobin in diabetic pregnancy: a sequential study. Am J Obstet Gynecol 1980;136:1024–1029.
77. Fadel HE, Hammond SD, Huff TA. Glycosylated hemoglobins in normal pregnancy and gestational diabetes mellitus. Obstet Gynecol 1979;54:322–326.
78. Mills JL, Jovanovic L, Knopp R. Physiological reduction in fasting plasma glucose concentration in the first trimester of normal pregnancy: the Diabetes in Early Pregnancy Study. Metabolism 1998;47: 1140–1144.
79. Morris MA, Grandis AS, Litton JC. Longitudinal assessment of glycosylated blood protein concentrations in normal pregnancy and gestational diabetes. Diabetes Care 1986;9:107–110.
80. Suhonen L, Hiilesmaa V, Teramo K. Glycaemic control during early pregnancy and fetal malformations in women with type 1 diabetes mellitus. Diabetologia 2000;43:79–82.
81. American Diabetes Association. Position statement: preconception care of women with diabetes. Diabetes Care 1998;21(Suppl 1):S56–S59.
82. Pedersen JF, Mølsted-Pederson L, Mortensen HB. Fetal growth delay and maternal hemoglobin A1C in early diabetic pregnancy. Obstet Gynecol 1984;64:351–352.
83. Rosenn B, Miodovnik M, Combs CA. Glycemic thresholds for spontaneous abortion and congenital malformations in insulin-dependent diabetes mellitus. Obstet Gynecol 1994;84:515–520.
84. Little RR, Rohlfing CL, Wiedmeyer HM. The National Glyochemoglobin Standardization Program: a five-year progress report. Clin Chem 2001;47:1985–1992.
85. Thomas A. Standardization of Hb A1C measurement: the issues. Diabet Med 2000;17:2–4.
86. Voss EM, Cembrowski GS, Haig B. Stability of mailed and couriered capillary Hb A1C samples. Diabetes Care 1993;16:665.
87. Schnedl WJ, Krause R, Halwachs-Baumann G. Evaluation of Hb A1C determination methods in patients with hemoglobinopathies. Diabetes Care 2000;23:339–344.
88. Roberts WL, McCraw M, Cook CB. Effects of sickle cell trait and hemoglobin C trait on determinations of Hb A1C by an immunoassay method. Diabetes Care 1998;21:983–986.
89. Johnson R. Standardization of hemoglobin A1C. Clin Chem 1998;44:1068–1069.
90. Kobold U. Response to Johnson. Clin Chem 1998;44:1068–1069.
91. Weykamp CW, Miedema K, de Haan T. Carbamylated hemoglobin interference in glycohemoglobin assays. Clin Chem 1999;45:438–440.

92. Roberts WL, Chiasera JM, Ward-Cook KM. Glycohemoglobin results in samples with hemoglobin C or S trait: a comparison of four test systems. Clin Chem 1999;45:906–908.

93. Cohen MP, Clements RS. Measuring glycated proteins: clinical and methodological aspects. Diabetes Technol Ther 1999;1:57–70.

94. Boulton AJ, Saudek CD. The need for standardization of glycated hemoglobin measurements. Report on an international workshop held in Dusseldorf, Germany. 17 January 2002.

95. Roberts NB, Amara AB, Morris M. Long-term evaluation of electrospray ionization mass spectrometric analysis of glycated hemoglobin. Clin Chem 2001;47:316–321.

96. Krishnamurti U, Steffes MW. Glycohemoglobin: a primary predictor of the development or reversal of complications of diabetes mellitus. Clin Chem 2001;47:1157–1165.

97. Roberts AB, Court DJ, Henley P. Fructosamine in diabetic pregnancy. Lancet 1983;2:998–999.

98. Smart LM, Howie AF, Young RJ. Comparison of fructosamine with glycosylated hemoglobin and plasma proteins as measures of glycemic control. Diabetes Care 1988;11:433–437.

99. Roberts AB, Baker JR, James AG. Fructosamine in the management of gestational diabetes. Am J Obstet Gynecol 1988;159:66–71.

100. Roberts AB, Baker JR. Serum fructosamine: a screening test for diabetes in pregnancy. Am J Obstet Gynecol 1986;154:1027–1030.

101. Schrader HM, Jovanovic-Peterson L, Bevier WC. Fasting plasma glucose and glycosylated plasma protein at 24 to 28 wk of gestation predict macrosomia in the general obstetric population. Am J Perinat 1995;12:247–251.

102. Ghosh G, Pildes RS, Richton S. Maternal and cord serum glycosylated protein in neonatal macrosomia and correlation with birth weight. Obstet Gynecol 1990;75:79–82.

103. Brown EM, Grunberger G. Usefulness of albumin-based and total protein-based fructosamine correction formulas in diabetes practice. Diabetes Care 1991;14:353–354.

104. Hom FG, Ettinger B, Lin MJ. Comparison of serum fructosamine vs glycohemoglobin as measures of glycemic control in a large diabetic population. Acta Diabetol 1998;35:48–51.

105. Go RC, Desmond R, Roseman JM. Prevalence and risk factors of microalbuminuria in a cohort of African-American women with gestational diabetes. Diabetes Care 2001;24:1764–1769.

106. Mogensen CE, Chachati A, Christensen CK. Microalbuminuria: an early marker of renal involvement in diabetes. Uremia Invest 1986;9:85–85.

107. Higby K, Suiter CR, Phelps JY. Normal values of urinary albumin and total protein excretion during pregnancy. Am J Obstet Gynecol 1994;171:984–989.

108. Knuppel RA, Sbarra AJ, Cetrulo CL. 24-hour urine creatinine excretion in pregnancy. Obstet Gynecol 1979;54:327–329.

109. Higby K, Suiter CR, Siler-Khodr T. A comparison between two screening methods for detection of microproteinuria. Am J Obstet Gynecol 1995;173:1111–1114.

110. Gordon M, Landon MB, Samuels P. Perinatal outcome and long-term follow-up associated with modern management of diabetic nephropathy. Obstet Gynecol 1996;87:401–409.

111. Goebelsman U, Freeman RF, Mestman J. Estriol in pregnancy. II. Daily urinary estriol assays in the management of the pregnant diabetic woman. Am J Obstet Gynecol 1973;115:795.

112. Bashyam MM, O'Sullivan NJ, Baker, HH. Microalbuminuria in NIDDM. Diabetes Care 1993;16:634–635.

113. Di Gilio AR, Greco P, Vimercati A. Incidence of thyroid diseases in pregnant women with type 1 diabetes mellitus (abstract). Acta Biomed Ateneo Parmense 2000;71(suppl 1):387–391.

114. Jovanovic-Peterson L, Peterson CM. De novo clinical hypothyroidism in pregnancies complicated by type 1 diabetes, subclinical hypothyroidism, and proteinuria: a new syndrome. Am J Obstet Gynecol 1988;159:442–446.

115. Burrow GN, Palackwich R, Donabedian R. The hypothalamic pituitary-thyroid axis in normal pregnancy. In: Fisher DA, Burrow GN, eds. Perinatal Thyroid Physiology and Disease. New York: Raven, 1975.

116. Laffel L. Ketone bodies: a review of physiology, pathophysiology and application of monitoring to diabetes. Diabetes Metab Res Rev 1999;15:412–426.

117. Wallace TM, Meston NM, Gardner SG. The hospital and home use of a 30-second hand-held blood ketone meter: guidelines for clinical practice. Diabet Med 2001;18:640–645.

118. Csako G, Elin RJ. Spurious ketonuria due to captopril and other free sulfhydryl drugs. Diabetes Care 1996;19:673–674.

119. Horton WE Jr, Sadler TW. Effects of maternal diabetes on early embryogenesis. alterations in morpho-genesis produced by the ketone body, B-hydroxybutyrate. Diabetes 1983;32:610–616.
120. Horton WE Jr, Sadler. TW, Hunter ESI. Effects of hyperketonemia on mouse embryonic and fetal glucose metabolism in vitro. Teratology 1985;31:227–233.
121. Sheehan EA, Beck F, Clarke CA. Effects of β-hydroxybutyrate on rat embryos grown in culture. Experientia 1985;42:273–275.
122. Wentzel P, Eriksson UJ. Insulin treatment fails to abolish the teratogenic potential of serum from diabetic rats. Eur J Endocrinol 1996;134:459–466.
123. Sadler TW, Hunter ES 3rd, Balkan W. Effects of maternal diabetes on embryogenesis. Am J Perinatol 1988;5:319–326.
124. Jovanovic L, Metzger BE, Knopp RH. The diabetes in early pregnancy study: β-hydroxybutyrate levels in type 1 diabetic pregnancy compared with normal pregnancy. Diabetes Care 1998;21:1978–1984.

18 Preeclampsia, Eclampsia, and Hypertension

Kee-Hak Lim, MD and
Melanie M. Watkins, MD

INTRODUCTION

Hypertensive disorders of pregnancy complicate approx 10% of pregnancies and are leading causes of maternal mortality *(1–3)*. Although preeclampsia occurs in 5 to 8% of pregnancies, it is a major contributor of premature deliveries and neonatal morbidity in the United States *(4)*. Despite the recognition of eclampsia since ancient times, it was not until the late 1800s when an association between hypertension, edema, proteinuria, and eclampsia was suggested *(5)*. The differentiation of preeclampsia–eclampsia from epilepsy, primary renal disease, and essential hypertension gained widespread acceptance only in the 1950s. Even today, distinguishing these clinical entities from preeclampsia can be difficult. More important, definition and classification of hypertensive diseases of pregnancy remain controversial.

Preeclampsia is characterized by new-onset hypertension and proteinuria after 20 wk gestation and is usually associated with edema. The clinical spectrum varies from mild to severe and can involve multiple end organs including the kidney, the liver (HELLP syndrome), the coagulation system, and the brain (eclampsia). Preeclampsia seems to occur only in the presence of placenta and usually remits dramatically after the delivery. Observations to date suggest that perhaps the earliest pathologic event is placental insufficiency. Eclampsia is characterized by convulsions and coma.

From: *Current Clinical Pathology: Handbook of Clinical Laboratory Testing During Pregnancy*
Edited by: A. M. Gronowski © Humana Press, Totowa, NJ

Because the etiology and pathogenesis of preeclampsia is poorly understood, our ability to distinguish between different hypertensive disorders of pregnancy remains limited. In addition, our ability to predict, diagnose, and prevent preeclampsia continues to be poor. In this chapter, we review the current classification for hypertensive diseases in pregnancy and discuss clinical and laboratory tests for preeclampsia.

CLASSIFICATION OF HYPERTENSIVE DISEASES IN PREGNANCY

Hypertensive disorders of pregnancy are divided into the following four major groups (1,4):

- *Chronic hypertension*: Presence of systolic pressure greater than 140 mmHg, diastolic pressure of greater than 90 mmHg or both before the pregnancy, before the 20th wk gestation, or after 12 wk postpartum.
- *Gestational hypertension*: Hypertension without proteinuria or other signs of preeclampsia developing in the latter part of pregnancy. If it resolves by 12 wk postpartum, the condition is termed transient hypertension of pregnancy.
- *Preeclampsia–eclampsia*: Onset of hypertension and proteinuria or symptoms of preeclampsia, usually after 20 wk gestation, in otherwise normotensive women.
- *Superimposed preeclampsia*: New-onset proteinuria or onset of symptoms of preeclampsia in women with chronic hypertension after 20 wk pregnancy. In women with preexisting proteinuria (before 20 wk), an exacerbation of blood pressure to severe range (systolic >160 mmHg or diastolic >110mmHg) in the last half of the pregnancy.

INCIDENCE AND RISK FACTORS

In the United States, chronic hypertension is found in 1–5% of pregnant women (6). The incidence of gestational hypertension is estimated to be 6% (7). As many as 25% of women with gestational hypertension will develop preeclampsia (8). The incidence of preeclampsia is 5–8%, and 10% of preeclampsia occurs in pregnancies less than 34 wk (9). The incidence of various hypertensive disorders of pregnancy rises with increasing maternal age. The incidence of chronic hypertension in women 40 to 49 yr of age is 30.5%, whereas in the 18- to 29-yr-old group, it is only 2% (10). The incidence of preeclampsia in women over 40 yr of age is roughly threefold higher than that of women in their early 20s (1). Table 1 summarizes the risk factors for preeclampsia.

PATHOPHYSIOLOGY OF PREECLAMPSIA

The etiology and pathogenesis of preeclampsia remain poorly understood. Available evidence suggests that preeclampsia is a disorder of the endothelium, with characteristic features of microangiopathic hemolytic anemia. A number of investigators showed that endothelial cell dysfunction precedes the development of symptoms of preeclampsia (Fig. 1). Studies in humans have found increased circulating cellular fibronectin and factor VIII antigen, both markers of endothelial cell injury, in women with preeclampsia before they develop the symptoms (4,7). Decreased production of endothelial-derived relaxing factors (such as nitric oxide and prostacyclin) and increased production of endothelin and thromboxane in women with preeclampsia also suggest abnormal endothelial function (2,7). This model of preeclampsia suggests that the appearance of pro-

Table 1
Risk Factors for Preeclampsia

Factor	Risk ratio
Nulliparity	3:1
Age >40 y African-American race	3:1
Family history	
of pregnancy-induced hypertension	1.5:1
Chronic hypertension	10:1
Chronic renal disease	20:1
Antiphospholipid syndrome	10:1
Diabetes mellitus	2:1
Twin gestation	4:1
High body mass index	3:1
Angiotensinogen gene T235	
Homozygous	20:1
Heterozygous	4:1

Adapted from ref. *1*.

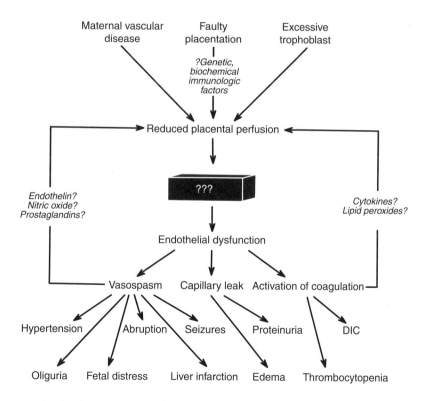

Fig. 1. The pathophysiology of preeclampsia. Reproduced from ref. *24*, with permission from Appleton and Lang.

teinuria and hypertension signals the end stage of the disease process and that involvement of other end organs may be imminent. More importantly, the model suggests that hypertension and proteinuria need not precede liver failure, coagulopathy, or seizure.

Several lines of evidence suggest that placental insufficiency plays an etiological role in the pathogenesis of preeclampsia: (1) successful animal models of preeclampsia involve creating placental insufficiency by disrupting uterine blood flow *(11)*; (2) preeclampsia has been associated with inadequate trophoblast invasion of maternal decidual arterioles *(12,13)*; (3) pathological examination of placentas from preeclamptic pregnancies reveals numerous placental infarcts and sclerotic narrowing of arterioles *(14,15)*; (4) maternal risk factors for preeclampsia include medical conditions that predispose a patient to underlying vascular insufficiency such as chronic hypertension, diabetes, systemic lupus erythematosus, and acquired and inherited thrombophilias *(1)*; and (5) obstetrical conditions such as multiple gestations or hydatidiform moles are associated with increased placental mass, which may result in a relative decrease in placental blood flow.

The mechanism by which placental insufficiency leads to diffuse endothelial cell injury remains poorly understood but is believed to involve production of putative factor(s) that can lead to endothelial cell dysfunction. Some of the candidate molecules include, but are not limited to, tumor necrosis factor-α, interleukin (IL)-6, IL-1α, IL-1β free fatty acid, and neurokinin-B (a close relative of substance P) *(16–18)*.

More recently, we published data showing that the soluble form of vascular endothelial cell growth factor receptor-1 (sVEGFR-1, or sFlt-1) is elevated in sera of patients with preeclampsia. sVEGFR-1 is a differentially spliced form of membrane-bound VEGFR-1 that is secreted into the serum. sVEGFR-1 can bind circulating vascular endothelial cell growth factor (VEGF) and placental growth factor and act as their antagonists. Placenta obtained from patients with preeclampsia had significantly higher VEGFR-1 mRNA. We also confirmed that the serum concentrations of free VEGF and free placental growth factor are decreased in patients with preeclampsia. Administration of exogenous sVEGFR-1 in rats induced proteinuria, hypertension, and the renal lesion that is thought to be consistent with preeclampsia (glomerular endotheliosis). Taken together, these data suggest that a balance between angiogenic and antiangiogenic factors could play a role in the pathogenesis of preeclampsia. Furthermore, in pregnancy, the placenta appears to be the main source of sVEGFR-1 and, for reasons not yet clear, placental production of sVEGFR-1 in preeclampsia is markedly increased *(19)*.

One of the consistent features of preeclampsia is an increased vascular responsiveness to angiotensin II. Recently, a German group confirmed this finding and suggested that the increased sensitivity of angiotensin II may be related to increased expression of bradykinin (B2) receptors *(20)*. The up-regulation of B2 receptors was found to lead to heterodimerization of B2 receptors with angiotensin II type I receptors (AT1), and this angiotensin II type I/B2 heterodimer increased responsiveness to angiotensin II. The fundamental causes of all these abnormalities described above still remain elusive.

DIAGNOSTIC CRITERIA FOR PREECLAMPSIA

Recently published criteria for preeclampsia are listed in Table 2. The increase in systolic pressure of 30 mmHg and diastolic pressure of 15 mmHg (30–15 rule) is no longer a part of the criteria for preeclampsia *(4)*. Although 24-h urine protein measure-

Table 2
Diagnostic Criteria for Preeclampsia

Hypertension:	Blood pressure ≥ 140/90 mmHg (or mean arterial pressure of ≥ 105 mmHg)
Proteinuria:	≥ 300 mg of protein in 24-h urine collection or ≥ 1+ protein on urine dipstick

Adapted from ref. *1*.

ment remains the standard for the diagnosis of preeclampsia, protein–creatinine ratio and urine dipstick analysis have gained popularity. Caution should be used when the protein–creatinine ratio and/or urine dipstick is used to exclude preeclampsia or to make the diagnosis of severe preeclampsia.

Meyer et al. showed that nearly 30% of women with trace protein on urine analysis had at least 300 mg of protein in a 24-h collection *(21)*. Adelberg et al. also showed a poor correlation between urine dipstick and 24-h collection *(22)*.

Similarly, a prospective study comparing protein–creatinine ratio and 24-h urine protein in women with suspected preeclampsia showed a poor negative predictive value (NVP;47.8%) and specificity (52.4%) for mild proteinuria. The positive predictive value (PPV) and sensitivity for mild proteinuria were 87.7 and 85.5%, respectively. Interestingly, the protein–creatinine ratio showed low PPV and sensitivity for severe proteinuria of 63.6 and 58.3%, respectively, whereas the NPV and specificity were 94.6 and 95.7%, respectively *(23)*. On the basis of on these data, the authors concluded that protein–creatinine ratio alone should not be used to exclude mild preeclampsia or diagnose severe preeclampsia.

The available data to date support the use of 24-h urine protein as the gold standard for diagnosis of preeclampsia. Adelberg et al. showed that there is a good correlation between 12-h and 24-h urine collection in 65 patients, raising the possibility that 24-h urine collection may not be necessary for the diagnostic accuracy *(22)*. However, this needs to be investigated in a larger cohort.

The clinical spectrum of preeclampsia varies widely. Although the severe form carries a higher incidence of maternal and perinatal mortality and morbidity, it can be difficult to distinguish the two. Complicating the clinical diagnosis of different forms of disease is the fact that the progression of the disease can be extremely rapid. According to one observational study, approx 20% of women with eclampsia (convulsions or coma) did not have proteinuria and 23% had minimal or relative hypertension *(25)*, emphasizing the fact that preeclampsia–eclampsia is a disorder of the endothelium rather than hypertension or renal disorder. Thus, eclampsia, which is the most severe form of the disease, may occur before the development of all or any of the classical symptoms and signs of preeclampsia. The criteria for severe preeclampsia are listed in Table 3. The presence of any one of the criteria in the setting of preeclampsia will be enough to diagnose severe preeclampsia. Occasionally, a patient may present with an atypical form of preeclampsia where one or more of the classic signs and/or symptoms of preeclampsia may be absent. In such a case, the presence of one of the criteria listed in Table 4 could strengthen the diagnosis of preeclampsia.

Table 3
Criteria for Severe Preeclampsia

Systolic blood pressure of ≥ 160 mmHg and/or
    diastolic of ≥ 110 mmHg on two occasions 6 h apart
Proteinuria > 5 g per 24 h
Oliguria (< 500 mL in 24 h)
Cerebral or visual disturbances
Pulmonary edema or cyanosis
Epigastric or right upper-quadrant pain
Impaired liver function
Thrombocytopenia
Fetal growth restriction

Adapted from ref. *1*.

Table 4
Other Signs That Increase the Certainty of the Diagnosis of Preeclampsia

Proteinuria of ≥ 2 g in 24-h period
Serum creatinine level of > 1.2 mg/dL (unless previously elevated)
Thrombocytopenia and/or elevated lactic acid dehydrogenase
    (signs of microangiopathic hemolytic anemia)
Persistent headache
Persistent epigastric pain
Systolic blood pressure of ≥ 160 mmHg
Diastolic blood pressure of ≥ 110 mmHg

Adapted from ref. *4*.

Most of the frequently seen laboratory abnormalities in preeclampsia are listed in Table 5. The most well-characterized values are for proteinuria, thrombocytopenia, and elevated serum transaminase values. However, even for these values, there is controversy regarding the abnormal threshold. Although various investigators reported different cutoff values for serum aspartate aminotransaminase, it has been suggested that a value that is 2 standard deviations away from the mean for a given laboratory should be used *(26)*. Abnormal values for coagulopathy and hemolysis may vary among different laboratories as well. The presence of hemolysis, elevated liver enzymes, and low platelets meet the criteria for diagnosis of HELLP syndrome, a severe form of preeclampsia that has been associated with increased maternal and perinatal mortality compared to mild preeclampsia *(26)*.

Hyperuricemia in preeclampsia has been well documented. However, it is not helpful in distinguishing preeclampsia from transient hypertension of pregnancy (likelihood ratio [LR] 1.4). In patients with chronic hypertension, a serum uric acid value of greater than 5.5 mg/dL has an LR of 2.5 for superimposed preeclampsia *(27)*.

Table 5
Laboratory Criteria for Preeclampsia and HELLP Syndrome

Renal

Proteinuria of $\geq$ 300 mg/24 h
Urine dipstick $\geq$ 1+
Protein/creatinine ratio $\geq$ 0.3[a]
Serum uric acid $\geq$ 5.6 mg/dL[a]
Serum creatinine >1.2 mg/dL[a]

Low Platelets/Coagulopathy

Platelet count < 100,000/mm^3
Elevated PT or PTT[a]
Decreased fibrinogen[a]
Increased d-dimer[a]

Hemolysis

Abnormal peripheral smear[a]
Total bilirubin $\geq$ 1.2 mg/dL[a]
Lactate dehydrogenase $\geq$ 600 U/L[a]

Elevated Liver Enzymes

Serum aspartate aminotransferase $\geq$ 70 U/L *(26)*
                                  $\geq$ 50 U/L *(29)*
                                  $\geq$ 40 U/L *(28)*
                                  $\geq$ 30 U/L *(30)*
Lactate dehydrogenase > 600 U/L[a]

[a]Not required for the diagnosis or classification of preeclampsia
PT, prothrombin time; PTT, partial thromboplastin time.
Adapted from ref. *4*.

SCREENING TESTS FOR PREECLAMPSIA

For several decades, investigators attempted to develop screening tests that would predict the onset of preeclampsia. Although the only definitive therapy is delivery, intensified maternal and fetal surveillance could be offered to women at high risk for developing the disease.

A screening test should be safe, valid, reliable, acceptable to the population, reproducible, appropriate for the population, and economical. Preeclampsia is an appropriate disease for which to screen, because it is common, important, and increases both maternal mortality and perinatal mortality. However, no specific tests are available that are proven to be appropriate screening tests for preeclampsia *(31)*. This is caused, in part, by the wide range of terminology used for hypertensive disorders in pregnancy. Researchers have sought to identify predictors of the development of gestational hypertension and/or preeclampsia in normotensive women, the development of severe preeclampsia in women with mild preeclampsia, and predictors of maternal morbidity and mortality in patients with severe preeclampsia. At the same time, researchers have different criteria for the diagnosis of these complex disorders and different measures of outcomes.

Table 6
Screening Tests for Preeclampsia

Test	Cutoff	Author	No. Pt.	SENS	SPEC	PPV	NPV
Serum βhCG	≥ 2 MOM	Sorensen (32)	426	69	70	7	99
	≥ 3 MOM		426	15	94	7	97
	≥ 2 MOM	Vaillant (33)	434	69	85	15	99
	≥ 2 MOM	Ashour (34)	2737	12	89	5	96
	≥ 3 MOM		2737	5	97	8	96
	Combined ≥ 2 MOM		3597	23	86	7	96
	Combined ≥ 3 MOM		3163	6	97	8	96
Uric Acid (plasma)	≥ 350 μmol/L (≥ 5.9 mg/dL)	Jacobson (35)	135	54	89	33	95
Uric Acid (serum)	Not specified	Conde-) Agudelo (36)	387	53	65	6	97
Urinary kallikrein	IUK:Cr ≤ 170 IUK: Cr ≤ 170	Millar (37) Kyle (38)	307 458	83 80	99.7 71	91 11	99 99
Urinary Calcium	≤ 195 mg/day Not specified	Sanchez-Ramos (39) Conde-Agudelo (36)	103 387	88 47	84 59	32 5	99 96
Fibronectin (plasma)	≥ 230 mg/L	Paarlberg (40)	376	69	59	12	96
Platelet Count	?	Conde-Agudelo (36)	387	47	59	5	96
Platelet Activation	Platelet CD63 2%	Konijnenberg (41)	244	47	76	13	95

Adapted from ref. 28.
MOM, multiple of the median; No. Pt., number of patients; NVP, negative predictive value; PPV, positive predictive value; SENS, sensitivity; SPEC, specificity.

Studies have evaluated laboratory markers for the prediction of preeclampsia, such as urinary kallikrein and creatinine, urine thrombomodulin–creatinine ratio, and urine calcium–creatinine ratio (Table 6). In addition, a number of clinical variables have been investigated, such as blood pressure measurements, weight gain, and response to angiotensin II infusion early in pregnancy. Currently, none of the screening tests are being used in clinical practice because there is no effective method of preventing preeclampsia.

REFERENCES

1. Diagnosis and management of preeclampsia and eclampsia. ACOG Practice Bulletin No. 33. Washington, DC: American College of Obstetricians and Gynecologists, 2000, pp. 1–2.
2. Walker JJ. Pre-eclampsia. Lancet 2000;356:1260–1265.
3. Koonin LM, MacKay AP, Berg CJ, Atrash HK, Smith JC. Pregnancy-related mortality surveillance: United States, 1987–1990. Morb Mort Wkly Rep CDC Surveill Summ 1997;46(4):17–36.
4. Report of the National High Blood Pressure Education Program Working Group on high blood pressure in pregnancy. Am J Obstet Gynecol 2000;183:S1–S22.
5. Lindheimer MD, Roberts JM, Cunningham FG, Chesley L. Introduction, history, controversies, and definitions. In: Lindheimer M, Cunningham FG, Roberts JM, ed. Chesley's Hypertensive Disorders in Pregnancy, 2nd ed. Stamford, CT: Appleton & Lange 1999, pp. 3–41.
6. Sibai BM. Treatment of hypertension in pregnant women. N Engl J Med 1996;335:257–265.
7. Lain KY, Roberts JM. Contemporary concepts of the pathogenesis and management of preeclampsia. JAMA 2002;287:3183.
8. Saudan P, Brown MA, Buddle ML, Jones M. Does gestational hypertension become preeclampsia? Br J Obstet Gynaecol 1996;105:1177–1184.
9. Saftlas AF, Olson DR, Franks AL, et al. Epidemiology of preeclampsia and eclampsia in the United States, 1979–1986. Am J Obstet Gynecol 1990;163:460.
10. Witlin A, Sibai BM. Epidemiology and classification of hypertension in women. In: Sibai BM, ed. Hypertensive Disorders in Women. Philadelphia: W.B. Saunders, 2001;pp.1–8.
11. Venuto RC, Lindheimer MD. Animal models. In: Lindheimer M, Cunningham FG, Roberts JM, ed. Chesley's Hypertensive Disorders in Pregnancy, 2nd ed, Stamford, CT: Appleton & Lange, 1999, pp. 487–515.
12. Robertson WB, Bronsens I, Dixon HG. The pathological response of the vessels of the placental bed to hypertensive pregnancy. J Pathol Bacteriol 1967;93:581–592.
13. Brosens IA, Robertson WB, Dixon HG. The role of the spiral arteries in the pathogenesis of preeclampsia. Obstet Gynecol Ann 1972;1:177–191.
14. Khong TY, De Wolf F, Robertson WB, Brosens I. Inadequate maternal vascular response to placentation in pregnancies complicated by pre-eclampsia and by small-for-gestational age infants. Br J Obstet Gynaecol 1986;93:1049–1059.
15. De Wolf F, Robertson WB, Brosens I. The ultrastructure of acute arthrosis in hypertensive pregnancy. Am J Obstet Gynecol 1975;123:164–174.
16. Benyo DF, Smarason A, Redman CW, Sims C, Conrad KP. Expression of inflammatory cytokines in placentas from women with preeclampsia. J Clin Endocrinol Metab 2001;86(6):2505–2512.
17. Conrad KP, Miles TM, Benyo DF. Circulating levels of immunoreactive cytokines in women with preeclampsia. Am J Reprod Immunol 1998;40(2):102–111.
18. Page NM, Woods RJ, Gardiner SM, et al. Excessive placental secretion of neurokinin B during the third trimester causes pre-eclampsia. Nature 2000;405(6788):797–800.
19. Maynard SE, Min J-Y, Merchan J, et al. Excess placental sFlt-1 may contribute to endothelial dysfunction, hypertension, and proteinuria in preeclampsia. J Clin Invest 2003;111(5):649–658.
20. AbdAlla S, Lother H, el Massiery A, Quitterer U. Increased AT(1) receptor heterodimers in preeclampsia mediate enhanced angiotensin II responsiveness. Nat Med 2001;7(9):1003–1009.
21. Meyer NL, Mercer BM, Friedman SA, Sibai BM. Urinary dipstick protein: a poor predictor of absent or severe proteinuria. Am J Obstet Gynecol 1994;10:137–141.
22. Adelberg AM, Miller J, Doerzbacher M, Lambers DS. Correlation of quantitative protein measurements in 8-, 12-, and 24-hour urine samples for the diagnosis of preeclampsia. Am J Obstet Gynecol 2001;185:804–807.
23. Durnwald C, Mercer B. A prospective comparison of protein/creatinine ratio and 24 hour urine protein in women with suspected preeclampsia. Abstract 569. Am J Obstet Gynecol 2002;187(suppl.)S215.
24. Friedman SA, Lindheimer MD. Prediction and differential diagnosis. In: Lindheimer M, Cunningham FG, Roberts JM, eds. Chesley's Hypertensive Disorders in Pregnancy, 2nd ed. Stamford, CT: Appleton & Lange, 1999, pp. 201–227.
25. Sibai BM. Eclampsia. VI. Maternal–perinatal outcome in 254 consecutive cases. Am J Obstet Gynecol 1990;163:1049–1054.
26. Sibai BM, Taslimi MM, El-Nazer A, et al. Maternal–perinatal outcome associated with the syndrome of hemolysis, elevated liver enzymes, and low platelets in severe preeclampsia–eclampsia. Am J Obstet Gynecol 1986;155:501–509.

27. Lim KH, Friedman SA, Ecker JL, et al. The clinical utility of serum uric acid measurements in hypertensive diseases of pregnancy. Am J Obstet Gynecol 1998;178:1067.

28. Martin JN Jr, Blake PG, Lowry SL, et al. Pregnancy complicated by preeclampsia–eclampsia with the syndrome of hemolysis, elevated liver enzymes, and low platelet count: how rapid is postpartum recovery? Obstet Gynecol 1990;76:737–741.

29. van Pampus MG, Wolf H, Ilsen A, et al. Maternal outcome following temporizing management of the (H)ELLP syndrome. Hypertens Pregn 2000;19:211–220.

30. Visser W, Wallenburg HCS. Temporizing management of severe pre-eclampsia with and without the HELLP syndrome. Br J Obstet Gynaecol 1995;102:111–117.

31. Friedman SA, Lubarsky SL, Lim KH. Mild gestational hypertension and preeclampsia. In: Sibai BM, ed. Hypertensive Disorders in Women. Philadelphia: W.B. Saunders, 2001, pp. 9–23.

32. Sorensen TK, Williams MA, Zingheim RW, Clement SJ, Hickok DE. Elevated second trimester human chorionic gonadotropin and subsequent pregnancy-induced hypertension. Am J Obstet Gynecol 1993;169:834–838.

33. Vaillant P, David E, Constant I, et al. Validity in nulliparas of increased β-human chorionic gonadotrophin at midterm for predicting pregnancy-induced hypertension complicated with proteinuria and intrauterine growth retardation. Nephron 1996;72:557–563.

34. Ashour AMN, Lieberman ES, Wilkins, Haug LE, Repke JT. The value of elevated second-trimester β-human chorionic gonadotropin in predicting development of preeclampsia. Am J Obstet Gynecol 1997;176:436–442.

35. Jacobson S-L, Imhof R, Manning N, et al. The value of Doppler assessment of the uteroplacental circulation in predicting preeclampsia or intrauterine growth retardation. Am J Obstet Gynecol 1990;167:110–114.

36. Conde-Agudelo A, Belizan JN, Lede R, Bergel E. Prediction of hypertensive disorders of pregnancy by calcium/creatinine ratio and other laboratory tests [letter]. Int J Gynecol Obstet 1994;47:285–286.

37. Millar JGB, Campbell SK, Albano JDM, et al. Early prediction of preeclampsia by measurement of kallikrein and creatinine on a random urine sample. Br J Obstet Gynaecol 1996;103:421–426.

38. Kyle P, Redman C, de Swiet M, Millar G. A comparison of the inactive urinary kallikrein:creatinine ratio and the angiotensin sensitivity test for the prediction of preeclampsia [letter reply]. Br J Obstet Gynaecol 1997;104:969–974.

39. Sanchez-Ramos L, Jones DC, Cullen MT. Urinary calcium as an early marker for preeclampsia. Obstet Gynecol 1991;77:685–688.

40. Paarlberg KM, DeJong CLD, Van Geijn HB, et al. Total plasma fibronectin as a marker of pregnancy-induced hypertensive disorders: a longitudinal study. Obstet Gynecol 1998;91:383–388.

41. Konijnenberg A, van der Post JAM, Mol BW, et al. Can flow   cytometric detection of platelet activation early in pregnancy predict the occurrence of preeclampsia? a prospective study. Am J Obstet Gynecol 1997;177:434–442.

19 Liver Diseases in Pregnancy

Jason D. Wright, MD and
Yoel Sadovsky, MD

CONTENTS

ANATOMICAL AND PHYSIOLOGICAL CHANGES DURING PREGNANCY

Understanding physiological changes that take place in the hepatobiliary system during gestation is obligatory for diagnosis and treatment of pregnant women with diseases of the liver and gallbladder. Because liver test abnormalities may occur during normal pregnancies as well as in pregnancy-specific nonhepatic diseases, caution during interpretation of these tests is warranted. Liver size, anatomy, and histology are minimally affected by pregnancy *(1)*. Several studies have evaluated hepatic blood flow using bromsulfalein and indocyanine green *(2,3)*, revealing that although absolute blood flow to the liver during pregnancy is unchanged, the fraction of cardiac output reaching the liver is diminished from 34% in nonpregnant females to 28% during pregnancy *(4)*. Compression of the inferior vena cava and increased flow to the azygous system frequently results in esophageal varices in pregnant women *(5)*.

Elevated concentrations of circulating estrogen and progesterone during pregnancy lead to significant changes in both hepatic and biliary physiology. The hyperestrogenic state of pregnancy has a myriad of effects on hepatic function during gestation. In general, estrogen does not influence hepatic conjugation but does inhibit canalicular excretion of anions, leading to a relative cholestasis. Hyperestrogenemia also increases hepatic cholesterol synthesis and excretion *(4)*. Interestingly, high circulating estradiol causes angiomata and spider nevi, seen in more than half of pregnant women, and therefore should not be used to suggest a liver disease. Gallbladder contractility is influenced by pregnancy. After the first trimester, both fasting and postcontraction residual gallbladder volume are higher than in nonpregnant women, reflecting delayed or incomplete emptying *(6)*. This has been attributed to smooth muscle relaxation by progesterone, perhaps

From: *Current Clinical Pathology: Handbook of Clinical Laboratory Testing During Pregnancy*
Edited by: A. M. Gronowski © Humana Press, Totowa, NJ

through the blunting of acetylcholine- and cholecystokinin-mediated smooth muscle contractions *(7)*. The increase in hepatic cholesterol synthesis results in altered bile composition, associated with increased concentration of bile acids and a decreased concentration of biliary water *(4)*. These changes lead to an increase in the biliary lithogenic index *(5)*. These alterations, coupled with a decrease in enterohepatic circulation, serve to promote cholelithiasis during pregnancy *(5)*.

HEPATIC BIOSYNTHETIC FUNCTION DURING PREGNANCY

This section examines key liver function tests that are commonly used to diagnose acute or chronic liver diseases. It is imperative to understand the influence of normal pregnancy on these laboratory tests before they are utilized to diagnose liver dysfunction during pregnancy *(8)*. Although the incidence of jaundice during pregnancy is diminishing, the majority of cases are caused by acute viral hepatitis or cholestasis of pregnancy. Many causes of chronic liver dysfunction are associated with infertility and consequently are not a part of the differential diagnosis of jaundice during pregnancy.

Transaminases

The transaminases aspartate aminotransferase (AST), also known as serum glutamate oxaloacetate (SGOT) and alanine aminotransferase (ALT), also known as serum glutamate pyruvate transaminase (SGPT) are commonly used as indicators of liver function. Both enzymes catalyze the transfer of an amino group to either aspartate or alanine. AST is a mitochondrial enzyme found ubiquitously throughout the body, whereas ALT is a cytosolic enzyme localized primarily to hepatocytes, with lower expression in the kidney. Hepatocellular damage results in the rapid release of aminotransferases. Peak concentrations of AST are reached 24–36 h after the initial insult and return to normal in 3–6 d. Although the concentrations of AST and ALT remain within normal limits throughout gestation *(9–11)*, serum concentrations of both aminotransferases are higher in late gestation than during the first trimester, with further increases during labor *(9)*. Although variations in aminotransferase concentrations may occur during gestation, any elevation that exceeds the upper limit of the normal reference range requires further evaluation.

Elevated serum concentration of either AST or ALT may reflect hepatocyte injury. Patients with acute hepatitis exhibit aminotransferase concentrations that commonly exceed 10–20 times the upper limit of normal. The ratio of AST to ALT is generally less than 1 in patients with acute viral hepatitis. The increase in serum concentrations of aminotransferases is less pronounced in patients with chronic hepatitis. Modest aminotransferase elevations are commonly seen in patients with alcoholic liver disease. In these patients, the AST to ALT ratio is generally greater than 1. Other causes of mild AST and ALT elevation include passive liver congestion, drug-induced hepatocellular damage, liver neoplasm, and systemic viral infections such as infectious mononucleosis. In patients with long-standing cirrhosis, AST and ALT concentrations may be near normal. Diverse pregnancy-specific diseases are associated with elevated aminotransferase concentrations. An increase in AST and ALT concentrations characterizes acute fatty liver of pregnancy (AFLP). The increase in aminotransferase concentrations in AFLP is usually moderate, with most patients exhibiting enzyme concentrations less than 1000 U *(12)*. Mild to moderate AST and ALT elevations are frequently seen in pregnant women with hyperemesis gravidarum or intrahepatic cholestasis *(13,14)*. Elevated aminotransferase concentrations characterize preeclampsia and HELLP syndrome (hemolysis, elevated liver enzymes, and low platelet count). Similar to alcoholic liver disease, serum concentrations of AST typically exceed those of ALT in these conditions.

Alkaline Phosphatase

Alkaline phosphatases (AP) are a group of enzymes that are expressed in diverse tissues including the liver and biliary tract, bone, gastrointestinal tract, and placenta *(15)*. Osteoblasts produce AP, and enzyme concentrations are commonly elevated in children and adolescents because of active bone growth and remodeling. Placental AP isozyme is heat stable, remaining active after heating to 60°C for 5 min, whereas the liver and bone forms are heat labile *(16)*.

The serum concentration of AP is elevated throughout pregnancy, peaking in the third trimester *(9,11,17–20)*. Near delivery, 50% of parturients have AP concentrations one to two times the upper normal range, 29% have concentrations two to three times the upper limit of normal, and 6% have concentrations greater than three times the upper limit of normal. The remaining 15% exhibit enzyme concentrations within the nonpregnant reference range *(21)*. Several sources contribute to elevated serum concentration of AP during pregnancy (Fig. 1). The most important source is placental AP *(9)*, which accounts for 40–60% of the increase in AP *(19,22,23)*. As expected, placental AP is almost undetectable within 6 wk after delivery *(23)*. Bone production of AP is also increased in pregnancy *(19,22,23)* and remains elevated by 6 wk postpartum *(23)*. In contrast, hepatic AP remains unchanged during pregnancy *(23)*.

Serum AP concentrations are commonly elevated in intrahepatic and extrahepatic biliary obstruction and in patients with hepatic tumors. Hepatic AP release is also elevated during liver congestion and viral infections such as infectious mononucleosis. Common causes of bone-derived AP elevations include fractures, bone growth during childhood and adolescence, tumors, and Paget's disease. The liver-specific γ-glutamyl-transferase (GGT) and 5'-nucleotidase (see below) can be used to distinguish hepatic and extrahepatic sources for elevated AP. Although the physiological increase in AP during pregnancy impedes its diagnostic utility, marked elevation characterizes conditions that typically occur late in pregnancy, such as intrahepatic cholestasis of pregnancy and AFLP. Interestingly, it has been reported that placental AP synthesis is lower in preeclamptic pregnancies than in normotensive controls *(19)*.

GGT

GGT, produced primarily in hepatocytes, catalyzes amino acid transport across cellular membranes. GGT activity has also been demonstrated in placental tissue *(24)*. Nevertheless, serum concentrations of GGT remain within normal limits during pregnancy *(10,11,24)* and even decline during the second and third trimesters of pregnancy *(9)*.

Determination of GGT concentrations is commonly utilized to further assess elevated AP. Elevated AP in the context of a normal GGT concentration suggests a non-hepatobiliary source. Disorders associated with GGT elevation include biliary tract disease, acute hepatocellular injury, hepatitis, and liver tumors. GGT is frequently elevated in patients with alcoholism, even without apparent hepatic disease *(21)*. Other etiologies for an elevated GGT concentration include acute myocardial infarction and ingestion of high amounts of acetaminophen or phenytoin. GGT determination during pregnancy can be used to distinguish between physiologic and pathologic elevations of AP. Whereas

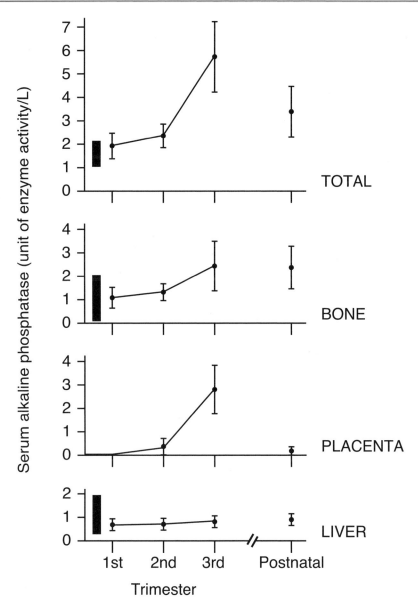

Fig. 1. Serial measurements of serum AP concentrations in 17 women during pregnancy and 6 wk after delivery. The solid bars indicate the range of values in normal women and men. (Reprinted with permission from the Endocrine Society [23].)

GGT may remain normal in women with intrahepatic cholestasis of pregnancy (5), women with preeclampsia often exhibit GGT elevations, along with elevated aminotransferases (10).

5'-Nucleotidase

The enzyme 5'-nucleotidase is produced primarily in the liver and biliary systems. Unlike AP, osseous structures produce little 5'-nucleotidase. Thus, 5'-nucleotidase can be helpful in determining the source of elevated AP. Although early studies of 5'-nucleotidase during pregnancy indicated that concentrations are unchanged *(18,25)*, recent data revealed that the concentration of 5'-nucleotidase is elevated from the midtrimester until delivery *(9)*. Although placental synthesis of 5'-nucleotidase has been documented, because of its large molecular weight, it is not clear if 5'-nucleotidase can diffuse into the maternal circulation *(9,25)*.

Lactate Dehydrogenase

The cytosolic enzyme lactate dehydrogenase (LDH) catalyzes the conversion of lactate to pyruvate. LDH is expressed in numerous tissues, including skeletal muscle, cardiac muscle, red blood cells, liver, lung, and kidney. Five isoenzymes of LDH have been isolated. The LDH_5 fraction is the most sensitive marker for hepatic disease. All five LDH isoforms are expressed in the placenta *(26)*. During pregnancy, LDH concentrations usually remain within normal limits, although some reports have documented slightly higher LDH concentrations during the third trimester *(27)*.

Because of its ubiquitous expression, LDH is a relatively nonspecific marker of hepatic disease. Hepatic LDH may be elevated by diverse inflammatory diseases and tumors *(15)*. The most common source of LDH elevation in pregnancy is severe preeclampsia and HELLP syndrome, where LDH concentrations reflect hepatocyte damage, red blood cell hemolysis, and higher production by the placenta *(26,28)*.

Bilirubin

Bilirubin is produced by metabolic breakdown of hemoglobin. Hemoglobin is released from senescent erythrocytes and degraded to heme and globin chains in the reticuloendothelial system. Oxidation of the porphyrin ring of heme results in the formation of biliverdin, which is further reduced to bilirubin by biliverdin reductase. The resulting unconjugated bilirubin is transported to the liver, predominantly bound to albumin, and extracted by hepatic cells. Unconjugated bilirubin is the substrate for glucuronyl transferase within hepatocytes, resulting in formation of conjugated bilirubin. Conjugated bilirubin is transported from the hepatocytes into the biliary tree and ultimately into the intestine, where a portion of the bilirubin is metabolized by local intestinal flora to urobilinogen. Although the majority of urobilinogen is excreted from the gastrointestional tract, some is reabsorbed and enters the portal circulation. Whereas most of the reabsorbed urobilinogen is re-excreted by the liver, a small fraction is excreted by the kidneys and appears in the urine. The kidneys in patients with conjugated hyperbilirubinemia also excrete conjugated bilirubin.

During pregnancy, serum bilirubin concentrations remain within normal limits *(9–11,17)*, with a small decrease identified by several groups *(8–10)*, likely reflecting the hemodilution that normally occurs during pregnancy *(9)*. Interestingly, Knopp et al. reported lower serum bilirubin concentrations in pregnant women and oral contraceptive users compared to nonpregnant females, suggesting a possible role for estrogen in the decrease of bilirubin concentrations observed during gestation *(8)*.

Diverse pathological processes may lead to an increase in blood bilirubin concentration. Hemolytic anemia is a common cause of hyperbilirubinemia. Typically, unconjugated bilirubin is elevated and exceeds the concentration of conjugated bilirubin. Intrahepatic and extrahepatic biliary obstruction also lead to hyperbilirubinemia. Cholelithiasis is the most common cause of elevated bilirubin in adults. Conjugated bilirubin predominates in obstructive hepatobiliary disease. Diseases that result in

heptocellular injury also may give rise to elevated bilirubin and are typically characterized by elevation of both conjugated and unconjugated fractions of bilirubin. Rare metabolic and transport diseases such as Gilbert's syndrome, Crigler-Najjar syndrome, and
Dubin-Johnson syndrome are also associated with hyperbilirubinemia. During pregnancy, women with severe preeclampsia or isolated HELLP syndrome may also display
abnormally high blood bilirubin concentrations. In addition, women with cholestasis of
pregnancy typically display an elevated serum bilirubin concentration, although bile acid
elevation (see below) is a more sensitive marker of the disease. Bilirubin concentrations
are also frequently elevated in AFLP pregnancy.

Bile Acids

Bile acids are derived from hepatic cholesterol metabolism. The primary bile acids
cholic acid and chenodeoxycholic acid are produced and conjugated with glycine and
taurine, and subsequently excreted into the bile. On entering the small intestine, the
conjugated bile acids are degraded by intestinal bacteria into the secondary bile acids
deoxycholic acid and lithocholic acid. Ninety to 95% of the bile acids are then reabsorbed
in the jejunum and ileum, enter the enterohepatic circulation, and return to the liver, with
a small proportion excreted via the kidneys.

During pregnancy, serum bile acids remain within normal limits (9,29–31). Several
studies have documented an increase in serum bile acid concentrations in late pregnancy
compared to first-trimester values (9,31). Specifically, Lunzer et al. reported an increase
in mean cholyglycine concentration from 0.3 μmol/L at 15 wk to 0.6 μmol/L at 40 wk,
yet these concentrations are within normal limits (31). Similarly, Heikkinen et al.
reported an increase in chenodeoxycholic acid near term but no change in cholic acid
or deoxycholic acid (30).

Because almost any disease of the hepatobiliary system results in an elevation of the
serum bile acids, serum bile acids are a sensitive yet nonspecific marker of hepatic and
biliary disease. Bile acids have been reported to remain elevated in inactive cirrhosis and
resolving hepatitis, when other tests of liver function are normal. The main application
for the measurement of serum bile acids during pregnancy is for the evaluation of pruritus
that commonly accompanies cholestasis of pregnancy (32). As described below, cholic
acid frequently exhibits the most dramatic change in this condition, with elevation of
nearly 70-fold (31).

Lipoproteins

Serum lipoproteins, composed of polypeptide apolipoproteins and lipid fractions,
transport serum cholesterol and lipids. Apolipoproteins serve to bind lipoproteins to cell
receptors and regulate lipase activity. Elevated serum concentrations of low-density
lipoprotein (LDL) cholesterol is a major cause of coronary heart disease in the United
States (33).

The blood concentration of most lipoproteins is increased during pregnancy (34–39).
In a prospective evaluation of 553 pregnant females, Knopp et al. demonstrated that,
compared to the prepregnancy period, total cholesterol increased by 46%, LDL increased
by 49%, high-density lipoprotein (HDL) increased by 23%, and very low-density lipoprotein increased by 36% (34). Interestingly, during early gestation, cholesterol concentrations decrease and then rise in the second and third trimesters until the time of delivery
(35) (Fig. 2A). During the postpartum period, cholesterol declines by 2 wk, yet the return

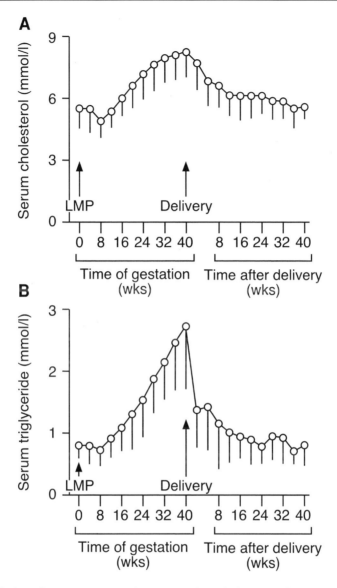

Fig. 2. (**A**) Variation of serum cholesterol concentrations during and after pregnancy (mean SD, $n = 34$). LMP, last menstrual period. (**B**) Variation in serum triglyceride concentration during and after pregnancy (mean SD, $n = 34$). LMP, last menstrual period. (Reprinted with permission from Elsevier Science [35].)

to preconception concentrations is variable (Fig. 2A). Estrogens enhance cholesterol synthesis, thus contributing to the hyperlipoproteinemia of pregnancy (4,38,40). Indeed, pregnancy-related changes in lipid profile are similar to those observed in women receiving exogenous estrogens (4,34). Similar to plasma lipoproteins, triglyceride concentrations are significantly elevated during pregnancy (34–36). After a small decrease in the first trimester, serum triglyceride concentrations increase during the midtrimester until term and return to pregestational concentrations after several weeks (35) (Fig. 2B). The hypertriglyceridemia of pregnancy is largely attributed to increased hepatic triglyceride production, likely secondary to estrogenic effect *(34,36)*. In parallel, the enzymatic activity of lipoprotein lipase, which catabolizes lipids in adipose tissue, is decreased *(36)*.

Elevated concentrations of plasma lipoproteins and free fatty acids have been implicated in the pathophysiology of preeclampsia and are associated with severity of the disease *(41–43)*. Hyperlipidemia may enhance endothelial cell dysfunction, perhaps by stimulation of oxidative stress in vessel walls *(44)*.

Serum Proteins

ALBUMIN

Albumin, the most abundant serum protein, is synthesized by the liver and accounts for two-thirds of total plasma protein content *(45)*. Albumin maintains plasma oncotic pressure and transports proteins, fatty acids, and steroids. Diverse acute and chronic disorders lead to hypoalbuminemia. Depressed albumin synthesis may occur in chronic liver disease, cirrhosis, malnutrition, malabsorption, and chronic debilitation. Decreased albumin concentrations also occur secondary to protein loss in patients with nephropathy or enteropathy *(45)*.

Serum albumin concentrations are decreased during pregnancy *(46–50)*. Albumin concentrations begin to decline early in pregnancy, and the decrease continues throughout gestation *(46,49)* (Fig. 3), with a rapid return to preconception concentrations in the puerperium *(46)*. This decline is attributed to the physiologic hemodilution of pregnancy *(46)*. Indeed, albumin mass in pregnant women is similar to that of controls *(49)*, and the rate of albumin synthesis and catabolism is unchanged during gestation *(49)*.

HORMONE-BINDING GLOBULINS

Sex hormone-binding globulin (SHBG) plays an important role in binding and transporting lipophilic steroid hormones in the blood, primarily testosterone and estrogen. During pregnancy, production of SHBG in the maternal liver is up-regulated beginning in the first trimester. This results in an increase in serum SHBG concentrations from a mean of 70 nmol/L early in pregnancy to a plateau late in the second trimester at a mean serum concentration of 392 nmol/L *(51)* (Fig. 4). Interestingly, reduced concentrations of SHBG are associated with hyperinsulinemia and insulin resistance in nonpregnant women. During pregnancy, reduced first-trimester SHBG was found to be associated with a higher incidence of preeclampsia *(52)*.

Similar to SHBG, corticosteroid-binding globulin (CBG) binds both progesterone and cortisol in the serum. Even though the two- to threefold increase in CBG concentration during pregnancy *(53)* diminishes the concentration of free hormones in the serum, the concentration of unbound progesterone and cortisol is still elevated during pregnancy. The concentration of thyroid-binding globulin is also elevated by two- to threefold during pregnancy, buffering the concentration of free thyroid hormone in the serum *(54)*. The increase in serum concentration of the three hormone-binding globulins is believed to be stimulated primarily by circulating estrogens.

α-1-ANTITRYPSIN

α-1-Antitrypsin is a plasma protease inhibitor, which neutralizes other serum proteases such as elastase. Rarely, hereditary deficiency of α-1-antitrypsin can lead to early-onset emphysema and cirrhosis. α-1-antitrypsin increases early in pregnancy and remains elevated throughout gestation (Fig. 5) *(48,49,55)*. In an evaluation of multiple serum

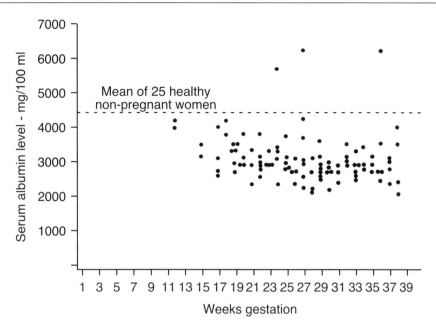

Fig. 3. Antepartum serum albumin concentrations ($n = 102$). (Reprinted with permission from Elsevier Science [49].)

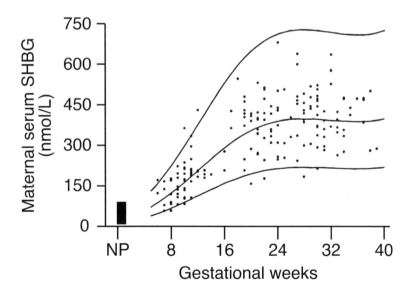

Fig. 4. Changes in maternal serum concentrations of SHBG during pregnancy. Nonpregnant (NP) reference interval for SHBG, 30–90 nmol/L, shown in shaded black area at the left. The mean curves are described by the equation for $\log(\text{SHBG}) = \exp(3.0751 - 0.6617 \times \text{week} + 0.0231 + \text{week}^2)$. (Reprinted with permission of the American Association for Clinical Chemistry [51].)

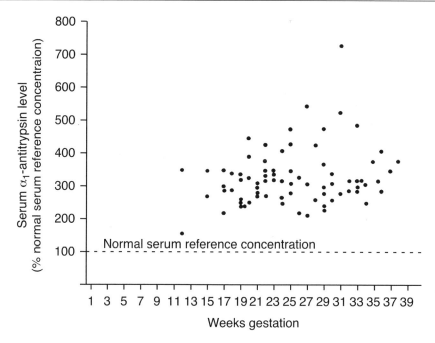

Fig. 5. Antepartum serum alpha$_1$-antitrypsin concentrations by gestational age ($n = 79$). (Reprinted with permission from Elsevier Science [49].)

proteins during pregnancy, Mendenhall et al. (49) noted that the rise in α-1-antitrypsin was greater than of any of the other proteins evaluated. A similar, but less dramatic increase in α-1-antitrypsin has been noted in users of estrogen-containing oral contraceptives, suggesting that estrogenic stimulation during pregnancy contributes to the gestational increase in serum concentrations of α-1-antitrypsin (50,56).

TRANSFERRIN

Transferrin is synthesized by the liver and transports ferric ions to the bone marrow for incorporation into erythrocytes. Transferrin is most commonly measured by assessing the total iron-binding capacity. Serum transferrin concentrations gradually increase during pregnancy (49). Interestingly, there is no increase in transferrin concentrations in women receiving estrogen-containing formulations (50,57).

CERULOPLASMIN

Ceruloplasmin is a copper-binding protein synthesized by the liver (45). The main clinical use of serum ceruloplasmin measurements is in the diagnosis of Wilson's disease (hepatolenticular degeneration), in which ceruloplasmin concentrations are depressed. Ceruloplasmin concentrations are elevated during pregnancy (48–50,58). As postulated for other hepatic proteins, administration of exogenous estrogens to women results in an increase in serum ceruloplasmin, thereby supporting a role for estrogen in that process (50,57,59,60).

HAPTOGLOBIN

Serum haptoglobin binds free hemoglobin from lysed erythrocytes. After binding hemoglobin, the haptoglobin–hemoglobin complex is rapidly taken up by the reticuloendothelial system. In a longitudinal study of normal pregnant women, Haram et al. demonstrated that haptoglobin exhibits a relative decrease during gestational weeks 24–27 *(48)*, although concentrations remain within nonpregnant references ranges *(48,57, 58,60)*.

IMMUNOGLOBULINS

In nonpregnant individuals, immunoglobins make up 20% of plasma proteins. During gestation, immunoglobulin concentrations decline slightly *(47,48,57)*, yet this decline does not exceed normal nonpregnant reference ranges *(48)*. A decrease in immunoglobulin concentration has been seen in women receiving synthetic estrogens, suggesting that the decrease during pregnancy may be estrogen mediated *(57)*.

C-REACTIVE PROTEIN

The serum protein C-reactive protein (CRP) is produced in response to a variety of inflammatory stimuli. CRP concentrations rise 4–6 h after an inflammatory insult and are used as a nonspecific marker of inflammation and tissue necrosis. CRP concentrations remain within normal limits in the majority of pregnant women *(48,58,61)*. In a longitudinal study of 81 gravid females, Watts et al. found that median CRP concentrations were higher in pregnancy, yet 74% of women sampled had blood CRP concentrations that were within the normal nonpregnant range. Interestingly, serum CRP concentrations tend to be higher during labor *(61)* and have been suggested as a marker for intra-amniotic infection *(62)*.

COMPLEMENT

The complement system is a group of serum proteins that play a role in the inflammatory response. More than 30 proteins are involved in the complement system. Complement activity is most commonly quantitated as total hemolytic complement (CH_{50}), which assesses the function of the entire complement system, as well as C3 and C4. During gestation, complement activity is mildly increased *(63–65)*. In serial measurements of CH_{50} throughout pregnancy, Baines et al. documented a small increase in CH_{50} activity from the midtrimester until term *(63)* (Fig. 6A). CH_{50} measurements rapidly decline during the peurperium *(64)*. C3 and C4 concentrations rise throughout pregnancy and are significantly elevated in the third trimester *(63,65)* (Fig. 6B).

The physiology of clotting factors, fibrinogen and endogenous anticoagulants during pregnancy is discussed in Chapter 10.

LABORATORY FINDINGS IN COMMON HEPATOBILIARY DISEASES DURING PREGNANCY

Preeclampsia, Eclampsia, and HELLP Syndrome

Preeclampsia, a most common obstetrical disease, as well as eclampsia and HELLP syndrome are discussed fully in Chapter 18.

AFLP

AFLP is a rare disorder that complicates 1 in 13,000–16,000 pregnancies *(12)*. AFLP usually occurs in the third trimester *(5,12,66)*. AFLP is more common in nulliparous women, as well as women with multifetal gestations *(12)*. AFLP is a life-threatening disorder, associated with an 18% maternal mortality and a 23% fetal mortality rate *(67)*.

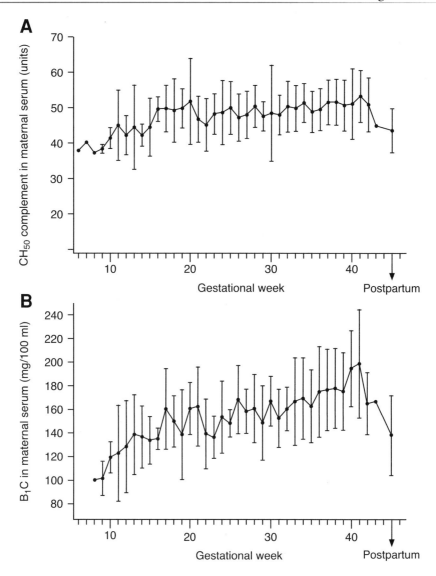

Fig. 6. (**A**) Total hemolytic complement (CH_{50}) concentrations (± 1 SD) by gestational age in normal pregnancies. (**B**) The concentration of B_1C, a component of the C3 complement, in maternal serum (mg/100 mL ± 1 SD) by gestational age in normal pregnancies. (Reprinted with permission from the American College of Obstetricians and Gynecologists *[63]*.)

The precise mechanism that leads to AFLP is unknown. Recent reports have linked fetal defects in the mitochondrial enzyme long chain 3-hydroxyl-acyl CoA dehydrogenase *(13,68–70)*. Heterozygosity for the enzyme defect in the mother is likely to play a role in the development of AFLP *(5)*. Histological examination of liver biopsies of women with AFLP typically reveals microvesicular fatty infiltration with displacement of central hepatocyte nuclei *(5)*. Electron microscopy reveals histological changes similar to those seen in Reye's syndrome *(68–70)*.

Pregnant women with AFLP initially present with malaise, nausea, vomiting, and weight loss *(5,12)*. Abdominal pain, hematemesis, and jaundice may accompany the initial symptoms. In contrast, pruritus is rare. Signs and symptoms of coexistent preeclampsia may also occur. Ascites may be present on physical examination, but hepatosplenomegaly is rare *(5)*. Complications of AFLP include fulminant hepatic failure, disseminated coagulopathy, hypoglycemia, pancreatitis, and terminally, encephalopathy and acute renal failure *(5,12)*. Less common complications include subcapsular hepatic hematomas, hepatic rupture, and fat emboli *(5)*.

Laboratory findings in patients with AFLP depend on the severity of the disease. The hallmark of AFLP is elevated concentrations of serum aminotransferases, although they usually remain less than 1000 U *(12,13)*, with AST typically higher than ALT. Serum AP exceeds the physiological increase during the third trimester of pregnancy *(5)*. Bilirubin may be markedly elevated *(5)*. Ammonia is elevated in 75% of patients, and creatinine and uric acid are abnormally increased in over 90% of patients *(71)*. Little data is available on either 5'-nucleotidase or GGT during the course of AFLP. Hematological abnormalities that indicate disseminated intravascular coagulation are common in women with AFLP, including elevated prothrombin time (PT) and partial thromboplastin times (PTT) *(12,71)*. Additionally, hypofibrinogenemia, low antithrombin III concentrations, and thrombocytopenia are common *(71)*. Other abnormalities include mild leukocytosis and hemolysis *(12)*. Laboratory findings from two series of pregnant women with AFLP are displayed in Table 1. Delivery is indicated for patients with AFLP and should be accompanied by aggressive supportive care for the mother. Platelet and clotting factor replacement should be undertaken to correct coagulopathy. A minority of survivors may exhibit persistent hepatic failure and benefit from liver transplantation *(12)*.

Intrahepatic Cholestasis of Pregnancy

Intrahepatic cholestasis of pregnancy (ICP) is a form of cholestatic jaundice that typically occurs in the third trimester of pregnancy *(72)*. The incidence of ICP is estimated at 0.5–1.0% of pregnancies, with a higher incidence in some countries, such as Chile and Scandinavia, suggesting a genetic predisposition *(5,73)*. The incidence of ICP is higher in families with progressive familiar intrahepatic cholestasis and associated with mutations in the multidrug resistance-3 gene (reviewed in Germain et al. *[73]*). ICP is more common in women with multiple gestations and in women of advanced maternal age *(72)*.

The etiology of ICP is incompletely understood. It is hypothesized that the pregnancy-related increase in estrogen concentration impairs biliary function *(5,72,74)*. This hypothesis is supported by the higher recurrence of ICP-like presentation when women who had this condition use estrogen-containing oral contraceptives. Decreased dehydro-epiandrosterone sulfate, a precursor for estriol, has also been implicated *(75)*. Abnormalities in progesterone metabolites have also been implicated in ICP *(13,72)*. Histological specimens reveal centrilobular cholestasis with accumulation of bile pigments in hepatocytes but without evidence of necrosis or inflammation.

The first symptom and commonly the hallmark of ICP is nocturnal pruritus, which begins on the palms and soles and progresses to the trunk and face *(72)*. Mild jaundice may follow pruritus, typically by 2 wk *(5)*. Right upper quadrant pain is less commonly observed. Although the disease is generally mild, a higher incidence of fetus-related complications has been attributed to ICP, including perinatal mortality, preterm delivery, and meconium-stained amniotic fluid *(72,76)*.

Table 1
Common Laboratory Findings in Women With Acute Fatty Liver of Pregnancy

| | Usta (71) (n = 14) | | Castro (100) (n = 28) |
	Mean (SD)	Abnormal (%)	Median (Range)
Creatinine (mg/dL)	2.4 (1.0)	100	2.5 (1.1–5.2)
Uric acid (mg/dL)	10.7 (1.0)	93	10.2 (6.3–20.4)
Platelets (10^3/mm^3)	126.0 (96)	64	113 (11–186)
Fibrinogen (mg/dL)	139.0 (79)	93	125 (32–446)
PT (sec)	19.5 (8.3)	86	NR
PT (% activity)	NR	—	36 (12–60)
PTT (sec)	50.6 (21.8)	79	98 (45–180)
AST (U/L)	1067.0 (1098)	100	210 (45–1200)
ALT (U/L)	NR	—	235 (20–1500)
Total bilirubin (mg/dL)	NR	—	8.6 (2.9–49.5)
Ammonia (μmol/L)	80.0 (91)	75	NR
Glucose (mg/dL)	61.0 (19)	71	45 (33–75)

NR, not reported; ALT, alanine aminotransferase; AST, aspartate aminotransferase; PT, prothrombin time; PTT, partial thromboplastin time; SD, standard deviation.

Diverse liver function abnormalities occur in women with ICP *(77)*. Mild elevations of the transaminases, typically less than 250 U, are common *(5,14,67)*. GGT, 5'-nucleotidase, and alkaline phosphatase may also be elevated *(13,72,78)*. Bilirubin is usually elevated with a predominance of the conjugated fraction *(13)*. The total bilirubin is typically less than 6 mg/dL *(72)*. These tests are useful primarily for excluding other causes of liver disease. The most sensitive and specific laboratory parameter for the evaluation of ICP is serum bile acid concentration *(72)*. Total serum bile acids may be elevated 10–25-fold during the course of ICP. An increase by 5-fold in chenodeoxycholic acid and 10-fold in cholic acid concentrations is found in women with ICP *(30)*. The most predictive bile acid profile of women with ICP includes a total bile acid concentration greater than 11.0 μmol, cholic to chenodeoxycholic acid ratio greater than 1.5, and glycine to taurine bile acid ratio less than 1.0 *(79)*.

Treatment of ICP is usually supportive. Symptomatic relief is frequently attempted with antihistamines or sedatives. Cholestyramine may be useful but is associated with malabsorption of fat-soluble vitamins. Ursodeoxycholic acid, in combination with S-adenosylmethionine, is a newer agent that has shown promise for the treatment of ICP *(72,80)*. Dexamethasone has also been tried but without clear benefit *(81)*. Importantly, there is no evidence that any of these approaches alter fetal outcome. ICP naturally disappears several days after delivery. The recurrence rate in subsequent pregnancies is typically 40–60% *(73)*.

Hyperemesis Gravidarum

Hyperemesis gravidarum is severe nausea, vomiting, and dehydration, frequently accompanied by weight loss, ketonuria, and electrolyte abnormalities. It usually occurs in the first and early second trimester. Mild elevations in the transaminases (< 250–300 U/L) and bilirubin (<4 mg/dL) are frequently observed *(5,82)*. Increased concentrations of serum cholesterol and HDL have also been reported in women with hyperemesis gravidarum when compared to controls *(83)*. Elevated human chorionic gonadotropin (hCG) concentrations are associated in women with hyperemesis gravidarum. Although hCG has a weak thyroid-stimulating hormone (TSH)-like activity, marked elevation may lead to suppression of TSH and erroneous diagnosis of hyperthyroidism. Elevations in the serum amylase concentration may also occur in women with severe vomiting *(82)*. Treatment requires aggressive hydration, prompt electrolyte replacement, and antiemetics.

Viral Hepatitis

Viral hepatitis during pregnancy may expose both the mother and fetus to substantial risk. The diagnosis of viral hepatitis relies on serologic confirmation, as performed for nonpregnant patients *(84)*. Acute hepatitis usually manifests as malaise, nausea, fatigue, anorexia, and abdominal pain. The most common physical finding is jaundice, which usually occurs several weeks after the development of subjective symptoms. Other physical findings include hepatomegaly, acholic stools and darkened urine. After initial infection, patients with hepatitis B, C, or D may progress to a chronic carrier state. One-third of chronic carriers will subsequently develop chronic active hepatitis, cirrhosis, or even end-stage liver disease *(85)*. The hallmark of acute hepatitis is an elevation of the transaminases. AST and ALT are generally more than 10–20 times the upper limit of normal. ALT is usually higher than AST. AP and LDH are often elevated but usually less dramatically than the transaminases. Total bilirubin, as well as the conjugated and unconjugated fractions of bilirubin, rise in patients with hepatitis. The elevation in bilirubin usually begins before the appearance of jaundice and then gradually declines. Additionally, 5'-nucleotidase and GGT are often elevated.

HEPATITIS A

Hepatitis A is caused by an RNA virus of the picornavirus family. Transmission of hepatitis A virus (HAV) is usually by fecal–oral contamination. The incubation period is 15–50 d. Viremia is usually short, and serious complications are uncommon. Perinatal transmission of HAV has not been demonstrated *(85,86)*.

Detection of hepatitis A relies on detection of HAV antibodies by radioimmunoassay or enzyme-linked immunosorbent assay (ELISA). Immunoglobulin M (IgM) antibodies coincide with development of symptoms, peak 3 to 4 wk after the onset of clinical disease, and resolve 3–4 mo afterward. The detection of HAV IgM indicates an acute HAV infection. HAV IgG appears 2–3 wk after IgM, remains elevated indefinitely, and provides immunity against future HAV infections *(21)*.

HEPATITIS B

Hepatitis B is caused by a DNA hepadenovirus. Acute hepatitis B accompanies 1–2/1000 pregnancies, whereas chronic hepatitis B is present in 5–15/1000 pregnancies *(87,88)*. Transmission of hepatitis B virus (HBV) is by parenteral and sexual contact *(85)*. After an acute infection, 10–15% of patients will become chronic carriers. Fifteen to 30% of chronic carriers demonstrate continued viral replication and are at risk for chronic active hepatitis, cirrhosis, and hepatocellular carcinoma *(89)*. HBV transmission may occur transplacentally, through exposure to contaminated blood or genital secretions at the time of delivery, or through breast-feeding. Transmission occurs in nearly 20% of pregnant women who are positive for hepatitis B surface antigen and is more common late in gestation *(85)*. The rate of fetal transmission of HBV is not proven to be influenced by the mode of delivery.

The laboratory evaluation of HBV relies on the detection of several antigens and antibodies. Three serum antigens and their corresponding antibodies are commonly determined: hepatitis B surface antigen (HBsAg), hepatitis B core antigen (HBcAg), and hepatitis B early antigen (HBeAg).

HBsAg is present on the outer surface of the HBV particle, appears 2–6 wk after exposure, and peaks around the time of onset of hepatitis symptoms. HBsAg can be detected by immunoassay or nucleic acid probe and is a marker for HBV activity. The antibody to HBsAg, hepatitis B surface antibody (HBsAb), appears 2–6 wk after the disappearance of HBsAg and persists indefinitely. HBsAb is a marker for immunity to HBV. Patients with chronic hepatitis remain positive for HBsAg in the absence of HBsAb. HBcAg is an antigen on the inner core of the HBV particle. The antibody to HBcAg, the hepatitis B core antibody (HBcAb), appears 3–4 wk after the appearance of HBsAg and remains elevated indefinitely. HBcAb IgM is usually present during acute infection. HBcAb IgG is present in chronic infection or after recovery. HBcAb may be the only positive serologic test during the interval when HBsAg has disappeared and HBsAb has not yet become detectable ("core window"). HBeAg is an antigen contained within the core of the HBV particle and appears 3–5 d after HBsAg and disappears while HBsAg is still detectable *(21)*. HBeAg is a marker for increased infectivity and approximately threefold increased fetal transmission. HBV DNA can also be measured in the serum and is a marker of active HBV replication.

HEPATITIS C

Hepatitis C is caused by an RNA virus from the flaviviridae family. Like hepatitis B, transmission of hepatitis C virus (HCV) occurs parenterally and through sexual contact. After initial infection, 50% of patients have persistence of HCV and 20% develop chronic hepatitis or cirrhosis *(85)*. Vertical transmission of HCV occurs in 7–8% of infected mothers *(90,91)*.

Laboratory detection of HCV relies on either antibody testing or viral load by polymerase chain reaction. Hepatitis C virus antibodies, measured by ELISA or recombinant immunoblot assay, are present in the serum 6–16 wk after the onset of symptoms. Antibody detection by ELISA is usually employed as a screening test and has sensitivity in excess of 95% but low specificity. HCV RNA may be detected 1 to 2 wk after the initial infection. Tests for HCV genotyping are also commercially available and useful in predicting treatment responsiveness *(92)*. Patients with chronic hepatitis C remain positive for HCV antibody.

Hepatitis G, an RNA virus disease, may occur as a coinfection with HCV. Transmission is bloodborne, and diagnosis rests on the documentation of hepatitis G antibody.

HEPATITIS D

Hepatitis D is caused by a defective RNA virus that requires the surface-antigen coat of hepatitis B virus for survival. Thus, hepatitis D virus (HDV) occurs only in patients who are infected with HBV *(93)*. Transmission of HDV occurs parenterally and through sexual contact. Patients who develop chronic hepatitis D typically have severe disease with hepatic failure and death in 25% of patients. Vertical transmission of HDV is uncommon *(85)*.

Assays for the measurement of hepatitis D antigen and antibodies are available. HDV antigen is detectable by immunoassay and nucleic acid probe. The window for the detection of HDV antigen is brief; the antigen appears shortly before symptoms from HDV infection and then rapidly declines. Immunoassays for HDV IgM and total HDV Ig are also available. HDV IgM appears 10 d after the onset of symptoms and becomes undetectable in 10–80 d. Total HDV Ig rises 50 d after the appearance of symptoms and becomes undetectable in 7 mo *(21)*. In patients with chronic HDV infection, HDV total antibody remains elevated and HDV IgM may be present in low titers. HDV antigen can be demonstrated in hepatocytes but is undetectable in the serum *(21)*.

HEPATITIS E

Hepatitis E is an RNA virus that is rare in the United States but endemic in several third-world countries. Transmission is enteric. Hepatitis E is self-limited and does not result in a carrier state. Mortality from hepatitis E infection during pregnancy is 10–18% in some third-world countries *(85,94)*. Laboratory documentation of hepatitis E requires identification of hepatitis E antibodies.

Chronic Liver Disease and Cirrhosis

Because amenorrhea and ovulatory dysfunction are common in women with chronic and end-stage liver diseases, these conditions are uncommon during pregnancy. The laboratory diagnosis and evaluation of chronic hepatic diseases in pregnant women is similar to that undertaken in nonpregnant patients. Wilson's disease results from the aberrant deposition of copper in multiple tissues. Its diagnosis rests on the measurement of serum ceruloplasmin and urinary copper. The physiologic increase in serum ceruloplasmin concentrations during pregnancy (discussed earlier) should be taken into account when interpreting ceruloplasmin concentrations. Hemochromatosis is characterized by excess iron absorption and deposition. A transferrin saturation of greater than 50% is commonly used for the detection of hemochromatosis. Autoimmune hepatitis and primary biliary cirrhosis have rarely been described in pregnancy *(45,95,96)*. Autoimmune hepatitis is usually accompanied by high titers of antismooth muscle antibodies, whereas patients with primary biliary cirrhosis often display elevated titers of antimitochondrial antibodies. The effect of pregnancy on antibody presence and titer is uncertain. The evaluation of porphyria during pregnancy is similar to that undertaken in nonpregnant individuals *(96)*.

Cirrhosis is the end result of diverse hepatocellular diseases, such as alcohol abuse, viral hepatitis, hemochromatosis, or biliary cirrhosis, and characterized by liver fibrosis and regenerative nodules. Complications from cirrhosis include portal hypertension with esophageal varices, coagulopathy, jaundice, ascites, and encephalopathy. Cirrhosis is commonly associated with amenorrhea and ovulatory dysfunction; however, successful pregnancies have been documented in a number of women *(5,97)*. When women with cirrhosis become pregnant, complications are relatively frequent and include gastrointestinal bleeding, worsening hepatic function, and even maternal death during gestation and the puerperium *(97)*. A wide variety of laboratory abnormalities depend on the severity of the underlying hepatic damage. Patients with early cirrhosis often have minimal laboratory changes. As cirrhosis progresses, the serum transaminases, GGT, AP, and bilirubin typically rise. Elevated prothrombin time and hypoalbuminemia characterize advanced-stage cirrhosis, and serum ammonia correlates with the degree of encephalopathy.

Cholelithiasis and Cholecystitis

More than 20% of women over the age of 40 in the United States have gallstones, the vast majority of which contain cholesterol *(66)*. Physiological changes in pregnancy enhance the formation of biliary sludge, alter bile acid composition, and decrease gallbladder contractility, thus predisposing women to the development of symptomatic cholelithiasis *(7,98)*. Symptoms of cholelithiasis include fatty-food intolerance, dyspepsia, and right upper quadrant and epigastric pain *(7)*. The symptoms of biliary colic are usually episodic. The diagnosis of cholelithiasis rests on the demonstration of gallstones by ultrasonography. Patients with biliary obstruction typically have markedly elevated concentrations of AP and bilirubin. Seventy-five percent of the total bilirubin is usually conjugated. AST and ALT are usually only minimally elevated *(21)*. Prolonged biliary obstruction will result in progressive elevation of the aminotransferases, reflecting hepatocellular damage *(21)*. Patients with cholelithiasis and episodic biliary colic are treated symptomatically, with more intensive medical or surgical management if symptoms are unremitting or if acute cholecystitis develops.

The distinction between acute cholecystitis and biliary colic from cholelithiasis is not always clear. Pregnant women with cholecystitis exhibit severe pain accompanied by nausea, vomiting, and fever *(7)*. In addition to the laboratory findings of cholelithiasis, patients with cholecystitis often display leukocytosis with a left shift. Treatment of cholecystitis is either medical, with analgesia, bowel rest, hydration, and antibiotics, or surgical, by cholecystectomy. This procedure can be performed during pregnancy if the disease is severe or recurrent, or performed postpartum *(66,67,99)*.

REFERENCES

1. Ingerslev M, Teilum B. Biopsy studies on the liver in pregnancy. II. Liver biopsy on normal pregnant women. Acta Obstet Gynecol Scand 1945;25:352–359.
2. Robson SC, Mutch E, Boys RJ, Woodhouse KW. Apparent liver blood flow during pregnancy: a serial study using indocyanine green clearance. Br J Obstet Gynaecol 1990;97:720–724.
3. Munnell EW, Taylor HC. Liver blood flow in pregnancy: hepatic vein catheterization. J Clin Invest 1947;26:952–956.
4. Van Thiel DH, Gavaler JS. Pregnancy-associated sex steroids and their effects on the liver. Semin Liver Dis 1987;7:1–7.
5. Burroughs AK. Liver disease and pregnancy. In: Bircher J, Benhamou JP, McIntyre N, Rizzetto M, Rodes J, eds. Oxford Textbook of Clinical Hepatology. Vol. 2. Oxford: Oxford University Press, 1999, pp. 1901–1912.
6. Braverman DZ, Johnson ML, Kern F Jr. Effects of pregnancy and contraceptive steroids on gallbladder function. N Engl J Med 1980;302:362–364.
7. Scott LD. Gallstone disease and pancreatitis in pregnancy. Gastroenterol Clin North Am 1992;21:803–815.
8. Knopp RH, Bergelin RO, Wahl PW, Walden CE, Chapman MB. Clinical chemistry alterations in pregnancy and oral contraceptive use. Obstet Gynecol 1985;66:682–690.
9. Bacq Y, Zarka O, Brechot JF, et al. Liver function tests in normal pregnancy: a prospective study of 103 pregnant women and 103 matched controls. Hepatology 1996;23:1030–1034.
10. Girling JC, Dow E, Smith JH. Liver function tests in pre-eclampsia: importance of comparison with a reference range derived for normal pregnancy. Br J Obstet Gynaecol 1997;104:246–250.
11. Carter J. Liver function in normal pregnancy. Aust N Z J Obstet Gynaecol 1990;30:296–302.
12. Riely CA. Acute fatty liver of pregnancy. Semin Liver Dis 1987;7:47–54.
13. Riely CA. Liver disease in the pregnant patient. Am J Gastroenterol 1999;94:1728–1732.
14. McDonald JA. Cholestasis of pregnancy. J Gastroenterol Hepatol 1999;14:515–518.
15. Chopra S, Griffin PH. Laboratory tests and diagnostic procedures in evaluation of liver disease. Am J Med 1985;79:221–230.
16. Fishman WH. Perspectives on alkaline phosphatase isoenzymes. Am J Med 1974;56:617–650.
17. Wetstone HJ, LaMotta RV, Middlebrook L, Tennant R, White BV. Studies of cholinesterase activity. IV. Liver function in pregnancy: values of certain standard liver function tests in normal pregnancy. Am J Obstet Gynecol 1958;76:480–490.

18. Seitanidis B, Moss DW. Serum alkaline phosphatase and 5'-nucleotidase levels during normal pregnancy. Clin Chim Acta 1969;25:183–184.
19. Adeniyi FA, Olatunbosun DA. Origins and significance of the increased plasma alkaline phosphatase during normal pregnancy and pre-eclampsia. Br J Obstet Gynaecol 1984;91:857–862.
20. McNair RD, Jaynes RV. Alterations in liver function during normal pregnancy. Am J Obstet Gynecol 1960;80:500–505.
21. Ravel R. Clinical laboratory medicine: clinical application of laboratory data. St. Louis: Mosby, 1995, pp. 1–688.
22. Valenzuela GJ, Munson LA, Tarbaux NM, Farley JR. Time-dependent changes in bone, placental, intestinal, and hepatic alkaline phosphatase activities in serum during human pregnancy. Clin Chem 1987;33:1801–1806.
23. Rodin A, Duncan A, Quartero HW, et al. Serum concentrations of alkaline phosphatase isoenzymes and osteocalcin in normal pregnancy. J Clin Endocrinol Metab 1989;68:1123–1127.
24. Walker FBt, Hoblit DL, Cunningham FG, Combes B. Gamma glutamyl transpeptidase in normal pregnancy. Obstet Gynecol 1974;43:745–749.
25. Alvi MH, Amer NA, Sumerin I. Serum 5-nucleotidase and serum sialic acid in pregnancy. Obstet Gynecol 1988;72:171–174.
26. Tsoi SC, Zheng J, Xu F, Kay HH. Differential expression of lactate dehydrogenase isozymes (LDH) in human placenta with high expression of LDH-A(4) isozyme in the endothelial cells of pre-eclampsia villi. Placenta 2001;22:317–322.
27. Shukla PK, Sharma D, Mandal RK. Serum lactate dehydrogenase in detecting liver damage associated with pre-eclampsia. Br J Obstet Gynaecol 1978;85:40–42.
28. Magann EF, Martin JN Jr. The laboratory evaluation of hypertensive gravidas. Obstet Gynecol Surv 1995;50:138–145.
29. Carter J. Serum bile acids in normal pregnancy. Br J Obstet Gynaecol 1991;98:540–543.
30. Heikkinen J, Maentausta O, Ylostalo P, Janne O. Changes in serum bile acid concentrations during normal pregnancy, in patients with intrahepatic cholestasis of pregnancy and in pregnant women with itching. Br J Obstet Gynaecol 1981;88:240–245.
31. Lunzer M, Barnes P, Byth K, O'Halloran M. Serum bile acid concentrations during pregnancy and their relationship to obstetric cholestasis. Gastroenterology 1986;91:825–829.
32. Walker IA, Nelson-Piercy C, Williamson C. Role of bile acid measurement in pregnancy. Ann Clin Biochem 2002;39:105–113.
33. NCEP. Executive summary of the third report of the National Cholesterol Education Program (NCEP) expert panel on detection, evaluation, and treatment of high blood cholesterol in adults (Adult Treatment Panel III). Jama 2001;285:2486–2497.
34. Knopp RH, Bergelin RO, Wahl PW, Walden CE, Chapman M, Irvine S. Population-based lipoprotein lipid reference values for pregnant women compared to nonpregnant women classified by sex hormone usage. Am J Obstet Gynecol 1982;143:626–637.
35. Darmady JM, Postle AD. Lipid metabolism in pregnancy. Br J Obstet Gynaecol 1982;89:211–215.
36. Brizzi P, Tonolo G, Esposito F, et al. Lipoprotein metabolism during normal pregnancy. Am J Obstet Gynecol 1999;181:430–434.
37. Svanborg A, Vikrot O. Plasma lipid fractions, including individual phospholipids, at various stages of pregnancy. Acta Med Scand 1965;178:615–630.
38. Desoye G, Schweditsch MO, Pfeiffer KP, Zechner R, Kostner GM. Correlation of hormones with lipid and lipoprotein levels during normal pregnancy and postpartum. J Clin Endocrinol Metab 1987;64:704–712.
39. Knopp RH, Warth MR, Carrol CJ. Lipid metabolism in pregnancy. I. Changes in lipoprotein triglyceride and cholesterol in normal pregnancy and the effects of diabetes mellitus. J Reprod Med 1973;10:95–101.
40. Feingold KR, Wiley T, Moser AH, Lear SR, Wiley MH. De novo cholesterogenesis in pregnancy. J Lab Clin Med 1983;101:256–263.
41. Wang J, Mimuro S, Lahoud R, Trudinger B, Wang XL. Elevated levels of lipoprotein(a) in women with preeclampsia. Am J Obstet Gynecol 1998;178:146–149.
42. Hubel CA, McLaughlin MK, Evans RW, Hauth BA, Sims CJ, Roberts JM. Fasting serum triglycerides, free fatty acids, and malondialdehyde are increased in preeclampsia, are positively correlated, and decrease within 48 hours post partum. Am J Obstet Gynecol 1996;174:975–982.

43. Endresen MJ, Lorentzen B, Henriksen T. Increased lipolytic activity and high ratio of free fatty acids to albumin in sera from women with preeclampsia leads to triglyceride accumulation in cultured endothelial cells. Am J Obstet Gynecol 1992;167:440–447.

44. Lorentzen B, Henriksen T. Plasma lipids and vascular dysfunction in preeclampsia. Semin Reprod Endocrinol 1998;16:33–39.

45. Pincus MR, Schaffner JA. Assessment of liver function. In: Henry JB, ed. Clinical Diagnosis and Management by Laboratory Methods. Philadelphia: W.B. Saunders, 1996, pp. 253–267.

46. Esbjorner E, Jarnerot G, Sandstrom B, Ostling G. Serum albumin reserve for bilirubin binding during pregnancy in healthy women. Obstet Gynecol 1989;73:93–96.

47. Reboud P, Groulade J, Groslambert P, Colomb M. The influence of normal pregnancy and the postpartum state on plasma proteins and lipids. Am J Obstet Gynecol 1963;86:820–828.

48. Haram K, Augensen K, Elsayed S. Serum protein pattern in normal pregnancy with special reference to acute-phase reactants. Br J Obstet Gynaecol 1983;90:139–145.

49. Mendenhall HW. Serum protein concentrations in pregnancy. I. Concentrations in maternal serum. Am J Obstet Gynecol 1970;106:388–399.

50. Mendenhall HW. Effect of oral contraceptives on serum protein concentrations. Am J Obstet Gynecol 1970;106:750–753.

51. O'Leary P, Boyne P, Flett P, Beilby J, James I. Longitudinal assessment of changes in reproductive hormones during normal pregnancy. Clin Chem 1991;37:667–672.

52. Wolf M, Sandler L, Munoz K, Hsu K, Ecker JL, Thadhani R. First trimester insulin resistance and subsequent preeclampsia: a prospective study. J Clin Endocrinol Metab 2002;87:1563–1568.

53. Nolten WE, Lindheimer MD, Rueckert PA, Oparil S, Ehrlich EN. Diurnal patterns and regulation of cortisol secretion in pregnancy. J Clin Endocrinol Metab 1980;51:466–472.

54. Burrow GN, Fisher DA, Larsen PR. Maternal and fetal thyroid function. N Engl J Med 1994;331:1072–1078.

55. Ganrot PO, Bjerre B. α_1-antitrypsin and α_2-macroglobulin concentration in serum during pregnancy. Acta Obstet Gynecol Scand 1967;46:126–137.

56. Robertson GS. Serum protein and cholinesterase changes in association with contraceptive pills. Lancet 1967;1:232–235.

57. Musa BU, Doe RP, Seal US. Serum protein alterations produced in women by synthetic estrogens. J Clin Endocrinol Metab 1967;27:1463–1469.

58. Kuvibidila S, Warrier RP, Yu L, Ode D, Mbele V. Reference levels of acute phase reactant proteins in healthy Zairean women in the reproductive age group. J Trop Med Hyg 1994;97:239–243.

59. Musa BU, Seal US, Doe RP. Elevation of certain plasma proteins in man following estrogen administration: a dose–response relationship. J Clin Endocrinol Metab 1965;25:1163–1166.

60. Doe RP, Mellinger GT, Swaim WR, Seal US. Estrogen dosage effects on serum proteins: a longitudinal study. J Clin Endocrinol 1967;27:1081–1086.

61. Watts DH, Krohn MA, Wener MH, Eschenbach DA. C-reactive protein in normal pregnancy. Obstet Gynecol 1991;77:176–180.

62. Asrat T. Intra-amniotic infection in patients with preterm prelabor rupture of membranes: pathophysiology, detection, and management. Clin Perinatol 2001;28:735–751.

63. Baines MG, Millar KG, Mills P. Studies of complement levels in normal human pregnancy. Obstet Gynecol 1974;43:806–810.

64. Kitzmiller JL, Stoneburner L, Yelenosky PF, Lucas WE. Serum complement in normal pregnancy and pre-eclampsia. Am J Obstet Gynecol 1973;117:312–315.

65. Gallery ED, Raftos J, Gyory AZ, Wells JV. A prospective study of serum complement (C3 and C4) levels in normal human pregnancy: effect of the development of pregnancy-associated hypertension. Aust N Z J Med 1981;11:243–245.

66. Cunningham FG, Gant NF, Leveno KJ, Gilstrap LC III, Hauth JC, Wenstrom KD. Gastrointestinal disorders. Williams Obstetrics. New York: McGraw Hill, 2001, pp. 1273–1306.

67. Hunt CM, Sharara AI. Liver disease in pregnancy. Am Fam Physician 1999;59:829–836.

68. Ibdah JA, Bennett MJ, Rinaldo P, et al. A fetal fatty-acid oxidation disorder as a cause of liver disease in pregnant women. N Engl J Med 1999;340:1723–1731.

69. Sims HF, Brackett JC, Powell CK, et al. The molecular basis of pediatric long chain 3-hydroxyacyl-CoA dehydrogenase deficiency associated with maternal acute fatty liver of pregnancy. Proc Natl Acad Sci USA 1995;92:841–845.

70. Strauss AW, Powell CK, Hale DE, et al. Molecular basis of human mitochondrial very-long-chain acyl-CoA dehydrogenase deficiency causing cardiomyopathy and sudden death in childhood. Proc Natl Acad Sci USA 1995;92:10496–10500.

71. Usta IM, Barton JR, Amon EA, Gonzalez A, Sibai BM. Acute fatty liver of pregnancy: an experience in the diagnosis and management of fourteen cases. Am J Obstet Gynecol 1994;171:1342–1347.

72. Mullally BA, Hansen WF. Intrahepatic cholestasis of pregnancy: review of the literature. Obstet Gynecol Surv 2002;57:47–52.

73. Germain AM, Carvajal JA, Glasinovic JC, Kato CS, Williamson C. Intrahepatic cholestasis of pregnancy: an intriguing pregnancy-specific disorder. J Soc Gynecol Investig 2002;9:10–14.

74. Schreiber AJ, Simon FR. Estrogen-induced cholestasis: clues to pathogenesis and treatment. Hepatology 1983;3:607–613.

75. Leslie KK, Reznikov L, Simon FR, Fennessey PV, Reyes H, Ribalta J. Estrogens in intrahepatic cholestasis of pregnancy. Obstet Gynecol 2000;95:372–376.

76. Alsulyman OM, Ouzounian JG, Ames-Castro M, Goodwin TM. Intrahepatic cholestasis of pregnancy: perinatal outcome associated with expectant management. Am J Obstet Gynecol 1996;175:957–960.

77. Reyes H. Review: intrahepatic cholestasis: a puzzling disorder of pregnancy. J Gastroenterol Hepatol 1997;12:211–216.

78. Berg B, Helm G, Petersohn L, Tryding N. Cholestasis of pregnancy: clinical and laboratory studies. Acta Obstet Gynecol Scand 1986;65:107–113.

79. Brites D, Rodrigues CM, van-Zeller H, Brito A, Silva R. Relevance of serum bile acid profile in the diagnosis of intrahepatic cholestasis of pregnancy in a high incidence area: Portugal. Eur J Obstet Gynecol Reprod Biol 1998;80:31–38.

80. Nicastri PL, Diaferia A, Tartagni M, Loizzi P, Fanelli M. A randomised placebo-controlled trial of ursodeoxycholic acid and S-adenosylmethionine in the treatment of intrahepatic cholestasis of pregnancy. Br J Obstet Gynaecol 1998;105:1205–1207.

81. Hirvioja ML, Tuimala R, Vuori J. The treatment of intrahepatic cholestasis of pregnancy by dexamethasone. Br J Obstet Gynaecol 1992;99:109–111.

82. Herbert WNP, Goodwin TM, Koren G, Phelan ST. Nausea and vomiting of pregnancy. APGO Educational Series on Women's Health Issues. Washington, DC: Association of Professors of Gynecology and Obstetrics (APGO), 2001, pp. 1–28.

83. Abell TL, Riely CA. Hyperemesis gravidarum. Gastroenterol Clin North Am 1992;21:835–849.

84. Mishra L, Seeff LB. Viral hepatitis, A though E, complicating pregnancy. Gastroenterol Clin North Am 1992;21:873–887.

85. American College of Obstetricians and Gynecologists (ACOG). ACOG Educational Bulletin 248 (1998): viral hepatitis in pregnancy. In: ACOG 2002 Compendium of Selected Publications. Washington, DC: American College of Obstetricians and Gynecologists, 2002, pp. 240–246.

86. CDC. Protection against viral hepatitis: recommendations of the Immunizations Practices Advisory Committee (ACIP). Morb Mort Wkly Rep 1990;39(RR-2):1–26.

87. Sweet RL. Hepatitis B infection in pregnancy. Obstet Gynecol Report 1990;2:128–139.

88. Snydman DR. Hepatitis in pregnancy. N Engl J Med 1985;313:1398–1401.

89. Hoofnagle JH. Chronic hepatitis B. N Engl J Med 1990;323:337–339.

90. Ohto H, Terazawa S, Sasaki N, et al. for the Vertical Transmission of Hepatitis C Virus Collaborative Study Group. Transmission of hepatitis C virus from mothers to infants. N Engl J Med 1994;330:744–750.

91. Silverman NS, Snyder M, Hodinka RL, McGillen P, Knee G. Detection of hepatitis C virus antibodies and specific hepatitis C virus ribonucleic acid sequences in cord bloods from a heterogeneous prenatal population. Am J Obstet Gynecol 1995;173:1396–1400.

92. Satyanarayana R, Lisker-Melman M. Liver diseases. In: Ahya SN, Flood K, Paranjothi S, Schaiff RA, eds. The Washington Manual of Medical Therapeutics. Philadelphia: Lippincott, Williams & Wilkins, 2001.

93. Hoofnagle JH. Type D (delta) hepatitis. JAMA 1989;261:1321–1325 [erratum in JAMA 1989; 261:3552].

94. Bradley DW, Maynard JE. Etiology and natural history of post-transfusion and enterically-transmitted non-A, non-B hepatitis. Semin Liver Dis 1986;6:56–66.

95. Heneghan MA, Norris SM, O'Grady JG, Harrison PM, McFarlane IG. Management and outcome of pregnancy in autoimmune hepatitis. Gut 2001;48:97–102.

96. Lee WM. Pregnancy in patients with chronic liver disease. Gastroenterol Clin North Am 1992;21:889–903.

97. Schreyer P, Caspi E, El-Hindi JM, Eshchar J. Cirrhosis–pregnancy and delivery: a review. Obstet Gynecol Surv 1982;37:304–312.

98. Valdivieso V, Covarrubias C, Siegel F, Cruz F. Pregnancy and cholelithiasis: pathogenesis and natural course of gallstones diagnosed in early puerperium. Hepatology 1993;17:1–4.

99. Davis A, Katz VL, Cox R. Gallbladder disease in pregnancy. J Reprod Med 1995;40:759–762.

100. Castro MA, Goodwin TM, Shaw KJ, Ouzounian JG, McGehee WG. Disseminated intravascular coagulation and antithrombin III depression in acute fatty liver of pregnancy. Am J Obstet Gynecol 1996;174:211–216.

Appendix

Published Reference Intervals
During Pregnancy

From: *Current Clinical Pathology: Handbook of Clinical Laboratory Testing During Pregnancy*
Edited by: A. M. Gronowski © Humana Press, Totowa, NJ

Table 1
Explanation of Appendix Reference Intervals

Other refs	Ref	Specimen type	Units	1st trim	n	2nd trim	n	3rd trim	n	Meth[1]	Nonpreg	n	Meth[1]
Other useful references	Source of given ref interval	Analyte	units	Reference interval Pregnant mean + nonpregnant mean*	Pregnancy weeks	Reference interval Pregnant mean + nonpregnant mean*	Pregnancy weeks	Reference interval Pregnant mean + nonpregnant mean*	Pregnancy weeks	Method for ref interval calculation. See list at end of table.	Ref interval for nonpreg controls	n	Method for nonpreg ref interval calculation. See list at end of each table.

[1]Methods for Reference Range Calculations.
A, Mean ± 2SD.
B, Central 95%.
C, Range.
*Indicates mean preg value ÷ mean nonpregnant value.

Note. Reference intervals are method- and laboratory-specific. Caution should be used in applying published reference intervals to patients tested using different assays in different laboratories. Each laboratory should establish its own reference intervals.

Table 2
Published Reference Intervals for Serum During Pregnancy

Other refs	Ref	Serum	Units		1st trim	n		2nd trim	n		3rd trim	n	Meth[1]	Nonpreg	n	Meth[1]
(1,2)	(3)	α-1 antitrypsin	g/L	12 wk	1.76–3.72 129*	29	24 wk	2.14–4.50 154*	29	36 wk	2.47–5.67 189*	29	A	1.35–3.10	121	B
(3–6)	(7)	α-fetoprotein	ng/mL	1st trim	18–119	22	2nd trim	96–302	10	3rd trim	160–550	18	C			
	(3)	α-tocopherol	µmol/L	12 wk	10–38 100	29	24 wk	19–43 129	29	36 wk	17–65 171	29	A	16–37	121	B
	(3)	α-tocopherol: cholesterol ratio		12 wk	2.6–8.3 104	29	24 wk	3.3–7.6 104	29	36 wk	1.8–10.4 117	29	A	3.8–7.1	121	B
	(3)	Activated partial thromboplastin time	s	12 wk	24.6–34.2 95	29	24 wk	25.0–31.7 91	29	36 wk	23.9–33.0 92	29	A	26.6–35.5	121	B
(8–11)	(3)	Alanine amino-transferase (ALT)	U/L	12 wk	4–28 89	29	24 wk	4–28 89	29	36 wk	0–28 78	29	A	5–29	121	B
(2,9–17)	(3)	Albumin	g/L	12 wk	33–43 93	29	24 wk	29–37 80	29	36 wk	28–36 78	28	A	36–46	121	B
	(19)	Aldosterone	fmol/mL							3rd trim	1095–2488 400	83	E	256–599	80	E
(9,10,12–15,20–22)	(3)	Alkaline phosphatase, total	U/L	12 wk	22–91 90	29	24 wk	33–97 105	29	36 wk	73–267 274	29	A	38–98	121	B
(21)	(20)	Alkaline phosphatase, bone	U/L	10–12 wk	1.3–6.1 160	11	18–20 wk	1.7–10.5 270	11	32–34 wk	4.4–10.8 330	16	A	0–4.7	12	A
(21)	(20)	Alkaline phosphatase, hepatic	U/L	10–12 wk	0.9–5.3 82	11	18–20 wk	0–7.3 55	11	32–34 wk	0–7 47	16	A	0.4–7.2	12	A
(21)	(20)	Alkaline phosphatase, intestinal	U/L	10–12 wk	0–1.8 24	11	18–20 wk	0.1–1.7 27	11	32–34 wk	0–1.5 15	16	A	0–8.1	12	A
(21)	(20)	Alkaline phosphatase,	U/L	10–12 wk	0–0.3	11	18–20 wk	0–6.6	11	32–34 wk	0.4–20	16	A	0	12	A
	(3)	Amylase	U/L	12 wk	11–97 108	29	24 wk	19–92 110	29	36 wk	27–97 124	29	A	27–82	121	B
(23)		Androstenedione	nmol/L	5 wk	3.5–18.8	60				40 wk	4.6–24.5	60	B	3–10		NI
	(3)	Anion Gap	mmol/L	12 wk	10–20 115	29	24 wk	10–18 108	29	36 wk	11–18 108	29	A	10–17	121	B
(24)	(25)	Apo-A-1	g/L	0–8 wk	1.19–2.01	39	17–24 wk	1.44–2.47	34	33–40 wk	1.47–2.66	44	C			

Reference	Analyte	Units	Period 1	Period 2	Period 3	n	Grade	Pooled interval	n	Grade
(24)	Apo B	g/L	0–8 wk: 0.52–1.34 (39)	17–24 wk: 0.98–1.85 (34)	33–40 wk: 1.02–2.06 (44)		C			
(25)(26)	Arginine vasopressin (AVP)	pg/mL			32–34 wk: 0.27–2.51 (111)	8	A	0.01–2.49	8	A
(8–11,14,15,22)	Aspartate aminotransferase (AST)	U/L	12 wk: 4–30 (85)	24 wk: 1–32 (80)	36 wk: 2–37 (100)	29	A	9–32	121	B
(12)	Bicarbonate	mmol/L	12 wk: 18–26 (85)	24 wk: 18–26 (85)	36 wk: 18–26 (85)	29	A	22–29	121	B
(27)	Bile acid	µmol/L	20 wk: 2.3–7.9 (50)		36 wk: 2.7–8.7 (48)		A			
(8,10,11,14,15)	Bilirubin (total)	µmol/L	1st trim: 1–13 (70)	2nd trim: 1–9 (61)	3rd trim: 1–7 (47)	33	C	2–20	103	C
(9)	Bilirubin (conjugated)	µmol/L	1st trim: 0–2 (63)	2nd trim: 0–2 (50)	3rd trim: 0–1 (38)	33	C	0–3	103	C
(9,12)	Bilirubin (unconjugated)	µmol/L	12 wk: 0–11 (56)	24 wk: 0–9 (56)	36 wk: 3–10 (67)	29	A	4–20	121	B
(12)	Blood Urea Nitrogen	mg/dL		25 wk: 6.1–12.1 (10)	37 wk: 5.4–15.8	25	A			
(11,13,14,22,28–30)	Calcium (total)	mmol/L	12 wk: 2.12–2.44 (98)	24 wk: 2.04–2.36 (95)	36 wk: 2.05–2.37 (95)	29	A	2.17–2.43	121	B
(11,28–30)	Calcium (ionized)	mmol/L	12 wk: 1.13–1.33 (99)	24 wk: 1.13–1.29 (98)	36 wk: 1.14–1.38 (102)	29	A	1.1–1.36	121	B
(31)	CA 125	kIU/L	6–9 wk: 7.95–17.7 (2)	20–24 wk: 6.5–54.3 (14)	35–40 wk: 6.2–49.3 (20)	20	C	<40	100	D
(31)	CA 15-3	kIU/L	6–9 wk: 12.2–14.3 (2)	20–24 wk: 10.0–22.8 (14)	35–40 wk: 5.1–27.0 (20)	20	C	<30	100	C
(31)	CEA	µg/L	6–9 wk: 1.4–2.4 (2)	20–24 wk: 0.6–2.8 (14)	35–40 wk: 0.7–3.3 (20)	20	C	<3	100	B
(1,2)	Ceruloplasmin	mg/L	12 wk: 205–586 (157)	24 wk: 342–586 (184)	36 wk: 360–624 (195)	29	A	198–340	121	B
(10,12,32)	Chloride	mmol/L	12 wk: 99–108 (98)	24 wk: 100–107 (99)	36 wk: 100–108 (99)	29	A	101–108	121	B
(12,24,25,33)	Cholesterol (total)	mmol/L	12 wk: 3.02–5.94 (100)	24 wk: 3.91–7.47 (127)	36 wk: 4.71–8.55 (148)	29	A	3.13–6.87	121	B
(34)	Cholic acid	µmol/L	20 wk: 0–1.47 (25)		36 wk: 0–1.12	29	A			
(4,35–41)	Chorionic gonadotropin (hCG)	IU/mL	8–11 wk: 59–161 (8)	20–23 wk: 2.2–45.2 (8)	36–39 wk: 3.9–43.5 (8)	8	A			
(3)	Colloid osmotic pressure	cm H$_2$O	12 wk: 19–31 (93)	24 wk: 19–27 (85)	36 wk: 19–27	29	A	22–33	121	B
(3)	Complement C3	g/L	12 wk: 0.44–1.16 (112)	24 wk: 0.58–1.18 (124)	36 wk: 0.60–1.26 (132)	29	A	0.47–0.92	121	B
(3)	Complement C4	g/L	12 wk: 0.09–0.45 (108)	24 wk: 0.10–0.42 (104)	36 wk: 0.17–0.37 (108)	29	A	0.14–0.41	121	B
(3)	Copper	µmol/L	12 wk: 10.8–37.9 (158)	24 wk: 21.8–38.4 (195)	36 wk: 22.0–43.0 (211)	29	A	11.7–20.5	121	B

continued

Table 2 (continued)

Other refs	Ref	Serum	Units	1st trim	n	2nd trim	n	3rd trim	n	Meth[1]	Nonpreg	n	Meth.
	(3)	Cortisol	nmol/L	12 wk 205–632 111	29	24 wk 391–1407 238	29	36 wk 543–1663 292	29	A	110–580	121	B
(12)	(3)	Creatine kinase	U/L	12 wk 0–111 87	29	24 wk 0–100 79	29	36 wk 0–145 90	29	A	20–137	121	B
(10,12,14, 15,22,42)	(3)	Creatinine	µmol/L	12 wk 25–79 71	29	24 wk 25–74 68	29	36 wk 23–93 79	29	A	50–90	121	B
	(43)	Cystatin C	mg/L					3rd trim 0.79–1.47 128	14	A	0.66–1.1	12	A
	(23)	DHEAS	µmol/L	5 wk 2.0–16.5	60	20 wk 0.9–7.8	60	40 wk 0.8–6.5	60	B	3.4–8.6		NI
	(44)	Deoxycorti- costerone (DOC)	pg/mL	10–14 wk 168–300 209	44	23–26 wk 48–308 694	44	39–42 wk 999–1619 1169	44	A	72–152		A
	(3)	Erythrocyte Count	× 10 12/L	12 wk 3.21–4.89 94	29	24 wk 3.20–4.28 86	29	36 wk 3.35–4.67 93	29	A	3.72–4.98	121	B
(45)	(46)	Erythropoietin	U/L	14–18 wk 10.4–46 100	57	23–26 wk 12.2–97 114	57	39–43 wk 14.7–222 156	57	C	15–30		NI
(35,47)	(23) (4)	Estradiol Estriol (unconjugated)	nmol/L ng/mL	5 wk 0.69–3.88	60	16 wk 11.13–26.40 20 wk 1.85	60 168	40 wk 22.53–127	60	B G	0.37–0.77		NI
	(48)	Factor VII	% of normal	11–15 wk 60–206 118	41	21–25 wk 80–280 160	47	36–40 wk 87–336 182	48	C	52–171	61	C
(49)	(48)	Factor X	% of normal	11–15 wk 62–169 114	41	21–25 wk 74–177 128	47	36–40 wk 72–208 141	48	C	54–149	61	C
	(49)	Factor XI	% of normal	15 wk 47–139 99	8			38 wk 48–80 68	7	A	64–124	20	A
	(48)	Factor V	% of normal	11–15 wk 46–188 115	41	21–25 wk 36–185 101	47	36–40 wk 39–184 105	48	C	42–155	61	C
	(48)	Factor II	% of normal	11–15 wk 70–224 118	41	21–25 wk 73–214 118	47	36–40 wk 68–194 108	48	C	68–165	61	C
	(48)	Factor III:C	% of normal	11–15 wk 53–283 128	41	21–25 wk 44–453 148	47	36–40 wk 79–570 223	48	C	46–193	61	C
(10,46, 50,51)	(3)	Ferritin	µg/L	12 wk 0–45 81	29	24 wk 0–24 37	29	36 wk 0–22 37	29	A	4–63	121	B
	(17,48)	Fibrinogen	g/L	12 wk 1.60–4.96 119	29	24 wk 2.22–4.98 131	29	36 wk 3.13–5.53 157	29	A	1.76–3.64	121	B
(52)	(53)	Folate, plasma	nmol/L	1st trim 2.7–24.3 113	38	2nd trim 1.2–22.8 100	37	3rd trim 0–29.6 103	25	A	4–20	20	A

Ref	Test	Units	1st trim (wk)	n	1st interval (obs)	2nd trim (wk)	n	2nd interval (obs)	3rd trim (wk)	n	3rd interval (obs)	Grade	Nonpregnant interval	n	Grade
(53)	Folate, red cell	nmol/L	12 wk	38	21–3597 (176)	24 wk	37	313–2713 (147)	36 wk	25	57–2709 (134)	A	542–1518	20	A
(3) *(8–11)*	Gamma-glutamyl transferase	U/L	12 wk	29	9–28 (86)	24 wk	29	4–28 (76)	36 wk	29	7–32 (95)	A	14–33	121	B
(3) *(12,15,26,54,55)*	Glucose (≥4h fast)	mmol/L	12 wk	29	3.7–5.5 (98)	24 wk	29	3.3–5.0 (89)	36 wk	29	3.5–5.0 (91)	A	3.9–5.5	121	B
(3)	Glutathione peroxidase	U/L	12 wk	29	467–1103 (79)	24 wk	29	494–1106 (81)	36 wk	29	435–1098 (77)	A	670–1312	121	B
(3)	Granulocyte count (automated)	×10⁹/L	12 wk	29	2.6–8.6 (170)	24 wk	29	3.9–10.3 (215)	36 wk	29	4.5–9.7 (215)	A	1.5–6.0	121	B
(1)	Haptoglobin	g/L	8–11 wk	18	0.52–2.28 (121)	20–23 wk	22	0.41–1.81 (131)	36–37 wk	24	0–2.84 (127)	A	0.25–2.5		NI
(3) *(24,25,56)*	HDL-Cholesterol	mmol/L	12 wk	29	1.20–2.24 (121)	24 wk	29	1.25–2.45	36 wk	29	1.21–2.37 (127)	A	0.87–1.99	121	B
(3) *(10,26,45,48,57)*	Hematocrit	%	12 wk	29	31.2–41.2 (94)	24 wk	29	30.1–38.5 (89)	36 wk	29	31.7–40.9 (94)	A	34.3–42.6	121	B
(3) *(10,46,48,51,52)*	Hemoglobin	g/L	12 wk	29	108–140 (95)	24 wk	29	100–132 (89)	36 wk	29	104–140 (93)	A	115–147	121	B
(52) *(58)*	Homocysteine, total (tHcy)	μmol/L	9–12 wk	39	6.9 (6.2–7.6) 31	20–22 wk	39	5.9 (5.4–6.3)	36–38 wk	38	6.6 (5.9–7.2)	D			
(2,59)	Immunoglobulin A	g/L	12 wk	29	0.21–3.17 (76)	24 wk	29	0.30–3.06 (76)	36 wk	29	0.43–3.19 (82)	A	0.68–4.08	121	B
(2,59)	Immunoglobulin G	g/L	12 wk	29	8.38–14.1 (85)	24 wk	29	6.54–12.9 (74)	36 wk	29	5.22–11.46 (63)	A	8.93–18.21	121	B
(2,59)	Immunoglobulin M	g/L	12 wk	29	0.01–3.09 (80)	24 wk	29	0.02–2.90 (75)	36 wk	29	0–3.61 (91)	A	0.69–3.51	121	B
(59) *(55)*	Immunoglobulin E	U/mL	11–13 wk	11	53–1412 (72)	23–25 wk	11	14–1243	38–40 wk	11	44–905 (134)	C	0–13.8	19	A
(54) *(50,51)*	Insulin (fasting)	μU/mL	10 wk	19	0–9 (72)	20 wk	19	0.6–7.8	38 wk	19	0.2–15.4 (134)	A			
(50,51)	Iron	μmol/L	12 wk	29	7–31 (112)	24 wk	29	4–29 (94)	36 wk	29	3–30 (94)	A	6–32	121	B
(3)	Iron-binding capacity	μmol/L	12 wk	29	42–73 (95)	24 wk	29	54–93 (121)	36 wk	29	68–107 (142)	A	45–76	121	B
(3) *(10–12)*	Lactate dehydrogenase	U/L	12 wk	29	217–506 (92)	24 wk	29	213–525 (94)	36 wk	29	227–622 (108)	A	25–525	121	B
(3) *(24,25,56)*	LDL-Cholesterol	mmol/L	12 wk	29	1.02–3.18 (80)	24 wk	29	1.07–4.57 (111)	36 wk	29	2.32–5.56 (150)	A	1.27–4.64	121	B
(60)	Leptin	ng/mL	12 wk	9	0–22				28 wk	9	0–58.4	A			
(61) *(3)*	Leukocyte count	×10⁹/L	12 wk	29	3.9–11.9 (144)	24 wk	29	5.0–12.6 (160)	36 wk	29	5.3–12.9 (165)	A			

continued

Table 2 (continued)

Other refs	Ref	Serum	Units		1st trim	n		2nd trim	n		3rd trim	n	Meth	Nonpreg	n	Meth
(61)	(3)	Lymphocyte count (automated)	× 10⁹/L	12 wk	0.4–3.2 / 100	29	24 wk	0.7–2.7 / 94	29	36 wk	0.7–2.7 / 94	29	A	1.1–2.7	121	B
(13,29)	(3)	Magnesium	mmol/L	12 wk	0.62–0.84 / 92	29	24 wk	0.59–0.87 / 92	29	36 wk	0.59–0.79 / 87	29	A	0.67–0.92	121	B
	(3)	Mean corpuscular hemoglobin	pg	12 wk	28.5–33.7 / 102	29	24 wk	28.7–33.9 / 102	29	36 wk	27.0–33.8 / 99	29	A	27.4–33.8	121	B
	(3)	Mean corpuscular hemoglobin concentration	g/L	12 wk	325–353 / 100	29	24 wk	324–352 / 100	29	36 wk	319–355 / 99	29	A	314–360	121	B
(10,52)	(3)	Mean corpuscular volume (MCV)	fL	12 wk	85.0–97.8 / 101	29	24 wk	85.8–99.4 / 103	29	36 wk	82.4–100.4 / 101	29	A	83.3–96.8	121	B
	(3)	Mean platelet volume	fL	12 wk	6.4–11.6 / 87	29	24 wk	6.6–11.4 / 87	29	36 wk	7.1–11.5 / 89	29	A	8.0–12.4	121	B
(61)	(3)	Monocyte count (automated)	× 10⁹/L	12 wk	0.2–0.6 / 200	29	24 wk	0.2–0.6 / 200	29	36 wk	0.3–0.7 / 250	29	A	0.1–0.5	121	B
	(3)	Neutrophil count (manual)	× 10⁹/L	12 wk	2.82–8.23 / 175	29	24 wk	3.4–9.36 / 202	29	36 wk	3.79–9.67 / 213	29	A	0.92–5.40	121	B
(11)	(9)	5'-Nucleotidase	IU/L	1st trim	2.9–8.3 / 98	34	2nd trim	2.2–10.0 / 113	36	3rd trim	3.4–11.7 / 114	33	C	2.6–14.2	103	C
(10,22,26, 42,62)	(12)	Osmolality	mOsm/kg				25 wk	259.3–301.7	8	37 wk	264.4–299.2	21	A			
(29,63,64)	(28)	Parathyroid hormone (intact)	ng/L	1st trim	2.9–22.9 / 52	20	2nd trim	4–28 / 65	32	3rd trim	0–27.5 / 54	29	A	6.8–42.8	11	A
(63)		Parathyroid hormone–related protein	pmol/L				17 wk	0–3.47	12	40 wk	0.036–2.56	10	A			
(13,14,22)	(3)	Phosphate	mmol/L	12 wk	0.93–1.42 / 108	29	24 wk	0.84–1.31 / 100	29	36 wk	0.87–1.35 / 103	29	A	0.82–1.37	121	B
	(65)	Plasminogen	%	1st trim	59.8–190.2 / 122	9	2nd trim	82.6–203.4 / 140	11	3rd trim	98–197.6 / 145	34	A	60.1–144.1	20	A
(48,66,67)	(3)	Platelet count	× 10⁹/L	12 wk	149–357 / 98	29	24 wk	135–375 / 98	29	36 wk	121–373 / 95	29	A	166–381	121	B
(10–12,14, 22,32,57)	(3)	Potassium	mmol/L	12 wk	3.4–4.8 / 95	29	24 wk	3.5–4.7 / 95	29	36 wk	3.7–4.7 / 98	29	A	3.7–4.8	121	B
(41)		Pregnancy-associated plasma protein A (PAPP-A)	IU/L	8 wk	1.0	640							G			

Table (continued) — laboratory reference values. Columns: citation reference(s), analyte, units, then three gestational/trimester data blocks (gestational age, n, value with % of non-pregnant), followed by the non-pregnant reference (n, grade, range) and a reference number with grade.

Ref	Analyte	Units	GA	n	Value (%)	GA	n	Value (%)	GA	n	Value (%)	n	Grade	Non-pregnant	Ref	Grade
(18,35) (3)	Prealbumin	mg/L	12 wk	29	85–329 (84)	24 wk	29	167–303 (96)	36 wk	29	88–280 (75)	29	A	161–342	121	B
(23)	Progesterone	nmol/L	5 wk	60	26–91	19 wk	60		40 wk	60	314–1087	60	B	12–90		
(23)	17-Hydroxy-progesterone	nmol/L	5 wk	60	5.2–28.5	19 wk	60	5.2–28.5	40 wk	60	15.5–84	60	B	0.8–8.7		
(35,36) (23)	Prolactin	mIU/L	5 wk	60	101–857	16 wk	60	379–3227	40 wk	60	1471–12,531	60	B	50–500	20	A
(65)	Protein C, Immunoreactive	%	1st trim	9	55–147 (101)	2nd trim	11	68–148 (108)	3rd trim	11	64–148 (106)	34	A	70.6–129.4	18	A
(65)	Protein C, Function	%	1st trim	9	74–126 (104)	2nd trim	11	65–129 (101)	3rd trim	11	72–128 (104)	34	A	68.7–124.3		A
(10,12,14,15) (3)	Protein, total	g/L	12 wk	29	58–72 (92)	24 wk	29	56–64 (85)	36 wk	29	52–65 (83)	29	A	63–78	121	B
(3)	Prothrombin time	s	12 wk	29	8.9–12.2 (99)	24 wk	29	8.6–12.1 (98)	36 wk	29	8.7–12.1 (98)	29	A	9.4–12.0	121	B
(3)	Red cell distribution width		12 wk	29	0.117–0.149 (103)	24 wk	29	0.123–0.147 (105)	36 wk	29	0.114–0.166 (109)	29	A	0.116–0.155	121	B
(52)	Red blood cell count	× 10^{12}/L	9–12 wk	31	4.4 (4.3–4.6) (97)	20–22 wk	39	4.1 (4.0–4.2)	36–38 wk		4.1 (3.9–4.4)	38	D			
(19) (18)	Renin activity (PRA)	ng/mL/h				13–26 wk	8	2–8.3	26–40 wk		1.5–26.6	11	C			
(3)	Retinol	µmol/L	12 wk	29	0.87–1.91 (99)	24 wk	29	1.07–1.71 (99)	36 wk	29	0.79–1.71 (89)	29	A	0.85–2.31	121	B
(3)	Retinol-binding protein	mg/L	12 wk	29	23–51 (95)	24 wk	29	27–55 (108)	36 wk	29	20–56 (100)	29	A	22–57	121	B
(3)	Selenium	µmol/L	12 wk	29	1.24–2.04 (97)	24 wk	29	1.08–2.08 (92)	36 wk	29	1.08–1.88 (87)	29	A	1.38–2.29	121	B
(68) (23)	Sex hormone-binding globulin (SHBG)	nmol/L	5 wk	60	39–131	25 wk	60	214–717	40 wk	60	216–724	60	B	30–90		NI
(10–12,14, 22,26,32, 42,57,62) (3)	Sodium	mmol/L	12 wk	29	131–139 (97)	24 wk	29	133–139 (98)	36 wk	29	133–139 (98)	29	A	136–142	121	B
(31)	Squamous cell carcinoma	µg/L	6–9 wk	2	0.3–2.9 (100)	20–24 wk	14	0.1–2.2 (44)	35–40		0.5–2.2 (75)	20	C	<40	100	B
(23)	Testosterone	nmol/L	5 wk	60	0.9–7.4	2nd trim	265		3rd trim		2.2–10.8 (100)	60	B	0.7–3.5		NI
(69) (40)	Thyroglobulin	µg/L	1st trim	230	0–91	2nd trim		0–97	3rd trim		0–115	370	A	<30		NI
(35,69–74) (3)	Thyroid-stimulating hormone (TSH)	mU/L	12 wk	29	0–4.4 (111)	24 wk	29	0–5.0 (122)	36 wk	29	0–4.2 (111)	29	A	0.4–4.6	121	B
(35,38,40, 69–77) (3)	Thyroxine, free (fT4)	pmol/L	12 wk	29	8.8–16.8 (98)	24 wk	29	4.8–15.2 (77)	36 wk	29	3.5–12.7 (62)	29	A	9.5–16.5	121	B

continued

Table 2 (continued)

Other refs	Ref	Serum	Units		1st trim	n		2nd trim	n		3rd trim	n	Meth[1]	Nonpreg	n	Meth
(15,35,38, 40,71–75)	(3)	Thyroxine, total (T4)	nmol/L	12 wk	61–153 103	29	24 wk	78–150 110	29	36 wk	59–147 99	29	A	77–141	121	B
(40,74,75)	(3)	Thyroxine-binding globulin (TBG)	mg/L	12 wk	10–40 114	29	24 wk	23–46 155	29	36 wk	19–49 155	29	A	16–28	121	B
	(65)	Tissue-type plasminogen activator (t-PA)	ng/mL	1st trim	3.68–15.64 110	9	2nd trim	0–25.74 118	11	3rd trim	3.21–15.09 105	34	A	5.19–12.31	14	A
(51)	(50)	Total iron binding capacity (TIBC)	µg/L	0–12 wk	2524–4141 101	62	12–24 wk	2658–4325 105	65	24–40 wk	2707–4609 110	56	A	2514–4108	64	A
(78)	(3)	Transferrin	g/L	12 wk	2.09–3.89 105	29	24 wk	2.61–5.01 134	29	36 wk	3.11–6.03 160	29	A	2.18–3.89	121	B
	(50)	Transferrin receptor, serum (sTfR)	mg/L	0–12 wk	1.49–3.61 106	62	12–24 wk	2.93–4.98 180	65	24–40 wk	3.52–5.94 2.18	56	B	1.34–3.27	64	A
(9,126,136)	(3)	Transferrin saturation		12 wk	0.16–0.52 136	29	24 wk	0.01–0.45 92	29	36 wk	0–0.43 76	29	A	0.08–0.49	121	B
(12,24,25, 33,56)	(3)	Triglycerides	mmol/L	12 wk	0.12–2.36 141	29	24 wk	0.32–3.32 207	29	36 wk	1.01–5.25 356	29	A	0.49–1.86	121	B
(38,40, 73,76)	(71)	Triiodothyronine, free (T3)	ng/dL	8–11 wk	0.08–0.43 101	8	20–23 wk	0.10–0.29 80	8	36–39 wk	0.13–0.35 97	8	A	0.16–0.33	15	A
(15,48,46, 50,71,78, 88,90)	(3)	Triiodothyronine, total (T3)	nmol/L	12 wk	1.1–2.7 100	29	24 wk	1.4–3.0 116	29	36 wk	1.6–2.8 116	29	A	1.3–2.4	121	B
	(71)	Triiodothyronine, reverse (T3)	ng/dL	8–11 wk	34.8–83.4 134	8	20–23 wk	18.2–74.7 105	8	36–39 wk	20.1–84.5 119	8	A	0–93.7	15	A
	(31)	Tumor-associated trypsin inhibitor (TATI)	µg/L	6–9 wk	11.0–13.0 48	2	20–24 wk	7.0–35.0 68	14	35–40 wk	9.0–65.0 107	20	C	<40	100	B
(10,14,26, 42,62)	(3)	Urea	mmol/L	12 wk	1.6–5.0 77	29	24 wk	1.6–4.3 70	29	36 wk	0.9–4.5 63	29	A	2.5–6.5	121	B
(10,12,79)	(3)	Uric Acid	µmol/L	12 wk	75–251 68	29	24 wk	118–250 77	29	36 wk	144–360 106	29	A	154–325	121	B
(52,58)	(53)	Vitamin B12 (cobalamin)	pmol/L	1st trim	139–515 66	38	2nd trim	76–480 57	37	3rd trim	73–449 53	25	A	238–746	20	A
	(13)	Vitamin D binding protein	g/L	8–14 wk	0.19–0.47 106	40	17–27 wk	0.19–0.55 119	40	29–35 wk	0.24–0.48 116	40	A	0.15–0.47	280	A

Ref.		Analyte	Units													
(29,80)	(81)	1,25-dihydroxy-vitamin D	ng/L				12–22 wk	32–132 182	24	39–41 wk	45–149 216	40	A	17–73	58	A
(80)	(81)	25-hydroxy-vitamin D	ng/L				12–22 wk	3.5–29.1 116	24	39–41 wk	3.5–23.5 96	40	A	1.2–26.8	58	A
(3)		Zinc	µmol/L	12 wk	7.8–15.4 89	29	24 wk	6.6–14.2 80	29	36 wk	7.0–13.4 78	29	A	10.0–16.5	121	B
(3)		Zinc protoporphyrin	µmol/ mol heme	12 wk	14–76 107	29	24 wk	19–68 100	29	36 wk	12–91 119	29	A	26–64	121	B

[1]Methods for Reference Range Calculations

A, Mean ± 2SD.
B, Central 95%.
C, Range.
D, Mean and 95% confidence interval.
E, Interquartile range (central 50%).
F, Mean.
G, Median.
NI, Not indicated.
*Indicates mean preg value ÷ mean nonpregnant value.

Table 3
Published Reference Intervals for Amniotic Fluid During Pregnancy

Other refs	Ref	Amniotic fluid	Units	1st trim	n	2nd trim	n	3rd trim	n	Meth
(3,5,78)	(6)	α-fetoprotein	mg/L	14 wk, 2.4–38.5	396	20 wk, 1.8–22.3	396			B
	(12)	Albumin	g/dL	7–12 wk, 0–0.3	24	25 wk, 0–1.1	26	37 wk, 0–0.4	16	A
	(82)	Alkaline phosphatase, total	IU/L	15 wk, 10–42	85	20–21 wk, 4–36	31	24–35 wk, 2–46	56	C
	(83)									D
	(83)	Alkaline phosphatase, placental	% of total	15 wk, <10	85	20–21 wk, <10	31	24–35 wk, 30	56	D
	(83)	Amylase	IU/L	15 wk, 4–19	85	20–21 wk, 11–40	31	24–35 wk, 6–76	56	D
	(84)	Androstenedione	ng/mL	13–21 wk, 0–2.71	77					C
	(83)	Aspartate-aminotransferase (AST)	IU/L	7–12 wk, 11–45 (37); 15 wk, 4–22	85	20–21 wk, 8–25	31	24–35 wk, 6–23	56	D
	(12)	Bicarbonate	mmol/L	15 wk, 12.7–19.9	24	25 wk, 13.7–21.7	7	37 wk, 6.4–24	21	A
	(82)	Bicarbonate	mmol/L							C
	(12)	Bilirubin	mg/dL	15 wk, 0.01–0.25	28	25 wk, 0.08–0.20	3	37 wk, 0–0.65	28	A
	(82)	Calcium	mmol/L	7–12 wk, 0–0.12	24					C
	(82)	Calcium	mmol/L	7–12 wk, 0.86–2.57	40					C
	(12)	Chloride	mmol/L	15 wk, 107–114.6	25	25 wk, 115.5–113.5	8	37 wk, 97–111.8	21	A
(85)	(82)	Chorionic gonadotropin	IU/mL	7–12 wk, 83–111	32					C
	(36)			8–10 wk, 26.8–109.4	6					A
(42,85)	(12)	Creatinine	mg/dL	7–12 wk, 0.24–0.75 (40); 15 wk, 0.6–1.0	29	25 wk, 0.5–1.3	12	37 wk, 1.1–3.1	31	A
	(84)	Dehydroepiandrosterone	ng/mL	13–21 wk, 0.19–1.77	77					C
	(83)	Gamma-glutamyl transferase (GGT)	IU/L	15 wk, 431–1338	85	20–21 wk, 127–922	31	24–35 wk, 9–83	56	D
(82)	(12)	Glucose	mg/dL	15 wk, 28.3–65.5	27	25 wk, 20.6–58.2	11	37 wk, 7.2–28.8	31	A
	(86)	Neuron-specific enolase	μg/L	16–20 wk, <0.2–4.5	22	21–25 wk, <2–4.5	22	36–40 wk, <2–5.0	22	C
	(83)	5'-Nucleotidase	IU/L	15 wk, 29–120	85	20–21 wk, 6–59	31	24–35 wk, 1–5	31	D
(42)	(12)	Osmolality	mOsm/kg	15 wk, 265.1–280.3	21	25 wk, 263.4–280.6	2	37 wk, 232.3–281.5	26	A
	(82)			7–12 wk, 268–280	7					C
	(63)	Parathyroid hormone	ng/L			17 wk, 0.06–23.34	15	40 wk, 0–14.0	20	A

Ref	Analyte	Units	n	GA	Reference interval	n	GA	Reference interval	n	GA	Reference interval	n	GA	Reference interval	n	Grade
(63)	Parathyroid hormone-related protein	pmol/L								17 wk	0–49.8	15	40 wk	0–43.3	20	A
(85)	Phosphate	mmol/L	34	7–12 wk	0.47–2.84											C
(82)	Phosphate	mmol/L										8	37 wk	3.5–5.5	21	A
(12)	Potassium	mmol/L	36	7–12 wk	3.7–4.4					25 wk	3.8–4.2					C
(82)	Potassium	mmol/L				25	15 wk	3.3–4.5								C
(84)	17-Hydroxyprogesterone	ng/mL				77	13–21 wk	0.21–4.96								A
(36)	Prolactin	ng/mL	7	12–14 wk	28.8–37.2	3	21 wk	2.4		18–20 wk	1418–6082	34	34–36 wk	217–702	8	G
(5)	Prostate-specific antigen (PSA)	μg/L	5	11 wk	0.022					≥40 wk	0.13	6				A
(42,85)	Sodium	mmol/L	36	7–12 wk	139–144	25	15 wk	131.6–140		25 wk	131–145.8	8	37 wk	111.5–141.1	22	C
(12)	Sodium	mmol/L														C
(82)																B
(84)	Testosterone	ng/mL				77	13–21 wk	0–0.5					27–39 wk	<0.1–0.4	127	C
(88)	Thyrotropin (TSH)	μIU/mL				201	16–19 wk	<0.15–1.7					27–39 wk	<0.1–0.4		C
(89)																B
(90,91)	Total thyroxine (tT4)	μg/mL											27–39 wk	2.3–3.9	129	B
(88)																A
(88)	Free thyroxine (fT4)	ng/dL											27–39 wk	<0.04–0.7	119	C
(88)																C
(12)	Total protein	g/dL	29	7–12 wk	0–0.4	29	15 wk	0.1–0.9	12	25 wk	0–1.6		37 wk	0.1–0.5	12	A
(82)	Urea	mmol/L	38	7–12 wk	2.0–5.4							26	>39 wk	2.7–8.0		A
(42)																A
(85)	Urea Nitrogen	mg/dL	27	15 wk	5.4–16.2		25 wk	6.7–15.9				11	37 wk	7.2–28.8	31	A
(12)	Uric Acid	mg/dL	28	15 wk	2.0–6.0		25 wk	3.9–7.5				12	37 wk	3.6–16.8	29	A
	AMINO ACIDS															
(92)	Taurine	μmol/L	9	10–13 wk	106–281		16–18 wk	62–117				10	>27 wk	70–142	12	C
(92)	Aspartic Acid	μmol/L	9	10–13 wk	3–13		16–18 wk	3–12				10	>27 wk	1–24	12	C
(92)	Hydroxyproline	μmol/L	9	10–13 wk	27–61		16–18 wk	25–55				10	>27 wk	23–60	12	C
(92)	Threonine	μmol/L	9	10–13 wk	192–273		16–18 wk	125–293				10	>27 wk	42–186	12	C
(92)	Serine	μmol/L	9	10–13 wk	18–41		16–18 wk	14–42				10	>27 wk	15–46	12	C
(92)	Asparagine	μmol/L	9	10–13 wk	84–121		16–18 wk	53–154				10	>27 wk	12–67	12	C
(92)	Glutamic acid	μmol/L	9	10–13 wk	86–212		16–18 wk	30–104				10	>27 wk	5–28	12	C
(92)	Glutamine	μmol/L	9	10–13 wk	157–287		16–18 wk	170–543				10	>27 wk	101–371	12	C
(92)	Proline	μmol/L	9	10–13 wk	173–340		16–18 wk	138–256				10	>27 wk	62–223	12	C
(92)	Glycine	μmol/L	9	10–13 wk	103–203		16–18 wk	114–233				10	>27 wk	72–237	12	C
(92)	Alanine	μmol/L	9	10–13 wk	266–689		16–18 wk	271–432				10	>27 wk	61–323	12	C
(92)	Citrulline	μmol/L	9	10–13 wk	6–19		16–18 wk	5–19				10	>27 wk	3–20	12	C
(92)	α-Aminobutyric	μmol/L	9	10–13 wk	8–24		16–18 wk	6–20				10	>27 wk	1–8	12	C

continued

Table 3 (continued)

Other refs	Ref	Amniotic fluid	Units		1st trim	n		2nd trim	n		3rd trim	n	Meth[1]
	(92)	Valine	µmol/L	10–13 wk	245–335	9	16–18 wk	131–298	10	>27 wk	28–167	12	C
	(92)	Half-cystine	µmol/L	10–13 wk	53–106	9	16–18 wk	51–91	10	>27 wk	38–91	12	C
	(92)	Methionine	µmol/L	10–13 wk	28–41	9	16–18 wk	17–33	10	>27 wk	4–21	12	C
	(92)	Isoleucine	µmol/L	10–13 wk	63–94	9	16–18 wk	25–61	10	>27 wk	3–40	12	C
	(92)	Leucine	µmol/L	10–13 wk	140–198	9	16–18 wk	44–150	10	>27 wk	8–68	12	C
	(92)	Tyrosine	µmol/L	10–13 wk	67–107	9	16–18 wk	28–88	10	>27 wk	8–51	12	C
	(92)	Phenylalanine	µmol/L	10–13 wk	79–109	9	16–18 wk	49–92	10	>27 wk	12–51	12	C
	(92)	Ornithine	µmol/L	10–13 wk	46–88	9	16–18 wk	17–58	10	>27 wk	7–32	12	C
	(92)	Lysine	µmol/L	10–13 wk	312–514	9	16–18 wk	205–406	10	>27 wk	63–191	12	C
	(92)	Histidine	µmol/L	10–13 wk	85–132	9	16–18 wk	56–139	10	>27 wk	14–74	12	C
	(92)	Arginine	µmol/L	10–13 wk	54–146	9	16–18 wk	31–74	10	>27 wk	8–45	12	C
	(92)	Homocysteine	µmol/L	10–13 wk	0–2.4	4	16–18 wk	0–3.8	7	>27 wk	0–4.0	4	C

[1]Methods for Reference Range Calculations.
A, Mean ± 2SD.
B, Central 95%.
C, Range.
D, Central 90%.

Table 4
Published Reference Intervals for Urine During Pregnancy

Other refs	Ref	Urine	Units	1st trim	n	2nd trim	n	3rd trim	n	Meth¹	Nonpreg	n	Meth
(93,94)	(95)	Albumin (24 h)	mg/24 h			1.8–15 (13–24 wk)		4.9–31.8 (25–36 wk)	7	13 C			
	(16)	Albumin excretion rate	µg/min	4.2–16.2; 130* (14 wk)	30	4.8–29; 159* (28 wk)	31	2.9–22.4; 119* (36 wk)	31	28 B	2.5–18	30	B
(10,16,57)	(96)	Creatinine clearance	mL/min	88–211; 152 (15–18 wk)	10	101–210; 158 (25–28 wk)	10	86–183; 137 (35–38 wk)	10	10 A	44–153	10	A
	(97)	Glucose, random	mmol/L	<2; 143 (10–20 wk)	158	<2.3; 164 (21–30 wk)	124	<2.7; 193 (31–42 wk)	124	245 B	<1.4	330	B
	(98)	γ-glutamyl transferase (random)	kU/mol creatinine	3.1–6.9; 117 (1st trim)	11	0.3–12.5; 112 (2nd trim)	34	0.9–25.4; 115 (3rd trim)	34	37 C	3.1–7.0	29	C
(96)	(99)	Insulin clearance	mL/min	114–183; 151 (16 wk)	25	117–188; 155 (26 wk)	25	87–214; 153 (36 wk)	25	25 A	62–135	25	A
	(40)	Iodine (random)	µg/L	0–122 (1st trim)	115	0–127 (2nd trim)	132	0–135 (3rd trim)	132	185 A	≤150		NI
(100)	(98)	Protein, Total (random)	g/mol creatinine	2.4–12.7; 151 (1st trim)	11	1.1–17.1; 171 (2nd trim)	34	1.1–24.9; 200 (3rd trim)	34	37 C	1.03–7.6	29	C
(94)	(101)	Protein, Total (24 h)	g/24 h	0–3.16 (1st trim)	16, 28	0–8.61 (2nd trim)	29, 58	0–17.56; 141 (3rd trim)	29	15 A	0–12.05	15	A
	(101)	Protein:Creatinine Ratio (random urine)		0–5; 39 (1st trim)	16	0–7; 62 (2nd trim)	29	0–13; 125 (3rd trim)	29	15 A	0–10	15	A
	(57)	Potassium excretion	mmol/day	9.4–40.9 (1st trim)	38	0–52.17 (2nd trim)	73	0–46.6 (3rd trim)	73	55 A			
	(57)	Sodium excretion	mmol/day	0–217 (1st trim)	38	0–225.52 (2nd trim)	73	0–204.49 (3rd trim)	73	55 A			
	(98)	Transferrin (random)	mg/mol creatinine	14.5–430; 203 (1st trim)	11	6.7–903; 449 (2nd trim)	34	12–55610; 1210 (3rd trim)	34	37 C	2.8–58.2	29	C
(57)	(62)	Volume	mL/day	631–2511; 122; 128 (10 wk)	9	991–2295 (16 wk)	9			A	1185–1375	9	A

¹Methods for Reference Range Calculations.

A. Mean ± 2SD.

B. Central 95%.

C. Range.

*Indicates preg value + mean nonpregnant value.

REFERENCES

1. Haram K, Augensen K, Elsayed S. Serum protein pattern in normal pregnancy with special reference to acute-phase reactants. Br J Obstet Gynaecol 1983;90:139–145.
2. Mendenhall HW. Serum protein concentrations in pregnancy. Am J Obstet Gynecol 1970;106(3): 388–399.
3. Lockitch G. Handbook of Diagnostic Biochemistry and Hematology in Normal Pregnancy. Boca Raton: CRC, 1993.
4. Benn PA, Clive JM, Collins R. Medians for second-trimester maternal serum a-fetoprotein, human chorionic gonadotropin, and unconjugated estriol; differences between races or ethnic groups. Clin Chem 1997;43(2):333–337.
5. Yu H, Diamandis E. Prostate-specific antigen immunoreactivity in amniotic fluid. Clin Chem 1995;41(2):204–210.
6. Johanasson SGO, Kjessler B, Sherman MS, Wahlstrom J. Alpha-fetoprotein (AFP) levels in maternal serum and amniotic fluid in singleton pregnant women in their 10th–25th week post last menstrual period. Acta Obstet Gynecol Scand 1977;69:20–24.
7. Seppala M, Ruoslahti E. Radioimmunoassay of maternal serum alpha fetoprotein during pregnancy and delivery. Am J Obstet Gynecol 1972;112(2):208–212.
8. Girling JC, Dow E, Smith JH. Liver function tests in pre-eclampsia: importance of comparison with a reference range derived for normal pregnancy. Br J Obstet Gynaecol 1997;104:246–250.
9. Bacq Y, Zarka O, Brechot J-F, et al. Liver function tests in normal pregnancy: a prospective study of 103 pregnant women and 103 matched controls. Hepatology 1996;23:1030–1034.
10. van Buul EJA, Steegers EAP, Jongsma HW, Eskes TKAB, Thomas CMG, Hein PR. Haematological and biochemical profile of uncomplicated pregnancy in nulliparous women: a longitudinal study. Netherland J Med 1995;46:73–85.
11. Berg B, Petersohn L, Helm G, Tryding N. Reference values for serum components in pregnancy. Acta Obstet Gynecol Scand 1984;63:583–586.
12. Benzie RJ, Doran TA, Harkins JL, et al. Composition of the amniotic fluid and maternal serum in pregnancy. Am J Obstet Gynecol 1974;119:798–810.
13. Ardawi MSM, Nasrat HAN, BA'Aqueel HS. Calcium-regulating hormones and parathyroid hormone-related peptide in normal human pregnancy and postpartum: a longitudinal study. Eur J Endocrinol 1997;137:402–409.
14. Moniz CF, Nicholaides KH, Bamforth FJ, Rodeck CH. Normal reference ranges for biochemical substances relating to renal, hepatic, and bone function in fetal and maternal plasma throughout pregnancy. J Clin Path 1985;38:468–472.
15. Knopp RH, Bergelin RO, Wahl PW, Walden CE, Chapman MB. Clinical chemistry alterations in pregnancy and oral contraceptive use. Obstet Gynecol 1985;66:682–690.
16. Wright A, Steele P, Bennett JR, Watts G, Polak A. The urinary excretion of albumin in normal pregnancy. Br J Obstet Gynaecol 1987;94:408–412.
17. Reboud P, Groulade J, Groslambert P, Colomb M. The influence of normal pregnancy and the postpartum state on plasma proteins and lipids. Am J Obstet Gynecol 1963;86(6):820–828.
18. Ledoux F, Genest J, Nowaczynski W, Kuchel O, Lebel M. Plasma progesterone and aldosterone in pregnancy. Can Med Assoc J 1975;112:943–947.
19. Brown MA, Zammit VC, Mitar DA, Whitworth JA. Renin–aldosterone relationships in pregnancy-induced hypertension. Am J Hypertens 1992;5:366–371.
20. Valenzuela GJ, Munson LA, Tarbaux NM, Farley JR. Time-dependent changes in bone, placental, intestinal, and hepatic alkaline phosphatase activities in serum during human pregnancy. Clin Chem 1987;33(10):1801–1806.
21. Rodin A, Duncan A, Quartero WPPG, et al. Serum concentrations of alkaline phosphatase isoenzymes and osteocalcin in normal pregnancy. J Clin Endocrinol Metab 1989;68:1123–1127.
22. Kametas N, McAuliffe F, Krampl E, Sherwood R, Nicolaides KH. Maternal electrolyte and liver function changes during pregnancy at high altitude. Clin Chim Acta 2003;238:21–29.
23. O'Leary P, Boyne P, Flett P, Beilby J, James I. Longitudinal assessment of changes in reproductive hormones during normal pregnancy. Clin Chem 1991;37(5):667–672.
24. Desoye G, Schweditsch MO, Pfeiffer KP, Zechner R, Kostner GM. Correlation of hormones with lipid and lipoprotein levels during normal pregnancy and postpartum. J Clin Endocrinol Metab 1987;64: 704–712.

25. Panteghini M, Pagani F. Serum concentrations of lipoprotein(a) during normal pregnancy and postpartum. Clin Chem 1991;37(11):2009–2010.

26. Davison JM, Gilmore EA, Durr J, Robertson GL, Lindheimer MD. Altered osmotic thresholds for vasopressin secretion and thirst in human pregnancy. Am J Physiol 1984;246:F105–F109.

27. Carter J. Serum bile acids in normal pregnancy. Br J Obstet Gynaecol 1991;98:540–543.

28. Davis OK, Hawkins DS, Rubin LP, Posillico JT, Brown EM, Schiff I. Serum parathyroid hormone (PTH) in pregnant women determined by an immunoradiometric assay for intact PTH. J Clin Endocrinol Metab 1988;67(4):850–852.

29. Mimouni F, Tsang RC, Hertzberg VS, Neumann V, Ellis K. Parathyroid hormone and calcitriol changes in normal and insulin-dependent diabetic pregnancies. Obstet Gynecol 2002;74:49–54.

30. Pitkin RM, Gebhardt MP. Serum calcium concentrations in human pregnancy. Am J Obstet Gynecol 1977;127(7):775–778.

31. Schlageter MH, Larghero J, Cassinat B, Toubert ME, Borschneck C, Rain J-D. Serum carcinoembryonic antigen, cancer antigen 125, cancer antigen 15-3, squamous cell carcinoma, and tumor-associated trypsin inhibitor concentrations during healthy pregnancy. Clin Chem 1998;44(9):1995–1998.

32. Isichei UP, Egwuata VE, Umez-Eronini EM. Serum and urine electrolytes in primgravid Africans during pregnancy and postnatal period. Clin Chim Acta 1978;90:115–120.

33. Darmady JM, Postle AD. Lipid metabolism in pregnancy. Br J Obstet Gynaecol 1982;89:211–215.

34. Heikkinen J, Maentausta O, Ylostalo P, Janne O. Changes in serum bile acid concentrations during normal pregnancy, in patients with intrahepatic cholestasis of pregnancy and in pregnant women with itching. Br J Obstet Gynaecol 1981;88:240–245.

35. Carranza-Lira S, Hernandez F, Sanchez M, Murrieta S, Hernandez A, Sandoval C. Prolactin secretion in molar and normal pregnancy. Int J Gynecol Obstet 1998;60:137–141.

36. Kletzky OA, Rossman F, Bertolli SI, Platt LD, Mishell, DR. Dynamics of human chorionic gonadotropin, prolactin, and growth hormone in serum and amniotic fluid throughout normal human pregnancy. Am J Obstet Gynecol 1985;151:878–884.

37. Braunstein GD, Rasor J, Adler D, Danzer H, Wade ME. Serum human chorionic gonadotropin levels throughout normal pregnancy. Am J Obstet Gynecol 1976;126:678–681.

38. Guillaume J, Schussler GC, Goldman J, Wassel P, Bach L. Components of the total serum thyroid hormone concentrations during pregnancy: high free thyroxine and blunted thyrotropin (TSH) response to TSH-releasing hormone in the first trimester. J Clin Endocrinol Metab 1985;60:678–684.

39. Varma K, Larraga L, Selenkow HA. Radioimmunoassay of serum human chorionic gonadotropin during normal pregnancy. Obstet Gynecol 1971;37:10–18.

40. Glinoer D, De Nayer P, Bourdoux P, et al. Regulation of maternal thyroid during pregnancy. J Clin Endocrinol Metab 1990;71:276–287.

41. Morssink LP, Kornman LH, Hallahan TW, et al. Maternal serum levels of free b-hCG and PAPP-A in the first trimester of pregnancy are not associated with subsequent fetal growth retardation or preterm delivery. Prenat Diagn 1998;18:147–152.

42. Lind T, Billewicz WZ, Cheyne GA. Composition of amniotic fluid and maternal blood through pregnancy. J Obstet Gynecol Br Commonw 1971;78:505–512.

43. Strevens H, Wide-Swensson D, Torffvit O, Grubb A. Serum cystatin C for assessment of glomerular filtration rate in pregnant and nonpregnant women: indications of altered filtration process in pregnancy. Scand J Clin Lab Invest 2002;62:141–148.

44. Parker CR, Everett RB, Whalley PJ, Quirk JG, Gant NF, MacDonald PC. Hormone production during pregnancy in the primigravid patient. Am J Obstet Gynecol 1980;138:262–631.

45. Harstad TW, Mason RA, Cox SM. Serum erythropoietin quantitation in pregnancy using an enzyme-linked immunoassay. Am J Perinatol 1992;9(4):233–235.

46. Milman N, Graudal N, Nielsen OJ, Agger AO. Serum erythropoietin during normal pregnancy: relationship to hemoglobin and iron status markers and impact of iron supplementation in a longitudinal, placebo-controlled study on 118 women. Int J Hematol 1997;66:159–168.

47. Berg FD, Kuss E. Serum concentrations and urinary excretion of "classical" estrogens, catecholestrogens and 2-methoxyestrogens in normal human pregnancy. Arch Gynecol Obstet 1992;251:17–27.

48. Stirling Y, Woolf L, North WRS, Seghatchian MJ, Meade TW. Haemostasis in normal pregnancy. Thromb Haemostas 1984;52(2):176–182.

49. Hellgren M, Blomback M. Studies on blood coagulation and fibrinolysis in pregnancy, during delivery and in the puerperium. Gynecol Obstet Invest 1981;12:141–154.

50. Choi JW, Im MW, Pai SH. Serum transferrin receptor concentrations during normal pregnancy. Clin Chem 2000;46(5):725–727.

51. Romslo I, Haram K, Sagen N, Augensen K. Iron requirement in normal pregnancy as assessed by serum ferritin, serum transferrin saturation and erythrocyte protoporphyrin determinations. Br J Obstet Gynaecol 1983;90:101–107.

52. Koebnick C, Heins UA, Dagnelie PC, et al. Longitudinal concentrations of vitamin B12 and vitamin B12-binding proteins during uncomplicated pregnancy. Clin Chem 2002;48(6):928–933.

53. Zamorano AF, Arnalich F, Sanchez Casas E, et al. Levels of iron, vitamin B12, folic acid and their binding proteins during pregnancy. Acta Haemat 1985;74:92–96.

54. Lind T, Billewicz WZ, Brown G. A serial study of changes occuring in the oral glucose tolerance test during pregnancy. J Obstet Gynecol Br Commonw 1973;80(12):1033–1039.

55. Taylor GO, Modie JA, Agbedana EO, Akande EO. Serum free fatty acids, insulin and blood glucose in pregnancy. Br J Obstet Gynaecol 1978;85:592–596.

56. Knopp RH, Bergelin RO, Wahl PW, Walden CE, Chapman M, Irvine S. Population-based lipoprotein lipid reference values for pregnant women compared to nonpregnant women classified by sex hormone usage. Am J Obstet Gynecol 1982;143:626–637.

57. Singh HJ, Mohammad NH, Nila A. Serum calcium and parathyroid during normal pregnancy in Malay women. J Matern Fetal Med 1999;8:95–100.

58. Pardo J, Peled Y, Bar J, et al. Evaluation of low serum viatamin B12 in the non-anaemic pregnant patient. Hum Reprod 2000;15(1):224–226.

59. Amino N, Tanizawa O, Miyai K, et al. Changes of serum immunoglobulins IgG, IgA, IgM, and IgE during pregnancy. Obstet Gynecol 1978;52:415–419.

60. Tamas P, Sulyok E, Szabo I, et al. Changes of maternal serum leptin levels during pregnancy. Gynecol Obstet Invest 1998;46:169–171.

61. Pitkin RM, Witte DL. Platelet and leukocyte counts in pregnancy. JAMA 1979;242:2692–2698.

62. Davison JM, Vallotton MB, Lindheimer MD. Plasma osmolality and urinary concentration and dilution during and after pregnancy: evidence that lateral recumbancy inhibits maximal urinary concentrating ability. Br J Obstet Gynaecol 1981;88:472–479.

63. Dvir R, Golander A, Jaccard N, et al. Amniotic fluid and plasma levels of parathyroid hormone-rlated protein and hormonal modulation of its secretion by amniotic fluid cells. Eur J Endocrinol 1995;133: 277–282.

64. Cushard WG, Creditor MA, Canterbury JM, Reiss E. Physiologic hyperparathyroidism in pregnancy. J Clin Endocrinol 1972;34:767–771.

65. Aznar J, Gilabert J, Estelles A, Espana F. Fibrinolytic activity and protein C in preeclampsia. Thromb Haemostas 1986;55(3):314–317.

66. O'Brien WF, Saba HI, Knuppel RA, Scerbo JC, Cohen GR. Alterations in platelet concentration and aggregation in normal pregnancy and preeclampsia. Am J Obstet Gynecol 1986;155:486–490.

67. Fenton V, Saunders K, Cavill I. The platelet count in pregnancy. J Clin Path 1977;30:68–69.

68. Cheng CY, Bardin CW, Musto NA, Gunsalas GL, Cheng SL, Ganguly M. Radioimmunoassay of testosterone–estradiol-binding globulin in humans: a reassessment of normal values. J Clin Endocrinol Metab 1983;56:68–75.

69. Eltom A, Elnagar B, Elbagir M, Gebre-Medhin M. Thyroglobulin in serum as an indicator of iodine status during pregnancy. Scand J Clin Lab Invest2000; 60:1–8.

70. Yoshikawa N, Nishikawa M, Horimoto M, et al. Thyroid-stimulating activity in sera of normal pregnant women. J Clin Endocrinol Metab 1989;69(4):891–895.

71. Yamamoto T, Amino N, Tanizawa O, et al. Longitudinal study of serum thyroid hormones, chorionic gonadotropin and thyrotropin during and after normal pregnancy. Clin Endocrinol 1979;10:459–468.

72. Bobrowski RA, Streicher P, Dzieczkowski JS, Dombrowski MP, Gonik B. Applicability of the third generation, thyroid-stimulating hormone assay in pregnancy. J Maternal Fetal Med 1998;7:65–67.

73. Pacchiarotti A, Martino E, Bartalena L, et al. Serum thyrotropin by ultrasensitive immunoradiometric assay and serum free thyroid hormones in pregnancy. J Endocrinol Invest 1986;9:185–188.

74. Skjoldebrand L, Brundin J, Carlstrom A, Petterson T. Thyroid associated components in serum during normal pregnancy. Acta Endocrinol 1982;100:504–511.

75. Boss M, Kingston D. Serum free thyroxine in pregnancy. Br Med J 1979;2:550.

76. Parker JH. Amerlex free triiodothyronine and free thyroxine levels in normal pregnancy. Br J Obstet Gynaecol 1985;92:1234–1238.

77. Ball R, Freedman DB, Holmes JC, Midgley JEM, Sheehan CP. Low-normal concentrations of free thyroxine in serum in late pregnancy: physiological fact, not technical artifact. Clin Chem 1989;34(9): 1891–1896.

78. Nwebube NI, Lockitch G, Halstead C, Johnson J, Wilson RD. Alpha-fetoprotein values in amniotic fluid obtained during early amniocentesis (11–13 weeks). Fetal Diagn Ther 2002;17:25–28.

79. Lind T, Godfrey KA, Otun H. Changes in serum uric acid concentrations during normal pregnancy. Br J Obstet Gynaecol 1984;91:128–132.

80. Whitehead M, Lane G, Young O, et al. Interregulations of calcium-regulating hormones during normal pregnancy. Br Med J 1981;283:10–12.

81. Bouillon R, VanAssche FA, VanBaelen H, Heyns W, DeMoor P. Influence of the vitamin D-binding protein on the serum concentration of 1,25-dihydroxy vitamin D3. J Clin Invest 1981;67:589–596.

82. Campbell J, Wathen N, Macintosh M, Cass P, Chard T. Biochemical composition of amniotic fluid and extraembryonic coelomic fluid in the first trimester of pregnancy. Br J Obstet Gynaecol 1992;99: 563–565.

83. Burc L, Guibourdenche J, Luton D, et al. Establishment of reference values of five amniotic fluid enzymes: analytical performances of the Hitachi 911: application to complicated pregnancies. Clin Biochem 2001;34:317–322.

84. Wudy SA, Dorr HG, Solleder C, Djalali M, Homoki J. Profiling steroid hormones in amniotic fluid of midpregnancy by routine stable isotope dilution/gas chromatography-mass spectrometry: reference values and concentrations in fetuses at risk for 21-hydroxylase deficiency. J Clin Endocrinol Metab 1999;84(8):2724–2728.

85. Doran TA, Bjerre S, Porter CJ. Creatinine, uric acid, and electrolytes in amniotic fluid. Am J Obstet Gynecol 1970;106(3):325–332.

86. Elimian A, Figueroa R, Patel K, Visintainer P, Sehgal PB, Tejani N. Reference values of amniotic fluid neuron-specific enolase. J Matern Fetal Med 2001;10:155–158.

87. Yoshida K, Sakurada T, Takakashi T, Furruhashi N, Kaise K, Yoshinaga K. Measurement of TSH in human amniotic fluid: diagnosis of fetal thyroid abnormality in utero. Clin Endocrinol 1986;25:313–318.

88. Singh PK, Parvin CA, Gronowski AM. Establishment of reference intervals for markers of fetal thyroid status in amniotic fluid. J Clin Endocrinol Metab 2003;88:4175–4179.

89. Kourides IA, Heath CV, Ginsberg-Fellner F. Measurement of thyroid-stimulating hormone in human amniotic fluid. J Clin Endocrinol Metab 1982;54:635–637.

90. Chopra IJ, Crandall BF. Thyroid hormones and thyrotropin in amniotic fluid. N Engl J Med 1975;293:740–743.

91. Klein AH, Murphy BEP, Artal R, Oddie TH, Fisher DA. Amniotic fluid thyroid hormone concentrations during human gestation. Am J Obstet Gynecol 1980;136:626–629.

92. Rabier D, Chadefaux-Vekemans B, Oury J-F, et al. Gestational age-related reference values for amniotic fluid amnio acids: a useful tool for prenatal diagnosis of aminoacidopathies. Prenatal Diag 1996;16:623–628.

93. Helkjaer PE, Holm J, Hemmingsen L. Intra-individual changes in concentrations of urinary albumin, serum albumin, creatinine, and uric acid during normal pregnancy. Clin Chem 1992;38:2143–2145.

94. Taylor A, Davison JM. Albumin excretion in normal pregnancy. Am J Obstet Gynecol 1997;177(6): 1559–1560.

95. Lopez-Espinoza I, Dhar H, Humphreys S, Redman CWG. Urinary albumin excretion in pregnancy. Br J Obstet Gynaecol 1986;93:176,181–181.

96. Davison JM, Hytten FE. Glomerular filtration during and after pregnancy. J Obstet Gynecol 1974;81:588–595.

97. Mortenson H, Molsted-Pedersen L, Schmolker L, Henrik O. Reference intervals for urinary glucose in pregnancy. Scand J Clin Lab Invest 1984;44:409–412.

98. Cheung CK, Lao T, Swaminathan R. Urinary excretion of some proteins and enzymes during normal pregnancy. Clin Chem 1989;35:1978–1980.

99. Dunlop W. Serial changes in renal haemodynamics during normal human pregnancy. Br J Obstet Gynaecol 1981;88(1):1–9.

100. Kuo VS, Koumantakis G, Gallery EDM. Proteinuria and its assessment in normal and hypertensive pregnancy. Am J Obstet Gynecol 1992;167(723):728.

101. Quadri KHM, Bernardini J, Greenberg A, Laifer S, Syed A, Holley JL. Assessment of renal function during pregnancy using a random urine protein to creatinine ratio and Cockcroft-Gault formula. Am J Kidney Dis 1994;24(3):416–420.

INDEX

	DATE DUE		

ID = 7815